Nuclear Medicine

THE ESSENTIALS

Nuclear Medicine

THE ESSENTIALS

Hossein Jadvar, MD, PhD, MPH, MBA, FACNM, FSNMMI

Professor of Radiology, Urology, and Biomedical Engineering
Division of Nuclear Medicine and Molecular Imaging Center
Departments of Radiology, Urology, and Biomedical Engineering
Keck School of Medicine and Viterbi School of Engineering
USC Kenneth Norris Jr. Comprehensive Cancer Center
University of Southern California
Los Angeles, California, USA

Patrick M. Colletti, MD, FACNM, FSNMMI

Professor of Radiology
Division of Nuclear Medicine
Department of Radiology
Keck School of Medicine
University of Southern California
Los Angeles, California, USA

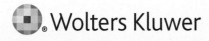

Philadelphia · Baltimore · New York · London
Buenos Aires · Hong Kong · Sydney · Tokyo

Acquisitions Editor: Nicole Dernoski
Development Editor: Eric McDermott
Editorial Coordinator: Remington Fernando
Marketing Manager: Kristin Ciotto
Production Project Manager: Bridgett Dougherty
Design Coordinator: Stephen Druding
Manufacturing Coordinator: Beth Welsh
Prepress Vendor: Lumina Datamatics

Copyright © 2022 Wolters Kluwer

9 8 7 6 5 4 3 2 1

Printed in China

Library of Congress Cataloging-in-Publication Data

ISBN-13: 978-1-4963-0064-5

Cataloging in Publication data available on request from publisher.

shop.lww.com

To Mojgan, Donya, Delara, (and Pepper).......with love

—**Hossein Jadvar**

To Heather and Alexandra.......with love

—**Patrick M. Colletti**

CONTRIBUTORS

Abass Alavi, MD (Hon), PhD (Hon), D.Sc. (Hon)
Professor of Radiology and Neurology
Director of Research Education
Department of Radiology
Perelman School of Medicine
University of Pennsylvania
Philadelphia, Pennsylvania

Kai Chen, PhD
Associate Professor of Research Radiology
Department of Radiology
Keck School of Medicine
University of Southern California
Los Angeles, California

Patrick M. Colletti, MD, FACNM, FSNMMI
Professor of Radiology
Division of Nuclear Medicine
Department of Radiology
Keck School of Medicine
University of Southern California
Los Angeles, California

James Connelly, FRCR, FEBNM, D.Phil
Consultant Nuclear Medicine Radiologist
Department of Nuclear Medicine
Oslo University Hospital
Oslo, Norway

Jan Fjeld, MD, MSc, PhD
Senior Consultant in Nuclear Medicine
Department of Nuclear Medicine
Oslo University Hospital
Oslo, Norway

Søren Hess, MD
Clinical Associate Professor in Nuclear Medicine
Department of Regional Health Research
University Hospital of Southern Denmark
and
Senior Consultant, Head of Section (Nuclear Medicine & PET),
    Head of Research (Imaging)
Department of Radiology of Nuclear Medicine
Hospital South West Jutland
Esbjerg, Denmark

Andrei H. Iagaru, MD
Professor of Radiology—Nuclear Medicine
Stanford University
Stanford, California

Hossein Jadvar, MD, PhD, MPH, MBA, FACNM, FSNMMI
Professor of Radiology, Urology, and Biomedical Engineering
Division of Nuclear Medicine and Molecular Imaging Center
Departments of Radiology, Urology, and Biomedical Engineering
Keck School of Medicine and Viterbi School of Engineering
USC Kenneth Norris Jr. Comprehensive Cancer Center
University of Southern California
Los Angeles, California

Hedieh Khalatbari, MD, MBA
Assistant Professor of Pediatric Radiology
Seattle Children's Hospital
University of Washington
Seattle, Washington

Kai Lee, PhD
Professor Emeritus
Division of Nuclear Medicine
Department of Radiology
University of Southern California
Los Angeles, California

Carina Mari Aparici, MD, FACNM
Clinical Professor of Radiology
Division of Nuclear Medicine and Molecular Imaging
Department of Radiology
Stanford University
Stanford, California

Erik S. Mittra, MD, PhD
Associate Professor of Diagnostic Radiology
Chief of Nuclear Medicine & Molecular Imaging
Oregon Health & Science University
Portland, Oregon

Farshad Moradi, MD, PhD
Clinical Assistant Professor, Radiology/Nuclear Medicine
Division of Nuclear Medicine and Molecular Imaging
Department of Radiology
Stanford University
Stanford, California

**Helen R. Nadel, MD FRCPC (Diag Rad) (Nuc Med),
ABR (Ped Rad), ABNM**
Director of Pediatric Nuclear Medicine
Lucile Packard Children's Hospital at Stanford
Clinical Professor of Radiology
Stanford University School of Medicine
Stanford, California

Hong Song, MD, PhD
Resident, PGY V
Dual Pathway Nuclear Medicine and Diagnostic Radiology
    Residency Program
Department of Radiology
Stanford University Medical Center
Stanford, California

Mona-Elisabeth Revheim, MD, PhD, MHA
Associate Professor
Institute of Clinical Medicine, Faculty of Medicine
University of Oslo
Chief Consultant
Department of Nuclear Medicine, Division of Radiology and
    Nuclear Medicine
Oslo University Hospital
Oslo, Norway

Barry L. Shulkin, MD, MBA
Adjunct Professor of Radiology
University of Tennessee Health Science Center
Member, Department of Diagnostic Imaging
Nuclear Medicine
St. Jude Children's Research Hospital
Memphis, Tennessee

Marguerite T. Parisi, MD, MS
Professor, Radiology; Adjunct Professor, Pediatrics
University of Washington School of Medicine
Seattle, Washington
Attending Radiologist and Division Chief, Nuclear Medicine
Department of Radiology, Seattle Children's Hospital
Seattle, Washington

SERIES FOREWORD

The Essentials Series is a collection of radiology textbooks following a standardized format. Each book in The Essentials Series is a practical tool for those wanting to quickly acquire a broad base of knowledge in a specialty area. The content is limited to the essentials of that specialty so as not to overwhelm the novice, yet provides enough detail that it can serve as a quick review for residents or practicing radiologists, a guide for those who teach the specialty, and a reference for specialty physicians and other health care professionals whose patients are referred for imaging in that specialty area. What sets Essentials texts apart from other similar texts is that they (a) are compact and of practical size for a resident to read during an initial 4-week rotational experience, (b) include learning objectives at the beginning of each chapter, and (c) provide an exercise for self-assessment. Each book includes citations from the most recent literature that are called out in the text.

Self-assessment is a key component of the Essentials texts. Multiple-choice items are included at the end of every chapter, and a self-assessment examination is included at the end of each text. This should be of particular benefit to those who are preparing for the new image-rich computer-based examinations that are a component of professional certification and maintenance of certification.

The series not only includes texts related to clinical specialties that are rich with radiologic images and illustrations but also texts related to noninterpretive subjects such as radiologic physics and quality and safety in medical imaging. The goal of The Essentials Series is to provide a collection of practical references to accompany a well-rounded education in diagnostic imaging and imaging-guided therapy.

JANNETTE COLLINS, MD, MED, FCCP, FACR

PREFACE

Nuclear medicine is thriving as one of the most exciting fields in clinical medicine. The recent acceleration in development and approval of radiopharmaceuticals for imaging and targeted therapy has contributed meaningfully to the care of patients with a variety of illnesses in the domains of cardiology, neurology, oncology, and inflammatory and infectious diseases. The innovations in imaging technology including digital and time-of-flight PET/CT, total-body PET/CT, PET/MRI, SPECT/CT, theranostics, and current research in incorporating sophisticated radiomics and artificial intelligence–deep learning algorithms have all provided unprecedented insights into health and disease, which is the foundation for precision health and precision medicine.

The objective of this book to provide a concise yet comprehensive overview of nuclear medicine in a manner aligned with the intent of The Essentials Series. All major clinical topics are covered including additional information on the basics of nuclear medicine physics, instrumentation technology and quality assurance, radiochemistry, radiation safety, plus content on specialized topics of pregnancy, lactation, pediatrics, and SARS-CoV-2 (COVID-19) infection. Self-assessment questions and answers are embedded in each chapter. This book will be of interest to nuclear medicine professionals, including physicians, technologists, and scientists, whether they are trainees, early in their career, or who are experienced and need a refresher for updated information. We thank all the contributing authors and the publication and editorial staff at Wolters Kluwer.

HOSSEIN JADVAR
PATRICK M. COLLETTI

CONTENTS

Chapter 13 — Renal Scintigraphy

Basics of Nuclear Medicine Physics and Radiation Safety

1

Kai Lee

LEARNING OBJECTIVES

1. Review of atomic structure.

2. Recognize the mechanisms of radioactivity and radiation.

3. Summarize the principles of radiation safety for compliant nuclear medicine practice.

THE ATOMIC STRUCTURE

An atom consists of a nucleus surrounded by layers of electrons (Fig. 1.1). The nucleus is made up of positively charged protons and electrically neutral neutrons. Electrons are negatively charged.

Atomic number (Z) is the number of protons. The mass number (A) is the sum of the number of protons and neutrons. Isotopes of an element have atoms with the same Z but different A and similar chemical properties. The convention for isotope nomenclature is shown in Figure 1.1 with X representing the chemical element.

The atomic number Z is often absent as the elemental symbol defines the number of protons. An isotope is referenced by its symbol followed by its mass number (e.g., Ga-67).

Chemical elements may have many isotopes. Nuclide refers to any atom with specific nuclear components. The term isotope refers to different nuclides of the same element. Nuclides may be radioactive (radionuclide) or stable.

Radioactive decay

Unstable radionuclides achieve stability through radioactive decay, which may be through alpha, beta, or positron emissions, and electron capture.

Alpha decay occurs in radionuclides with Z of 83 or higher. Alpha particle is a high kinetic energy (5–8 MeV), positively charged helium ion that travels a short distance (50–80 um) with high linear energy transfer of about 80 keV/um. The first approved alpha particle emitting radionuclide for treatment of bone metastases in men with castrate resistant prostate cancer is Ra-223 dichloride. Through alpha decay the parent Ra-223 transforms to daughter Rn-219 with emission of an alpha particle with a physical half-life of 11.4 days. The half-life of a radionuclide is the period during which 50% of the atoms of the parent radionuclide decays to the daughter nuclide.

$$^{223}_{88}\text{Ra} \rightarrow ^{219}_{86}\text{Rn} + ^{4}_{2}\alpha$$

Rn-219 has two less neutrons and two less protons than Ra-223 (i.e., mass number A of Rn-219 is 4 less than Ra-223).

Beta particle emission typically occurs in radionuclides having a high neutrons to protons (N/P) ratio. An example of beta decay is the decay of P-32 to S-32 with the emission of a beta particle and an anti-neutrino.

$$^{32}_{15}\text{P} \rightarrow ^{32}_{16}\text{S} + _{-1}\beta + \tilde{\nu}$$

In beta decay, the mass number A of the daughter radionuclide remains the same since the atomic number Z increases by 1 and the neutron number decreases by 1. When the parent and daughter radionuclides have the same mass number A, they are referred to as isobars, and therefore beta decays are isobaric transitions. Figure 1.2 shows the decay of P-32 in a decay diagram that entails more detail than a decay equation. The horizontal axis in a decay diagram represents the atomic number Z, with Z increasing from left to right. The vertical axis represents the nuclide's energy state. Each horizontal bar in the diagram represents a unique radionuclide.

Figure 1.2 demonstrates the decay scheme for P-32 as it becomes S-32 with the emission of a beta particle of maximum energy 1.71 MeV with a physical half-life of 14.3 days. Because the daughter, S-32 has one more proton than the parent P-32 the horizontal bar representing the daughter is to the right of P-32 as the atomic number Z of the daughter S-32 is increased by 1. The S-32 representation bar is below the P-32 bar because of the lower energy of the daughter nucleus. The mean beta energy is approximately one third of its maximum energy E_{max} (i.e., $E_{avg} = E_{max}/3$). With beta decay, the subatomic particle, neutrino that is also produced captures about two thirds of the released energy, and has infinitesimally small mass and no electrical charge.

Some radionuclide also produce gamma radiation along with beta decay (e.g., Cs-137). The decay equation for Cs-137 is as follows:

$$^{137}_{55}\text{Cs} \rightarrow ^{137}_{56}\text{Ba} + _{-1}^{0}\beta + \tilde{\nu} + \gamma$$

Figure 1.3 shows the decay diagram for Cs-137. Cs-137 decays with a half-life of 30 years emitting a beta particle with a maximum energy E_{max} of 1.17 MeV in 5% of the decays, and a beta particle with $E_{max} = 0.51$ MeV in 95% of the decays. The unstable daughter Ba-137 releases its excess energy of 0.662 MeV as

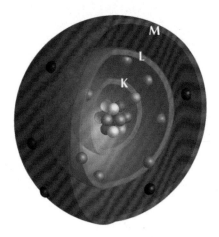

FIG 1.1 ● A simple model of the atom has a nucleus of protons and neutrons surrounded by layers of electrons. Reprinted with permission from Lee (5).

gamma photon emission (vertical line; no change in Z, and A) and has one more proton than Cs-137 (horizontal line). It should be noted that there are no radionuclides that decay only through gamma emission. Gamma emissions are preceded by either electron capture, positron mission, and alpha or beta particle emission.

Isomeric transition

Figure 1.4 shows the decay scheme for Mo-99 with 12.5% of the decays through beta emission to yield Tc-99, and in the remaining 87.5% of the decays to produce Tc-99m, both daughters with the A and Z, but differ in the amount of nucleus energy. Tc-99m is a meta-stable radionuclide (hence the letter m after 99) that stays in transient high-energy state with half-life of 6 h emitting 140 KeV gamma photon to decay to Tc-99. Isomeric transition is the transition of a meta-stable nuclide from high-energy to low-energy state without change in A or Z.

Positron decay

Positrons (anti-matter) are similar to electrons (matter) except for their positive electrical charge. Radionuclides with low N/P ratio and sufficient excess energy (at least 1.02 MeV) may decay by positron emission by converting a proton to a neutron and generation of a neutrino as kinetic energy.

$$^{+1}_{1}P \rightarrow ^{1}_{1}N + ^{+1}_{0}\beta + \nu$$

In the process of positron emission, the Z of the parent radionuclide decreases by 1, the A's for both the parent and daughter

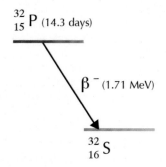

$$^{32}_{15}P \text{ (14.3 days)}$$

$$\beta^{-} \text{ (1.71 MeV)}$$

$$^{32}_{16}S$$

FIG 1.2 ● The decay diagram is a graphical display of the series of events that occurs during the decay of a radionuclide. The atomic number Z increases from left to right in the horizontal axis, energy increases in the vertical axis. Each horizontal bar represents a nuclide. Reprinted with permission from Lee (5).

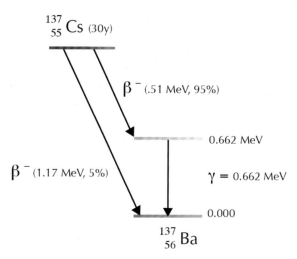

$$^{137}_{55}Cs \text{ (30y)}$$

$$\beta^{-} \text{ (.51 MeV, 95%)}$$

0.662 MeV

$$\beta^{-} \text{ (1.17 MeV, 5%)}$$

$$\gamma = 0.662 \text{ MeV}$$

0.000

$$^{137}_{56}Ba$$

FIG 1.3 ● The decay scheme of Cs-137. Reprinted with permission from Lee (5).

remain the same, and the N/P ratio of the daughter nucleus is increased. F-18 decay is an example of positron decay.

$$^{18}_{9}F \rightarrow ^{18}_{8}O + ^{0}_{+1}\beta + \nu$$

In the decay scheme for F-18, the positron is emitted with E_{max} = 633 KeV and E_{avg} of about 250 KeV, with the neutrino representing the remaining kinetic energy (Fig. 1.5).

Positrons ejected from the nucleus lose their kinetic energy and collide with the electrons in the environment. The anti-matter and matter annihilate each other, converting their masses to two 511 KeV annihilation photons emitted at approximately 180° from each other (Fig. 1.6). The mean free path is the average distance that is traveled by the positron from its origin before exhausting its kinetic energy and meeting an electron to annihilate with. The mean free path varies for different positron-emitting radionuclides. The mean free path for F-18 is about 1 mm, which is the theoretical resolution limit on imaging.

Electron capture

Electron capture is the mode of decay for radionuclides with low N/P ratios that do not have excess kinetic energy above 1.02 MeV. In electron capture, a neutron is generated by a proton capturing an electron from the atomic shell electron.

$$^{1}_{+1}P + ^{0}_{-1}e \rightarrow ^{1}_{0}n + \tilde{\nu}$$

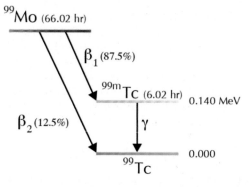

$$^{99}Mo \text{ (66.02 hr)}$$

$$\beta_1 \text{ (87.5%)}$$

$$^{99m}Tc \text{ (6.02 hr)} \quad 0.140 \text{ MeV}$$

$$\beta_2 \text{ (12.5%)}$$

$$\gamma$$

0.000

$$^{99}Tc$$

FIG 1.4 ● Mo-99 in 87.5% of the beta decays goes to the metastable state Tc-99m. Tc-99m decays to Tc-99 in 6.02 h with emission of a 140 KeV photon. Reprinted with permission from Lee (5).

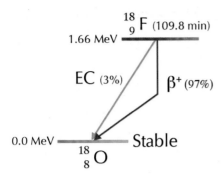

FIG 1.5 ● F-18 decays either by positron emission or electron capture, 97% of the decays are by positron emission, and 3% by electron capture. Reprinted with permission from Lee (5).

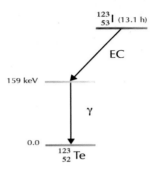

FIG 1.7 ● The decay diagram of I-123. Notice that the arrow points to the left because the daughter Te-123 has one fewer proton than I-123. Reprinted with permission from Lee (5).

An example of electron capture decay is Iodine-123 (I-123) with the decay scheme shown in Figure 1.7. The decay of parent I-123 results in daughter Te-123 with a release of 159 KeV excess energy.

Characteristic X-rays

A characteristic x-ray (florescent x-ray) is released when an outer shell electron fills in an inner shell electron vacancy that occurs during electron capture by the nucleus. This released excess energy is due to the fact that the outer shells possess more energy than electrons in inner shell. This emitted x-ray is unique to a given atom therefore is called as characteristic x-ray. As an example, Tl-201 decay through electron capture emits characteristic x-rays spectrum of the daughter Hg-201 with a broad peak energy of 60 to 85 KeV (Fig. 1.8).

Radioactivity

The decay of a radionuclide is a random process and thus cannot be predicted in a moment of time, but a constant fraction of decay will occur over a specific unit of time at a decay rate called "radioactivity." Radioactivity is defined as the product of this constant fraction decaying per unit time and the number of atoms present in the sample:

$$A = \lambda N \tag{1.1}$$

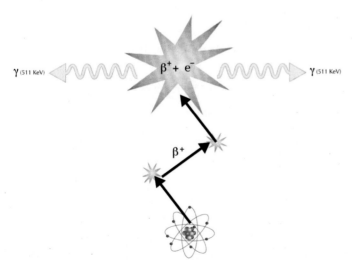

FIG 1.6 ● The positron loses its kinetic energy after going through a series of interactions in a tortuous path and undergoes annihilation reaction with an electron. Reprinted with permission from Lee (5).

where A is the symbol for radioactivity, or the rate of decay, λ is the decay constant, and N is the number of atoms in the sample. The fundamental unit for radioactivity is the number of atoms disintegrating per second (dps), which is the same as a Becquerel. The radioactivity unit Curie (Ci) is defined as follows:

$$1\,\text{Ci} = 3.700 \times 10^{10}\,\text{dps} = 3.7 \times 10^{10}\,\text{Bq}$$

A millicurie (mCi) and a microcurie (uCi) are one-thousandth and one-millionth of a curie, respectively.

The decay constant λ, which is characteristic for a given radionuclide, is the fraction of the radioactive atoms in a sample decayed per unit time. The half-life of a radionuclide is the amount of time for 50% of the radioactive atoms in the sample to decay. Tc-99m has a half-life of 6.02 h, thus after 12.04 h, 25% remains, after 18.06 h 12.5%, and so on.

The relationship between the decay constant λ and $T_{\frac{1}{2}}$ can be derived from the equation describing the amount of radioactivity remaining in the sample at a given time. The radioactivity A_t at time t in a sample of radionuclide behaves according to the exponential equation as follows:

$$A_t = A_0 e^{-\lambda t} \tag{1.2}$$

In the previous equation, A_0 is radioactivity in the sample initially. After one half-life $t = T_{\frac{1}{2}}$, we get

$$A_t = 0.5 A_0$$

Substituting the previous equation into Equation (1.2), and solving for λ the relationship between λ and $T_{\frac{1}{2}}$ is

$$\lambda = 0.693/T_{\frac{1}{2}} \tag{1.3}$$

The half-life $T_{\frac{1}{2}}$ of radionuclides are tabulated in references.

Universal decay table

The universal decay table is a table of the fractions that remain at selected time intervals since the time of calibration. The table is constructed using the equations in radioactivity calculations

$$A = A_0 e^{-\lambda t} \tag{1.4}$$

$$\lambda = 0.693/t_{\frac{1}{2}} \tag{1.5}$$

Substituting the relationship in Equation (1.5) between λ and $t_{\frac{1}{2}}$ into Equation, (1.4) we get

$$A = A_0 e^{-(0.693/t_{\frac{1}{2}})t}$$

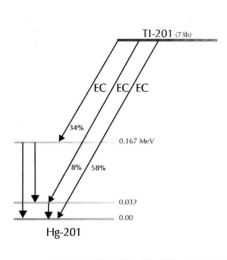

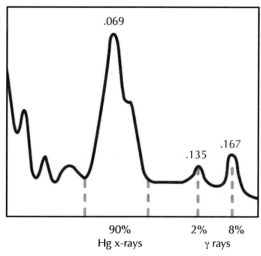

FIG 1.8 ● Tl-201 decays by electron capture. The daughter is Hg-201 (left). The broad peak between 60 and 85 KeV are characteristic x-rays of Hg-201. The two small peaks at 135 and 169 KeV are gamma photons. Reprinted with permission from Lee (5).

Rearranging the previous equation, the expression becomes

$$A = A_0 \left[e^{-0.693} \right]^{t/t_{1/2}}$$
$$= A_0 \left[\tfrac{1}{2} \right]^{t/t_{1/2}}$$
$$A = A_0 \left[\tfrac{1}{2} \right]^{y} \tag{1.6}$$

where $y = t/t_{1/2}$

The exponenty in Equation (1.6) represents the ratio of the elapsed time t to the half-life $t_{1/2}$ of the radionuclide. Equation (1.6) is called the universal decay equation and is used to construct decay tables in radiopharmacies for drawing doses for delivery to the nuclear medicine clinics.

RADIOACTIVITY EQUILIBRIUM

Transient equilibrium occurs when the parent half-life is at the most about 10 times longer than the daughter half-life. Transient equilibrium is best exemplified by the activity relationship of Mo-99 and Tc-99m in the Mo-99/Tc-99m generator (Fig. 1.9). Mo-99 decays to Tc-99m which then decays to Tc-99 by isomeric transition. In a mixture of M-99 and Tc-99m, the Tc-99m activity is a balance between the loss of Tc-99m atoms due to its decay and the birth of new Tc-99m atoms by the decay of Mo-99. The

dynamics of the Tc-99m activity in the mixture can be described using a single compartment model.

Figure 1.9 shows that the Tc-99m activity starts from zero, rises to a maximum, and then decays in parallel with the Mo-99 activity. The condition in which a constant relationship is established between activities of the parent and daughter radionuclides is called radioactivity transient equilibrium; in the generator, the pool of Tc-99m decays with an apparent half-life equal to that of Mo-99 at 66.7 h, but in isolation, the sample of Tc-99m decays with a half-life of 6.02 h.

In secular equilibrium the daughter activity equals parent activity (Fig. 1.10). The Sr-82/Rb-82 generator is an example of secular equilibrium. Sr-82 decays with a half-life of 25 days while the daughter Rb-82 decays with a half-life of 75 s. With a fresh sample of Sr-82, the daughter Rb-82 achieves secular equilibrium with the parent in about 10 min.

Interaction of radiation with matter

Radionuclide imaging is achievable through interaction of the emitted radiation with the detector material to create ions. Charged particles such as positrons and beta particles interact with matter by ionization and excitation. Ionization occurs when a charged particle collides with an electron along its path and

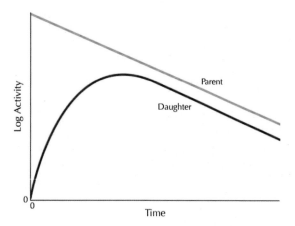

FIG 1.9 ● The parent and daughter activity relationship in Mo-99/Tc-99 generator after equilibrium is established. Reprinted with permission from Lee (5).

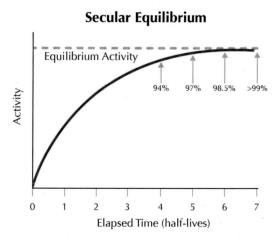

FIG 1.10 ● After secular equilibrium is reached, the daughter activity equals the parent activity. Reprinted with permission from Lee (5).

knocking it loose from the atom. The collision creates a positively charged atom and an energetic free electron ejected to the environment. The energetic electron may produce additional ionizations by colliding and ejecting other electrons in atoms along its path. As the electron loses energy and is unable to produce additional ionizations, it interacts with other electrons through excitation. Excitation is the process in which the incident electron shifts a resting electron to a higher energy state without knocking out the electron from the atom.

Gamma rays and x-rays interact with matter predominantly via photoelectric effects and Compton interactions, which are best described by treating these emitted rays as photon packets of energy instead of waves. During photoelectric effect, the photon disappears leaving behind an energetic electron and a positively charged ion, through liberating an inner shell electron of an atom. Compton interaction occurs between the incident photon and a loosely held outer shell electron; some of the photon energy is imparted to the orbital electron and the balance of the energy is carried away by the recoil photon, termed as scattered photon, Figure 1.11 illustrates the differences between photoelectric effect and Compton interaction.

Radiation safety

Only authorized users (AUs) are approved by the government through a licensing process to use radioactive material for diagnosis and therapy. The Nuclear Regulatory Commission (NRC) is the federal agency in charge of overseeing the safe use of radioactive materials. The NRC sets the regulations in the Code of Federal Regulations 10 CFR 20 on the use of radioactive materials and dose limits for human exposure to radiation. State governments have radiological health departments to enforce regulations of the NRC. The Agreement States have entered agreements with the NRC to enforce the NRC regulations.

All activities with radioactive materials require a current radioactive materials license. The two types of radioactive materials licenses are called "broad scope" or "specific licenses." Facilities such as universities may obtain a broad scope license to allow for transitioning AUs, use locations, and novel investigational radionuclides. Each facility must establish a Radiation Safety Committee for the management of a radiation safety program with a

Radiation Safety Officer (RSO) and a radiation safety committee chairman. A broad scope license allows the radiation safety committee to issue use permits to authorized personnel for the use of radioactive materials in specified locations. Specific licenses are issued to private practice physicians and nonuniversity hospitals. While a radiation safety committee is not required for private practice clinics but it is required for nonuniversity hospitals. An Radiation Safety Officer (RSO) is still designated on the license to oversee compliance with the safety regulations. Human use of radioactive materials is authorized only to AU physicians named on the license for very specific categories of use, regardless license type. Physicians in training may use radioactive materials under direct supervision of an AU physician. The different categories of human use of radioactive materials are given in the Code of Federal Regulations 10 CFR 35. Groups 10 CFR 35.100, 10 CFR 35.200, and 10 CFR 35.300 authorize physicians to use radiopharmaceuticals for diagnostic imaging, in vitro studies, and therapeutic treatments with unsealed radionuclides, respectively. The AUs are free to use any FDA-approved radiopharmaceuticals. Users participating in a clinical trial for a new radioactive drug must submit an Investigative New Drug (IND) to the FDA.

Radiation exposure limits

The NRC sets forth in 10 CFR 20 the limits to radiation workers not to exceed 50 mSv (5,000 mrems) annually to their whole body. The users of radioactive materials and x-ray devices are required to ensure radiation to the general public arising from their licensed operations not to exceed 1 mSv (0.1 rem) annually. Maximum permissible dose (MPD) are these two annual limits of radiation exposure to the occupational workers and the general public. The NRC defines the MPD as the amount of radiation with the benefits that outweigh its possible theoretical risks. The MPD is based on the "linear no threshold (LNT)," model which postulates that exposure to radiation no matter how little always carries risks—higher the dose, higher the risks of somatic or genetic damage to the exposed individual. Therefore, we have to make every reasonable effort to reduce radiation exposure to ourselves and to others as low as practicable, taking into account the technical, economic, and social considerations, in a guiding principle that is termed "As Reasonably Achievable (ALARA)"

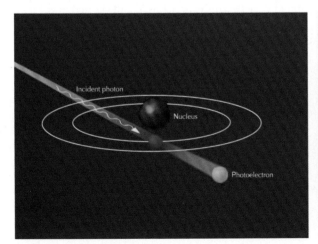 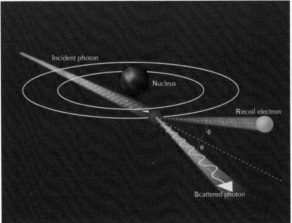

FIG 1.11 ● In photoelectric effect, the incident photon is absorbed by an inner shell electron. Having absorbed the photon energy, the electron is ejected with high energy. In compton interaction, the incident photon collides with an outer shell electron. After the collision, the incident photon recoils with a lower energy and an electron acquires the energy lost by the photon and moves away from the interaction. Reprinted with permission from Lee (5).

principle. NRC mandates that all licensees of radioactive materials adhere to the ALARA principle.

A special consideration is the potential radiation to the human fetus from medically warranted procedures that involve radioactive agents. The NRC sets the exposure limit to the unborn child to no more than 5 mSv (500 mrem) throughout the gestation period, with the exception of 500 mSv fetal dose only applied to occupational personnel after formal declaration of pregnancy by the health radiation worker. The pregnant personnel are permitted at their discretions to undeclared their pregnancy at any time. There have been propositions to lower the fetal exposure limit to 1 mSv (100 mrem) to align with the MPD to the general public. Of note, proponents of the hormesis model think that exposure to small amounts of radiation is actually beneficial. Although this has been a matter of rather heated debates, the current MPD for the radiation workers and general public appear to be overly restrictive and should be considered to be relaxed to a higher radiation exposure level.

Release of patients following I-131 therapy

The NRC in 10 CFR 35.75 permits a patient to release from inpatient confinement if the treated individual would not impart greater than 5 mSv (500 mrem) to people in contact with. The default release criteria are (1) if the administered activity is less than 33 mCi, or (2) if the exposure rate at 1 m from the patient is less than 7 mR/h. Outpatient treatment of patients with greater than 33 mCi of I-131 is permitted if in the judgment of the physician the following conditions are met for at least the first 2 days after I-131 therapy:

- The patient is capable of self-care.
- The patient can keep at least 1 m from others.
- No pregnant woman or children are present at home.
- Not to travel by airplane or mass transit.
- Sleep in a separate bed.
- Have sole use of a bathroom.

The licensee may use the following equation to assure that the released patient would not expose other persons in contact with greater than 5 mSv.

$$D = 1.44\,T_{\text{eff}} \times R_0 \times \text{OF}$$

where
D = cumulative dose to others at 1 m from patient
T_{eff} is the effective half-life of I-131 taking into account bioexcretion.
R_0 is the dose rate measured at 1 m at time of considering discharge.
OF is the occupancy factor. Use OF = 0.25 if the previously provided bulleted conditions are met in the first 2 days after discharge. Use OF = 0.75 if any one of the conditions are not met.

I-131 is excreted in urine, saliva, and perspiration. Therefore, the written instructions to the patient on minimizing radiation to others are required before patient discharge. There are, however, some concerned groups urging NRC to revert to the traditional guidelines that mandate hospital confinement for doses above 33 mCi because of cited incidents in which radiation safety instructions were willfully ignored by the patients, and the physicians did not do due diligence to fully verify the conditions for outpatient treatments are met. However, this is a matter of debate that can potentially confine patients to hospitals which may be unnecessary and increase the overall health care cost to the society.

RADIATION SAFETY FUNDAMENTALS
Radiation monitoring

A personal radiation dosimeter should be employed in those personnel with the potential to receive 10% or more of the MPD in one quarter. Individual dosimeter radiation readings of whole-body exposure and body regions exposures may be recorded, depending on the number of badges in use. In order to monitor radiation to the hands during radiopharmaceutical injection, ring badges are appropriate. Pregnant radiation workers may wear a belt-level badge as a measure of fetal radiation exposure. Upon changes of employment location, a summation of the radiation worker's lifetime radiation exposure should be submitted to the new employer. Dosimeter badges are usually exchanged monthly or quarterly. Valid measurement of a radiation worker's occupational radiation exposure depends on consistent dosimeter use and reliable dosimeter submission for radiation recording. The radiation worker is notified by the RSO if their dosimeter badge readings exceeded accepted levels as

Level I: 1.25 mSv / quarter

Level II: 3.75 mSv / quarter

Level I notices advise the radiation worker regarding recommended methods for exposure reduction. Level II notices require the radiation worker to respond in writing with an explanation for the high radiation exposure. The worker and the RSO then create a plan of corrective actions to take to minimize future radiation exposure.

Radiation exposure to pregnant personnel

A radiation worker with confirmed pregnancy has the option to inform her superior and the RSO, and sign a written statement called "Declaration of Pregnancy." The pregnant worker assumes all risks of radiation until she signs the Declaration of Pregnancy. She may also undeclare her pregnancy at any time. Pregnant radiation workers may sign a Declaration of Pregnancy and continue working as before, but with additional monitoring. An additional fetal dose badge should be worn at waist level. In the event of the use of a lead apron, the additional badge is worn behind the lead. Facilities must ensure that the duties of the pregnant personnel do not result in more than 5 mSv (500 mrem) to the fetal dose monitor between the declaration and the end of the pregnancy. It is also illegal for the employer to assign a worker to a different job classification that results in lower monetary compensation because of her pregnancy.

Area designation and posting

Specific warning signs are required by law to alert people to take precautions when entering an area where radiation may be present. Radiation and radioactivity related signage are shown in Figure 1.12.

Controlled area

A controlled area is any area whose access is limited and supervised for risks either of radiation, security, privacy, or theft.

Restricted area

"Restricted Area" posting is required if a person continually present in that area might receive 20 μSv/h (2 mrem/h), but not greater than 50 uSV/h (100 mrem/h). Access to a restricted area is supervised and in nuclear medicine includes places where an

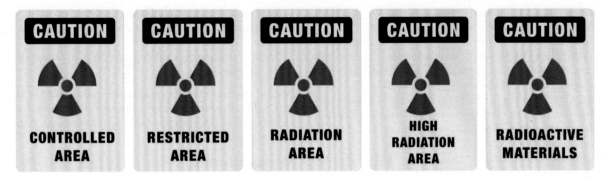

FIG 1.12 ● Caution signs that may be found in areas where radioactive materials are used. Reprinted with permission from Lee (5).

individual may by chance come into contact with radioactive materials, or objects may be contaminated with radioactivity (e.g., the hot lab, imaging rooms, waste storeroom, corridors).

Radiation area

A radiation area is an area within which an individual may receive an equivalent dose of 50 uSv/h (5 mrem/h), or a dose equivalent in excess of 1.0 mSv (100 mrem) to the whole body in 5 consecutive days. The "Caution: Radiation Area" sign is typically posted, although this is not required by the NRC.

High radiation area

An individual in a high radiation area could receive a dose equivalent to the whole body in excess of 1 mSv/h (100 mrem/h). Posting of the sign "Caution: High Radiation Area" is required including an audible and a flashing red light at the entrance (e.g., the entrance to a cyclotron vault). It is unlikely for any area in a clinical nuclear medicine environment to qualify as a high radiation area.

Radioactive materials

Rooms or containers where radioactive materials are used or stored must post the sign "Caution: Radioactive Materials."

Ordering, receipt, and disposal of radioactive materials

Radioactive materials must be ordered by AUs only. Commercial radiopharmacies and other suppliers are required to review the radioactive materials license to document that the ordering AU may legally receive the type and quantity of radionuclides requested. Radiopharmaceuticals are typically ordered by licensed nuclear medicine technologists under the supervision of an AU physician. Upon receipt of the radioactive material, the carton is logged in, inspected, and opened in a timely manner to exclude package damage, contamination, or leakage. A carton surface wipe test must be performed to assure that surface counts do not exceed background counts. The package is surveyed to ensure the exposure rate is less than 2 mSv/h (200 mR/h) on the surface, and less than 0.1 mSv/h (10 mR/h) at 1 m or twice the transport index shown on the package. An example of the label put on a package containing radioactive materials is shown in Figure 1.13.

Radiation safety surveys

Locations where radioactive materials are used have to be surveyed each day of use, and wipe-tested weekly for removable contamination. Decontamination is required if the exposure rates in the unrestricted areas are greater than 0.5 μSv/h (i.e., background level), or greater than 0.2 mSv/h (2.0 mR/h) in the restricted areas. The bathroom used by the patients most likely shows dose rates above background. Action level for area wipe tests is set to 2000 dpm/100 cm^2 (200 dpm/100 cm^2 for iodine). Scintillation detectors such as survey meters and well counters based on sodium iodide are needed.

Waste disposal

The sign "Radioactive Materials" should be placed on all containers that hold radioactive waste. Both the radioactive materials

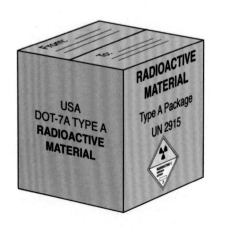
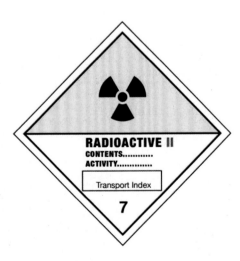

FIG 1.13 ● Markings on package containing radioactive materials. Symbol of the radionuclide is written on the line labeled "Contents" (e.g., Tc-99m). Activity of the contents is stated in SI or traditional units of radioactivity (e.g., MBq or mCi). The transport Index is the dose rate at 1 m from the surface of the package. Reprinted with permission from Lee (5).

and biohazardous signs should be used for used syringes and needles stained with radioactive blood.

Additional radioactive waste may be stored for decay or managed by a licensed radioactive waste disposal service. Radioactive waste with a half-life of up to 120 days may be safely stored until the container surface exposure exposure rate measures at background activity level. Upon decay to background level, formerly radioactive waste may be managed as ordinary trash. All radiation labels must be removed or destroyed prior to disposal. This is known as "disposal by decay."

It is erroneous to assume that upon storage for 10 half-lives that radioactive waste can be considered as ordinary trash. While after 10 half-lives radiation levels are reduced by a factor of 1000, residual measurable radiation above background may be readily detected in some settings. Consider that an initial sample of 1 mCi of I-131 would result in a measurable residual of 1uCi of activity.

Other than human waste and liquids from washing of contaminated laboratory apparatus, liquid waste must be stored for decay or be solidified for disposal by a licensed radioactive waste service. Contaminated radioactive patient bedding after radionuclide therapy must be retained for radioactivity decay to background level laundering.

Spill of radioactive materials

Radioactive spillage may be considered either a minor spill or a major spill. As each radioactive spill is different, a logical approach is recommended. Some initial considerations are as follows:

- Are there patients, visitors, or workers at risk?
- How much of what radioactive material has spilled?
- How extensive is the spill?
- What supplies are available to contain the spill?
- How easy or difficult will the decontamination be?
- Decide if it is a minor spill or a major spill.

Minor spills

- Radiation exposure is minimal.
- The amount of radioactive spill is small and in a contained area.
- Qualified personnel with proper equipment and decontamination supplies are available to contain and efficiently remove the contamination without assistance.

Major spills

- Larger amounts of radioactive material were spilled.
- The spill involves high-risk radionuclides (e.g., I-131, alpha emitters, or radioactive gases).

- Large areas or a large number of people were contaminated.
- The contamination appears to be rapidly spreading to other areas.
- Decontamination may risk high exposure to workers or require special equipment.

Nuclear medicine facility radioactive spills rarely are associated with high radiation exposure to the workers or occupants in the vicinity. Reassuring everyone after a spill is as important as area decontamination.

Medical events

The NRC* criteria for a nuclear medicine "medical event" are as follows:

(1) The dose of radiopharmaceutical administrated to the patient resulted in a whole-body dose greater than 0.05 Sv (5 rem), or an organ dose greater than 0.5 Sv (50 rem), and
(2) One or more of the following events also occurred:
    (a) The wrong radiopharmaceutical was administered.
    (b) The radiopharmaceutical was administered to the wrong patient.
    (c) The dose administered to the patient was either 20% higher or lower than the prescribed dose.
    (d) The radiopharmaceutical was administered by the wrong route.

When a medical event occurs, the user has to report to the NRC or their local regulatory agency within 24 h of the occurrence.

*https://www.nrc.gov/reading-rm/doc-collections/cfr/part035/part035-3045.html

Wrong route of radiopharmaceutical administration and administration of the radiopharmaceutical to the wrong patient are two most reported incidents in nuclear medicine. Currently, in these cases, a medical event occurs only if the patient received a whole-body dose greater than 0.05 Sv (5 rem), or an organ dose greater than 0.5 Sv (50 rem) assuming a diagnostic nuclear medicine dose was administered. The referring physician and the patient are to be informed of the error. In-service training and enforcement of the policies and procedures for safe use of radioactive materials can minimize the occurrence of medical events (1–16).

References

1. Bailey DL, Humm JL, Todd-Pokropek A, van Aswegen A, (Eds.). *Nuclear medicine physics a handbook for teachers and students.* https://www.iaea.org/MTCD/Publications/PDF/Pub1617web-1294055.pdf. Last accessed: May 20, 2020.
2. Chandra R, Rahmim A. *Nuclear medicine physics: the basics.* 8th ed. LWW; 2017.
3. Cherry SR, Sorenson JA, Phelps ME. *Physics in nuclear medicine.* 4th ed. Saunders; 2012.
4. Khalil MM (Ed). *Basic sciences of nuclear medicine.* Springer-Verlag; 2011.
5. Lee, KH. *Basic science of nuclear medicine: the bare bone essentials.* 1st ed. Society of Nuclear Medicine and Molecular Imaging; 2015.
6. Maher K, et al., Basic Physics of Nuclear Medicine. https://en.wikibooks.org/wiki/Basic_Physics_of_Nuclear_Medicine. Last accessed: May 20, 2020.
7. McCollough CH, Schueler BA, Atwell TD, et al. Radiation exposure and pregnancy when should we be concerned? *Radiographics.* 2007;27:909–918.
8. Mettler FA, Guiberteau M. *Essentials of nuclear medicine imaging.* 8th ed. Saunders; 2018.
9. NCRP Report No. 54. Medical Radiation Exposure of Pregnant and Potentially Pregnant Women. National Council on Radiation Protection and Measurements; 1977.
10. Noz M, Maguire GQ. *Radiation protection in the health sciences (with problem solutions manual).* 2nd ed. World Scientific Pub Co Inc; 2007.
11. Powsner RA, Palmer MR, Powsner ER. *Essentials of nuclear medicine physics and instrumentation.* 3rd ed. Wiley-Blackwell; 2013.
12. Saha GB. *Physics and radiobiology of nuclear medicine.* 4th ed. Springer-Verlag; 2013.

13. Shapiro J. *Radiation protection: A guide for scientists, regulators, and physicians*. 4th ed. Harvard University Press; 2002.
14. U.S. NRC Regulatory Guide. Release of patients administered radioactive materials. https://www.nrc.gov/docs/ML0833/ML083300045.pdf, 1997, Accessed June 26, 2020.
15. U.S. NRC, Part 20 – Standards for Protection Against Radiation, http://www.nrc.gov/reading-rm/doc-collections/cfr/part020/, Accessed June 26, 2020.
16. Waterstram-Rich KM, Gilmore D. *Nuclear medicine and PET/CT: Technology and techniques*. 8th ed. Mosby; 2016.

CHAPTER SELF-ASSESSMENT QUESTIONS

1. For the radioactive decay of Tc-99m, what fraction remains after 19 h?

A. 6/19

B. $(6/19)^2$

C. $(0.5)^{6/19}$

D. $(0.5)^{19/6}$

2. Which sign should be posted on the door at the entrance of an operating nuclear medicine department?

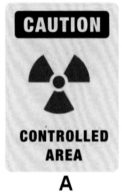
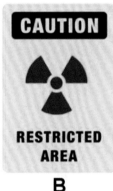
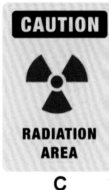
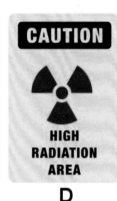
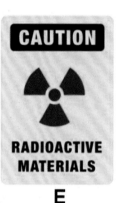

A   B   C   D   E

Answers to Chapter Self-Assessment Questions

1. In order to answer this question, you must first know that the $T_{1/2}$ for Tc-99m is 6.03 h. We will use 6 h for our calculations. As 18 h is 6×3 half-lives, at 18 h we will have $100\% \times 0.5 \times 0.5 \times 0.5 = 12.5\%$ remaining. As 19 h is longer than 18 h, we expect the answer to question 1 to be less than 12.5%. While it is useful to be able to readily estimate the answer, the exact answer is

$$A(t) = A_0 e^{-(0.693/T_{1/2}) * \text{time}}$$
$$A(t)/A_0 = e^{-(0.693/6) * 19}$$
$$A(t) = 0.111 \text{ or } 11.1\%$$

where $A(t)$ is the activity at a given time and A_0 is the initial activity.

Alternatively:

$$A(t)/A_0 = (0.5)^{\text{time}/T_{1/2}}$$
$$A(t)/A_0 = (0.5)^{19/6}$$
$$A(t)/A_0 = 0.111 \text{ or } 11.1\%$$

Most internet browsers can solve this easily if you type in $.5 \wedge (\text{time}/T_{1/2})$ as .5^(19/6) yielding "0.11136233976."

Thus, the correct answer to Question 1 is **D.** $(0.5)^{19/6}$.

2. Which sign should be posted on the door at the entrance of an operating nuclear medicine department?

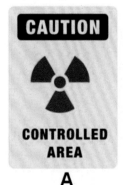
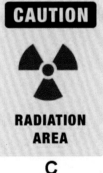
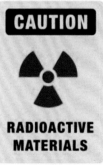

A   B   C   D   E

A controlled area (A) is any area whose access is limited and supervised, not necessarily for radiation safety.

Posting of the sign "Restricted Area" (B) is required if a person continually present in that area might receive 20 μSv/h (2 mrem/h), but not greater than 50 μSv/h (5 mrem/h).

A radiation area is an area within which an individual may receive an equivalent dose of 50 μSv/h (5 mrem/h), or a dose equivalent in excess of 1.0 mSv (100 mrem) to the whole body in 5 consecutive days. Although not required by the NRC, the sign "Caution: Radiation Area" (C) is usually posted.

An individual in a high radiation area could receive a dose equivalent to the whole body in excess of 1 mSv/h (100 mrem/h). Posting of the sign "Caution High Radiation Area" (D) is required. An audible and a flashing red light are required at the entrance to a high radiation area. One may find the High Radiation Area sign at the entrance to a cyclotron vault. It is unlikely for any area in a clinical nuclear medicine environment to qualify as a high radiation area.

Rooms or containers in which radioactive materials are used or stored are required to post the sign "Caution: Radioactive Materials" (E). Thus, the correct answer is (**E**).

Look for the "Caution: Radioactive Materials" signs in your nuclear medicine department.

Basics of Radiochemistry

2

Kai Chen

LEARNING OBJECTIVES

1. Describe the composition and behavior of atomic nucleus.
2. Describe different types of radiation.
3. List possible methods for producing radionuclides.
4. Describe different approaches for radiolabeling with positron emission tomography (PET) radionuclides.
5. Identify the difference between radiochemicals and radiopharmaceuticals.
6. List commonly used tests for quality control of radiopharmaceuticals.

INTRODUCTION

In this chapter, the basic concepts of radionuclide and radiochemistry are discussed, including the nuclear forces acting in the nucleus of the atoms, the kinds and source of nuclear radiations, the interactions of radionuclide with matter, the applications of radiochemistry approaches for radiolabeling of positron emission tomography (PET) tracers, and the development of radiopharmaceuticals. The fundamental role of radiochemistry in nuclear radiology is to synthesize radiopharmaceuticals for diagnostic and therapeutic applications in clinic.

BASIC CONCEPTS OF RADIONUCLIDE

Atomic nucleus

The atomic nucleus was discovered by Ernest Rutherford, an English physicist, on the basis of the Geiger–Marsden experiments (1). In their experiments, Marsden and Hans Geiger studied the backscattering of positively charged alpha rays from a gold plate and observed that very small portions (about 1 in 100,000) of these particles were scattered back at an angle of 180°. Because the backscattering of the alpha particles is directed by electrostatic forces, this is possible only if a very high portion of the positive charge of the atom is concentrated in very small volume. This part of the atom is the atomic nucleus. The backscattered portion of the alpha particles indicates that the radius of the nucleus is about 105 times smaller than the radius of the atom. In addition to the positive charge, the mass of the atom is concentrated in the nucleus. The density of any atomic nucleus is approximately the same, independent of the identity of the atoms. The mass of the nucleus is evenly distributed in the nucleus. The alpha-backscattering experiments proved that the atomic nucleus have mass, charge, and well-defined geometric size. According to the alpha-backscattering experiments, J.J. Thomson's atomic model was conceptualized where electrons must be present in the nucleus in order to neutralize the positive charge of the protons (2). Later on, it was proved that electrons cannot be present in the nucleus due to their high energy. Electrons would leave the nucleus instantly if they were restricted in the nucleus. Subsequently, in 1920, Rutherford conceptualized that the nucleus contains neutral particles that explain the difference between the charge and the mass of the nucleus. These particles, as called "neutrons," were experimentally demonstrated by James Chadwick in 1932 (3). Atomic nucleus consists of protons and neutrons. The number of protons is the atomic number (Z), and the sum of the number of protons (Z) and neutrons (N) is the mass number (A). The particles composing the nuclei are called "nucleons." The nuclei are classified as isotope, isobar, isotone, or isodiaphere based on the number of nucleons (Table 2.1).

Table 2.1 CLASSIFICATION OF NUCLEI ON THE BASIS OF THE NUMBER OF NUCLEONS				
Term	Atomic Number (Z)	Number of Neutrons (N)	Number of Nucleons (A)	Number of Extra Neutrons (N–Z)
Isotope	Equal	Different	Different	
Isobar	Different	Different	Equal	
Isotone	Different	Equal	Different	
Isodiaphere				Same

Forces in the nucleus

The masses of free protons, neutrons, and electrons are listed in Table 2.2. The sum of the mass of the free nucleons is always greater than the mass of the corresponding nucleus in the atom. This difference will be equal to the binding energy of the nucleus (ΔE). The stability of a given nucleus can be characterized by the ΔE value per nucleon. The characteristic ΔE per nucleon for the most stable nuclei is in the range of 7 to 9 MeV. The binding energy is often expressed in millions of electron volts. One electron volt is the amount of energy gained by an electron when it is accelerated through an electric potential of 1 V. The energy of an atomic mass unit (931 MeV) is about 10^{13} J (joule, the SI unit of energy). The binding energy per nucleon (7-9 MeV) is about 10^8 kJ, and the binding energy of the nuclei is about 10^8 kJ/mol. The energy of primary ionic and covalent bonds is a few hundred kJ/mol (an amount of electron volts). Therefore, the binding energy of the nuclei is about a million times higher than the energy of the chemical bonds.

Table 2.2 **THE MASSES OF THE ATOMIC PARTICLES**			
Particle	kg	Atomic mass unit (a.m.u.)	Million electron volts (MeV)
Proton	1.6726×10^{-27}	1.0078	938.2
Neutron	1.6749×10^{-27}	1.0086	939.5
Electron	9.1072×10^{-31}	5.48×10^{-4}	0.511

An interpretation of the nature of the forces in the atomic nuclei was provided by Yukawa using quantum mechanics in 1935 (4). Yukawa constructed a model similar to the one for electrostatic forces, where two charged particles interact through the electromagnetic field. The total nuclear ΔE can be approximately calculated on the basis of nuclear forces, by the summation of the interaction energies of the nucleon pairs at a certain distance. In general, nuclei with the equal number of protons and neutrons should be stable. For heavier nuclei, with the increase of the electrostatic repulsion of the positively charged protons, extra neutrons are needed for stability.

Isotopes and radioactive decay

The term "isotope" was coined by a Scottish doctor and writer Margaret Todd in 1913 in a suggestion to chemist Frederick Soddy, who postulated that elements consist of atoms with the same number of protons but different numbers of neutrons (5). If the ratio of the neutrons and protons is not optimal as the stable state of an atom, the nucleus decomposes and emits radiation. This process is known as "radioactive decay." The rest mass of the parent nucleus is greater than the total rest mass of the daughter nucleus and the emitted particle(s). The difference in the masses can be accounted for as the energy of the emitted radiation or particles. The emitted energy is usually not released in the form of thermal energy but rather as the energy of the radiation and high-energy particles.

Absolution activity (A) is defined as the number of decompositions in a unit time. Radioactivity is in proportion to the initial quantity of the radioactive nuclei:

$$A = A_0 e^{-\lambda t}$$

The unit of radioactivity is the becquerel (Bq), which describes the number of decomposition/disintegrations that take place in 1 s (1 Bq = dps = disintegrations per second). An earlier unit of radioactivity was the curie (Ci), which is the number of decompositions in 1 g of radium in 1 s. The relation between the two activity units is 1 Ci = 3.7×10^{10} Bq. For a significant number of identical atoms, the overall decay rate can be expressed as a decay constant or half-life.

The mechanism of radioactive decay can be generally categorized into the following groups: (i) alpha decay, (ii) beta decay, (iii) gamma decay, (iv) neutron emission, (v) electron capture, (vi) spontaneous fission, and (vii) exotic decay. Alpha decay occurs when the nucleus ejects an alpha particle. Alpha particles consist of two protons and two neutrons. The energy of alpha radiation is in the range of 4 to 10 MeV. Beta decay occurs in two ways: (i) beta-plus decay, when the nucleus emits a positron and a neutrino in a process that changes a proton to a neutron, or (ii) beta-minus decay, when the nucleus emits an electron and an antineutrino in a process that changes a neutron to a proton. In gamma decay, a radioactive nucleus first decays by the emission of an alpha or beta particle. The resulting daughter nucleus is usually left in an excited state and it can decay to a lower-energy state by emitting a gamma ray photon.

Interaction of radiation with matter

Radiation can partially or completely transfer its energy to matter. It can also be absorbed, scattered elastically, or inelastically. As a consequence, the matter undergoes excitation or ionization. Nuclear resonance or nuclear reactions can be induced. The interactions between radiation and matter can be weak or strong. The interaction possibilities are summarized in Figure 2.1.

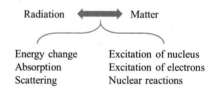

FIG 2.1 ● Interaction of radiation with matter.

The interaction of ionizing radiation with matter is the foundation for radiation detection and measurement. Radiation is either particulate or electromagnetic. Particulate radiation includes charged particles, such as alpha particles, beta particles, and neutral particles. Electromagnetic radiation includes X-rays and gamma rays, which are high-energy photons that interact with matter in the same manner as particles. The most important types of ionizing radiation in nuclear medicine are alpha particles, beta particles, X-rays, and gamma rays.

Alpha particles can interact with orbital electrons, leading to ionization or other chemical changes. They can be scattered with the nuclear field or initiate nuclear reactions with the nucleus. When beta particle interacts with matter, the electrons in the matter may be excited or ionized, and the direction of the pathway of the beta particle may change as a result of elastic and inelastic collisions. A summary of interaction of beta particles with matter is shown in Figure 2.2. Because gamma radiation has no mass or charge, it is very different from alpha and beta radiation. The major type of the interaction of gamma radiation with matter is strongly affected by the energy of gamma photons. Depending

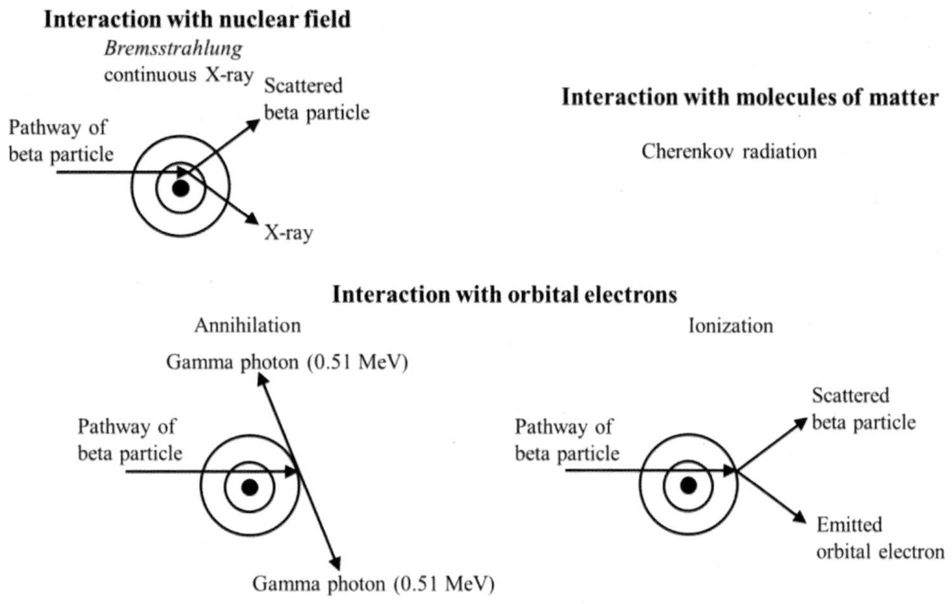

Interaction with nuclear field

Bremsstrahlung
continuous X-ray

Scattered
beta particle

Pathway of
beta particle

X-ray

Interaction with molecules of matter

Cherenkov radiation

Interaction with orbital electrons

Annihilation

Gamma photon (0.51 MeV)

Pathway of
beta particle

Gamma photon (0.51 MeV)

Ionization

Scattered
beta particle

Pathway of
beta particle

Emitted
orbital electron

FIG 2.2 ● Interaction of beta particle with matter.

on the energy, the gamma photons can interact with the orbital electrons, the nuclear field, and the nucleus.

Production of radionuclides

Radionuclides used in nuclear medicine are usually produced by either a nuclear reactor or an accelerator. Some radionuclides are available from radionuclide generators to supply the desired radionuclide when it is needed. The production of medically useful radionuclides involves a nuclear reaction between stable target nuclei and bombarding high-energy particles.

A nuclear reactor contains fuel rods of enriched fissionable ^{235}U positioned in the reactor core. The fuel rods are surrounded by a moderator such as heavy water (D_2O). When the uranium atoms fission, they release more neutrons, which sustain the chain reaction. The fission process generates heat that is carried off by water or other coolants through heat exchangers. Nuclear reactors are designed with different purposes. Isotope production reactors have specialized ports where target material may be introduced into the neutron flux, causing neutron activation of stable nuclides into radionuclides.

A cyclotron is a type of particle accelerator, which accelerates charged particles outward from the center along a spiral path (6). The basic construction of a cyclotron consists of two hollow, semicircular chambers called Dees placed in a magnetic field. The Dees are coupled to a high-frequency electrical system that alternates the electrical potential on each Dee during cyclotron operation. When the proton is accelerated into the opposite Dee, the radius of the proton circular path will increase as a result of its increased kinetic energy. This process is repeated until the proton acquires great energy. Then the proton is deflected onto a target where the desired nuclear reaction takes place. Cyclotrons for producing medically useful radionuclides usually operate between 11 MeV and 17 MeV.

A generator consists of a long-lived parent nuclide that decays to a short-lived daughter. The daughter nuclide can be chemically separated from the parent nuclide. Radionuclide generators are a convenient means of supplying good amounts of short-lived radionuclides for use in the hospital. For example, a $^{68}Ge/^{68}Ga$

generator is used to extract the positron-emitting isotope ^{68}Ga from a source of decaying ^{68}Ge with a 271-day half-life. After its production in a cyclotron by the proton bombardment of stable gallium, ^{68}Ge is adsorbed on various columns containing alumina, titanium oxide, or stannic oxide. Then, the accumulated ^{68}Ga activity in the generator can be eluted with 0.1 M to 1.0 M hydrochloric acid as gallium chloride.

BASIC CONCEPTS OF RADIOLABELING

Isotopic labeling

Isotopic labeling involves the substitution of a stable atom in a compound with its radioisotope, producing a radioactive analogue. The radioactive analogue has similar chemical and biologic properties to the parent compound, and thus it is a true physiologic tracer. A good example of this in nuclear medicine is radioactive iodide ($^{131}I-$ or $^{123}I-$) as a radioactive analogue of stable iodide ^{127}I. Although isotopic labeling is a good approach to the preparation of radioactive analogues, it has practical limitations. Biologic molecules of interest are composed mostly of the elements carbon, hydrogen, oxygen, nitrogen, phosphorus, and sulfur. Their radioisotopes generally have undesirable radioactive properties for clinical use, such as unsatisfactory half-life and photon energy.

Nonisotopic labeling

Nonisotopic labeling involves incorporating a radioactive atom that is not native to the compound being labeled. Nonisotopic labeling is not ideal because the presence of a nonisotopic atom in a molecule may change its biochemical properties. If the radionuclide is located at a site involved with biological target binding, the biological properties of the radiolabeled molecule can be altered.

Specific activity

Specific activity is the ratio of the radioactivity to the mass of a radionuclide or a radioactive compound. Typical units might be curies per millimole (Ci/mmol) or microcuries per microgram (µCi/µg). The mass of a radionuclide in a given amount of activity can be determined from the number of radioactive atoms present. For small capacity and high affinity receptor binding, a high specific activity of radioligands is demanded, whereas a low specific activity of radiotracers may be acceptable for large capacity and low affinity biological systems.

Radiochemistry for positron emission tomography tracers

PET is a noninvasive functional imaging technique with good resolution and high sensitivity. In PET, the radionuclide decays and the resulting positrons subsequently interact with nearby electrons after travelling a short distance (~1 mm) within the body. Each positron–electron transmutation produces two 511-KeV gamma photons in opposite trajectories, and these two gamma photons may be detected by the detectors surrounding the subject to precisely locate the source of the decay event. Subsequently, the "coincidence events" data can be processed by computers to reconstruct the spatial distribution of the radiotracers (7).

PET imaging can provide quantitative information of physiological, biochemical, and pharmacological processes in living subjects. It is possible to synthesize PET probes with the same chemical structure as the parent unlabeled molecules without altering their biological activity. PET has been widely applied not only in the field of oncology, cardiology, and neurology (8–10), but also in the process of drug development (11,12). The potential of PET in clinical setting heavily relies on the availability of suitable PET tracers, and radiochemistry is a challenging factor for clinical applications of PET.

Radionuclide selection

Several positron-emitting radionuclides can be used in the development of a PET radiotracer. These radionuclides include, but are not limited to, ^{18}F (E_{max} 635 KeV, $t_{1/2}$ 109.8 min), ^{11}C (E_{max} 970 KeV, $t_{1/2}$ 20.4 min), ^{15}O (E_{max} 1.73 MeV, $t_{1/2}$ 2.04 min), ^{13}N (E_{max} 1.30 MeV, $t_{1/2}$ 9.97 min), ^{64}Cu (E_{max} 657 KeV, $t_{1/2}$ 12.7 h), ^{68}Ga (E_{max} 1.90 MeV, $t_{1/2}$ 68.1 min), and ^{124}I (E_{max} 2.13 MeV; 1.53 MeV; 808 KeV, $t_{1/2}$ 4.2 days). The selection of the PET radionuclide is depended on its physical and chemical characteristics, availability, and the studied time course of biological process (7,13). The half-life of the PET radionuclide determines whether the radiolabeling procedure of incorporating the radionuclide into the target compound is appropriate and/or feasible. For instance, if a relatively lengthy radiolabeling procedure is required, or the tracers need to be transported from the radiolabeling sites to imaging sites, it may not be possible to use short-lived isotopes such as ^{11}C. Due to the very short half-lives of ^{15}O and ^{13}N, the tracers containing ^{15}O or ^{13}N are usually prepared in the chemical forms directly from a cyclotron target, or their derivatives that can be obtained by reactions in a very high radiochemical yield. Other factors for the radionuclide selection include the radiolabeling conditions, tracer specific activity, and radionuclide production. In addition, the physical half-life of the PET radionuclide should match the biological half-life of the corresponding tracer in order to achieve good target-to-background ratio, that is, high contrast images. For small molecules and peptides exhibiting fast clearance, ^{18}F with a short half-life may be a better choice. For antibodies who have the binding equilibrium of several hours or days in the body after intravenous injection of the tracer, radionuclides such as ^{64}Cu or ^{89}Zr with relatively longer half-lives may be optimal.

Radiochemistry with positron emission tomography radionuclides

Radiolabeling is a chemical process during which a radionuclide is incorporated into a desired molecule. For PET radiochemistry, radiation safety and radiolabeling effectiveness are essential when dealing with high-energy short-lived radioactive compounds. Traditional bench-top organic synthesis approaches may not be applicable for radiochemistry. In order to reduce radiation exposure to radiochemists, radiolabeling is often performed in radiosynthesis modules located in lead-shielded hot cells. In addition, the development of rapid radiosynthetic methods for introducing short-lived positron-emitting isotopes into the molecule of interest is also a challenge for radiochemists. PET tracers must be radio synthesized, purified, formulated, and analyzed within a few half-lives of the radionuclide to ensure that enough radiation doses can be administered into a subject undergoing PET scans. The radiochemical approaches are very limited for PET probes based on the extremely short-lived radionuclides, such as ^{15}O and ^{13}N. Radiolabeling with ^{18}F and ^{11}C is usually carried out using organic chemistry approaches. Although a single-step reaction with a high yield is preferred, it is necessary in some cases to protect reactive groups of the target molecule or perform the radiolabeling using prosthetic agents. For radiometals, such as ^{64}Cu, ^{89}Zr, and ^{68}Ga, the radiolabeling reaction is often performed using coordination chemistry. Biomolecules are commonly modified with a suitable metal-chelating group prior to the chelation of the radiometal. Recently, a wide range of new technologies, including solid-phase extraction (SPE) and microfluidics, have been adapted into radiolabeling procedure to further speed up radiolabeling, enhance radiolabeling efficiency, and facilitate product purification.

Radiolabeling with F-18

Fluorine-18 appears to be an ideal radionuclide for routine PET imaging because of its almost perfect chemical and nuclear properties (7). Compared with other short-lived radionuclides, such as ^{11}C, ^{18}F has a half-life of 109.8 min, which is long enough to allow for time-consuming multistep radiosynthesis as well as imaging procedures to be extended over several hours. In addition, the low β^+-energy of ^{18}F, 635 KeV, promises a short positron linear range in tissue, contributing to high spatial resolution PET images. There are varieties of chemical methods to incorporate the ^{18}F isotope into target molecules. The synthetic strategies generally fall into two categories: (i) direct fluorination, including nucleophilic and electrophilic reactions: the ^{18}F isotope is directly incorporated into the target molecule of interest (Fig. 2.3); and (ii) indirect fluorination: the ^{18}F isotope is introduced using ^{18}F-containing prosthetic agents where a multistep synthetic approach is usually involved in radiolabeling (Fig. 2.4).

Nucleophilic reactions

Nucleophilic ^{18}F-fluorination reactions are extensively used to produce the most important PET tracers, such as [^{18}F]-fluorodeoxyglucose ([^{18}F]FDG). In nucleophilic fluorination, F-18 fluoride ion (^{18}F$^-$) is obtained as an aqueous solution from the cyclotron target. After trapping on an ion exchange column, ^{18}F$^-$ is then eluted using potassium carbonate in a water/acetonitrile solution. A phase transfer reagent kryptofix-222 (K222) is added to enhance the fluoride nucleophile, followed by the removal of water. Mannose triflate is commonly used precursor in the production of [^{18}F]FDG (Fig. 2.3). The [^{18}F]fluoride ion is a nucleophile that reacts at carbon atom number 2 of mannose triflate

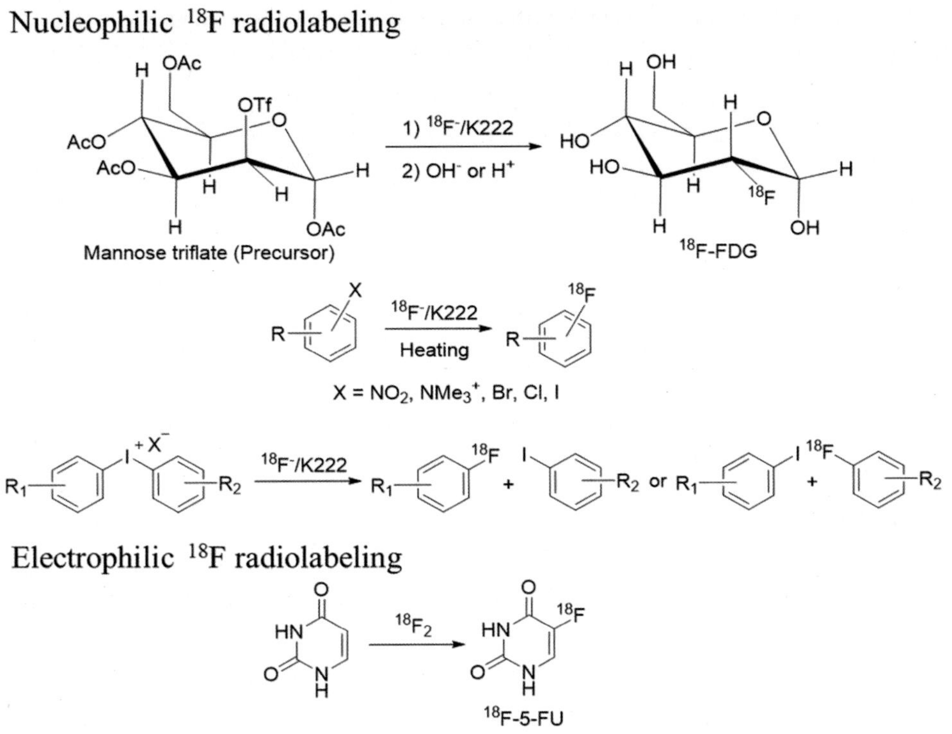

Nucleophilic ¹⁸F radiolabeling

Mannose triflate (Precursor)

1) ¹⁸F⁻/K222
2) OH⁻ or H⁺

¹⁸F-FDG

X

R——

¹⁸F⁻/K222

Heating

¹⁸F

R——

X = NO₂, NMe₃⁺, Br, Cl, I

R₁——I⁺X⁻——R₂

¹⁸F⁻/K222

R₁——¹⁸F + I——R₂   or   R₁——I + ¹⁸F——R₂

Electrophilic ¹⁸F radiolabeling

¹⁸F₂

¹⁸F-5-FU

FIG 2.3 ● Representative nucleophilic and electrophilic ¹⁸F radiolabeling.

with "inversion of stereochemistry" thereby converting "mannose" substrate into a "glucose" product.

Aliphatic nucleophilic substitutions with ¹⁸F⁻ are highly efficient. The requirement for aliphatic nucleophilic ¹⁸F reactions to

occur is a favorable leaving group in the radiolabeling precursor, such as a sulfonate (e.g., triflate, tosylate, mesylate, or nosylate) or other halides (13). Substrate reactivity follows a pattern of typical SN2 type reactions with substitution at the primary carbon

[¹⁸F]FPA [¹⁸F]NPFP [¹⁸F]SFB

[¹⁸F]FBA [¹⁸F]FBzA [¹⁸F]FPyME

[¹⁸F]FBEM [¹⁸F]FBBO

FIG 2.4 ● Representative prosthetic agents for ¹⁸F radiolabeling.

Click Chemistry Approach

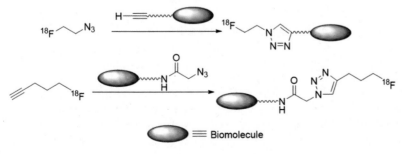

● ≡ Biomolecule

favored for a high yield. Substitution at a secondary carbon may be accompanied with significant amount of elimination from the precursor as a side reaction. The drawback of this method is the need to chemically protect any competing sites of nucleophilic attack in the molecule, such as acid, alcohol, and amine groups, which would result in radiolabeling failure or a low yield without the protection. Aliphatic nucleophilic substitutions with ^{18}F$^-$ are usually performed in a polar aprotic solvent such as acetonitrile, dimethyl sulfoxide, tetrahydrofuran, and N,N-dimethylformamide. Among these solvents, acetonitrile is a suitable and effective solvent for many aliphatic nucleophilic ^{18}F reactions and it is easy to be removed from the reaction. Protic solvents, such as alcohols, are generally not suitable for nucleophilic substitution reactions because of their ability to solvate the nucleophile and reduce reactivity of radiofluoride.

Direct nucleophilic substitutions with ^{18}F can also be applied to the radiolabeling of aromatic compounds. The reactions typically require that the aryl ring has been activated by at least one electron-withdrawing substituent on the ortho or para position. In general, the reaction conditions for direct fluorination of aromatic compounds are harsh with a high temperature (>100°C). Since heteroarenes present a wide array of biological activities, the radiosynthesis of ^{18}F-labeled heteroaromatic compounds is receiving increasing interest. For example, the radiolabeling of 2-position of a pyridinyl ring with ^{18}F has been utilized in the production of PET radiotracers for imaging nicotinic and mGluR5 receptors (14). In order to overcome the limitation of aromatic nucleophilic substitutions with ^{18}F on electron-rich arenes, a reaction using diaryliodonium salts as the radiolabeling precursor was introduced (15,16). Radiochemical yields of the substituted ^{18}F-fluoroarene increase as more substituents are presented in the ring.

Electrophilic reactions

Direct electrophilic fluorination of aromatic rings has been accomplished using a variety of ^{18}F-labeled electrophilic fluorinating agents. The most common reagent for electrophilic fluorination is ^{18}F$_2$. As ^{18}F$_2$ is very reactive, the fluorination reactions must be controlled either at a low temperature or using highly diluted solutions in an inert solvent. An alternative is to convert fluorine into a slightly less reactive form, such as acetyl hypofluorite (17). In fact, the first synthesis of [^{18}F]FDG was employed the method of direct electrophilic substitution (18). In general, electrophilic ^{18}F-fluorination methods, such as using the reagent ^{18}F$_2$, are less favorable because of limited availability, nonspecific labeling, and low specific activity of the labeled products. The lack of labeling regiospecificity has resulted in the use of demetallation reactions with ^{18}F$_2$, where organometallic intermediates are produced and subsequent demetallation form the corresponding fluorinating compound. A good example is the radiolabeling of L-[^{18}F]FDOPA (19).

Radiolabeling using prosthetic agents

Direct incorporation of ^{18}F into biomolecules, such as peptides and proteins, is very challenging due to the lack of functional groups in the biomolecules required for a nucleophilic ^{18}F-fluorination. In addition, the harsh ^{18}F-labeling reaction conditions with high temperature and strong base may cause the decomposition and denaturation of the biomolecules. In order to circumvent this obstacle, biomolecules labeling with ^{18}F has to be performed using prosthetic agents, which can be coupled to specific functional groups within peptides and proteins. A summary of ^{18}F-labeled prosthetic agents is shown in Figure 2.4.

The most common reaction for ^{18}F-labeling of peptides and proteins is the formation of a stable amide linkage between the biomolecule and the prosthetic agent. A large number of ^{18}F-labeled prosthetic agents have been developed for coupling to peptides and proteins. For example, the activated ester N-succinimidyl 4-^{18}F-fluorobenzoate (^{18}F-SFB) (20–23) is one of the widely used prosthetic agents for protein labeling via an acylation reaction. In addition to ^{18}F-SFB, other frequently used ^{18}F-labeled active esters include 2-^{18}F-fluoroacetic acid (24), methyl 2-^{18}F-fluoropropionate (25), N-succinimidyl 4-(^{18}F-fluoromethyl)benzoate (26,27), 3-^{18}F-fluoro-5-nitrobenzimidate,[28] 4-^{18}F-fluorophenacyl bromide (^{18}F-FPB) (28). The amide formation using an ^{18}F-labeled amine and an activated carboxylic group in the targeting molecule is an alternative strategy. However, the targeting molecule should not have free amino groups. Otherwise, inter- and intra-molecular cross-linking would produce undesired products.

Thiol group in biomolecules is another widely used functional group capable of forming conjugates with prosthetic agents. The free thiol group is only present in cysteine residues. Therefore, thiol reactive agents have been used to modify peptides and proteins at specific sites, providing a means of conjugation with high chemo-selectivity. Two N-substituted maleimides, N-(p-^{18}F-fluorophenyl) maleimide and m-maleimido-N-(p-^{18}F-fluorobenzyl) benzamide, have been reported for antibody coupling (29). As an ^{18}F-fluoropyridine-based maleimide reagent, 1-[3-(2-fluoropyridin-3-yloxy) propyl]pyrrole-2,5-dione) (^{18}F-FPyME) was developed for the prosthetic labeling of proteins via selective conjugation with a thiol group (30). As compared to the nonselective carboxylate and amine-reactive ^{18}F-labeled agents, ^{18}F-FPyME offers excellent chemo-selectivity for the development of new peptide and protein-based PET tracers.

Recent advances in chemistry offer novel strategies for robust radiolabeling of compounds with ^{18}F. For instance, bio-orthogonal chemical reactions between two exogenous moieties have powerful applications in ^{18}F radiolabeling. In one example, the rapid formation of triazole rings by the 1,3-dipolar Huisgen cycloaddition of alkynes to azides ("click chemistry") (31) has recently been exploited for the radiosynthesis of ^{18}F-labeled peptide (32,33). There are two routes to conjugate ^{18}F prosthetic agents with the peptides via click chemistry: [^{18}F]fluoroalkynes reacting with peptide azides, and the reverse, [^{18}F]-azide coupling with peptide alkyne (Fig. 2.4). In general, click chemistry provides chemists a platform for general, modular, and high-yielding synthetic transformations for constructing highly diverse molecules. Because click chemistry is a modular approach, it is possible to fine-tune the new PET probes and enhance their pharmacokinetic and pharmacodynamic profiles. Click chemistry has proven itself to be superior in satisfying many criteria, such as biocompatibility, selectivity, yield, and stereo-specificity; thus, one can expect it will become a routine strategy in the near future for a wide range of applications for the development of PET tracers (34).

Automation radiosynthesis

Fast implementation of PET into clinical studies has resulted in high demands in the automated synthesis modules for the preparation of PET tracers in a safe and reproducible manner. The design of automated synthesis modules is based on the principle of performing all the necessary chemical operations with radionuclide in one unit. This concept works well for one-step labeling synthetic strategies. In complex multistep synthesis, it is necessary to use two or more different reactors to conduct the separated stages of the process, to eliminate carryover of impurities and solvents. An approach to provide a compact solution to multistage synthesis is the modular concept. Within this concept, compact identical modules are placed within the same hot-cell and connected in a way that allows use of each module for one step with an automatic transfer of resulting radiolabeled intermediates from one stage to another. The entire process is controlled by one computer program. This method allows for virtually unlimited flexibility in use of the systems and enables production of a variety of radiotracers using standardized single-use kits. Recently, a new type of automated synthesizer has been developed by means of exchanging disposable cassette on one base unit. This approach eliminates the possibility of cross contamination and facilitates the clean procedure after radiosynthesis. The development of flexible multipurpose automated apparatus is important to meet the needs for complex radiolabeling procedures and standardization of radiotracer production.

Radiolabeling with C-11

Carbon-11 is an attractive and important positron-emitting isotope for labeling molecules of biological interest. Although the half-life of ^{11}C is short (20.4 min) and multiple step syntheses are not generally applicable for the radiosynthesis of ^{11}C-containing molecules, a diverse array of reactions to introduce ^{11}C into target molecules has been investigated and developed (35). Almost all C-11 radiosynthesis utilizes CH_4 or CO_2 as the starting material. Various ^{11}C-containing precursors have also been developed, which are shown in Figure 2.5.

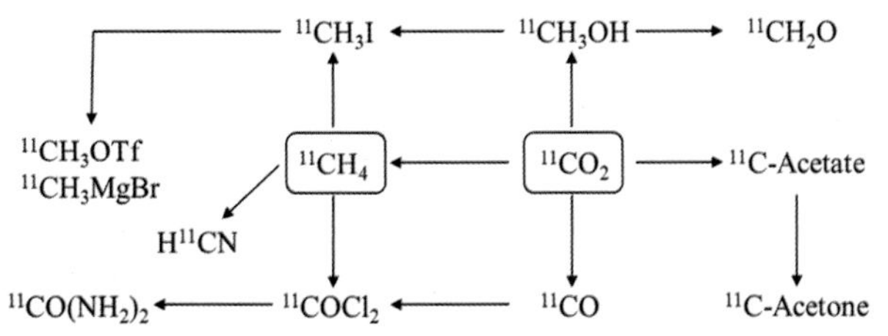

FIG 2.5 ● Representative ^{11}C-labeled precursors.

Alkylation with $^{11}CH_3I$ or $^{11}CH_3OTf$ is the most widely used method for introducing carbon-11 into target molecules. Various compounds have been prepared via N-, O-, and S-methylation reactions. There are two common ways to prepare $^{11}CH_3I$, that is, the "wet" method and the "gas phase" method. In the "wet" method, $^{11}CO_2$ is reduced to ^{11}C-methanol by LiAlH4, followed by treatment with HI (36). In the "gas phase" method, $^{11}CH_3I$ is directly prepared from ^{11}C-methane in the presence of iodine vapor (37–40). The use of $^{11}CH_3OTf$ in methylation reactions has several advantages over the use of $^{11}CH_3I$. Because $^{11}CH_3OTf$ is more reactive than $^{11}CH_3I$, methylations can be conducted using lower reaction temperatures, smaller amounts of precursor, and shorter reaction times. The synthesis of $^{11}CH_3OTf$ can be readily prepared as an online process by passing $^{11}CH_3I$ through a column containing silver triflate that is preheated at 200°C to 300°C.

The alkylation reactions can either be carried out in solution, on solid-phase support, or in micro reactors. Methylations on a solid support are very convenient for automation purposes. The precursor is coated on a solid support, such as a high-performance liquid chromatography (HPLC) loop or a SPE cartridge. The advantages of this method include simple operation, no significant loss of radioactivity, and rapid process. According to this method, various C-11-labeled tracers have been developed, such as ^{11}C-Choline (41), ^{11}C-WAY100635 (42), and L-[S-methyl-^{11}C]methionine (43).

Radiolabeling with other positron emission tomography radionuclides

Several metallic radionuclides are applicable for preparing PET tracers as well. These metallic PET isotopes include, but not limit to, ^{64}Cu, ^{68}Ga, ^{86}Y, and ^{89}Zr. Copper-64 can be effectively produced by both reactor-based and accelerator-based methods. During the last decade, there has been considerable research interest in the development of ^{64}Cu-labeled PET tracers for targeting specific receptors. ^{64}Cu is conjugated to targeting molecules by a chelator that is attached through a functional group (44). The chemical structures of selected bifunctional chelators are shown in Figure 2.6. These chelators are efficient to react with the radiometals through the coordination reaction. While several carboxylate groups might involve in the complex formation, the remaining ones can be activated in situ with

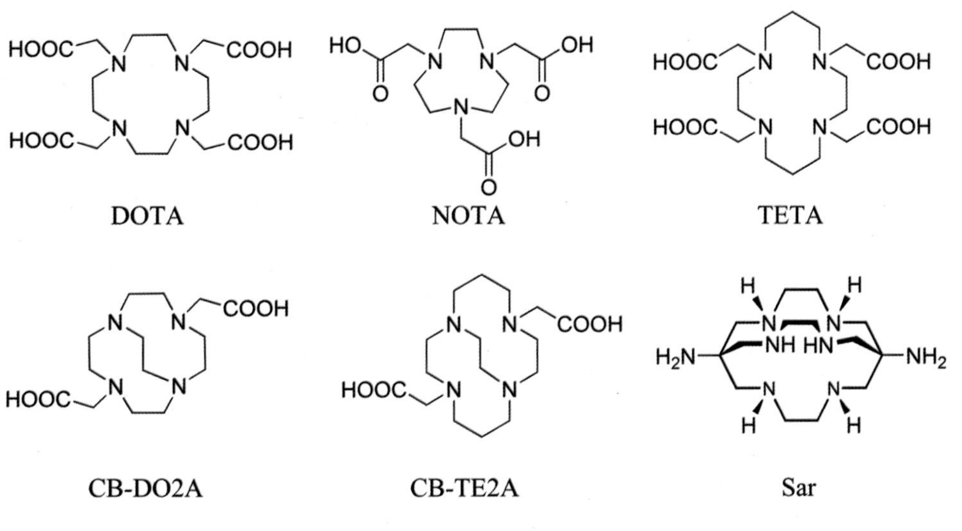

FIG 2.6 ● Representative macrocyclic chelators.

1-ethyl-3-(3-dimethylaminopropyl) carbodiimide hydrochloride (EDC) and *N*-hydroxysuccinimide (NHS), affording an intermediate that is reactive toward formation of amide bond with primary amine group (45). Some chelators containing the activate form of carboxylate group are now commercially available, facilitating the coupling into a single-step reaction. Recently, a new class of bifunctional chelators has been developed based on the structure of hexaazamacrobicyclic sarcophagine cage (Sar). The resulting Cu–Sar complex is extraordinarily stable under physiological conditions, and resists metal transchelation to copper-binding biomolecules (46).

Recently, the application of ^{68}Ga-labeled PET tracers has attracted considerable interest because of the physical characteristics of ^{68}Ga (47–52). ^{68}Ga decays by 89% through positron emission of 1.92 MeV (max energy) and is available from an in-house ^{68}Ge/^{68}Ga generator. With a half-life of 68 min, ^{68}Ga is also suitable for the pharmacokinetics of many biomolecules. ^{68}Ga is labeled with biomolecules through macrocyclic chelators. Both DOTA and NOTA (Fig. 2.6) can be used as bifunctional chelators for ^{68}Ga labeling. However, DOTA has a larger cavity than NOTA, which results in lower stability of the ^{68}Ga complex. In addition, the ^{68}Ga labeling of NOTA complex can be carried out at room temperature within short time, while the DOTA complex needs a higher temperature. Various ^{68}Ga-labeled PET tracers have been constructed, including ^{68}Ga-PSMA[LD1] (53).

RADIOPHARMACEUTICALS

A radiopharmaceutical is defined by the U.S. Food and Drug Administration (FDA) as "a drug that exhibits spontaneous disintegration of unstable nuclei with the emission of nuclear particles or photons." Essentially, a radiopharmaceutical is a radiochemical that has undergone a series of tests in animals and humans and has been shown to be safe and effective for a particular diagnostic or therapeutic application.

Unlike traditional drugs, radiopharmaceuticals possess a few unique characteristics. The risk of chemical toxicity from radiopharmaceuticals is essentially nil because only trace amounts are administered. Therefore, radiopharmaceuticals do not produce a pharmacologic effect in the body. However, radiopharmaceuticals possess an inherent radiation risk, limiting the amount of radioactivity that can be administered.

Radiopharmaceuticals can be prepared by a drug manufacturer, at a nuclear pharmacy, or at the site of use. Before a radiotracer can be administered to humans, reaction mixtures after radiolabeling need to be purified in order to isolate the radiotracer from the precursor and other reagents, which should not be present in the final product. The obtained radiotracer can be sterilized by sterile membrane filtration and formulated to produce a compound that is of pharmaceutical quality. The physicochemical forms of radiopharmaceuticals are diverse, including radiolabeled elemental forms, simple ions, small molecules, macromolecules, and particles. Radiopharmaceuticals are administered mainly by intravenous injection, but also as oral dosage forms, such as capsules or solutions, and by inhalation, as gases and aerosols.

New radiotracers deemed worthy of commercial investment require full evaluation via the traditional investigational new drug (IND) application. IND applications contain details that are reviewed by FDA prior to approval. The major areas described in the IND application are manufacturing information, pharmacology and toxicology data, clinical protocol, and investigator information. The manufacturing information regarding composition, manufacture, stability, and controls is provided to ensure that the drug can be produced and supplied in a consistent manner. Clinical trials must be reviewed and approved by the local institutional review board. Upon successful completion of a Phase 3 clinical trial, the sponsor may submit a new drug application (NDA) to FDA. If the data are sufficient to demonstrate safety and efficacy, the NDA will be approved by FDA, and then the sponsor has the legal right to market the radiopharmaceutical.

QUALITY CONTROL OF RADIOPHARMACEUTICALS

All radiopharmaceuticals must be tested to assure acceptable quality prior to administration to human subjects. In the United States, the FDA regulates the drug manufacturing process and develops the necessary requirements for good manufacturing practices (GMP). Manufacturing practices are the methods, facilities, and controls used in the preparation, processing, packaging, or storing of a drug. A current good manufacturing practice (cGMP) is a minimum standard, which ensures that the drug meets the requirements of safety and has the identity strength, quality, and purity characteristics. The FDA Modernization Act of 1997 (FDAMA) directs the FDA to establish cGMP requirements for radiopharmaceuticals.

The U.S. Pharmacopoeia (USP) describes the general guidelines for the safety, quality assurance (QA), and quality control (QC) of radiopharmaceuticals. The QA requirements for any drug product include QC test procedures, acceptance criteria, and test schedule. QC tests are performed in the manufacturing process of every single batch of a radiopharmaceutical. Due to the relatively short half-lives of radionuclides, each batch of the radiopharmaceutical may be released for administration into human subjects based on QC tests performed on the final batch preparation. Routine radiopharmaceutical QC tests can be broken down into the following categories: radiation tests, chemical tests, pharmaceutical tests, and biologic tests.

The safe use of radiopharmaceuticals requires that their radionuclide be of the highest purity. Half-life is a unique property of each radioisotope, and thus the radionuclidic identity can be determined by measuring the half-life of the radioactivity using a dose calibrator. Radionuclidic purity is defined as the fraction of total radioactivity that is present as the specified radionuclide in the final drug product. The nature and levels of radionuclidic impurities depend on the type of nuclear reaction. Determination of the nature and energy of the emitted electromagnetic radiation is usually carried out by gamma spectrometry using a multichannel analyzer equipped with either a sodium iodide thallium-activated [NaI(Tl)] or lithium-drifted germanium [Ge(Li)] detector. In addition, the concentration of radioactivity in every batch of the radiopharmaceutical must be determined and expressed as GBq/mL or mCi/mL at the end of synthesis. Furthermore, the radiopharmaceutical identity must be established by demonstrating that the chromatographic behavior of the radiolabeled drug product is similar to that of a non-radiolabeled drug product. The analytical methods include electrophoresis, gas chromatography

(GC), liquid chromatography (LC), paper chromatography, SPE, and thin-layer chromatography (TLC). A reference standard should be used in conjunction with the test sample during the radiochemical identification process to accurately identify and differentiate the desired radiochemical from radiochemical impurities. The radiochemical purity of a radiopharmaceutical is defined as the ratio, expressed as a percentage, of the radioactivity in the desired chemical form to the total radioactivity in the radiopharmaceutical preparation. Because of the undesirable distribution of the radiochemical impurities in human subjects, the amount of the total radiochemical impurities must be minimal in the final drug product. For receptor-targeted radiopharmaceuticals, specific activity is a critical specification, where the uptake of the radiopharmaceutical at receptors is significantly affected by the mass of radiotracer injected. Therefore, the specific activity may be included in the QC acceptance criteria.

The chemical purity test is a measurement of the presence of any undesirable chemical species in the final drug product. The chemical impurities may result from the breakdown of a precursor or other chemicals in the reaction mixture after the reaction. The mass of chemical impurities may cause undesirable pharmacological side effects or interfere with the radiopharmaceutical. Similar to the chemical purity assessment, any residual solvents present in the final drug product must be determined and below USP limits. A GC system with flame ionization detection is the instrument of choice in the determination of residual solvents.

Regarding the pharmaceutical aspects of a radiopharmaceutical, the basic considerations include appearance and color, pH, osmolality, and stability of the final drug product. The radiopharmaceutical is visually inspected to check for the color and presence of any particulate matter. The visual inspection should be carried out through leaded glass shielding that is not tinted or fogged and under adequate light so that the radiopharmaceutical observed is not obscured. All radiopharmaceuticals have an optimal pH range for stability, and most radiopharmaceuticals are within a pH range of 4 to 8. Since the pH of the final product may vary from batch to batch, it is important that the actual pH of the radiopharmaceutical is tested using pH paper or a suitably calibrated pH-measuring device. In addition, the final drug product of a radiopharmaceutical must be isotonic, meaning that the ionic strength of the drug formulation is the same or close to that of blood. Most radiopharmaceutical preparations are generally formulated using physiological saline or a phosphate buffered saline solution. Routine test of osmolality for each batch of the drug product may not be necessary. However, periodic test on the decayed drug product is appropriate. While the radiopharmaceutical product is being stored for administration, it should remain stable. Appropriate parameters should be evaluated to establish and document the stability of a drug product under proposed storage conditions. According to the stability data, the expiration of the radiopharmaceutical can be determined.

Radiopharmaceuticals must be prepared by aseptic processing to ensure that the drug product is free of microorganisms and toxic microbial byproducts. The drug products with a long enough half-life should be subjected to the sterility test before use. The sterility test uses fluid thioglycolate medium to test bacterial contamination and soybean casein digest medium to test fungi. Since the sterility test is completed retrospectively for most radiopharmaceuticals, the membrane filter integrity test (bubble point test) can be considered as an indicator of the microbiologic purity of the drug product. All membranes used for product sterilization must pass an integrity test prior to product release. Pyrogens are metabolic products of microorganisms that cause a pyretic response upon injection. Endotoxin is the most common pyrogen. All radiopharmaceutical products are required to be pyrogen free or below the endotoxin limit. For radiopharmaceuticals not administered intrathecally, the endotoxin limit is set at 175 endotoxin units (EUs) per V, where V is the maximum recommended dose in milliliters.

It is very important to emphasize that the patient safety should never be compromised under any circumstances; therefore, the quality of a radiopharmaceutical must meet all the QC acceptance criteria to assure safety and efficacy (Table 2.3).

Table 2.3 **RADIOPHARMACEUTICAL QUALITY ASSURANCE**			
	Radionuclide: ^{99}**Mo Breakthrough**	**Chemical:** **Al**$_3^{+++}$ **Breakthrough**	**Radiochemical:** **Free pertechnetate**
Method	Differential Attenuation 740–780 keV vs. 140 keV Or spectral analyzer	*Aurin Tricarboxylic* Acid test paper	Thin-layer chromatography
Limits	0.15/µCi ^{99}Mo/ mCi ^{99m}Tc at administration	10 µgm Al/mCi ^{99}Tc (10 ppm)	5–10% (typically, <3%)
Effects	Beta radiation to liver	Colloid formation, precipitation, agglutination	Thyroid, stomach, salivary activity
Required by NRC ?	Yes	No	Usually
Required for unit doses?	No	No	No

References

1. Andrade ENdC. *Rutherford and the nature of the atom.* Garden City, NY: Peter Smith Pub Inc; 1964.

2. Thomson JJ. On the structure of the atom: an investigation of the stability and periods of oscillation of a number of corpuscles arranged at equal intervals around the circumference of a circle; with application of the results to the theory of atomic structure. *Philosophical Magazine Sixth.* 1904;7(39):237–265.

3. Chadwick J. Possible existence of a neutron. *Nature.* 1932;129(3252):312.

4. Yukawa H. On the interaction of elementary particles. *Proc Phys-Math Soc Jpn.* 1935;17(48[LD2]).

5. Freedman MI. Frederick soddy and the practical significance of radioactive matter. *Br J Hist Sci.* 2009;12(3):257–260.

6. Close F, Marten M, Sutton C. *The particle odyssey: a journey to the heart of matter.* New York City, NY: Oxford University Press Inc; 2002.

7. Chen K, Conti PS. Target-specific delivery of peptide-based probes for PET imaging. *Adv Drug Deliv Rev.* 2010;62(11):1005–1022.

8. Chen K, Chen X. Positron emission tomography imaging of cancer biology: current status and future prospects. *Semin Oncol.* 2011;38(1):70–86.

9. Anderson CJ, Bulte JW, Chen K, et al. Design of targeted cardiovascular molecular imaging probes. *J Nucl Med.* 2010;51 Suppl 1:3s–17s.

10. Xiong KL, Yang QW, Gong SG, Zhang WG. The role of positron emission tomography imaging of β-amyloid in patients with Alzheimer's disease. *Nucl Med Commun.* 2010;31(1):4–11.

11. Tsukada H. Application of pre-clinical PET imaging for drug development. *Nihon Shinkei Seishin Yakurigaku Zasshi.* 2011;31 (5–6):231–237.

12. Murphy PS, McCarthy TJ, Dzik-Jurasz AS. The role of clinical imaging in oncological drug development. *Br J Radiol.* 2008;81(969): 685–692.

13. Li Z, Conti PS. Radiopharmaceutical chemistry for positron emission tomography. *Adv Drug Deliv Rev.* 2010;62(11):1031–1051.

14. Dolle F. Fluorine-18-labelled fluoropyridines: advances in radiopharmaceutical design. *Curr Pharm Des.* 2005;11(25):3221–3235.

15. Pike VW, Aigbirhio FI. Reactions of cyclotron-produced [^{18}F]fluoride with diaryliodonium salts – a novel single-step route to no-carrier-added [^{18}F]fluoroarenes. *J Chem Soc, Chem Commun.* 1995: 2215–2216.

16. Shah A, Pike VW, Widdowson DA. The synthesis of [^{18}F]fluoroarenes from the reaction of cyclotron-produced [^{18}F]fluoride ion with diaryliodonium salts. *J Chem Soc, Perkin Trans 1.* 1998:2043–2046.

17. Namavari M, Bishop A, Satyamurthy N, Bida G, Barrio JR. Regioselective radiofluorodestannylation with [^{18}F]F$_2$ and [^{18}F]CH$_3$COOF: a high yield synthesis of 6-[^{18}F]fluoro-*L*-DOPA. *Int J Rad Appl Instrum A.* 1992;43(8):989–996.

18. Ehrenkaufer RE, Potocki JF, Jewett DM. Simple synthesis of F-18-labeled 2-fluoro-2-deoxy-*D*-glucose: concise communication. *J Nucl Med.* 1984;25(3):333–337.

19. Luxen A, Guillaume M, Melega WP, Pike VW, Solin O, Wagner R. Production of 6-[^{18}F]fluoro-*L*-DOPA and its metabolism in vivo – a critical review. *Int J Rad Appl Instrum B.* 1992;19(2):149–158.

20. Wester HJ, Hamacher K, Stocklin G. A comparative study of N.C.A. fluorine-18 labeling of proteins via acylation and photochemical conjugation. *Nucl Med Biol.* 1996;23(3):365–372.

21. von Guggenberg E, Sader JA, Wilson JS, et al. Automated synthesis of an ^{18}F-labelled pyridine-based alkylating agent for high yield oligonucleotide conjugation. *Appl Radiat Isot.* 2009;67(9):1670–1675.

22. Vaidyanathan G, Zalutsky MR. Improved synthesis of N-succinimidyl 4-[^{18}F]fluorobenzoate and its application to the labeling of a monoclonal antibody fragment. *Bioconjug Chem.* 1994;5(4):352–356.

23. Vaidyanathan G, Zalutsky MR. Synthesis of N-succinimidyl 4-[^{18}F] fluorobenzoate, an agent for labeling proteins and peptides with ^{18}F. *Nat Protoc.* 2006;1(4):1655–1661.

24. Ponde DE, Dence CS, Oyama N, et al. ^{18}F-Fluoroacetate: a potential acetate analog for prostate tumor imaging--in vivo evaluation of ^{18}F-fluoroacetate versus ^{11}C-acetate. *J Nucl Med.* 2007;48(3):420–428.

25. Block D, Coenen HH, Stöcklin G. N.C.A. ^{18}F-fluoroacylation via fluorocarboxylic acid esters. *J Labelled Compd Radiopharm.* 1988(25):185–200.

26. Lang L, Eckelman WC. Labeling proteins at high specific activity using N-succinimidyl 4-[^{18}F](fluoromethyl) benzoate. *Appl Radiat Isot.* 1997;48(2):169–173.

27. Aloj L, Lang L, Jagoda E, Neumann RD, Eckelman WC. Evaluation of human transferrin radiolabeled with N-succinimidyl 4-[fluorine-18] (fluoromethyl) benzoate. *J Nucl Med.* 1996;37(8):1408–1412.

28. Kilbourn MR, Dence CS, Welch MJ, Mathias CJ. Fluorine-18 labeling of proteins. *J Nucl Med.* 1987;28(4):462–470.

29. Shiue CY, Wolf AP, Heinfeld JF. Synthesis of ^{18}F-labelled N-(p-[^{18}F] fluorophenyl)maleimide and its derivatives for labelling monoclonal antibody with ^{18}F. *J Label Compd Radiopharm.* 1988;26:287–289.

30. de Bruin B, Kuhnast B, Hinnen F, et al. 1-[3-(2-[^{18}F]Fluoropyridin-3-yloxy)propyl]pyrrole-2,5-dione: design, synthesis, and radiosynthesis of a new [^{18}F]fluoropyridine-based maleimide reagent for the labeling of peptides and proteins. *Bioconjug Chem.* 2005;16(2):406–420.

31. Kolb HC, Finn MG, Sharpless KB. Click chemistry: diverse chemical function from a few good reactions. *Angew Chem Int Ed Engl.* 2001;40(11):2004–2021.

32. Hausner SH, Marik J, Gagnon MK, Sutcliffe JL. In vivo positron emission tomography (PET) imaging with an alphavbeta6 specific peptide radiolabeled using ^{18}F-"click" chemistry: evaluation and comparison with the corresponding 4-[^{18}F]fluorobenzoyl- and 2-[^{18}F]fluoropropionyl-peptides. *J Med Chem.* 2008;51(19):5901–5904.

33. Li ZB, Wu Z, Chen K, Chin FT, Chen X. Click chemistry for ^{18}F-labeling of RGD peptides and micropet imaging of tumor integrin α$_v$β$_3$ expression. *Bioconjug Chem.* 2007;18(6):1987–1994.

34. Nwe K, Brechbiel MW. Growing applications of "click chemistry" for bioconjugation in contemporary biomedical research. *Cancer Biother Radiopharm.* 2009;24(3):289–302.

35. Miller PW, Long NJ, Vilar R, Gee AD. Synthesis of ^{11}C, ^{18}F, ^{15}O, and ^{13}N radiolabels for positron emission tomography. *Angew Chem Int Ed Engl.* 2008;47(47):8998–9033.

36. Conti PS, Alauddin MM, Fissekis JR, Schmall B, Watanabe KA. Synthesis of 2'-fluoro-5-[^{11}C]-methyl-1-β-*D*-arabinofuranosyluracil ([^{11}C]-FMAU): a potential nucleoside analog for in vivo study of cellular proliferation with PET. *Nucl Med Biol.* 1995;22(6):783–789.

37. Link JM, Krohn KA, Clark JC. Production of [^{11}C]CH$_3$I by single pass reaction of [^{11}C]CH$_4$ with I$_2$. *Nucl Med Biol.* 1997;24(1):93–97.

38. Mock BH, Mulholland GK, Vavrek MT. Convenient gas phase bromination of [^{11}C]methane and production of [^{11}C]methyl triflate. *Nucl Med Biol.* 1999;26(4):467–471.

39. Kniess T, Rode K, Wuest F. Practical experiences with the synthesis of [^{11}C]CH$_3$I through gas phase iodination reaction using a tracerlabfxc synthesis module. *Appl Radiat Isot.* 2008;66(4):482–488.

40. Andersson J, Truong P, Halldin C. In-target produced [^{11}C]methane: increased specific radioactivity. *Appl Radiat Isot.* 2009;67(1):106–110.

41. Pascali C, Bogni A, Itawa R, Cambiè M, Bombardieri E. [^{11}C]methylation on a C18 sep-pak cartridge: a convenient way to produce [N-methyl-^{11}C]choline,. *J Label Compds Radiopharm.* 2000;43: 195–203.

42. Wilson AA, DaSilva JN, Houle S. Solid-phase radiosynthesis of [^{11}C] WAY100635. *J Label Compds Radiopharm.* 1996;38:149–154.

43. Pascali C, Bogni A, Iwata R, Decise D, Crippa F, Bombardieri E. High efficiency preparation of *L*-[S-methyl-^{11}C]methionine by on-column [^{11}C]methylation on C18 sep-pak. *J Label Compds Radiopharm.* 1999;42:715–724.

44. Sun X, Anderson CJ. Production and applications of copper-64 radiopharmaceuticals. *Methods Enzymol.* 2004;386:237–261.

45. Sosabowski JK, Mather SJ. Conjugation of dota-like chelating agents to peptides and radiolabeling with trivalent metallic isotopes. *Nat Protoc.* 2006;1(2):972–976.

46. Voss SD, Smith SV, DiBartolo N, et al. Positron emission tomography (PET) imaging of neuroblastoma and melanoma with ^{64}Cu-SarAr immunoconjugates. *Proc Natl Acad Sci U S A.* 2007;104(44):17489–17493.

47. Banerjee SR, Pullambhatla M, Byun Y, et al. ^{68}Ga-Labeled inhibitors of prostate-specific membrane antigen (PSMA) for imaging prostate cancer. *J Med Chem.* 2010;53(14):5333–5341.

48. Dimitrakopoulou-Strauss A, Hohenberger P, Haberkorn U, Macke HR, Eisenhut M, Strauss LG. ^{68}Ga-Labeled bombesin studies in patients with gastrointestinal stromal tumors: comparison with 18F-FDG. *J Nucl Med.* 2007;48(8):1245–1250.

49. Sathekge M. The potential role of ^{68}Ga-labeled peptides in PET imaging of infection. *Nucl Med Commun.* 2008;29(8):663–665.

50. Schottelius M, Berger S, Poethko T, Schwaiger M, Wester HJ. Development of novel [68]Ga- and ^{18}F-labeled GnRH-I analogues with high GnRHR-targeting efficiency. *Bioconjug Chem.* 2008;19(6):1256–1268.

51. Ujula T, Salomaki S, Virsu P, et al. Synthesis, ^{68}Ga labeling and preliminary evaluation of dota peptide binding vascular adhesion protein-1: a potential PET imaging agent for diagnosing osteomyelitis. *Nucl Med Biol.* 2009;36(6):631–641.

52. Velikyan I, Beyer GJ, Bergstrom-Pettermann E, Johansen P, Bergstrom M, Langstrom B. The importance of high specific radioactivity in the performance of ^{68}Ga-labeled peptide. *Nucl Med Biol.* 2008;35(5):529–536.

53. Han S, Woo S, Kim YJ, Suh CH. Impact of ^{68}Ga-PSMA PET on the management of patients with prostate cancer: a systematic review and meta-analysis. *Eur Urol.* 2018;74(2):179–190.

CHAPTER SELF-ASSESSMENT QUESTIONS

1. During the [^{18}F]FDG synthesis, [^{18}F]fluoride ion reacts with the mannose triflate precursor through the nucleophilic substitution reaction.

   A. True

   B. False

2. In the case of radiometal labeling of biomolecules, chemical reactions take place when a radiometal reacts with a chelator in biomolecules. What type of the chemical reaction is called?

   A. Substitution

   B. Elimination

   C. Coordination

   D. Rearrangement

Answers to Chapter Self-Assessment Questions

1. B   [^{18}F]fluoride ion is a nucleophile that reacts at carbon atom number 2 of the mannose triflate precursor during the [^{18}F]FDG synthesis. In the nucleophilic substitution reaction, the triflate group is replaced by a radioactive fluorine atom (^{18}F) with "inversion of stereochemistry."

2. C   In the case of radiometal labeling of biomolecules, the chelator in biomolecules and the radiometal form a complex through the coordination reaction, where the chelator is attached to the radiometal by dative bonds, also known as coordinate bonds.

Basics of Instrumentation

3

Kai Lee

LEARNING OBJECTIVES

1. Recognize and explain how gas radiation detector works.

2. Recognize and explain how scintillators work.

3. Describe how the components of a gamma camera function.

4. Describe how single-photon emission computed tomography is acquired.

5. Describe how positron emission tomography is acquired.

INTRODUCTION

The most conspicuous equipment in nuclear medicine is the large gamma cameras and positron emission tomography/computed tomography (PET/CT) scanners for producing images of radionuclide distribution in the patient. The less conspicuous but indispensable instruments are the radiation survey meters, dose calibrators, and well counters for radiation safety survey and assay of radioactivity. Regardless of the diverse purposes and constructions, all nuclear medicine instruments rely on the photoelectric effects and Compton interactions to detect the presence of radiation. Therefore, grasping the mechanisms of interaction between radiation and matter is a prerequisite for selecting and fully utilizing the plethora of nuclear medicine instruments.

Nuclear medicine instruments can be broadly classified into two categories—gas detectors and scintillation detectors. Gas detectors measure the electric signal produced by interactions between the electrons and positively charged ions (ion pairs) created by the interaction of radiation with the gas atoms in the tube. The dose calibrators and Geiger survey meters as shown in Figure 3.1 exemplify the gas detectors. These ion pairs are attracted to the electrodes where they create a small electric current and a voltage pulse. The amplitude and frequency of voltage pulses represent the radiation exposure and radiation exposure rate.

Scintillation detectors use scintillator crystals coupled to photomultiplier tubes (PMTs) where photons are converted to electrical pulses. Gamma cameras typically use sodium iodide (NaI) crystals. PET scanners use other crystals including bismuth germanate and lutetium oxyorthosilicate. Scintillation detectors are unable to detect beta particles as they are markedly attenuated in the crystal's aluminum covering. These crystals are known as scintillators because they create a pulse of light upon photoelectric interactions with radiation. These pulse amplitudes are proportional to the energy and number of the incident photons, produced per unit time. Each light pulse is converted to an electrical signal in the PMT and sent on for processing. Figure 3.2 shows scintillators used for thyroid uptake counting and gamma camera imaging.

Gas detectors

A gas detector uses an air- or gas-filled chamber. Detector sensitivity is proportional to chamber volume. Larger chambers have more gas molecules available to interact with the incident radiation, improving the sensitivity of the detector. High-sensitivity gas detectors may be pressurized to as much as eight atmospheres to maximize the gas molecule density in the chamber for maximal photon interactions. Interior chamber walls are coated with an electrical conductor such as graphite that is maintained at a potential difference with the center wire as shown in Figure 3.3.

Radiation within the detector causes gas molecule ion pair formation. The positively charged, center wire anode attracts the electrons, and the negatively charged, chamber wall attracts the positively charged ions. This creates an electrical current. If the voltage between the center wire and the chamber wall is low, many of the negatively charged electrons and positively charged ions can recombine soon after they are formed, resulting in little or no detectible signal. As the voltage between the electrodes is increased, the signal increases because more of the electrons and positive ions are pulled apart before they have a chance to recombine.

Figure 3.4 shows the increasing output electric current as the applied electrode voltage increases. Due to the low potential difference between the electrodes in the recombination region (Region 1), many of the electrons and positive ions recombine immediately after they are created. This reduces the detectible signal. As the voltage increases, more electrons and positive ions are produced before they can recombine. Thus, increasing the applied voltage generally increases the signal. Region 2 is known as the saturation or ionization region. In the saturation region, applied voltage changes result in very little changes in the output signal. This occurs because the electrode is sufficiently high that all the ion pairs created by the radiation were separated and collected before they could recombine. The signal output reached a steady state because the detector is current limited by the inability of incident radiation to create more ion pairs.

Gas Detectors Used in Nuclear Medicine

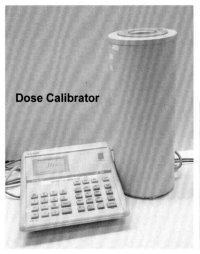

Dose Calibrator

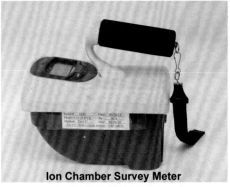

Ion Chamber Survey Meter

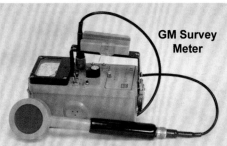

GM Survey Meter

FIG. 3.1 ● Typical gas detectors. Reprinted with permission from Lee, K. *Basic science of Nuclear Medicine: The Bare Bones Essentials.* Reston, VA: Society of Nuclear Medicine and Molecular Imaging; 2015.

GM, Geiger–Muller.

As shown in Figure 3.5, ionization chamber survey meters and dose calibrators are examples of gas instruments that operate in the ionization or saturation region. Ion chamber survey meters measure radiation exposure rate in μR/hour, mR/hour or R/hour (μSv/h, mSv/h, or Sv/h—in SI units). Ionization chambers are relatively independent of photon energy. These instruments produce the same reading for the same exposures of Tc-99m and I-131 even though the photon energy of Tc-99m (140 keV) is much lower than that of I-131 (360 keV).

The electric signal generated in an ionization chamber as in Figure 3.5 is low due to a limited number of ion pairs created by the incident radiation. Ionization chambers are most appropriate for high-activity radiation measurements. Dose calibrators are examples of low-sensitivity ionization chambers designed for measuring high levels of radioactivity. Dose calibrator scales are calibrated in microCuries (μCi). The dose calibrator scales are calibrated in microCurie (μCi), milliCurie (mCi), and Curie (Ci).

Geiger–Muller survey meters

Geiger–Mueller (GM) counters or survey meters are high-sensitivity gas detectors most commonly used for detecting low-level radioactivity. Like ionization chambers, GM meters use a gas mixture instead of air. The voltage applied to GM detectors is much higher than that applied to the ionization chambers. Ion pairs produced within a GM tube accelerate toward the electrodes with much greater energy with the production of many

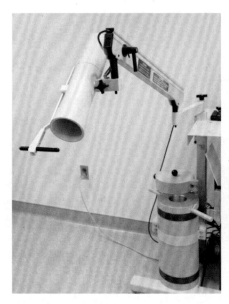

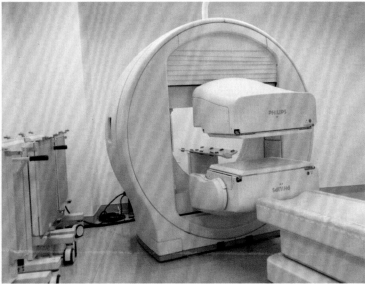

FIG. 3.2 ● Scintillation detectors are used in thyroid uptake probes, well counters, and gamma cameras. Reprinted with permission from Lee, K. *Basic science of Nuclear Medicine: The Bare Bones Essentials.* Reston, VA: Society of Nuclear Medicine and Molecular Imaging; 2015.

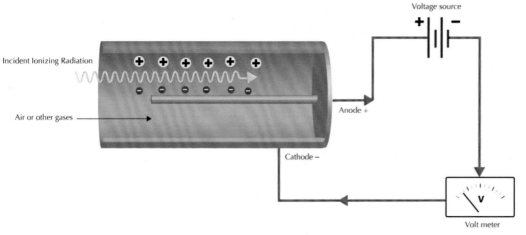

Voltage source

Incident Ionizing Radiation

Air or other gases

Anode +

Cathode −

Volt meter

FIG. 3.3 ● A simplified diagram of the basic components of a gas detector. Reprinted with permission from Lee, K. *Basic science of Nuclear Medicine: The Bare Bones Essentials*. Reston, VA: Society of Nuclear Medicine and Molecular Imaging; 2015.

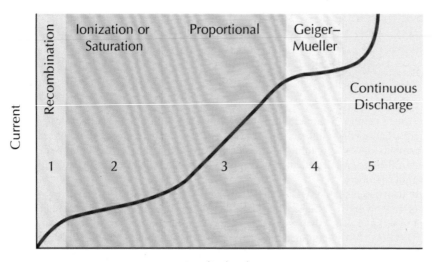

Ionization or Saturation

Proportional

Geiger–Mueller

Continuous Discharge

Recombination

Current

Applied Voltage

1   2   3   4   5

FIG. 3.4 ● The electric current generated as a function of the applied voltage between the electrodes. Reprinted with permission from Lee, K. *Basic science of Nuclear Medicine: The Bare Bones Essentials*. Reston, VA: Society of Nuclear Medicine and Molecular Imaging; 2015.

secondary ionizations upon interactions with the gas atoms. These secondary ion pairs also accelerate at high energy to the charged electrodes with the creation of more ion pairs. Thus, a single photon or beta particle can produce an avalanche of secondary ions. This avalanche of ions creates a strong electric signal suitable for display. GM survey meters are the appropriate choice for detecting low-level countertop radioactivity contamination. GM survey meters generally display radiation in counts per second (cps), counts per minute (cpm), or mR/hour.

It is important to note that GM instruments can fail to accurately detect and measure high levels of radioactivity. For example, a GM counter will underestimate true count rates for samples with greater than 10,000 disintegrations per second or a GM survey meter will present falsely low exposure rates if the true exposure rate exceeds 20 mR/hour. The cause of this GM tube failure in high count situations is the continued formation of excessive avalanche-produced ions which must be stopped or quenched so that the GM is prepared to react to subsequent radiation pulses. After a single ionization event, the time required for a GM detector to return to the quiescent state and be prepared for the detection of the second pulse of radiation is known as the resolving time. Typical GM tube resolving times are about 100 µs. Thus, the GM detector can count at the most one disintegration every 100 µs, or 10,000 cps. Disintegrations that occur in <100 µs after

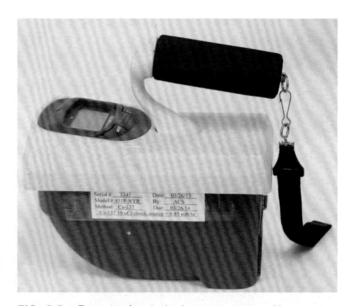

FIG. 3.5 ● Example of an ionization survey meter with a pressurized air chamber to increase the sensitivity. Reprinted with permission from Lee, K. *Basic science of Nuclear Medicine: The Bare Bones Essentials*. Reston, VA: Society of Nuclear Medicine and Molecular Imaging; 2015.

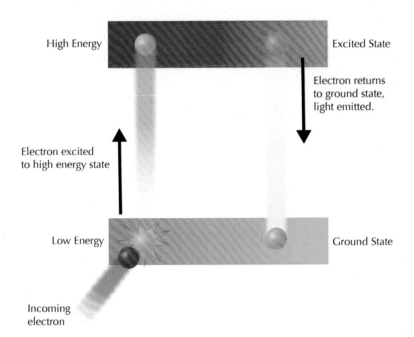

FIG. 3.6 ● An electron in the ground state is elevated to the excited states upon colliding with an energetic electron. Electrons in the high energy state are unstable and return to the ground state by releasing their excess energy as light. Reprinted with permission from Lee, K. *Basic science of Nuclear Medicine: The Bare Bones Essentials.* Reston, VA: Society of Nuclear Medicine and Molecular Imaging; 2015.

the preceding one will not be counted. Thus, GM counters are not suitable for counting samples with >10,000 cps.

Because of the long GM detector ionizing event recovery time, GM survey meters are inappropriate for measuring exposure rates from patients treated with I-131. This is especially true immediately after dose administration when the radiation exposure is highest. Undetected photons in the GM chamber result in falsely low radiation measurements. In the early days of the nuclear industry, some radiation overexposure accidents were caused by workers inappropriately relying on GM survey meters to measure radiation levels before inappropriately entering high-radiation areas. Misled by low instrument reading, workers entered the high-radiation area believing it was safe to do so.

Scintillation detectors

Scintillation detectors work by taking advantage of certain crystals that produce a flash of light upon absorbing a photon. NaI doped with a trace quantity of thallium is the most common scintillator used in radiation detection instruments. Photons interacting with NaI crystal create energetic electrons by photoelectric and Compton interactions as described in Chapter 1. Energetic electrons distribute their energy to other electrons in the NaI crystal by ionizations and excitations. In an excitation event,

the electron energy in a NaI atom is not sufficient to dislodge it from the atom but is sufficient to elevate the electron to the high-energy excited state as illustrated in Figure 3.6.

Electrons in the excited state are unstable, rapidly returning to the lower energy ground state with the release of light energy. The amplitude of the emitted light is characteristic for the crystal and is proportional to the amount of energy deposited in the crystal by the incident photon. NaI is hygroscopic and must be hermetically sealed to keep moisture from dissolving the crystal. Thus, scintillation detectors can only detect photons. Beta and alpha particles are unable to penetrate the metal casing to interact with the crystal to get detected. The next step is to convert the emitted light into an electrical signal using a PMT such as the ones shown in Figure 3.7.

A PMT is a glass vacuum tube with a photocathode, a series of dynodes, and an anode as in Figure 3.8. A PMT has a glass window with a photocathode and an optically transparent semiconductor coating. Electrons in the photocathode are weakly bound. Light transmitted from the NaI crystal causes the emission of electrons from the photocathode surface. The first dynode is charged at several hundred volts more positive than the photocathode. This attracts the electrons emitted from the photocathode toward the dynode. Electrons from the photocathode accelerate to the dynode with enough energy such that every

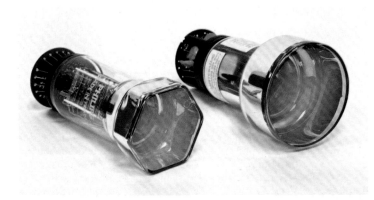

FIG. 3.7 ● Two types of end-window photomultiplier tubes used to convert flashes of light to electrical pulses in a gamma camera. Reprinted with permission from Lee, K. *Basic science of Nuclear Medicine: The Bare Bones Essentials.* Reston, VA: Society of Nuclear Medicine and Molecular Imaging; 2015.

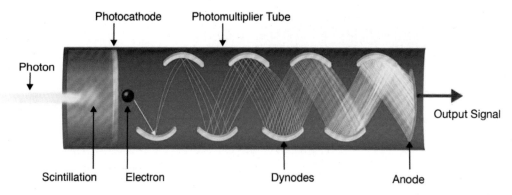

FIG. 3.8 ● Basic components of a scintillation detector. Light entered the photomultiplier tube causes the photocathode to release free electrons. The free electrons are accelerated toward a series of dynodes and multiply. Reprinted with permission from Lee, K. *Basic science of Nuclear Medicine: The Bare Bones Essentials.* Reston, VA: Society of Nuclear Medicine and Molecular Imaging; 2015.

electron striking the dynode releases three to five additional electrons that are emitted from the first dynode surface. This augmented electron cloud then accelerates to the second dynode, which has a greater positive voltage than the first dynode. More electrons are emitted from the second dynode. A typical PMT has a cascade of 10 dynodes that accelerate and amplify the electron cloud. The number of electrons collected by the anode at the end of the series of dynodes is about a million times that of at the photocathode. The final electrical pulse is easily measured.

The emitted light brightness in a NaI crystal is proportional to the incident photon energy. The number of electrons produced in the photocathode is proportional to the brightness of light transmitted from the crystal. The output pulse voltage at the PMT anode is proportional to the electron amplification factor of the dynode series. The output voltage from the PMT is, therefore, proportional to the photon energy deposited in the NaI crystal. This proportionality is the principle behind gamma-ray spectroscopy and the pulse height analyzer (PHA).

Pulse height analyzer

The principle behind pulse height analysis is that the PMT voltage pulse is proportional to the energy deposited by the photon in the scintillation crystal. Assume we place a 0.1µCi Cs-137 principle behind pulse height scintillation well counter and measure the voltage of each pulse exiting from the PMT. We will find that some pulses have higher voltages and some lower, indicating that different amounts of photon energy were absorbed in the NaI crystal. The term *pulse height* came from the old days when a voltage pulse was measured by the height of its blip on the oscilloscope screen. If we plot in a histogram of the number of pulses according to their pulse height, we obtain a pulse height spectrum as shown in Figures 3.9 and 3.10.

Gamma cameras

Figure 3.11 demonstrates the four components of a gamma camera. These include the collimator, a large flat NaI crystal, an array of PMTs, and a position and energy logic computer. Not shown in Figure 3.11 is an external computer that processes the signals from the camera to construct the images for viewing or quantitative analyses.

The collimator attached to the front of the gamma camera is a slab of lead with one or more holes in it. The collimator serves the following two essential functions:

1. Define the field of view.
2. Reject unwanted photons.

The collimator transmits only those photons traveling parallel to the open channels to pass through and absorbs those photons entering the channels at an oblique angle. The collimator wall thickness

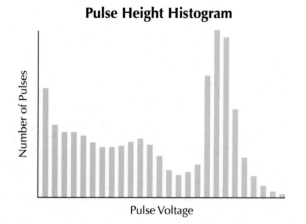

FIG. 3.9 ● A histogram of pulses received from Cs-137. Reprinted with permission from Lee, K. *Basic science of Nuclear Medicine: The Bare Bones Essentials.* Reston, VA: Society of Nuclear Medicine and Molecular Imaging; 2015.

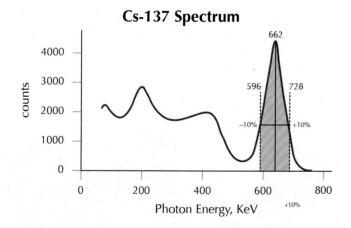

FIG. 3.10 ● Gamma-ray spectrum of Cs-137. A gamma-ray spectrum is a histogram of pulses produced by photons of different energies. A 20% window placed symmetrically on the 662 keV photopeak of Cs-137. Reprinted with permission from Lee, K. *Basic science of Nuclear Medicine: The Bare Bones Essentials.* Reston, VA: Society of Nuclear Medicine and Molecular Imaging; 2015.

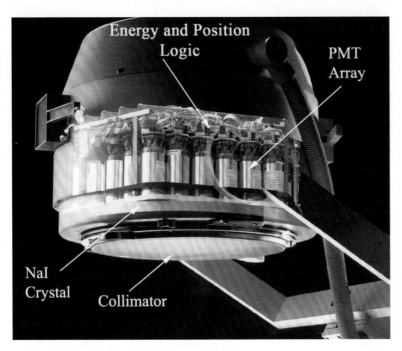

FIG. 3.11 ● Major components of a gamma camera. Reprinted with permission from Lee, K. *Basic science of Nuclear Medicine: The Bare Bones Essentials*. Reston, VA: Society of Nuclear Medicine and Molecular Imaging; 2015.

PMT, photomultiplier tube; NaI, sodium iodide.

limits what photon energies can be imaged. The size, shape, height, and angular orientation of the holes in the collimator affect the data input rate, the field of view, the magnification, contrast, and resolution of the acquired image. Collimator geometry affects the image resolution and count rate capability of the gamma camera.

Collimators are classified by their energy rating. The three major energy ratings of collimators are:

Energy Rating Energy Range Radionuclides

High energy—360 to 400 keV, I-131
Medium energy—200 to 300 keV, Ga-67 and In-111
Low energy—60 to 140 keV, Xe-133 and Tc-99m

The walls of the channels are called septa which have to be of sufficient thickness to absorb the oblique entry photons. Septal penetration is an image artifact resulting from the septa unable to block the oblique entry photons. In order to achieve a reasonable sensitivity, the medium- and high-energy collimators have relatively large channel openings to permit more photons to go through and spread to blur out the collimator hole pattern in the image. These collimator characteristics explain why Ga-67 and I-131 images have poorer resolution than that of Tc-99m.

Collimator geometry

The vast majority of nuclear medicine imaging procedures are done using the parallel-hole collimator, while the pinhole collimator is primarily used for imaging of the thyroid and other small body parts. The geometric shape of the parallel-hole and pinhole collimators is shown in Figure 3.12.

The parallel-hole collimator projects an image that is the same size as the source being imaged as shown in Figure 3.12. The field of view of a parallel-hole collimator is the same at all distances from the collimator because the incident photons are restricted to those entering parallel to the channel opening and perpendicular to the NaI crystal. The pinhole collimator produces superior image resolution compared with the parallel-hole collimator. Because the pinhole collimator limits photons to pass through a small aperture, the sensitivity is poor. As with the parallel-hole collimator, the smaller the pinhole opening, the better the image resolution, at the expense of sensitivity. We always have to contend with the inverse relationship between sensitivity and resolution. Pinhole collimator images are inverted as shown in Figure 3.12. Unlike the parallel hole collimator, magnification of the object in the image changes

FIG. 3.12 ● The parallel- and pinhole collimators are the two most commonly used collimators. Reprinted with permission from Lee, K. *Basic science of Nuclear Medicine: The Bare Bones Essentials*. Reston, VA: Society of Nuclear Medicine and Molecular Imaging; 2015.

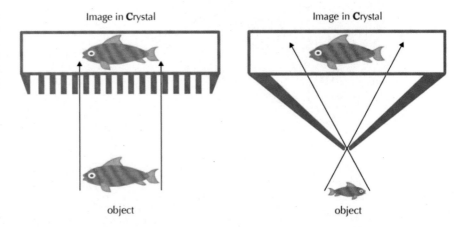

with distance from the aperture, closer the object to the pinhole, bigger the magnification.

Scintillation crystal

Photons passed through the collimator channels encounter a large flat NaI crystal. Whole-body gamma cameras use a 15 × 20 inches and 3/8-inch thick NaI crystal. Crystals of about 10 × 15 inches and ¼-inch thick are used in gamma cameras for cardiac imaging using Tc-99m. Thinner crystal reduces the distance available for light to diffuse and enables better scintillation event localization. Within the crystal, photons interact with the NaI atoms through the photoelectric effect and Compton scatter. The electrons liberated from Compton and photoelectric interactions in turn interact with other electrons in the NaI atoms by excitation and ionization. When the excited electrons return to their low-energy ground state, they release their excess energy by light emission. The emitted light brightness is proportional to the energy of the incident photon. This NaI characteristic allows photons of the desired energy to form the radionuclide image.

Photomultiplier tubes

The light produced in the NaI crystal is collected by an array of PMTs as shown in Figure 3.13. The PMT array serves to locate the site where the incident photon interacted with the NaI crystal. Each PMT in the array is assigned a pair of X- and Y-coordinates relative to the crystal center. Whenever a scintillation event occurs as the result of a photon striking the NaI crystal, the amount of light detected by each PMT depends on the proximity of the PMT to the origin of the light. The position and logic computer determines the location of the scintillation event by taking a weighted average of the X- and Y-coordinates of all the PMTs. The weighting factor is the amount of light a PMT receives. Thus, a PMT farther away from the photon source receives less light and produces less output voltage. Low voltage addresses are given lower weighting factors compared to the voltage from a PMT closer to the event. The location where the scintillation event occurs is determined as the average X- and Y-coordinates of all the PMTs in the array weighted by their respective output voltages.

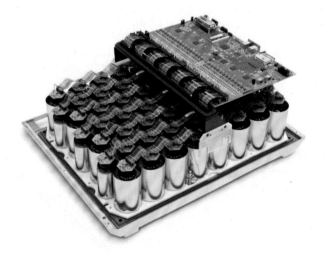

FIG. 3.13 ● Array of photomultiplier tubes covering the surface of the NaI crystal. Reprinted with permission from Lee, K. *Basic science of Nuclear Medicine: The Bare Bones Essentials.* Reston, VA: Society of Nuclear Medicine and Molecular Imaging; 2015.

Energy and position logic computer

The energy and position logic computer above the array of PMT adds the voltage output of each PMT in the array. The summed output voltage is proportional to the amount of light emitted by the NaI which in turn is proportional to the amount of energy deposited in the crystal by the incident photon. The pulse is then sent to a PHA in the external computer for processing. The PHA allows only those photons within the range of desired energy to form the radionuclide image and discards those photons with energies outside the desired range. The selection of appropriate scintillation events for radionuclide imaging is necessary because there is a considerable number of scattered photons that can pass through the collimator. Scattered photons are not desirable as they degrade the contrast of the image.

Single-photon emission computed tomography

A single-photon emission computed tomography (SPECT) system usually has two gamma cameras mounted on a gantry. For body or head imaging, the cameras are placed at 180° opposite each other. For cardiac imaging, the cameras are rotated to 90° relative to each other. The cameras rotate around the patient and stop to acquire images typically at 3° intervals over a 90° arc for cardiac, and 180° for non-cardiac studies. The images acquired at the various stops are called projection images. The projection images are then mathematically reconstructed to form a stack of cross-sectional images using an algorithm called filtered back projection. The picture elements, or pixels, in the reconstructed cross-sectional images can in turn be reformatted to produce images in coronal, sagittal, or any oblique angle views.

Single-photon emission computed tomography image quality

The quality of the reconstructed images depends strongly on the filter applied to the back-projection algorithm. For SPECT studies, the ramp filter convoluted with a Butterworth window was found to be the most satisfactory compromise between noise and resolution in the reconstructed images. Approximately, image resolution is the sharpness of the image, and noise is the graininess in the image. When applying the Butterworth window, we need to specify two parameters—the cut-off frequency and the order. The cut-off frequency is the threshold at which the image reconstruction begins to include less detail to suppress the rising image noise. The cut-off frequency at 0.5 means the filter starts to deal with the image graininess at 50% of the maximum sharpness that the camera or computer system can produce. The order is the rapidity at which the filter suppresses the inclusion of image details beyond the cut-off frequency to bring down the image noise. In Figure 3.14 (A), the image of a phantom was reconstructed using the ramp filter without the Butterworth window. The image in Figure 3.14 (B) was reconstructed with the ramp filter plus a Butterworth window with cut-off frequency at 0.5 and order 5. The image in Figure 3.14 (C) was reconstructed using the Butterworth window with cut-off frequency at 0.25 and order 10. Very little noise is evident in Figure 3.14 (C), but over-smoothing practically eliminated the image details.

How do we know which reconstruction filter to select for a given set of SPECT data? one may start the reconstruction with a high cut-off frequency to obtain a high-resolution image. If the reconstructed image appears grainy and fuzzy, use a lower cut-off

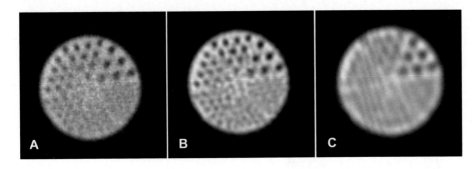

FIG. 3.14 • Transverse image of a phantom constructed with (**A**) Ramp filter, (**B**) Ramp + Butterworth with cut-off 0.5 and order 5, (**C**) Ramp filter + Butterworth with cut-off 0.25 and order 10. Image in (**A**) appears sharp but grainy; (**C**) appears smooth but devoid of detail; and (**B**) appears to be the best compromise between noise and resolution. Reprinted with permission from Lee, K. *Basic science of Nuclear Medicine: The Bare Bones Essentials.* Reston, VA: Society of Nuclear Medicine and Molecular Imaging; 2015.

frequency. If eliminating too many high frequencies results in over-smoothing, increase the cut-off frequency and reprocess. The filter selection is a subjective decision of the reader. Ultimately, there is a compromise between the amount of noise tolerated and the resolution desired in the reconstructed images. The Butterworth window with cut-off frequency at 0.5 and order 5 appears to be the best compromise between noise and resolution for SPECT reconstruction.

Positron emission tomography

The basis behind PET imaging is the labeling of a metabolically important molecule, such as glucose, to a positron-emitting radionuclide to study the metabolic processes in the patient. When a positron undergoes annihilation with an electron, two photons of 511 keV are simultaneously emitted at almost 180° relative to each other. The two photons interacting with two opposing detectors in the PET scanner produce a coincidence event and form a line of response (LOR) as shown in Figure 3.15. In a PET study, millions of LORs are acquired in about 20 min.

The LORs are reconstructed into cross-sectional images in two stages. The first stage is called rebinning. In rebinning, the LORs are sorted into parallel sets; each set is rotated a few degrees from the preceding set. Referring to Figure 3.16 (A), the number of counts in a LOR is proportional to the positron activity along the line through the patient. A set of such parallel LORs thus gives a projection profile at a given angle of coincident events through one slice of the patient. The count profiles are stored in a row of pixels in a matrix as shown in Figure 3.16 (B). The top row of the matrix is by convention the projection profile at zero-degree gantry angle. Each succeeding row in the matrix is the projection profile from a parallel set of LORs at a certain angular increment from the previous row. The angular increment between the rows of the projection profile depends on the reconstruction software. The last row is the count profile at 180° opposite the top row. PET imaging requires projection profiles 180° around the patient because the two opposing detectors for coincidence events provide the same information. The image formed by the rows of projection profiles in the matrix is called a sinogram. Each transverse image has its own sinogram. As the arm activity in Figure 3.16 (B) demonstrates, a sinogram traces a sine wave in the display. In summary, a pixel in the sinogram contains the counts measured along a LOR. Each row of pixels in the sinogram is a projection profile at a given angle around the patient. All the data for the reconstruction of a slice of a PET image are contained in the sinogram.

In the second stage of reconstruction, the sinogram is put through an iterative reconstruction algorithm to form a cross-sectional image as shown in Figure 3.16 (C). Upon reconstructing a series of contiguous cross-sectional images, the display software can rearrange pixels in the image volume to form coronal, sagittal, and other desired angular views.

Problems with reconstruction of positron emission tomography images

Are all the LORs acquired in a study useful for image reconstruction? The answer is a resounding no. A LOR can form from a true coincidence, a scatter coincidence, or a random coincidence. True coincidence events produce the ideal LORs in that the two 511 keV photons from the site of positron–electron annihilation are completely absorbed in opposite detectors. The number of true coincidence counts is proportional to the amount of positron-labeled pharmaceutical in the patient. True coincidence events provide accurate positional information, with higher spatial resolution and lower noise in the reconstructed image. In a scatter coincidence event, one or both annihilation photons underwent scatter in the patient's body before reaching the detectors. The LOR connecting the two detectors does not pass through the actual location of the annihilation event. Inaccurate geometric information from scatter coincident events increases the background counts and reduces the image contrast. Random coincidences arise from completely separate positron annihilation events; two totally unrelated photons just happened to strike opposing detectors simultaneously. The system mistakenly assumes the photons came from

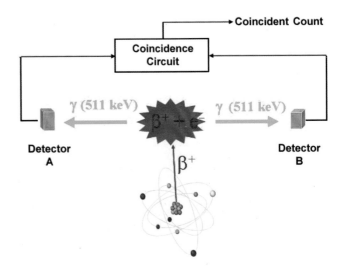

FIG. 3.15 • A coincident count is recorded when signals from Detector A and B arrive in the coincidence circuit within 5 to 10 ns of each other. Reprinted with permission from Lee, K. *Basic science of Nuclear Medicine: The Bare Bones Essentials.* Reston, VA: Society of Nuclear Medicine and Molecular Imaging; 2015.

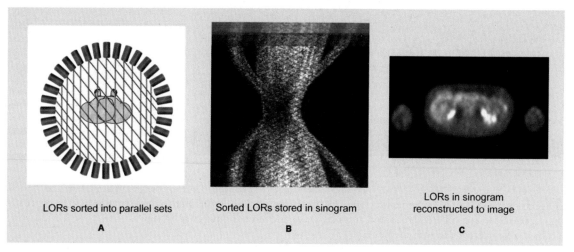

FIG. 3.16 ● (**A**) Coincident events are sorted or rebinned into parallel sets of LOR. The counts in each parallel set of LORs form the activity profile at a given angle. Two sets of parallel LORs are shown in the illustration. (**B**) The parallel sets of LORs are stored in an image matrix as rows of counts. There is one row of counts for each parallel set of LORS. The stack of parallel sets of LORs in the matrix forms image of a sinogram. (**C**) A reconstruction algorithm applied to the sinogram transformed the rows of counts (activity profiles) in the sinogram to a transverse image. Reprinted with permission from Lee, K. *Basic science of Nuclear Medicine: The Bare Bones Essentials*. Reston, VA: Society of Nuclear Medicine and Molecular Imaging; 2015.

LOR, lines of response.

a coincidence event and creates an erroneous LOR. Similar to scatter coincidences, random coincidences elevate the background noise and reduce the image contrast. High levels of random coincidence can paralyze the computer electronics, reduce the system's count rate capability, and substantially degrade the image resolution. Hardware and software solutions have been devised to reduce the contribution of random and scatter coincidences to the PET images.

Photon attenuation is a greater problem in PET than in SPECT. As shown in Figure 3.17, the two 511 keV photons in PET imaging must travel the entire width of the patient to get detected, while only one photon in SPECT needs to travel half the width of the patient to reach the gamma camera. With a longer travel distance for the annihilation photons, there is a greater chance that one of the two photons is scattered or absorbed, resulting in coincidence event loss. Problems presented by photon attenuation can be mitigated by performing a transmission scan to generate a map of correction factors to compensate for the loss of counts. In dedicated PET-only scanners, a radioactive source such as Ge-68 or Cs-137 provides the radiation source to perform the transmission scan. With the advent of PET/CT, transmission scans are done much more quickly using a CT scanner mounted in front of the PET scanner.

Positron emission tomography/computed tomography instrumentation

The most common configuration of a hybrid PET/CT scanner is a 16-slice CT mounted in tandem with a PET scanner as shown in Figure 3.18. Even though the CT and the PET scanners are built into one unit, the two scanners function independently. In a typical PET/CT exam, the CT transmission scan is acquired first. Photons from radioactivity in the patient do not affect the CT data because the gamma-ray intensity is much less than that of the X-ray. After completion of the CT scan, the patient is moved into

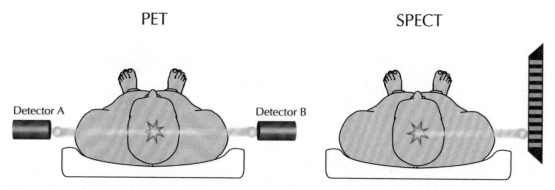

FIG. 3.17 ● In SPECT, only a single photon needs to travel across half the width of the patient to reach the gamma camera. In PET, the two annihilation photons have to travel the whole width to produce a coincident count. The likelihood for one of the two annihilation photons to get absorbed or scattered is increased in the longer path of travel. Reprinted with permission from Lee, K. *Basic science of Nuclear Medicine: The Bare Bones Essentials*. Reston, VA: Society of Nuclear Medicine and Molecular Imaging; 2015.

PET, positron emission tomography; SPECT, single-photon emission computed tomography.

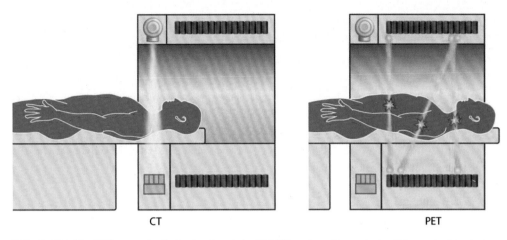

CT   PET

FIG. 3.18 ● The CT is mounted in the front end of a PET/CT system. Transmission CT scan is done before the emission PET scan. Reprinted with permission from Lee, K. *Basic science of Nuclear Medicine: The Bare Bones Essentials*. Reston, VA: Society of Nuclear Medicine and Molecular Imaging; 2015.

CT, computed tomography; PET, positron emission tomography.

the PET gantry for the emission scan. The CT serves two major functions. One function is to acquire high-resolution images to fuse with the PET images to provide anatomical landmarks for the sites of metabolic activities. The other function is to acquire data for the computation of correction factors to compensate for the loss of counts due to attenuation. CT tissue attenuation correction works by applying a database stored look-up table for each CT number with a corresponding attenuation coefficient for 511 KeV photons in the tissue. The correction factor for any pixel in the PET image is computed using the look-up table and the CT number in the corresponding pixel in the CT image.

Time of flight positron emission tomography/computed tomography

A time of flight (TOF) PET/CT uses fast electronics and scintillation crystals to detect the difference in time between the arrival of the 511 keV photons at opposing detectors. The time for an annihilation photon to travel from the site of annihilation to a detector is called TOF. If we could accurately measure the small difference in the TOF of the two annihilation photons, we could pinpoint the site of the annihilation event along their LOR without having to process the data through an image reconstruction algorithm.

Unfortunately, the timing resolution in current PET scanners is about 500 psec which gives us an uncertainty of 7.5 cm ([500 × 10^{-12} s][30 × 10^9 cm/s]/2). So our current technology limits our ability to identify the location of an annihilation event with an uncertainty of ±3.5 cm (7.5/2 cm). In spite of the inadequacy of our current technology, the TOF information put into the reconstruction algorithm helps to better localize an annihilation event. Figure 3.19 illustrates the difference between a TOF and a conventional PET scanner in placing coincident counts along the LOR.

With original PET scanners, reconstruction algorithms positioned counts received by two opposing detectors uniformly along the LOR as there was no information on where along the LOR the counts originated. With a current TOF scanner, differences in photon arriving time allowed the location of an annihilation event to within 7.5 cm in the LOR. Reducing the location uncertainty of annihilation events leads to less image noise and improvement in the image contrast. The contrast improvement increases with the size of the patient because the noise reduction applies not only to the true coincidence counts, but to the random and scattered coincidence counts which increase with the size of the patient. The interested reader on the topics presented in this chapter is referred to the following publications for further information (1–12).

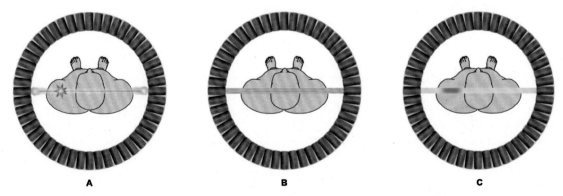

A   B   C

FIG. 3.19 ● The location of true event is shown in **A**. In conventional PET imaging (**B**) the coincident counts acquired between two opposing detectors are spread evenly along the LOR in the image matrix. In TOF PET imaging (**C**), the counts are localized to a segment of the LOR in the image matrix. Reprinted with permission from Lee, K. *Basic science of Nuclear Medicine: The Bare Bones Essentials*. Reston, VA: Society of Nuclear Medicine and Molecular Imaging; 2015.

LOR, lines of response; PET, positron emission tomography: TOF, time of flight.

References

1. Bailey DL, Townsend DW, Valk PE, Maisey MN. (eds). *Positron emission tomography: Basic sciences.* Springer-Verlag; 2005.
2. Buck AK, Nekolla S, Ziegler S, et al. SPECT/CT. *J Nucl Med.* 2008; 49:1305–1319.
3. Goldman LW. Principles of CT and CT technology. *J Nucl Med Technol.* 2007;35:115–128.
4. Goldman LW. Principle of CT: multislice CT. *J Nucl Med Technol.* 2008;36:57–68.
5. Kapoor V, McCook BM, Torok FS. An introduction to PET-CT imaging. *Radiographics.* 2004;24:523–543.
6. Lyra M, Ploussi A. Filtering in SPECT image reconstruction. *Int J Biomed Imaging.* 2011;1–14.
7. Patton JA, Turkington TG. SPECT/CT physical principles and attenuation correction. *J Nucl Med Technol.* 2008; 36:1–10.
8. Phelps ME. *PET: Physics, instrumentation, and scanners.* Springer-Verlag; 2006.
9. Prekeges J. *Nuclear medicine instrumentation.* 2nd ed. Jones & Bartlett; 2012.
10. Ranger NT. The AAPM/RSNA physics tutorial for residents: radiation detectors in nuclear medicine. *Radiographics* 1999;19:481–502.
11. Seibert AJ. X-ray imaging physics for nuclear medicine technologists. Part 1: basic principles of X-ray production. *J Nucl Med Technol.* 2004;32:139–147.
12. Seibert JA, Boone JM. X-ray imaging physics for nuclear medicine technologists. Part 2: X-ray interactions and image formation. *J Nucl Med Technol.* 2005;33:3–18.

CHAPTER SELF-ASSESSMENT QUESTIONS

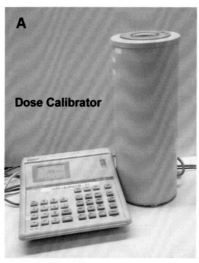

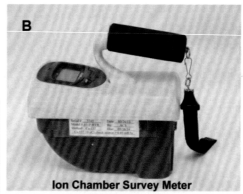

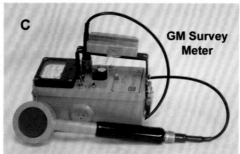

1. Which instrument would be best for examining a room for low-level radiation?

2. Which instrument would be better to measure the radioactivity of a patient receiving 200 mCi of I-131?

3. Which instrument is best suited to determine dosage in millicuries?

4. Which display is the smoothest?

5. Which display is the sharpest?

6. Which display has the best overall appearance?

Answers to Chapter Self-Assessment Questions

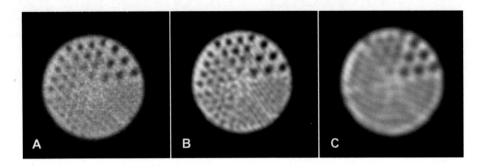

1. Which instrument would be best for examining a room for low-level radiation? The best choice is (**C**), the Geiger–Mueller survey meter due to its high sensitivity for low-level radiation.

2. Which instrument would be better to measure the radioactivity of a patient receiving 200 mCi of I-131? As the Geiger–Mueller survey meter (C) would likely saturate and thus underreport the actual dose rate, the Ion Chamber Survey Meter (**B**) would be the best choice.

3. Which instrument is best suited to determine dosage in millicuries? The appropriate instrument for measuring dosage in millicuries is the Dose Calibrator (**A**).

4. Which display is the smoothest? Display (**C**) applied a Ramp filter + Butterworth with cut-off 0.25 and order 10. The overall display is too smooth with no detail.

5. Which display is the sharpest? Display (**A**) is sharpened with a Ramp filter yielding a detailed but grainy image.

6. Which display has the best overall appearance? Display (**B**) applied Ramp plus Butterworth filtration with cut-off 0.5 and order 5, offering the best compromise between noise and resolution.

Thyroid Imaging and Therapy

4

Erik S. Mittra and Hong Song

LEARNING OBJECTIVES

1. Understand the role of nuclear radiology in the evaluation and treatment of patients with hyperthyroidism.
2. Understand the role of nuclear radiology in the evaluation and treatment of patients with thyroid cancer.

INTRODUCTION

Radioiodine therapy of hyperthyroidism is the origin of the field of Nuclear Medicine with the first treatments in 1941 (1), followed by the official publications documenting their efficacy in 1946 (2,3). Since then, of course, radioiodine imaging has also come to play an integral role both independent of and as an adjunct to radioiodine therapy both for hyperthyroidism and thyroid cancer. The difference between the latter two indications cannot be overemphasized, and is often a source of confusion for those new to the field. While it is true that the diagnostic and therapeutic radiopharmaceuticals I-123 and I-131, respectively, are the same for both hyperthyroidism and thyroid cancer, every other aspect of their use is different including the pathology, diagnostic algorithms, treatment algorithms, preparation for and types of scans, the doses used for therapy and how to determine the dose, and the radiation precautions associated with each therapy. As such, the role of radioiodine in hyperthyroidism and thyroid cancer will be described separately in this chapter.

By way of brief background, the thyroid is a small endocrine gland located in the low-anterior neck, overlying the thyroid cartilage, and is responsible for the production of the thyroid hormones triiodothyronine (T3) and thyroxine (T4), as well as the hormone calcitonin. These hormones influence metabolic rate and protein synthesis, and calcium homeostasis, respectively. The production of these hormones is in turn controlled by thyroid-stimulating hormone (TSH) production from the anterior pituitary gland and thyrotropin-releasing hormone (TRH) by the hypothalamus (4).

HYPERTHYROIDISM

Background

Hyperthyroidism is a syndrome caused by higher than normal levels of serum thyroid hormone (T4 and/or T3). Usually, this causes suppression of TSH, which then becomes a reliable marker of the disease. There are many causes of hyperthyroidism, but broadly, it is either due to overstimulation of the thyroid epithelium causing overproduction of hormones, or else destruction of the thyroid follicles and epithelium resulting in release of stored thyroid hormones, termed "thyroiditis." The most common cause of overproduction is either diffuse toxic goiter (Graves' disease) or nodular toxic goiter, and these tend to be a permanent issue in most patients. Less common causes include hyperfunctioning thyroid tumors, hashitoxicosis, secondary and tertiary hyperthyroidism, struma ovarii, or other tumors causing overproduction of TSH or TRH. There are many etiologies of thyroiditis including subacute, mechanical destruction of the thyroid, medications such as amiodarone, related to pregnancy, silent, and others (5). The broad divide between overproduction versus destruction as a cause of hyperthyroidism is important for imaging and therapy with radioiodine because overproduction results in increased uptake of radioiodine and therefore can be used to treat it, whereas destruction results in low uptake of radioiodine and therefore cannot be used to treat it (6).

General diagnostic and treatment algorithm

Once hyperthyroidism is biochemically confirmed, the next step is typically a radioiodine uptake and scan (6). A neck ultrasound (with or without fine needle aspiration [FNA]) may also be done if there are palpable nodules or if the radioiodine scan demonstrates hyper- or especially hypofunctioning nodules. If the cause of the hyperthyroidism is due to thyroiditis, typically only symptomatic management is needed, as the disease is self-limited. If the cause is due to overproduction of thyroid hormone, typically the first step is medical management with propylthiouracil (PTU) or methimazole (MMI). However, these medications can be difficult to manage and have significant potential side effects including agranulocytosis, liver failure, and birth defects (7), so they typically cannot be used in the long term. Definitive treatment options are either surgical removal of part or all of the thyroid gland or radioiodine ablation of the thyroid. Both have various pros and cons (8) which should be carefully discussed with the patient prior to a decision for therapy.

Role of nuclear imaging

As mentioned, the main indication for a radioiodine thyroid uptake and scan is for further evaluation of biochemically confirmed hyperthyroidism (9) (Figs. 4.1–4.6). Less commonly, it can be used to evaluate the functional status of a nodule seen on ultrasound even in the face of normal labs. The rationale being that hypofunctioning nodules are more likely to be cancerous than hyperfunctioning ones and so merit biopsy (10) Nowadays, ultrasound features rather than radioiodine uptake often makes this determination although it remains a consideration.

Preparation for an uptake and scan involves being off of thyroid medications (PTU or MMI) for at least 5 days and ensuring that no exogenous iodine (most commonly from a diagnostic computed tomography (CT) with intravenous-iodinated contrast) has been administered in the 6 weeks prior to therapy (11). For the same reason, it is ideal if the patient does not have an iodine-rich meal (i.e., seafood or seaweed) in the 48 h prior to imaging. A true low-iodine diet, however, is typically not necessary.

The procedure is composed of two distinct parts: an uptake measurement (non-imaging using a thyroid probe) and a scan

(imaging using a gamma camera). Both parts can be done using a single administration of I-123. The uptake can also be done separately using a smaller (half) dose of I-123. After oral administration of the pill, the patient returns 24 h afterward for the uptake measurement. And optional 4-h measurement is also done at some centers and can be useful for patients with high turnover to know whether the uptake is increasing or decreasing over time. There are several ways to do the uptake measurement. A common way is as follows. The thyroid probe is set a fixed distance away from the patient's neck to record the uptake. The patient's background counts are also measured by the thyroid probe pointed toward the mid-thigh. An equivalent standard dose of I-123 is then placed in a lucite scattering neck phantom and measured by the thyroid probe, and lastly the room background is measured. The patient's neck counts minus their thigh counts is divided by the standard counts minus the room background (11).

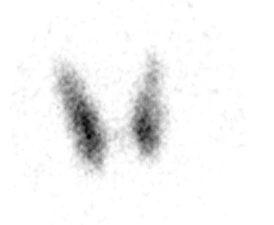

FIG. 4.1 ● I-123 scan showing physiologic uptake in the bilateral thyroid lobes. The 24-h radioiodine uptake (RAIU) is 16.6% (normal 10%–30%).

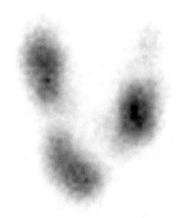

FIG. 4.3 ● I-123 scan showing multiple hyperfunctioning nodules, with relative suppression of the remaining normal thyroid gland. The 24-h RAIU is 35.9%.

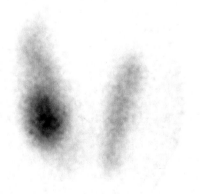

FIG. 4.2 ● I-123 scan showing a solitary hyperfunctioning nodule in the inferior right thyroid lobe, with relative suppression of the remaining normal thyroid gland. The 24-h RAIU is 39.3%.

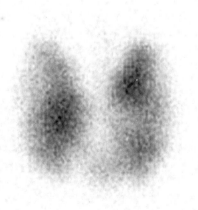

FIG. 4.4 ● I-123 scan showing hyperfunctioning nodules in the mid-right and upper-left thyroid lobes as well as hypofunctioning nodule in the mid-left thyroid lobe. The 24-h RAIU is 41.4%.

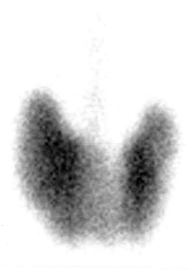

FIG. 4.6 ● I-123 scan showing almost no uptake in the bilateral thyroid lobes. The gland is barely visible above background. The 24-h RAIU is 1.1%.

FIG. 4.5 ● I-123 scan showing diffusely increased uptake in the bilateral thyroid lobes with visualization of the pyramidal lobe as well as the thyroid isthmus. The 24-h RAIU is 74.0%.

Normal radioiodine uptake is 6% to 18% at 4 h and 10% to 30% at 24 h (12).

The scan using a gamma camera is typically done with a pinhole collimator, focused on the neck. If there is low uptake, a Technetium-99m marker is useful to mark the top of the thyroid cartilage as well as the sternal notch, as the anatomy is otherwise unclear. If the patient has a palpable nodule, or known nodules >1 cm by ultrasound, it is also useful to try and mark where these are located while the patient is being imaged, so a direct correlation of nodule uptake can be made. In practice, this can be challenging unless the nodule is superficial, large, or the patient is thin.

Interpretation of the scan and uptake is relatively straightforward. Uptake values below the normal range suggest thyroiditis as the gland has released its stored thyroid hormone, which subsequently suppresses the TSH and the gland. In this case, the scan will show limited or no uptake in the thyroid. Uptake values higher than the normal range suggest either Graves' disease, disease or toxic nodular goiter as the gland is active despite a low TSH. In this case, the scan will show diffuse uptake for Graves', often with visualization of the thyroid isthmus and pyramidal lobes. For toxic nodule(s), the scan will typically show high uptake in the nodule(s) with variable suppression of the surrounding thyroid gland. Because of the latter issue, the uptake value may actually be in the normal range for nodular goiter if the uptake in the nodule is balanced by the low uptake in the suppressed gland. If the scan and uptake results are clear, then obtaining thyroid function tests at the time of the scan has limited added value. If, however, the uptake and scan is normal, then obtaining concurrent thyroid function tests is useful to know if the thyroid labs are also normal or abnormal at the time of the study (9).

Radioiodine therapy

A hyperthyroidism patient would be amenable to therapy with I-131 if the following conditions are met: (1) The radioiodine uptake at 24 h is greater than 30%, (2) the scan shows either diffusely increased uptake or solitary or multiple hyperfunctioning

nodules, and (3) there are no hypofunctioning nodules seen which have not already been evaluated by ultrasound and/ or biopsy to confirm they are not malignant. Other factors to consider are to ensure the patient has had a thorough discussion with their endocrinologist regarding alternative treatment options, a negative urine or serum pregnancy test within 48 h of the planned therapy, and appropriate counseling about radiation precautions including avoiding pregnancy. If the uptake is high normal, but the patient is otherwise a good candidate for radioiodine therapy and had proper preparation, then it may be beneficial to have the patient undergo a low iodine for 1 or 2 weeks and return for an uptake measurement. The idea is to further stimulate the thyroid gland and increase the uptake value above normal. This is beneficial to enhance the efficacy of the therapy.

The dose of I-131 for therapy of hyperthyroidism can either be chosen empirically or by calculation (13). For Grave's disease, empiric doses are typically in the range of 10 to 15 mCi and for hyperfunctioning nodule(s) in the range of 10 to 20 mCi as the latter can be more radioresistant. Alternatively, the dose can be calculated to deliver a specific radiation dose to the gland or nodule(s). For Grave's disease, the formula is 50 to 200 µCi/g of tissue, divided by the radioiodine uptake. For hyperfunctioning nodules, the formula is 150 to 200 µCi/g of tissue, divided by the radioiodine uptake. That is, the dose is directly related to the gland size and indirectly related to the uptake. To use the formula, then, the gland size must be known. Here, again, there are two methods. The most accurate is to use the measurements from a recent thyroid ultrasound. In this case, the formula for gland size is that of an oval (length × width × height/2). When an ultrasound is not available, a physical exam can be used to estimate the gland size. In this case, one must know that the average total gland size in an adult is 20 g (10 g/side). A gland that can easily be palpated but not seen is approximately 40 g in size. A gland that can easily be seen is 60 g. And a large goiter may be 80 to 100 g in size. This method is prone to error in larger patients in whom a large portion of the gland is hidden behind overlying soft tissue.

The goal of the therapy is not necessarily to achieve an euthyroid state, but rather to destroy the gland completely and render the patient hypothyroid. When that happens, they will require thyroid hormone replacement for the remainder of their life. Even with this approach, up to 20% of patients may require a second treatment to be fully effective (8). Lower doses are correlated to greater treatment failure (13) but this should be balanced by not giving high-radiation doses to everyone, which may increase the risk of side effects (see "Side effects and radiation precautions") as well as their life time radiation burden.

The timeline of therapy should be clarified with patients as many believe the I-131 will be immediately effective. Once the I-131 is localized to the thyroid gland, the emitted beta radiation will cause mostly single-stranded deoxyribonucleic acid (DNA) damage which ultimately cannot be effectively repaired by the cell, causing it to die (14). This process can take many weeks or months to have an effect on the whole thyroid gland. During this time, the patient's thyroid function should be checked periodically and symptomatic patients should continue their PTU or MMI and other medications such as beta-blockers for palpitations. Over time, the patient will slowly transition from hyperthyroid to euthyroid to hypothyroid (13).

Side effects and radiation precautions

Side effects of radioiodine treatment can be divided into those which are short and long term (14). Short-term side effects typically begin and also resolve within the first several days after the therapy. They include nausea (rarely strong enough to cause emesis), sialadenitis, swelling of the thyroid gland, change in taste, and generalized malaise. Ensuring the patient is well hydrated and controlling symptoms with non steroidal anti-inflammatory medications and/or antiemetics can mitigate these effects. Sialagogues such as sour candies or lemon have been advocated to reduce the risk of sialadenitis, but the timing of their use is not well understood (15). Several studies show that starting sialagogues immediately after I-131 administration (and continuing for several days) can reduce the uptake of I-131 in the salivary gland (16,17). However, one study showed that starting within 24 h of the I-131 administration can actually increase uptake in the salivary gland (so called "rebound effect") resulting in greater side effects (18).

Long-term side effects of radioiodine therapy include prolonged or permanent damage to the salivary glands causing persistent dry mouth. Infrequently, this can present itself several months after the therapy even in patients who did not initially experience sialadenitis. Again, the use of sialagogues has been shown to reduce these effects. Also, rarely, alteration in taste can be more prolonged or rarely permanent. There is a theoretical risk of developing a second malignancy from the radiation, but this is more of a concern at the higher doses used for thyroid cancer, not with the low doses used for hyperthyroidism.

Radiation precautions associated with radioisotope therapies of any type are a source of great confusion for physicians and patients alike and there is variability based on geography, institution, and organization (19). The US Nuclear Regulatory Commission (NRC) provides guidance on this but their interpretation can vary. The reason for this is most likely because the effects of such low-level radiation exposure are not well known and mostly safe. With any radioisotope therapy, the two types of radiation to consider is emitted radiation and cleared radiation (primarily from the urine). The NRC guidelines for release of radioactive patients from the hospital are three fold, (1) if the administered dose is less than 33 mCi, (2) if the emitted radiation is less than 7 mR/h

at 1 m from the patient, and (3) if the total radiation exposure to a caregiver or family member is less than 500 mrem. Given the doses discussed for hyperthyroidism, the first two criteria are always met and so the patient does not need to be admitted. Having said that, it is probably advisable for the patient to keep some distance from others (especially children less than 11 years of age, or pregnant women) for the first several days after therapy to allow for the majority of the clearance to happen. The cleared radiation is of slightly greater concern primarily to avoid contamination at home. To that end, good bathroom hygiene for the first week after therapy is advised. This includes avoiding spills (men should sit when urinating), flushing (with the lid down) 2 to 3 times after using the toilet, cleaning up any spills, washing hands thoroughly after using the bathroom, and taking daily showers to minimize the radiation in sweat.

THYROID CANCER

Background

Thyroid cancer incidence has steadily been increasing over time, although the mortality has been relatively stable except for advanced-stage disease (20,21). Possibilities for this discrepancy include increased detection of subclinical thyroid cancer such as microcarcinomas (less than 1 cm in size), increased radiation exposure to the general population, as well as other endocrinological, and environmental factors such as increasing obesity. There are several pathologic subtypes of thyroid cancer, although the most common are the differentiated thyroid cancers including papillary and follicular, together accounting for greater than 90% of thyroid cancers. This is fortuitous both because these cancers have a favorable prognosis and because they are amenable to radioiodine therapy. Other subtypes such as medullary thyroid cancer, anaplastic thyroid cancer, and other poorly differentiated thyroid cancers have a worse prognosis and do not take up radioiodine. The remainder of this chapter only pertains to differentiated thyroid cancers.

The most commonly used staging classification for differentiated thyroid cancer is the American Joint Committee on Cancer Tumor Node Metastasis (AJCC/TNM) staging system was revised in October 2016 as the eighth edition. The primary change in the new edition was the downstaging of a significant number of patients into lower stages, reflecting their low risk of thyroid cancer-related death (22,23).

A variety of mutations can also affect differentiated thyroid cancer. The ones of greatest importance for papillary thyroid cancer include RET, BRAF, tyrosine kinase, and TP53. But their importance for prognosis remains incompletely understood. For instance, one study found that the BRAFV600E mutation predicted a worse prognosis (24), while another did not (25). The RAS mutations or PAX8/PPAR gamma rearrangements are more related to development of follicular thyroid cancer.

Treatment overview

Thyroid cancers do not typically cause symptoms and are often found incidentally during a physical exam or by imaging of the neck done for other reasons. However, a suspicious nodule is first identified, the next step is ultrasound-guided FNA followed by a core biopsy. Once differentiated thyroid cancer is confirmed by pathology, the next step is typically total thyroidectomy, although this does vary based on size of the primary tumor (26). Papillary microcarcinomas (those smaller than 1 cm) may undergo lobectomy or active surveillance (27,28). Based on the pre surgical imaging, a central or lateral neck dissection is also done at the time of the thyroidectomy to sample and remove any metastatic lymph nodes. This surgery is complex given the proximity of the thyroid gland to important vasculature and nerves (e.g., recurrent laryngeal nerve) structures in this area. As such, it is not uncommon for some normal thyroid tissue to be left behind either inadvertently or on purpose.

The next step in treatment is potential radioiodine treatment to be discussed in the remainder of the chapter. Subsequently, the mainstay of therapy is proper suppression of any residual thyroid tissue/cancer by thyroid hormone supplementation, which is also needed given the patient's thyroidectomy (29–31). The goal for TSH suppression varies depending on the risk of the patient.

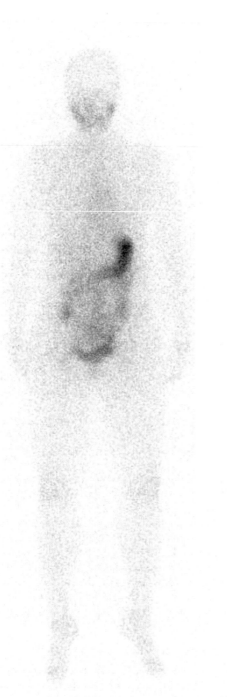

FIG. 4.7 ● I-123 pre-therapy whole-body scan in the anterior project showing physiologic uptake in the salivary glands, stomach, bowel, and clearance in the bladder. No focal uptake in the neck is seen to suggest residual thyroid tissue or cancer. The 24-h RAIU in the neck is 0.5%.

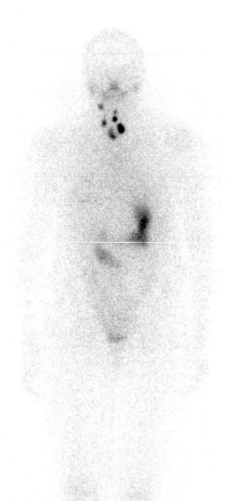

FIG. 4.8 ● I-123 pre-therapy whole-body scan in the anterior project showing multiple foci of uptake in the neck which likely represents a combination of residual thyroid tissue or cancer and nodal metastases. 24-h RAIU in the neck is 1.4%.

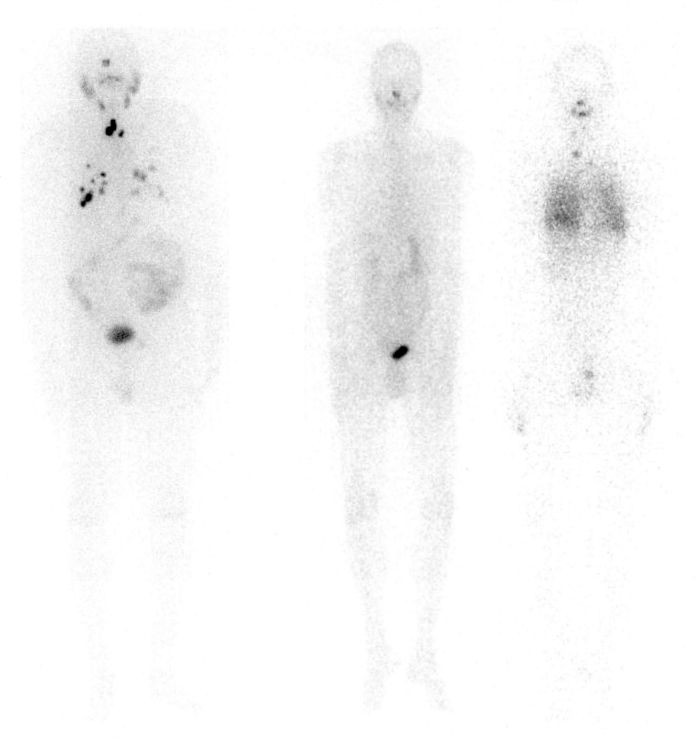

FIG. 4.9 ● I-123 pre-therapy whole-body scan in the anterior project showing several foci of uptake in the neck as well as multiple foci of uptake in the bilateral lungs corresponding to known lung metastases. The 24-h RAIU in the neck is 8.5% and in the chest is 17.5%.

FIG. 4.10 ● I-123 pre-therapy whole-body scan in the anterior project (left image) showing only physiologic uptake, with a 24-h RAIU in the neck of 0.6%. I-131 post-therapy whole-body scan in the anterior projection (right image) shows diffuse uptake in the bilateral lungs representing miliary pulmonary metastases. This was subsequently confirmed by high-resolution CT chest.

Thyroid labs are the mainstay for thyroid cancer surveillance. Thyroglobulin (Tg) is produced only by thyroid tissue. As such, after total thyroidectomy and radioiodine ablation of remnant tissue, the Tg level should be undetectable. If that does not happen or a subsequent rise in Tg would suggest residual/recurrent disease and this can be used to predict outcomes (32–34). It is important to clarify that Tg levels when the patient is on thyroid hormone suppression (so called suppressed Tg, with low TSH levels) cannot be directly compared with Tg levels when the patient is stimulated (has high TSH levels). Another complication

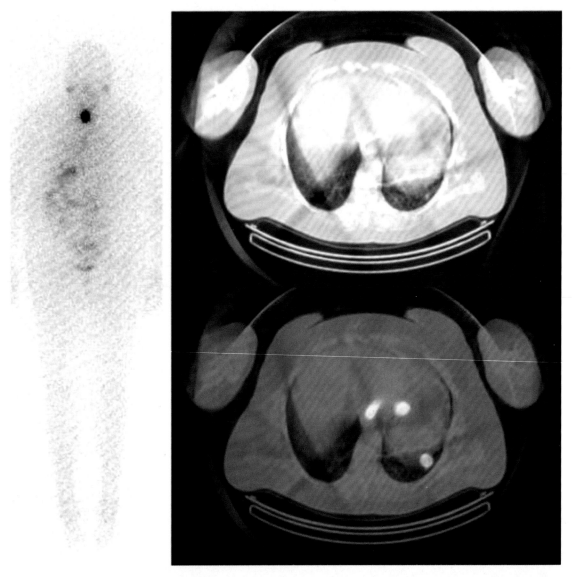

FIG. 4.11 ● I-123 pre-therapy whole-body scan in the posterior project (left image) showing a prominent focus of uptake in the mid-neck, with a 24-h RAIU in the neck of 14.3%. The remainder of the uptake seen is physiologic. Specifically, the lungs were felt to be normal, but the I-131 post-therapy SPECT/CT scan (axial images on the right; low-dose CT image on the top, fusion SPECT/CT image on the bottom) shows focal uptake corresponding to a small left lung base pulmonary nodule. Bowel uptake is also seen on this slice.

for many patients is the presence of antibodies to Tg (TgAb). These antibodies can interfere with the assay for Tg, artificially altering the measured value. In these patients, the TgAb itself can be followed to assess for cancer risk (35). As such, one needs to evaluate TSH, Tg, and TgAb together for each patient.

Role of nuclear imaging and therapy

In general, radioiodine whole-body scans are done in conjunction with a possible I-131 therapy (Figs. 4.7–4.13), either after initial thyroidectomy for the purpose of remnant ablation or adjuvant therapy, or subsequently to treat residual/recurrent disease. Routine surveillance radioiodine scans in patients without rising Tg levels is generally not recommended (36).

The use of a pre-therapy radioiodine scan at the time of the initial I-131 therapy is one of several controversies in the imaging and therapy of differentiated thyroid cancer (37). Some centers will routinely treat all thyroid cancer patients with a 100 to 150

mCi dose of I-131 after thyroidectomy in which case doing a pre-therapy scan is arguably of limited utility. But other centers base the dose of the initial therapy on the results of the pre-therapy scan (38). There are some other advantages as well. Sometimes, the amount of residual thyroid tissue is high enough to warrant a repeat surgery to ensure the effectiveness of the therapy. Also, sometimes, (usually young) female patients will have prominent physiologic uptake in breast tissue, during which time it is not advisable to do the therapy as the radiation exposure to the breast tissue may be too high. These are examples of issues, which would not be known if the pre-therapy scan is not done.

Of note, I-131 therapy itself has several controversies related to the necessity and dose of radioiodine for remnant ablation, adjuvant treatment, or treatment for known persistent or recurrent disease (37,39). Particularly, there is the issue of ablation of low-risk patients (40–42). Some of these issues are discussed in the following sections.

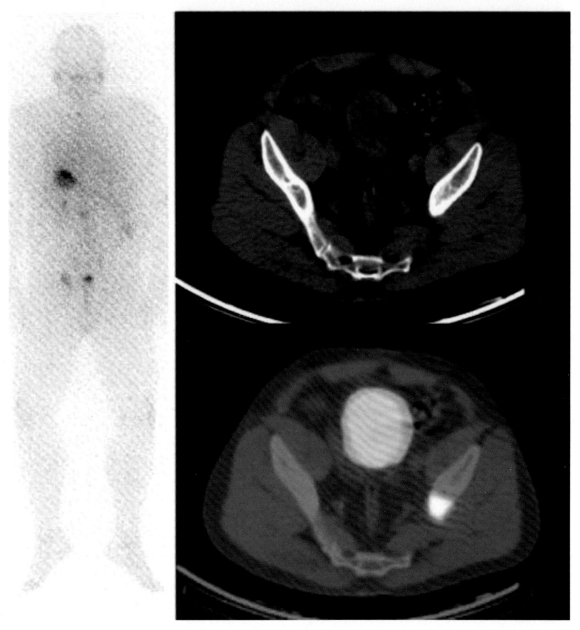

FIG. 4.12 ● I-123 pre-therapy whole-body scan in the posterior project (left image) showing minimal uptake in the neck, but scattered foci of uptake elsewhere in the body corresponding to bone metastases. The 24-h RAIU in the neck is 0.9%. SPECT/CT imaging of the pelvis (axial images on the right; low-dose CT image on the top, fusion SPECT/CT image on the bottom) confirms focal uptake corresponding to a mildly sclerotic lesion in the left ilium. Bladder uptake is also seen on this slice.

Radioiodine scans

Regardless of the specific indication for a radioiodine whole-body scan, the preparation and technique is generally the same. The preparation is critical to properly increase the sensitivity of the scan. As these patients are all post-thyroidectomy, the primary goal of preparation involves stimulating the residual normal thyroid tissue/recurrent thyroid cancer by either withdrawing the patient from T4 (levothyroxine/Synthroid) for 4 weeks and T3 (liothyronine/Cytomel) for 2 weeks to stimulate the patient's own TSH, or else giving exogenous TSH in the form of recombinant TSH (rTSH) injections (Thyrogen). The effect of this preparation is confirmed by checking the patient's TSH on the day the I-123 is given. It is largely superfluous if rTSH is used as the TSH level is always elevated (typically >200 mIU/L). But it is very important to check in the case of thyroid hormone withdrawal. The TSH should be at least 30 mIU/L , ideally greater than 50 mIU/L. Of note, if the patient has significant functioning thyroid tissue (either in the neck or in metastases), then the TSH may never rise appropriately despite following the preparation guidelines.

In addition to stimulating the patient's thyroid tissue, the patient's normal supply of non radioactive iodine is depleted by undergoing a low-iodine diet for 1 to 2 weeks in advance of the imaging/therapy (43). In theory, circulating non radioactive iodine may compete with the radioiodine for the sodium iodide symporter on thyroid cells although this has not been rigorously proven (44–46). Serum and urine iodine measurements can be

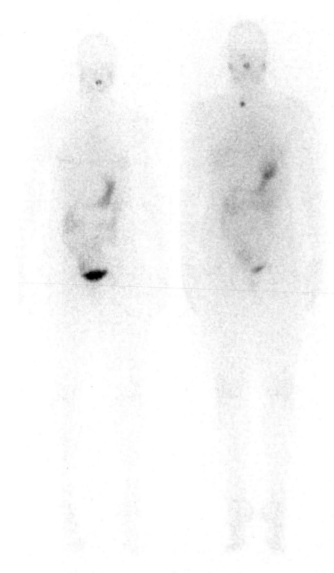

Thyroid Cancer Association (ThyCa.org) has a very thorough low-iodine diet cookbook with a wealth of details and recipes.

Once the preparation has been successfully done and confirmed, the radioiodine pill is given and the patient is usually asked to get thyroid labs done as well. In addition to checking the TSH level (primarily important for those stimulated with thyroid hormone withdrawal), the stimulated Tg and TgAb are helpful to make a final decision for therapy. The next morning, the patient returns for a whole-body iodine scan, and together with the lab results, a final treatment decision is made.

The radioiodine of choice for a pre-therapy scan is typically I-123, with a dose range of 2 to 4 mCi. However, traditionally, I-131 itself has also been used and can be given at low-dose of 1 to 5 mCi. I-123 is generally preferred given the favorable gamma photon energy, and lack of any beta particle emission. The latter can theoretically cause damage to the thyroid tissue resulting in reduced uptake of the therapeutic I-131 given subsequently (so called stunning). However, at doses below 5 mCi, stunning is typically not observed (47,48). And for those patients requiring pre-therapy dosimetry (see "Radioiodine therapy"), I-131 must be used for its longer half-life.

Radioiodine therapy

As mentioned previously, not every thyroid cancer patient needs I-131 therapy. The treatment decision is based on the pathology, molecular features, surgical findings, stage, and other medical conditions and comorbidities. If done, concurrent lab results, I-123 pre-therapy scan findings, and other imaging (i.e., chest CT) is also incorporated. Patients with very low-risk disease may defer treatment until their Tg level starts rising. For patients who will be treated, the next step is to decide on a dose.

As for the treatment of hyperthyroidism, there are two ways to choose a dose of I-131, either empirically or based on the extent of disease (49). Empiric dosing is typically done in the initial post-thyroidectomy setting for remnant ablation or adjuvant therapy in the range of 100 to 150 mCi. Some centers, primarily in Europe, also utilize this empiric/fixed dose on subsequent treatments even for patients with metastatic disease, but treat those patients more frequently. If based on the extent of disease, it is helpful to incorporate other imaging such as the pre-therapy I-123 scan and other conventional imaging.

The rationale for not using a fixed dose of 100 to 150 mCi is two fold. In support of using a lower dose is to limit the radiation exposure to patients who have low-risk disease if it will be equally efficacious (49–51). This is theoretically beneficial for that specific treatment, as well as for reducing the cumulative exposure with respect to potential future therapies. For instance, there is some evidence that side effects are increased with respect to dose (52). Also, the cumulative lifetime limit for I-131 therapy for a single patient is in the range of 1000 mCi or 1 Ci.

On the other hand, a higher dose will be more efficacious for patients with higher-risk disease. This is especially of concern in that repeated therapies may become less effective as each treatment selects for the radioresistant clones of cancer. Using this rational, the typical range for doses is 30 to 250 mCi based on the extent of disease: (1) 30 to 50 mCi for ablation of residual normal thyroid tissue, (2) 75 to 150 mCi if there is the possibility of residual cancer in the neck (extracapsular extension, lymphovascular invasion, or lymph node metastases), (3) 100 to 200 mCi if there are lung metastases, and (4) 200 to 250 mCi for bone metastases. Of note, solitary bone metastasis is usually best treated by external beam radiation.

FIG. 4.13 ● Two I-123 pre-therapy whole-body scan in the anterior project in the same patient. The images were taken one month apart without any in-between intervention. The left panel image is after stimulation with rTSH (Thyrogen) and the right panel image is after stimulation with thyroid hormone withdrawal. The left panel image shows only physiologic radioiodine uptake, while the right panel image shows abnormal uptake in the right low neck, corresponding to a known lymph node at this location. This case highlights the increased sensitivity of thyroid hormone withdrawal compared to rTSH stimulation. For more complicated or advanced cases, thyroid hormone withdrawal is favored if the patient can tolerate it. Whereas for the initial therapy after surgery, rTSH is sufficient.

done, but it takes a number of days to get the results, so it is only done under special circumstances (i.e., if the patient had a recent contrast-enhanced CT). Of note, this is a low-iodine diet, not a no-iodine diet, or a low- or no-salt diet. The basic tenant of the diet is to stay away from the most common source of dietary iodine, which is iodized salt. In practice, this means that eating processed foods from the grocery store and at most restaurants is excluded. Also, any type of seafood and seaweed is not allowed. A small amount of meat straight from a butcher is allowed in small amounts. Certain dyes, mostly red, are also restricted. The

With respect to high doses for patients with extensive metastases, ultimately a limit must be reached so radiation to normal surrounding tissues is not harmful. The two primary areas of concern are bone marrow suppression and radiation pneumonitis resulting in pulmonary fibrosis. For these patients, pretherapeutic dosimetry should be used to calculate an individual patient's maximum-tolerated dose (MTD) or maximum-tolerated activity (MTA). Based on each patient's biology, renal function, and distribution and burden of metastases, the same dose of I-131 will have different residence times in that individual and therefore different radiation exposure to normal organs. It should be noted, however, that this is another area of controversy as some studies show that pre-therapy dosimetry is helpful (53), while others do not (54).

There are a large number of ways of doing patient-specific dosimetry, and they vary considerably in complexity. The most basic concept of calculating MTA is based on seminal empiric work done at Memorial Sloan Kettering Cancer Center in the 1950s and 1960s looking at the long-term outcomes in some of the first patient's treated with I-131. Based on those observations, a surprisingly simple concept has withstood the test of time which is to limit the administered dose such that the patient's *whole body* retention of I-131 at 48 h after ingestion does not exceed 120 mCi to prevent bone marrow suppression or 80 mCi to prevent pulmonary toxicity in those patients with extensive pulmonary metastases. This is typically termed "simplified whole-body dosimetry" (55,56). Doing this requires one whole-body measurement (either using a gamma camera or a thyroid probe placed 2.5 m away from the patient) approximately 1 to 2 h after ingestion of I-131 before voiding (so that a baseline value is obtained), and then another similar measurement 48 h after ingestion just after voiding (to know the percent retained at this time). There are many other more complex algorithms for performing dosimetry, which involve many additional time points for these measurements in conjunction with blood and urine samples to more thoroughly understand the clearance. The majority of this discussion is beyond the scope of this textbook and the reader is encouraged to seek many good references on the topic.

To restress the point, however, if one is using a lower-fixed dose of 100 to 150 mCi, then dosimetry is not needed as all patients will be safe. But if one wants to give higher doses to patients with extensive disease, then dosimetry may be of benefit to prevent unwanted and hard to treat complications. Another group of patients in whom dosimetry should be considered are those with impaired renal function. Since that is the primary clearance route of I-131, poor or absent renal function will increase the residence time of I-131.

Post-therapy scans

Unlike hyperthyroidism patients treated with I-131, thyroid cancer patients also need to return for a post-therapy scan 5 to 8 days after the treatment is given. The reason for this is to take advantage of the very sensitive iodine scan that results from the high-dose I-131 therapy. The expectation is that the post-therapy scan will show uptake in the neck, in the same distribution as the pre-therapy I-123 scan (if done) although the uptake in the residual thyroid tissue or cancer will be much more intense. But the greater goal is to look for any distant metastases that were not known about. If additional metastases are seen, there is nothing further to be done at the moment as the therapy has already been given, but the information would tailor future management and affect prognosis.

If there is functioning thyroid tissue, the radioactive iodine also gets incorporated into thyroid hormone and released into the circulation. This ultimately gets trapped in the liver such that homogenous uptake in the liver is often seen on the post-therapy scan. There are also many examples of (potentially confusing) physiologic iodine uptake that can be seen on both the pre- and post-therapy scans, which have been reported (57–59). Single photon compute tomography (SPECT)/CT imaging can always be added to any whole body for the incremental gain it provides (60,61).

Side effects and radiation precautions

The side effects from I-131 therapy of thyroid cancer is the generally the same as for I-131 therapy of hyperthyroidism. As noted before, some studies show a dose relationship to side effects such that these side effects may be more prevalent in patients treated for thyroid cancer (15).

The primary concern for long-term side effects of radioiodine therapy for differentiated thyroid cancer is the development of second cancers due to the radiation. Overall, there is increased risk of secondary cancer in thyroid cancer survivors and the type of cancer depend on whether patients receive radioiodine therapy, age of diagnosis and treatment, and latency since treatment (62). Leukemia is the most well-established link for those who have received radioiodine treatment (63,64). Most of the leukemia cases occur within 10 years of initial diagnosis. The link to other cancers is less strong, but some that have been reported include renal and colorectal cancer since radioiodine is secreted through the kidney and gastrointestinal tracts. Additionally, breast and prostate cancer have been suggested although there are conflicting since the risk is not statistically different in thyroid cancer patients who received or did not receive radioiodine treatment. Some of the increased detection of secondary cancer can be attributed to genetic, environmental factors as well as sampling bias due to increased surveillance.

The radiation precautions for this therapy are also similar to that for hyperthyroidism. This is due to the fact that while the doses are much larger, the uptake is low (typically 1%–3% after thyroidectomy). As such, the emitted radiation will be initially high, but will drop off quickly (typically around 50% each day). Recalling the criteria for release from the hospital mentioned in the radiation precaution section under hyperthyroidism therapy, the thyroid cancer patients almost always have been treated with greater than 33 mCi, and therefore emit greater than 7 mR/h at 1 m. Yet, the vast majority of these patients are not admitted to the hospital (at least in the United States) because of the last rule that no caregiver or family member will be exposed to more than 500 mrem in total. Using the patient's uptake value, I-131 dose, and an occupancy factor to account for their living situation, the dose calculator on the RADAR website (https://www.doseinfo-radar.com/ExposureCalculator.html) will calculate this exposure which can be documented for release. Because of the higher doses, these patients will definitely need to be isolated for a few days in their room and use good bathroom hygiene. A separate bathroom is ideal but not absolutely necessary. Other recommendations are found on the SNMMI website (www.snmmi.org).

Non-iodine avid disease

Although not very common, in the natural course of disease, aggressive forms of differentiated thyroid cancer may dedifferentiate into non-iodine avid disease. These patients are typically identified by rising Tg or TgAb levels, or findings worrisome for recurrent disease on conventional imaging, but with a negative

I-123 pre-therapy or I-131 post-therapy scans. These patients create a management dilemma since radioiodine refractory disease portends a worse outcome and treatment options become limited. If only the I-123 pre-therapy scan is negative, one approach is to do an empiric I-131 therapy to see if the post-therapy scan will be positive, or perhaps it will simply have an effect on reducing the Tg or TgAb levels. If neither of those outcomes is seen, then I-131 therapy is no longer considered an option for these patients, and they would move to chemotherapy. An interesting exception to this is the use of the mitogen-activated protein kinase (MAPK) (MEK 1 and 2) inhibitor selumetinib to reverse refractoriness to radioiodine (65,66). Similar work has been done with BRAF inhibitor vemurafenib for patients who are BRAFV600E mutant (67). While initial results are promising, these approaches are still under investigation at this time and not widely adopted.

This group of patients (as well as those who have non-differentiated thyroid cancers to begin with) are best imaged with 18F-fluorodeoxyglucose positron-emission tomography (18F-FDG PET) (68,69). Typically, differentiated thyroid cancers have variable or low-18F-FDG uptake, but dedifferentiated and more aggressive histologies have higher uptake. Interestingly, it has been shown that TSH stimulation (whether by thyroid hormone withdrawal or rTSH), increases the sensitivity of the 18F-FDG scan as well so it is often ideal to plan for this in advance.

CONCLUSION

Different isotopes of radioiodine have a long history of use for both imaging and therapy of thyroid disease. I-123 uptake and scans are critical for the proper diagnosis of hyperthyroidism and I-131 therapy of hyperthyroidism is the origins of the field of Nuclear Medicine and thus very well established in its efficacy with limited side effects. For differentiated thyroid cancers, I-123 imaging can help stage the patient and show whether the disease is iodine avid such that it can be treated with I-131. The role of I-131 therapy is also well established, but especially for patients with more advanced, iodine-avid disease. There are many controversies in the nuclear imaging and therapy of differentiated thyroid cancer as a result of limited prospective-controlled studies on the topics. For all types of therapies, radiation safety and precautions must be ensured, but these are generally well accepted by the majority of patients as a straightforward outpatient treatment.

References

1. Sawin CT, Becker DV. Radioiodine and the treatment of hyperthyroidism: the early history. *Thyroid*. United States; 1997;7(2):163–176.
2. Hertz S, Roberts A. Radioactive iodine in the study of thyroid physiology; the use of radioactive iodine therapy in hyperthyroidism. *J Am Med Assoc*. United States; 1946;131:81–86.
3. Chapman EM, Evans RD. The treatment of hyperthyroidism with radioactive iodine. *J Am Med Assoc*. United States; 1946;131:86–91.
4. Hall J. *Guyton and Hall textbook of medical physiology*. 12th ed. Saunders/Eslevier: Philadelphia, PA; 2011.
5. LiVolsi VA, Baloch ZW. The pathology of hyperthyroidism. *Front Endocrinol* (Lausanne). Switzerland; 2018;9:737.
6. Sarkar SD. Benign thyroid disease: what is the role of nuclear medicine? *Semin Nucl Med*. United States; 2006;36(3):185–193.
7. Andersen SL, Olsen J, Laurberg P. Antithyroid drug side effects in the population and in pregnancy. *J Clin Endocrinol Metab*. United States; 2016;101(4):1606–1614.
8. Torring O, Tallstedt L, Wallin G, et al. Graves' hyperthyroidism: treatment with antithyroid drugs, surgery, or radioiodine–a prospective, randomized study. Thyroid Study Group. *J Clin Endocrinol Metab*. United States; 1996;81(8):2986–2993.
9. Meller J, Becker W. The continuing importance of thyroid scintigraphy in the era of high-resolution ultrasound. *Eur J Nucl Med Mol Imaging*. Germany; 2002;29 Suppl 2:S425–S438.
10. Carnell NE, Valente WA. Thyroid nodules in Graves' disease: classification, characterization, and response to treatment. *Thyroid*. United States; 1998;8(8):647–652.
11. ACR-SNM-SPR practice guideline for the performance of thyroid scintigraphy and uptake measurements. 2009. https://s3.amazonaws.com/rdcms-snmmi/files/production/public/docs/Thyroid_Scintigraphy_1382732120053_10.pdf (accessed July 15, 2021)
12. Society of nuclear medicine procedure guideline for thyroid uptake measurement. 2006. https://s3.amazonaws.com/rdcms-snmmi/files/production/public/docs/Thyroid%20Uptake%20Measure%20v3%200.pdf (accessed July 15, 2021).
13. Ross DS, Burch HB, Cooper DS, et al. 2016 American thyroid association guidelines for diagnosis and management of hyperthyroidism and other causes of thyrotoxicosis. *Thyroid*. United States; 2016;26(10):1343–1421.
14. Mumtaz M, Lin LS, Hui KC, Mohd Khir AS. Radioiodine I-131 for the therapy of graves' disease. *Malays J Med Sci*. Malaysia; 2009;16(1):25–33.
15. Haugen BR, Alexander EK, Bible KC, et al. 2015 American thyroid association management guidelines for adult patients with thyroid nodules and differentiated thyroid cancer: The American thyroid association guidelines task force on thyroid nodules and differentiated thyroid cancer. *Thyroid*. United States; 2016;26(1):1–133.
16. Kulkarni K, Van Nostrand D, Atkins F, Mete M, Wexler J, Wartofsky L. Does lemon juice increase radioiodine reaccumulation within the parotid glands more than if lemon juice is not administered? *Nucl Med Commun*. England; 2014;35(2):210–216.
17. Van Nostrand D, Atkins F, Bandaru VV, et al. Salivary gland protection with sialagogues: a case study. *Thyroid*. United States; 2009;19(9):1005–1008.
18. Nakada K, Ishibashi T, Takei T, et al. Does lemon candy decrease salivary gland damage after radioiodine therapy for thyroid cancer? *J Nucl Med*. United States; 2005;46(2):261–266.
19. Silberstein EB, Alavi A, Balon HR, et al. The SNMMI practice guideline for therapy of thyroid disease with 131I 3.0. *J Nucl Med*. United States; 2012;53(10):1633–1651.
20. Milano AF. Thyroid Cancer: 20-Year comparative mortality and survival analysis of six thyroid cancer histologic subtypes by age, sex, race, stage, cohort entry time-period and disease duration (SEER*Stat 8.3.2) a systematic review of 145,457 cases for diagnosis year. *J Insur Med*. United States; 2018;47(3):143–158.
21. Lim H, Devesa SS, Sosa JA, Check D, Kitahara CM. Trends in thyroid cancer incidence and mortality in the United States, 1974–2013. *JAMA*. United States; 2017;317(13):1338–1348.
22. Tam S, Boonsripitayanon M, Amit M, et al. Survival in differentiated thyroid cancer: comparing the AJCC cancer staging seventh and eighth editions. *Thyroid*. United States; 2018;28(10):1301–1310.
23. Casella C, Ministrini S, Galani A, Mastriale F, Cappelli C, Portolani N. The new TNM Staging system for thyroid cancer and the risk of disease downstaging. *Front Endocrinol* (Lausanne). Switzerland; 2018;9:541.
24. Elisei R, Ugolini C, Viola D, et al. BRAF(V600E) mutation and outcome of patients with papillary thyroid carcinoma: a 15-year median follow-up study. *J Clin Endocrinol Metab*. United States; 2008;93(10):3943–3949.
25. Damiani L, Lupo S, Rossi R, et al. Evaluation of the role of BRAFV600E somatic mutation on papillary thyroid cancer disease persistence: a prospective study. *Eur Thyroid J*. Switzerland; 2018;7(5):251–257.
26. Owens PW, McVeigh TP, Fahey EJ, et al. Differentiated thyroid cancer: how do current practice guidelines affect management? *Eur Thyroid J*. Switzerland; 2018;7(6):319–326.

27. Leboulleux S, Tuttle RM, Pacini F, Schlumberger M. Papillary thyroid microcarcinoma: time to shift from surgery to active surveillance? *Lancet Diabetes Endocrinol*. England; 2016;4(11):933–942.

28. Brito JP, Moon JH, Zeuren R, et al. Thyroid cancer treatment choice: a pilot study of a tool to facilitate conversations with patients with papillary microcarcinomas considering treatment options. *Thyroid*. United States; 2018;28(10):1325–1331.

29. Freudenthal B, Williams GR. Thyroid stimulating hormone suppression in the long-term follow-up of differentiated thyroid cancer. *Clin Oncol* (R Coll Radiol). England; 2017;29(5):325–328.

30. Fussey JM, Khan H, Ahsan F, Prashant R, Pettit L. Thyroid-stimulating hormone suppression therapy for differentiated thyroid cancer: the role for a combined T3/T4 approach. *Head Neck*. United States; 2017;39(12):2567–2572.

31. Schmidbauer B, Menhart K, Hellwig D, Grosse J. Differentiated thyroid cancer-treatment: state of the art. *Int J Mol Sci*. Switzerland; 2017;18(6):1292.

32. Heemstra KA, Liu YY, Stokkel M, et al. Serum thyroglobulin concentrations predict disease-free remission and death in differentiated thyroid carcinoma. *Clin Endocrinol* (Oxf). England; 2007;66(1):58–64.

33. Aldawish M, Jha N, McEwan AJB, Severin D, Ghosh S, Morrish DW. Low but measurable stimulated serum thyroglobulin levels <2 microg/L frequently predict incomplete response in differentiated thyroid cancer patients. *Endocr Res*. England; 2014;39(4):157–163.

34. Wong KCW, Ng TY, Yu KS, et al. The use of post-ablation stimulated thyroglobulin in predicting clinical outcomes in differentiated thyroid carcinoma–what cut-off values should we use? *Clin Oncol (R Coll Radiol)*. 2019;31(2):e11–e20.

35. Doggui R. Immunoanalytical profile of thyroglobulin antibodies. *Ann Biol Clin* (Paris). France; 2018;76(6):695–704.

36. Lamartina L, Grani G, Durante C, Borget I, Filetti S, Schlumberger M. Follow-up of differentiated thyroid cancer–what should (and what should not) be done. *Nat Rev Endocrinol*. England; 2018;14(9):538–551.

37. Van Nostrand D. selected controversies of radioiodine imaging and therapy in differentiated thyroid cancer. *Endocrinol Metab Clin North Am*. United States; 2017;46(3):783–793.

38. Song H, Mosci C, Akatsu H, Basina M, Dosiou C, Iagaru A. Diagnostic 123I whole body scan prior to ablation of thyroid remnant in patients with papillary thyroid cancer: implications for clinical management. *Clin Nucl Med*. United States; 2018;43(10):705–709.

39. Tuttle RM. Controversial issues in thyroid cancer management. *J Nucl Med*. United States; 2018;59(8):1187–1194.

40. Schlumberger M, Leboulleux S, Catargi B, et al. Outcome after ablation in patients with low-risk thyroid cancer (ESTIMABL1): 5-year follow-up results of a randomised, phase 3, equivalence trial. *Lancet Diabetes Endocrinol*. England; 2018;6(8):618–626.

41. Schlumberger M, Catargi B, Borget I, et al. Strategies of radioiodine ablation in patients with low-risk thyroid cancer. *N Engl J Med*. United States; 2012;366(18):1663–1673.

42. Bal C, Ballal S, Soundararajan R, Chopra S, Garg A. Radioiodine remnant ablation in low-risk differentiated thyroid cancer patients who had R0 dissection is an over treatment. *Cancer Med*. United States; 2015;4(7):1031–1038.

43. Lee M, Lee YK, Jeon TJ, et al. Low iodine diet for one week is sufficient for adequate preparation of high dose radioactive iodine ablation therapy of differentiated thyroid cancer patients in iodine-rich areas. *Thyroid*. United States; 2014;24(8):1289–1296.

44. Morris LF, Wilder MS, Waxman AD, Braunstein GD. Reevaluation of the impact of a stringent low-iodine diet on ablation rates in radioiodine treatment of thyroid carcinoma. *Thyroid*. United States; 2001;11(8):749–755.

45. Li JH, He ZH, Bansal V, Hennessey J V. Low iodine diet in differentiated thyroid cancer: a review. *Clin Endocrinol* (Oxf). England; 2016;84(1):3–12.

46. Sawka AM, Ibrahim-Zada I, Galacgac P, et al. Dietary iodine restriction in preparation for radioactive iodine treatment or scanning in well-differentiated thyroid cancer: a systematic review. *Thyroid*. United States; 2010;20(10):1129–1138.

47. Kalinyak JE, McDougall IR. Whole-body scanning with radionuclides of iodine, and the controversy of "thyroid stunning." *Nucl Med Commun*. 2004;25(9):838–847.

48. McDougall IR, Iagaru A. Thyroid stunning: fact or fiction? *Semin Nucl Med*. United States; 2011;41(2):105–112.

49. Bal CS, Kumar A, Pant GS. Radioiodine dose for remnant ablation in differentiated thyroid carcinoma: a randomized clinical trial in 509 patients. *J Clin Endocrinol Metab*. United States; 2004;89(4):1666–1673.

50. Hommel I, Pieters GF, Rijnders AJM, van Borren MM, de Boer H. Success rate of thyroid remnant ablation for differentiated thyroid cancer based on 5550 MBq post-therapy scan. *Neth J Med*. Netherlands; 2016;74(4):152–157.

51. Cai XY, Vijayaratnam N, McEwan AJB, Reif R, Morrish DW. Comparison of 30 mCi and 50 mCi I-131 doses for ablation of thyroid remnant in papillary thyroid cancer patients. *Endocr Res*. England; 2018;43(1):11–14.

52. Cherk MH, Kalff V, Yap KSK, Bailey M, Topliss D, Kelly MJ. Incidence of radiation thyroiditis and thyroid remnant ablation success rates following 1110 MBq (30 mCi) and 3700 MBq (100 mCi) post-surgical 131I ablation therapy for differentiated thyroid carcinoma. *Clin Endocrinol* (Oxf). England; 2008;69(6):957–962.

53. Klubo-Gwiezdzinska J, Van Nostrand D, Atkins F, et al. Efficacy of dosimetric versus empiric prescribed activity of 131I for therapy of differentiated thyroid cancer. *J Clin Endocrinol Metab*. United States; 2011;96(10):3217–3225.

54. Deandreis D, Rubino C, Tala H, et al. Comparison of empiric versus whole-body/-blood clearance dosimetry-based approach to radioactive iodine treatment in patients with metastases from differentiated thyroid cancer. *J Nucl Med*. United States; 2017;58(5):717–722.

55. Atkins F, Van Nostrand D, Moreau S, Burman K, Wartofsky L. Validation of a simple thyroid cancer dosimetry model based on the fractional whole-body retention at 48 hours post-administration of (131)I. *Thyroid*. United States; 2015;25(12):1347–1350.

56. Van Nostrand D, Atkins F, Moreau S, et al. Utility of the radioiodine whole-body retention at 48 hours for modifying empiric activity of 131-iodine for the treatment of metastatic well-differentiated thyroid carcinoma. *Thyroid*. United States; 2009;19(10):1093–1098.

57. Chudgar AV, Shah JC. Pictorial review of false-positive results on radioiodine scintigrams of patients with differentiated thyroid cancer. *Radiographics*. United States; 2017;37(1):298–315.

58. Glazer DI, Brown RKJ, Wong KK, Savas H, Gross MD, Avram AM. SPECT/CT evaluation of unusual physiologic radioiodine biodistributions: pearls and pitfalls in image interpretation. *Radiographics*. United States; 2013;33(2):397–418.

59. Carlisle MR, Lu C, McDougall IR. The interpretation of 131I scans in the evaluation of thyroid cancer, with an emphasis on false positive findings. *Nucl Med Commun*. England; 2003;24(6):715–735.

60. Maruoka Y, Abe K, Baba S, et al. Incremental diagnostic value of SPECT/CT with 131I scintigraphy after radioiodine therapy in patients with well-differentiated thyroid carcinoma. *Radiology*. United States; 2012;265(3):902–909.

61. Spanu A, Solinas ME, Chessa F, Sanna D, Nuvoli S, Madeddu G. 131I SPECT/CT in the follow-up of differentiated thyroid carcinoma: incremental value versus planar imaging. *J Nucl Med*. United States; 2009;50(2):184–190.

62. Brown AP, Chen J, Hitchcock YJ, Szabo A, Shrieve DC, Tward JD. The risk of second primary malignancies up to three decades after the treatment of differentiated thyroid cancer. *J Clin Endocrinol Metab*. United States; 2008;93(2):504–515.

63. Molenaar RJ, Sidana S, Radivoyevitch T, et al. Risk of hematologic malignancies after radioiodine treatment of well-differentiated thyroid cancer. *J Clin Oncol*. United States; 2018;36(18):1831–1839.

64. Molenaar RJ, Pleyer C, Radivoyevitch T, et al. Risk of developing chronic myeloid neoplasms in well-differentiated thyroid cancer patients treated with radioactive iodine. *Leukemia*. England; 2018;32(4):952–959.

65. Larson SM, Osborne JR, Grewal RK, Tuttle RM. Redifferentiating thyroid cancer: selumetinib-enhanced radioiodine uptake in thyroid cancer. *Mol Imaging Radionucl Ther.* Turkey; 2017;26(Suppl 1):80–86.

66. Ho AL, Grewal RK, Leboeuf R, et al. Selumetinib-enhanced radioiodine uptake in advanced thyroid cancer. *N Engl J Med.* United States; 2013;368(7):623–632.

67. Dunn LA, Sherman EJ, Baxi SS, et al. Vemurafenib redifferentiation of BRAF mutant, RAI-Refractory thyroid cancers. *J Clin Endocrinol Metab.* 2019;104(5):1417–1428.

68. Mosci C, Iagaru A. PET/CT imaging of thyroid cancer. *Clin Nucl Med.* United States; 2011;36(12):e180–e185.

69. Iagaru A, Kalinyak JE, McDougall IR. F-18 FDG PET/CT in the management of thyroid cancer. *Clin Nucl Med.* United States; 2007;32(9):690–695.

CHAPTER SELF-ASSESSMENT QUESTIONS

1. What is the proper range for an empiric dose of I-131 for Graves' disease?

   A. 5–10 mCi

   B. 10–15 mCi

   C. 15–20 mCi

   D. 20–25 mCi

2. What is the best diagnosis based on this image, with a 24-h radioiodine uptake of 20.6% (normal 10%–30%)?

   A. Physiologic uptake

   B. Graves' disease

   C. Solitary nodular toxic goiter

   D. Multinodular toxic goiter

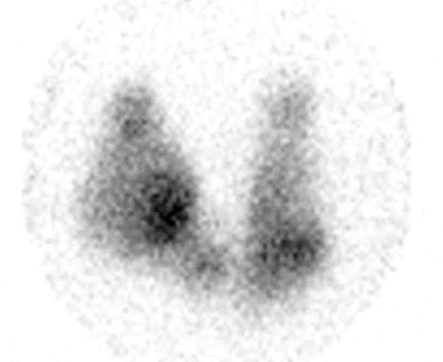

3. Which is the proper preparation for I-131 therapy for thyroid cancer?

   A. High-iodine diet

   B. Low-iodine diet

   C. Low-salt diet

   D. Dietary iodine is irrelevant

4. Given the findings in the pre-therapy I-123 whole-body scan on the left, and the axial SPECT/CT image of the same scan on the right, what is the next best step?

   A. MRI scan of the pelvis for further evaluation of these findings.

   B. Pre-therapy dosimetry before proceeding with treatment.

   C. Treat with 100 mCi of I-131.

   D. Treat with 200 mCi of I-131.

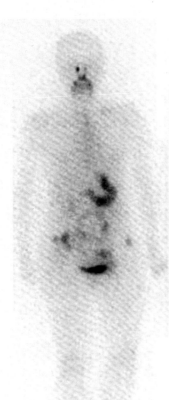

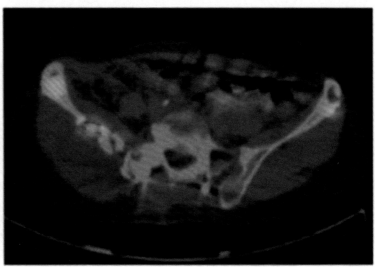

Answers to Chapter Self-Assessment Questions

1. B The recommended empiric dose of I-131 for Graves' disease is in the range of 10 to 15 mCi. Solitary or multiple toxic nodules typically require doses closer to 20 mCi. Doses higher than 30 mCi are reserved for thyroid cancer only.

2. D The scan shows two focal areas of increased uptake in the mid-right thyroid lobe and inferior left thyroid lobe consistent with hyperfunctioning nodules. There is relative suppression of the remainder of the normal gland, resulting in a normal 24-h radioiodine uptake value.

3. B To avoid theoretical competition for the sodium iodide symporters on thyroid cells, it is recommended to undergo a low-iodine diet for 1 to 2 weeks prior to the therapy. The strength of this evidence is not strong given lack of prospective studies on this topic. This is not a low-salt diet because of the availability of non-iodized salt.

4. D The whole-body scan shows several foci of abnormal iodine uptake in the region of the pelvis, bilaterally. The SPECT/CT image shows that this uptake corresponds to osseous metastases. Further evaluation with MRI is not needed. The number of metastases is limited enough not to warrant pre-therapeutic dosimetry, but a higher-dose would be recommended over a lower-dose given the osseous metastases.

Parathyroid Scintigraphy

5

Patrick M. Colletti

LEARNING OBJECTIVES

1. Explain the basic principles of hyperparathyroidism.
2. Describe the methods of parathyroid scintigraphy.
3. Compare the results of five different parathyroid scintigraphy techniques.

BACKGROUND

Primary hyperparathyroidism (pHPT) is associated with one or more abnormally active parathyroid gland. Secondary hyperparathyroidism (sHPT) is associated with chronic hypocalcemia results in reactive overproduction of parathyroid hormone (PTH). sHPT is often directly related to chronic renal failure. Tertiary hyperparathyroidism (tHPT) is the result of untreated sHPT, with continuously elevated PTH levels.

Parathyroidectomy for hyperparathyroidism is typically planned on the basis of medical imaging and performed via a scope or small incision with intraoperative PTH (IOPTH) monitoring. Given the biological half-life of PTH of 5 min, successful excision of target parathyroid lesions should result in a 50% or greater reduction in IOPTH compared with preoperative baseline levels at 5 min and a normal or near-normal IOPTH level at 10 min post-excision (1–3).

There are several effective methods for locating parathyroid adenoma and parathyroid hyperplastic glands, including ultrasound, 4D contrast-enhanced computed tomography (CT), selective angiography with venous sampling, and radionuclide parathyroid imaging. This chapter presents the methods and results of parathyroid scintigraphy.

Parathyroid scintigraphy

While there are alternative radiopharmaceuticals that may be used for parathyroid localization, including ^{11}C-choline positron emission tomography (PET)/CT (4), ^{99m}Tc sestamibi is reliable and effective as applied in a variety of techniques (5–10):

- [99m]Tc sestamibi alone with delayed views, with or without pinhole imaging, single photon emission computed tomography (SPECT), or SPECT/CT.

- [99m]Tc sestamibi with subtraction of the ^{99m}Tc-pertechnetate or ^{123}I-labeled thyroid with or without pinhole imaging, SPECT, or SPECT/CT.

Table 5.1 compares the clinical performance of these techniques [11]. Parathyroid scintigraphy detects 50% to 75% of parathyroid adenomas.

Interpretation may be as simple as visually comparing pertechnetate images with sestamibi images, looking for differences on the sestamibi images not seen on the pertechnetate images. In general, delayed ^{99m}Tc sestamibi images will increase the contrast between parathyroid adenomas and thyroid tissue, as the thyroid activity washes out faster than parathyroid adenomas.

Figure 5.1 demonstrates differences in activity seen on ^{99m}Tc sestamibi as compared with ^{99m}Tc-pertechnetate images along with differential thyroid washout.

Figure 5.2 demonstrates the advantage of SPECT/CT for the 3D location of mediastinal parathyroid adenoma.

Figure 5.3 shows how sestamibi and pertechnetate comparison with differential washout demonstrates all four hyperplastic parathyroid glands in a patient with renal failure.

Figure 5.4 presents examples from patients with secondary and tertiary hyperparathyroidism.

While ultrasound and four-phase contrast-enhanced CT are effective in detecting parathyroid adenomas, parathyroid imaging with sestamibi is reliable for guiding surgery in most patients. Parathyroid scintigraphy is particularly helpful in identifying and localizing ectopic adenomas. Occasionally, handheld gamma probe assisted surgery may be helpful for locating lesions in the operating room.

Table 5.1 **PERFORMANCE OF DIFFERENT ^{99M}TC-MIBI PARATHYROID PLANAR SCINTIGRAPHY PROTOCOLS IN SECONDARY HYPERPARATHYROIDISM**

Tracers Used	Pinhole Collimator	Studies/Patients/Number of Lesions	Sensitivity (%)
A ^{99m}Tc-MIBI only "dual-phase"	No	15/308/899	56.2 (505/899)
B ^{99m}Tc-MIBI only "dual-phase"	Yes	4/60/196	63.2 (124/196)
C ^{99m}Tc-MIBI + 123I (simultaneous acquisition plus subtraction)	Yes	2/31/126	75.4 (95/126)
D ^{99m}Tc-MIBI + 99mTcO$_4$ (non-simultaneous)	No	2/51/178	51.7 (92/178)
E ^{99m}Tc-MIBI + 99mTcO$_4$ (non-simultaneous)	Yes	1/21/78	62.8 (49/78)

Comparisons between imaging protocols were performed using chi-squared test: A versus B ($P = 0.082$); A versus C ($P = 0.001$); B versus C ($P = 0.031$).

Reprinted with permission from Taïeb et al. (9).

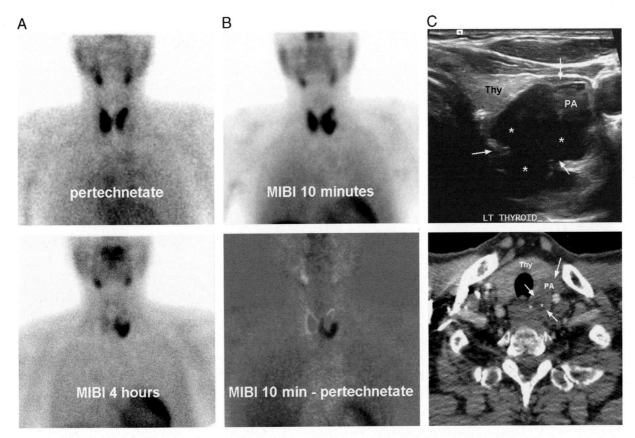

FIG. 5.1 ● Left lower-posterior parathyroid adenoma with MIBI retention at 4 h. **A:** Planar anterior views demonstrating a medially deviated left thyroid lobe on ^{99m}TcO$_4$ imaging with left lower-MIBI activity and physiologic washout of the thyroid at 4 h. **B and C:** Subtraction of the ^{99m}TcO$_4$ image from the 10-min MIBI image demonstrating deferential activity in the 4.0 × 4.5-cm necrotic left lower-pole parathyroid adenoma (arrows) seen extending posterior to the trachea on axial ultrasound (B) and contrast-enhanced CT scan (C). Asterisk (*) indicates necrotic portion; PA, parathyroid adenoma (solid portion); Thy, thyroid. With permission from Taïeb et al. (8).

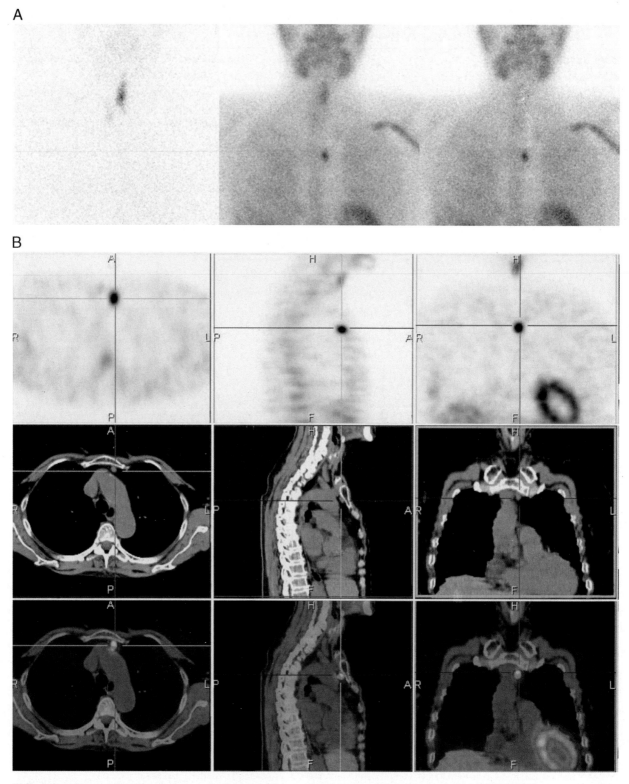

FIG. 5.2 ● One-centimeter anterior mediastinal ectopic parathyroid adenoma demonstrated with SPECT/CT.
A: Planar anterior $^{99m}TcO_4$ image (left), early planar anterior-MIBI image (middle), and late planar anterior-MIBI image (right) demonstrating MIBI retention in the ectopic parathyroid adenoma. **B:** Localization to the anterior mediastinum by axial, sagittal, and coronal SPECT/CT; SPECT (top row), CT (middle row), and hybrid SPECT/CT (bottom row) images. With permission from Taïeb et al. (8).

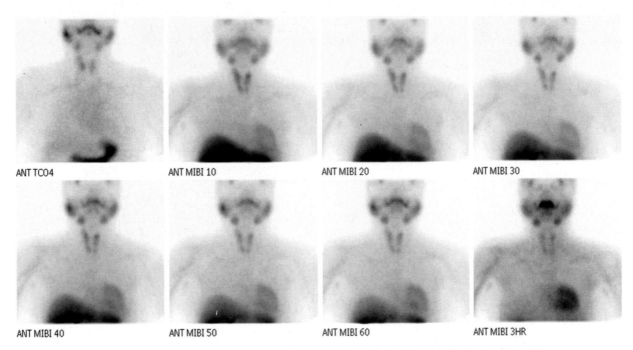

ANT TCO4   ANT MIBI 10   ANT MIBI 20   ANT MIBI 30

ANT MIBI 40   ANT MIBI 50   ANT MIBI 60   ANT MIBI 3HR

FIG. 5.3 ● Parathyroid hyperplasia with MIBI retention in four parathyroid glands at 3 h. MIBI 10 indicates MIBI image 10 min after injection; MIBI 3HR, MIBI image 3 h after injection; TCO4, $^{99m}TcO_4$. With permission from Taïeb et al. (8).

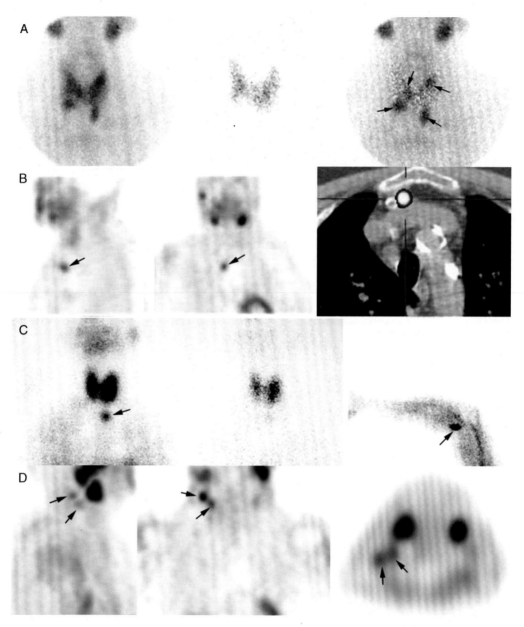

FIG. 5.4 ● Case examples of parathyroid scintigraphy in secondary (sHPT) and tertiary hyperparathyroidism. **A:** Parathyroid scintigraphy prior to initial surgery for secondary HPT. Subtraction protocol: [123]I at 2 h post-administration of 12 MBq from 740 MBq of ^{99m}Tc-sestamibi at time 0, simultaneous dual-tracer image recording (planar + pinhole), digital subtraction of images (^{99m}Tc-sestamibi minus ^{123}I). Four enlarged parathyroid glands are seen on pinhole subtraction images in this patient, with asymmetrical gland locations (arrows). **B–D:** Parathyroid scintigraphy for persistent or recurrent sHPT. **B:** Recurrent tertiary HPT related to a supernumerary ectopic gland (left and middle: SPECT images; right: fusion SPECT/CT image). **C:** Recurrence caused by supernumerary ectopic upper-mediastinal parathyroid gland and forearm graft hyperplasia (arrows). Left: planar static cervicomediastinal ^{99m}Tc-sestaMIBI; middle: planar static cervicomediastinal ^{123}I image; right: ^{99m}Tc-sestaMIBI planar image centered over the graft. **D:** Recurrent sHPT related to parathyromatosis. The patient had total thyroid ablation during one of the previous parathyroid surgeries. Multiple foci of ^{99m}Tc-sestaMIBI uptake, corresponding to hyperfunctioning parathyroid tissue are seen in upper lateral right neck. With permission from Taïeb et al. (9).

References

1. Richards ML, Thompson GB, Farley DR, Grant CS. An optimal algorithm for intraoperative parathyroid hormone monitoring. *Arch Surg.* 2011;146(3):28.
2. Bergenfelz AO, Hellman P, Harrison B, et al. Positional statement of the European Society of Endocrine Surgeons (ESES) on modern techniques in pHPT surgery. *Langenbecks Arch Surg.* 2009;394:761–764.
3. Bilezikian JP, Khan AA, Potts JT Jr. Guidelines for the management of asymptomatic primary hyperparathyroidism: summary statement from the third international workshop. *J Clin Endocrinol Metab.* 2009;94:335–339.
4. Vellani C, Hodolič M, Chytiris S, Trifirò G, Rubello D, Colletti PM. Early and delayed 18F-FCH PET/CT imaging in parathyroid adenomas. *Clin Nucl Med.* 2017;42:143–144.
5. Hindie E, Ugur O, Fuster D, et al. 2009 EANM parathyroid guidelines. *Eur J Nucl Med Mol Imaging.* 2009;36:1201–1216.
6. Taillefer R, Boucher Y, Potvin C, et al. Detection and localization of parathyroid adenomas in patients with hyperparathyroidism using a single radionuclide imaging procedure with technetium-99m-sestamibi (double-phase study). *J Nucl Med.* 1992;33:1801–1807.
7. Martin D, Rosen IB, Ichise M. Evaluation of single isotope technetium 99m sestamibi in localization efficiency for hyperparathyroidism. *Am J Surg.* 1996;172:633–636.
8. Taieb D, Hindie E, Grassetto G, Colletti PM, Rubello D. Parathyroid scintigraphy when, how, and why? a concise systematic review. *Clin Nucl Med.* 2012;37:568–574.
9. Taïeb D, Ureña-Torres P, Zanotti-Fregonara P, et al. Parathyroid Scintigraphy in renal hyperparathyroidism: the added diagnostic value of SPECT and SPECT/CT. *Clin Nucl Med.* 2013;38:630–635.
10. Fuster D, Depetris M, Torregrosa JV, Squarcia M, Paschoalin RP, Mayoral M, Granados U, Colletti PM, Rubello D, Pons F. Advantages of pinhole collimator double-phase scintigraphy with 99mTc-MIBI in secondary hyperparathyroidism. *Clin Nucl Med.* 2013;38:878–881.
11. Caldarella C, Treglia G, Pontecorvi A, et al. Diagnostic performance of planar scintigraphy using (99m)Tc-MIBI in patients with secondary hyperparathyroidism: a meta-analysis. *Ann Nucl Med.* 2012;26:794–803.

CHAPTER SELF-ASSESSMENT QUESTIONS

1. What is the most likely diagnosis?

   A. Lymphoma

   B. Parathyroid adenoma

   C. Parathyroid cancer

   D. Sarcoidosis

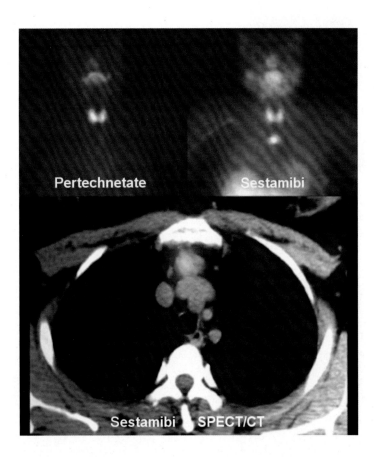

2. What is the most likely diagnosis?

   A. Parathyroid adenoma

   B. Parathyroid cancer

   C. Parathyroid dysplasia

   D. Parathyroid hyperplasiaa

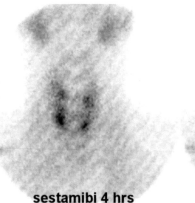

sestamibi 4 hrs

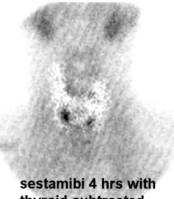

sestamibi 4 hrs with thyroid subtracted

Answers to Chapter Self-Assessment Questions

1. While sestamibi may not accumulate in sarcoidosis (D), it is a potential tumor agent that can localize breast and thyroid cancer. Thus, choices lymphoma (A) and parathyroid carcinoma (C) are possible but are less likely as sestamibi imaging is much more commonly done for the correct answer, parathyroid adenoma (**B**). Note that this is a mediastinal parathyroid adenoma located within the thymus.

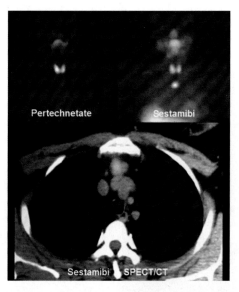

2. As there are four separate lesions on the 4-h sestamibi exam, parathyroid adenoma (A) and parathyroid cancer (B) are unlikely. Parathyroid dysplasia (C) is not a reasonable consideration. Thus, the correct answer is parathyroid hyperplasia (D). Primary hyperparathyroidism (pHPT) is associated with abnormally active parathyroid glands. Secondary hyperparathyroidism (sHPT) is associated with chronic hypocalcemia results in reactive overproduction of PTH. Tertiary hyperparathyroidism (tHPT) is the result of untreated sHPT, with continuously elevated PTH levels.

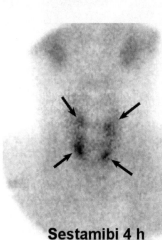

Sestamibi 4 h

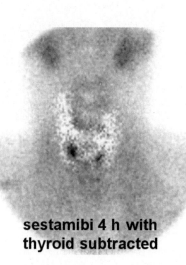

sestamibi 4 h with thyroid subtracted

Neuroendocrine Tumor Imaging and Therapy

6

Erik S. Mittra and Hong Song

LEARNING OBJECTIVES

1. Understand the background of neuroendocrine tumors and physiologic basis for theranostics.
2. Describe the technique and interpretation of somatostatin receptor (SSTR) and metaiodobenzylguanidine (mIBG) imaging.
3. Understand the practical aspects of SSTR and mIBG therapy.

INTRODUCTION

Imaging of neuroendocrine tumors (NETs) has a long history in Nuclear Medicine (NM). Because NETs constitute a diverse group of tumor types, this field is broad. Earlier, however, there were only limited options for imaging and no food and drug administration (FDA)-approved therapies. Recently, there has been a resurgence of this area due to the FDA approval of one new imaging (in 2016) and two new therapeutic radiopharmaceuticals (both in 2018). This area is also an excellent example of the concept of theranostics, which has received much attention in NM over the last decade.

BACKGROUND

NETs include a wide range of tumors that arise from cells of the endocrine or nervous system and are well known for being heterogenous. They can arise from a variety of different organs, may be benign or malignant, are well-, moderately-, or poorly differentiated (e.g., their grade), have variable metastatic potential, and are either functional or nonfunctional (i.e., overproduce hormones causing symptoms or not) (1). Beyond disease progression, these symptoms can significantly reduce the quality of life (QoL) and are an important consideration for the need for therapy. NETs have low incidence, but a high prevalence given the relatively lower mortality associated with these tumors.

Regarding anatomic site or organ of origin, the most common site is the bowel (either foregut, midgut, or hindgut), followed by the pancreas, and by the lung. The first two are often grouped as gastro-entero-pancreatic (GEP) NETs and account for approximately two thirds of NETs. Those originating in the lungs can be further subdivided into bronchial, pulmonary carcinoid, small-cell lung cancer, and large-cell neuroendocrine carcinomas (NECs) of the lung. Other NETs include pheochromocytomas, paragangliomas, neuroblastoma, medullary thyroid cancer, and Merkel cell cancer.

The World Health Organization grading of NETs is based on cellular proliferation, either mitotic count (per 10 high-powered field) or the Ki-67 proliferation index (%). Low-grade (G1) tumors have a mitotic count of <2 or a Ki-67 of <3%. Intermediate-grade (G2) tumors have a mitotic count between 2 and 20 or a Ki-67 of 3% to 20%. And high-grade (G3) carcinomas have a mitotic count of >20 or a Ki-67 of >20%. It has been suggested that G3 be further subdivided into well- and poorly differentiated neoplasms to better reflect prognosis.

Nuclear imaging and therapy of NETs are based primarily on one of two features of these cell types. The first is somatostatin receptors (SSTRs) and the second is norepinephrine. The former is the basis of Indium-111 pentetreotide (OctreoScan) and Gallium-68 DOTATATE (NetSpot) imaging, and Lu-177 DOTATATE (Lutathera) therapy. The latter is the basis of I-123 metaiodobenzylguanidine (mIBG) imaging and I-131 mIBG or I-131 iobenguane (Azedra) therapy. Each of these is discussed in greater detail further in this chapter.

While not the focus of this chapter, it should also be noted that two other radiopharmaceuticals have a role in the imaging of NETs, which include ^{18}F-fluorodeoxyglucose (FDG) and ^{18}F-fluorodopa (FDOPA). As a glucose analog, ^{18}F-FDG crosses the cell membrane via the glucose transporter and evaluates the glycolytic pathway of the cell. It is primarily useful for high-grade NECs which typically do not have high SSTR expression. Well-differentiated NECs (Ki-67 values in the range of 20%–50%) may need both ^{68}Ga-DOTATATE and ^{18}F-FDG imaging for full staging given the variable expression of SSTRs. FDOPA is a fluorinated form of levodopa and is taken up by NETs based on their ability to store biogenic amines and crosses the cell membrane via the large amino acid transporter. Studies have shown that ^{18}F-FDOPA may have higher sensitivity than SSTR scintigraphy (2).

Somatostatin receptors

A primary commonality among many NETs (especially lung and GEP-NETs, more variable for other NETs) is their expression of the G protein-coupled SSTRs, of which there are five known subtypes in humans. Several peptides have been developed to bind with SSTRS, with variable affinity. Table 6.1 shows the relative binding affinity of a subset of these, focused on the imaging compounds.

Table 6.1   **RELATIVE BINDING AFFINITY (IC$_{50}$ IN NMOL/L) OF DIFFERENT SOMATOSTATIN RECEPTOR ANALOGS TO THE FIVE KNOWN SUBTYPES OF THE HUMAN SOMATOSTATIN RECEPTOR, HIGHLIGHTING THE DIFFERENCE BETWEEN PEPTIDES AS WELL AS THE EFFECT OF CHELATORS AND ISOTOPES (71)**

	Somatostatin-Receptor Subtype				
	1	2	3	4	5
Somatostatin-28	5.2+0.3	2.7+0.3	7.7+0.9	5.6+0.4	4.0+0.3
Octreotide	>10,000	2.00.7	18755	>1000	22+6
DTPA-octreotide	>10,000	122	37684	>1000	29950
In-DTPA-octreotide	>10,000	223.6	18213	>1000	23752
DOTATOC	>10,000	142.6	880324	>1000	39384
Ga-DOTATOC	>10,000	2.50.5	613140	>1000	7321
In-DTPA-octreotate	>10,000	1.30.2	>10,000	43316	>1000
Ga-DOTATATE	>10,000	0.20.04	>1000	300140	37718

Reprinted with permission from Brabander et al. (71). Copyright © 2015 Karger Publishers, Basel, Switzerland.

The human somatostatin molecule is a hormone used by neuroendocrine cells for neurotransmission and cell proliferation. It has two active forms, one composed of 28 amino acids and the other 14 amino acids. An abbreviated version of the human somatostatin molecule, composed of 8 amino acids, with a much longer plasma half-life, is octreotide (Sandostatin®). Octreotide was FDA-approved in 1988 for symptom control in patients with functional NETs (3). However, it is also known to have antiproliferative effects and is practically used in that way for patients with low- or intermediate-grade, metastatic, inoperable NET (4). A slight variation of this peptide is lanreotide (Somatuline®), which is also used for the same indications.

To allow imaging and therapy of NETs, several variations of the octreotide peptide have been developed and labeled with gamma-, positron-, or beta-emitting isotopes for these various applications (5). The isotope connects to the peptide with one of two structural linkers, either diethylenetriaminepentaacetic acid (DTPA) or tetraazocyclodecanetetraacetic acid (DOTA). Aside from octreotide, the other peptide used is octreotate. These different radiopharmaceuticals (peptide-linker-isotope combinations) have different binding affinities to the various subtypes of SSTRs as well as dosimetry in normal organs (Table 1) (6–9). Ultimately, the images as well as lesional dosimetry are similar but not the same (4,7,10).

Somatostatin receptor imaging

Historically, the first approach to both nuclear imaging and therapy of NETs was with Indium-111 DTPA-octreotide (or In111-pentetreotide; Octreoscan™) (5). In-111 allows for gamma-imaging and this has been the mainstay of nuclear imaging of NETs since the 1980s. The imaging protocol is somewhat cumbersome as the radiopharmaceutical injection is followed 24 and (often) 48 h afterward with whole-body planar imaging with or without SPECT/CT. Even further delayed imaging is sometimes necessary and the patient is requested to have regular bowel movements during this time (with the use of over-the-counter laxatives if needed) to increase the specificity of the scan.

The next generation of imaging agents used the positron-emitting isotope Gallium-68 (^{68}Ga) bound to either octreotide or octreotate using the DOTA-linker (6). Three peptides based on this concept include DOTA-TATE, DOTA-TOC, and DOTA-NOC. In June 2016, ^{68}Ga-DOTATATE (NetSpot, Advanced Accelerator Applications [AAA]) was FDA approved, thereby providing a PET-imaging alternative to the long-used ^{111}In-pentetreotide

(Figs. 6.1–6.3). Aside from the improved resolution of positron emission tomography (PET) over planar as well as SPECT gamma camera imaging, the imaging protocol is also much more favorable as the whole-body scan is done at 60 min post injection. In fact, in all key aspects (resolution, imaging time, radiation dose, sensitivity, and resultant change in clinical management), ^{68}Ga-DOTATATE is superior to ^{111}In-pentetreotide and should, therefore, be used whenever possible. There are still some areas that are struggling with the availability of Ga68-DOTATATE locally, or insurance denials, but these issues will become less in the future.

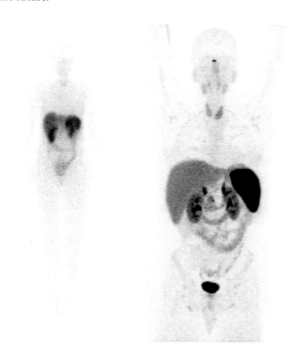

FIG 6.1 ● Examples of normal ^{111}In-DTPA-octreotate gamma-camera (left, planar whole-body images in the anterior projection) and ^{68}Ga-DOTATATE PET (right, MIP image from the vertex-to-mid-thighs) scans in the same patient. In both cases, there is normal biodistribution to the liver and spleen, and clearance through the kidneys (into the bladder) and bowel. Primarily because of its higher resolution, the DOTATATE scan shows additional physiologic glandular uptake in the pituitary, salivary, thyroid, and bilateral adrenals. [68]Ga, Gallium-68; ^{111}In-DTPA, Indium-111 diethylenetriaminepentaacetic acid; MIP, maximum intensity projection; PET, positron emission tomography.

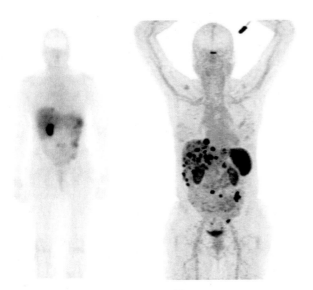

FIG 6.2 ● Examples of an abnormal ^{111}In-DTPA-octreotate gamma-camera (left, planar whole-body images in the anterior projection) and ^{68}Ga-DOTATATE PET (right, MIP image from the vertex-to-mid-thighs) scan in the same patient. In both cases, there are seen multiple liver metastases as well as nodal metastases in the abdomen and pelvis. The much higher resolution of the PET scan is clear. ^{68}Ga, Gallium-68; ^{111}In-DTPA, Indium-111 diethylenetriaminepenta-acetic acid; MIP, maximum intensity projection; PET.

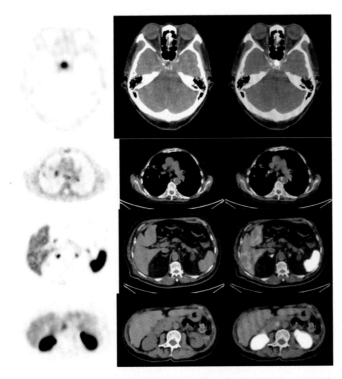

FIG 6.3 ● Composite axial PET (left column), CT (middle column), and fused PET/CT (right column) images showing physiologic or benign uptake on a ^{68}Ga-DOTATATE PET/CT scan, including pituitary uptake (top row), reactive lymphadenopathy (2nd row), adrenal glands (3rd row), and uncinate process of the pancreas (4th row). CT, computed tomography; ^{68}Ga, Gallium-68; PET, positron emission tomography.

There is some controversy about the proper preparation for these scans, with regard to stopping octreotide or lanreotide therapy. Since those medications will compete with the same SSTRs

for imaging, they can theoretically cause a reduction in uptake and, therefore, decrease the sensitivity of the scan. Results are somewhat mixed, but the general guidance is to stop short-acting medications for 24 h before imaging, and long-acting medications for 1 month before imaging, if possible.

Somatostatin receptor therapy

Therapy is also possible with In-111 from the auger electrons that are produced by the photons, which results in DNA damage, and this was the first therapeutic approach tried. However, efficacy was low. As such, the next generation of therapeutic radionuclides used were the beta-emitting isotopes Yttrium-90 (Y-90) and Lutetium-177 (Lu-177) bound to the same linker and peptide combinations described earlier for imaging. Both of these therapeutic isotopes are still in use today (more so in Europe than in the United States) although Lu-177 is the only one that has both FDA and European medicines agency (EMA) approval and is commercially available.

While both Y-90 and Lu-177 are primarily beta-emitting radioisotopes, there are some differences between them. Y-90 has a half-life of 2.7 days, energy of 935 keV, a path length of 12 mm in soft tissue, and no primary gamma emission. Lu-177 has a half-life of 6.7 days, energy of 133 keV, path length of 2 mm in soft tissue, and additional 113 keV (6.6%) and 208 keV (11%) gamma emission. Primarily, it is theorized that the higher energy (and the resulting longer path length) of Y-90 will provide greater efficacy for larger tumors (11). This has been investigated in several clinical trials (12). Unfortunately, the longer path length can also result in greater toxicity to surrounding normal tissue such as bone marrow or the kidneys, although this is still limited (11). As such, Lu-177 was chosen for commercialization given similar efficacy but lower toxicity, as compared to Y-90.

The use of a radionuclide attached to a peptide for the purpose of therapy is generally termed peptide receptor radionuclide therapy (PRRT). It is not specific to NETs, but NET therapy using a somatostatin analog attached to Lu-177 is currently the most advanced and only FDA-approved example of PRRT. Furthermore, this combination of imaging and therapeutic isotopes utilizing the same target is a good example of theranostics, which is a portmanteau of the words therapy and diagnostics, and is a powerful concept in the field of NM.

CLINICAL TRIALS OF PEPTIDE RECEPTOR RADIONUCLIDE THERAPY

Phase I or II experience

Because of regulatory and funding differences between the United States and Europe, much of the initial work on PRRT for NETs has been done in Europe, primarily in the Netherlands and Germany, as well as a few other places in the world. The first patient treated with ^{177}Lu-DOTATATE was in 1997, and since then, various sites in Europe have gained considerable experience with this therapy. While valuable, the majority of the studies have been smaller Phase I and II trials.

Even very early prospective studies on ^{177}Lu-DOTATATE with only 35–50 patients showed partial response rates of 10% to 25%, as well as improvements in QoL measures in those with metastatic NET who were refractory to traditional therapies (13,14). Follow-up studies in much larger (500–600 patients, but single institution) cohorts continued to show favorable outcomes with 30% objective response rates, 40-month progression-free survival

(PFS), and low G3 and G4 toxicities (15). Recent publications from these groups focus on long-term tolerability and outcomes (again in larger groups of 400–800 patients), showing favorable toxicity profiles regarding the kidneys and bone marrow (with greater renal toxicity in those treated with Y-90 vs. Lu-177) and low levels of significant toxicity otherwise, with the suggestion for individual predilections toward radiation (16). The worst outcomes were very small percentages of patients developing acute leukemia (<1%) or myelodysplastic syndrome (<2%), in the context of PFS of 29 months and overall survival (OS) of 63 months (17,18).

Neuroendocrine tumors therapy trial

Based on many favorable Phase I/II results, AAA funded the registry trial (neuroendocrine tumors therapy trial [NETTER-1]) for ^{177}Lu-DOTATATE, with the brand name Lutathera. This was the first Phase III multicenter, randomized, controlled, trial of Lutathera (19). It was simultaneously launched in both Europe and the United States, with a goal of both EMA and FDA approval, respectively.

The study design for the NETTER-1 trial is as follows. Eligibility was for adult participants with biopsy-proven, low-grade (Ki-67 <20%), metastatic or locally advanced, midgut NET, which was inoperable and radiographically progressing on standard dose (30–40 mg) octreotide therapy. Confirmation of SSTR expression was based on planar OctreoScan imaging since ^{68}Ga-DOTATATE PET was not available in most centers at this time.

Participants randomized to the experimental arm received four doses of 200 mCi (7.4 GBq) of Lutathera once every 2 months. Importantly, long-acting octreotide was held for 1 month before each dose of Lutathera, but could be given 4 to 24 h after completion of the Lutathera infusion. Participants randomized to the control arm did not receive placebo. Rather, they received high-dose (60 mg) octreotide, which has a potential therapeutic benefit as well. The primary endpoint of the trial was PFS, with multiple secondary endpoints including OS, objective response rate, toxicity, and QoL measures.

A total of 229 patients were enrolled in the study; 116 on the experimental arm, and 113 on the control arm. Overall, the results were very favorable. The primary endpoint was reached with a strong difference between the two arms. Subjects receiving Lutathera had a 79% reduction in risk of progression (hazard ratio of 0.21, $p < 0.001$), with an estimated PFS of 40 months, compared to 8.4 months on high-dose octreotide therapy.

At the time of the initial NETTER-1 publication (as well as this study), the OS data were not finalized, as the 5-year follow-up phase is still ongoing. But the interim analysis showed a 60% lower risk of death with Lutathera (hazard ratio of 0.40, $p < 0.004$). The objective response rate was also significantly different between the two arms, with 1 complete response and 17 partial responses with Lutathera, and no complete response and 3 partial responses with high-dose octreotide. Lastly, the QoL measures showed improvements overall, as well as specifically for diarrhea, flushing, and abdominal pain.

^{177}Lu-DOTATATE THERAPY

Patient selection

The FDA approval of Lutathera is for the treatment of SSTR-positive GEP-NETs, including foregut, midgut, and hindgut NETs in adults (20). It should be noted again that this therapy can also be used for other NETs such as those arising from the

lung, as well as pheochromocytomas, paragangliomas, medullary thyroid cancer, and Merkel cell carcinomas, but the data are much more limited, and so is not the focus of this chapter. However, these applications are indicated in the joint International Atomic Energy Agency (IAEA), European Association of Nuclear Medicine (EANM); Society of Nuclear Medicine and Molecular Imaging (SNMMI) guidelines for this therapy (21). The primary considerations for patient selection for this therapy are the tumor grade, SSTR density based on nuclear imaging, operability, distribution of disease, progression, and laboratory values.

Tumor grade and SSTR density based on imaging are linked concepts. The therapy is most effective in patients who have high expression of SSTRs on their tumor cells (22). This is typically true for well-differentiated tumors (23,24), which is why the NETTER-1 trial required patients to have either low- or intermediate-grade tumors (Ki-67 <20%). Poorly differentiated or high-grade carcinomas (Ki-67 >20%) are more variable in their SSTR expression. Those in the Ki-67 range of 20% to 50% may have high-enough SSTR expression to warrant PRRT, while those above 50% generally do not. The assessment of SSTR expression is based on ^{111}In-pentetreotide (OctreoScan) gamma-camera and SPECT imaging or, preferably, ^{68}Ga-DOTATATE PET imaging. The majority of the patient's lesions should have uptake greater than the liver background to be eligible for the therapy. There are ongoing studies on specific standardized uptake value (SUV) values or cutoffs to use for therapy and how it relates to outcomes (25). It is also worthwhile to note that because of those issues, ^{18}F-FDG PET may also have a role in the determination of proper patient selection and response assessment for these patients (26), especially those with high-grade tumors.

Since partial or complete surgical removal of tumors is always preferred when possible, PRRT is reserved for patients with locally aggressive and inoperable diseases. Furthermore, the disease is typically metastatic to multiple sites making other approaches such as liver-directed therapy, or external beam radiation, less appealing. Disseminated metastases within the liver are another example where PRRT should likely be favored over liver-directed therapies alone. Lastly, the disease needs to be progressing on standard-dose SSTR therapy with either Octreotide or Lanreotide. In the clinical trials, progression was typically confirmed radiographically (with either CT or MR) using response evaluation criteria in solid tumors (RECIST) criteria. Another area of consideration here is the role of OctreoScan or 68Ga-DOTATATE PET to show progression (e.g., when the disease is radiographically stable or only slightly enlarging, but the SUVs on PET imaging have increased significantly). This is presently an area of ongoing research.

Patients should meet certain laboratory values to ensure that potential transient collateral damage to the bone marrow and the kidneys will not be an issue. The laboratory cutoffs from the NETTER-1 and early access program (EAP) trials were as follows, and it would be reasonable to continue to check these same values for clinical patients at screening, and during the therapy. Patients should have a serum creatinine <1.7 mg/dL (or a creatinine clearance >50 mL/min calculated by the Cockroft–Gault method), hemoglobin >8 g/dL, white blood cell count >2000/mm^3, platelets >75,000/mm^3, total bilirubin less than three times the upper limits of normal, and a serum albumin >3 g/dL, unless the prothrombin time is within the normal range.

Sequencing therapy

Even if a patient is eligible for PRRT based on the previously provided guidelines, it may not be the best choice relative to other therapeutic options such as surgery, mTOR inhibitors, chemotherapy, external beam radiation, or a variety of liver-directed therapies (bland embolization, chemoembolization, or radioembolization) for those with liver dominant disease. This area is an active area of discussion and research, and the consideration is not only what will have great therapeutic benefit, but also which will have less toxicity now and in the future (23). Another possibility is combination therapies, which may have a greater benefit than the sum of their parts, for instance, by using radiosensitizing chemotherapies in conjunction with radioembolization or PRRT (27).

The European Neuroendocrine Tumor Society guidelines have long recommended PRRT as a second-line therapy after progression on SSTR therapy, and this is a very reasonable approach to consider, with the caveats provided earlier. Ultimately, the therapy sequencing decision should ideally be done in the context of a multidisciplinary conference with experts from all the disciplines (oncology, surgery, radiation oncology, NM, radiology, and pathology) represented (1). Since in many places it is difficult to have so many NET experts, progressive NET patients should be referred to a NET Center of Excellence (aka NET Advanced Care Center), at least once in their care.

Performing the therapy

As compared to other radioisotope therapies such as I-131, Ra-223 dichloride (Xofigo), and I-131 ibritumomab tiuxetan (Zevalin), PRRT is significantly more involved. Having said that, once the therapy program has been set up at an institution, it is relatively straightforward and requires only a reasonable amount of input.

As mentioned earlier for imaging, but even more important for therapy, is to stop octreotide/lanreotide therapy for the appropriate amount of time (24 h for short-acting and 1 month for long-acting formulations) before treatment. The Lutathera is shipped from a radiopharmacy (either in Italy or in New Jersey) to the clinical site either the day before or on the day of the therapy and arrives as a clear liquid in a glass vial. The ^{177}Lu-DOTATATE is then administered over 30 minutes, with another 10 to 20 minutes for infusion of saline to minimize the residual. There are two main recommended methods for administration. The first is referred to as the gravity method and requires the use of two needles inserted into the vial. The instillation of saline (either running via gravity or through a pump) through one needle increases the pressure within the vial and pushes the Lutathera out the other needle, which is attached to the patient. The second method is to manually draw out the contents of the vial into the syringe and then using a shielded, automated syringe-pump to administer the therapy to the patient.

The ^{177}Lu-DOTATATE needs to be given in conjunction with an amino acid (AA) formulation, which is given intravenously through either the same or a second IV line. AAs reduce the residence time of ^{177}Lu-DOTATATE in the kidneys thereby reducing radiation toxicity. Recently, there are various AA formulations available with different amounts of AAs, as well as different osmolalities. The only two necessary AAs are lysine and arginine. More pure formulations of just these two AAs, together with a lower osmolality solution, significantly reduce the nausea associated with their infusion. Depending upon which AAs are used (and their emetogenic potential) and the patient's sensitivity, a variable amount of anti-nausea pre medication needs to be given before starting the AAs. Additional PRN anti-nausea medication may also have to be given during the infusion.

There is a low (1%–10%) but documented risk of hormone crisis either during or within a few days of PRRT administration (28,29). Principally based on prior experiences with similar crises which can occur with anesthetics or surgery, recommendations for management center around identifying patients at risk for hormone crisis, giving subcutaneous octreotide either as a bolus or as an infusion either prophylactically (for high-risk patients) or if a crisis happens (for low-risk patients), parenteral H1 or H2 blockers, and resuming short- or long-acting octreotide after PRRT. It should be noted, however (again based on the surgical literature), that there is some controversy to the utility of giving octreotide in this setting (30,31).

On the day of the therapy, most people would agree that the most important person is the nurse who manages all the supportive care including placing the IV(s), giving the anti-nausea medication and AAs, and monitoring the patient for any adverse effects. This nurse can be trained in either oncology or radiology. The latter would require special training for this therapy. Beyond this, the technologist gets the Lutathera dose ready and is responsible for administering it to the patient. The physician's (who must be an authorized user (AU)) role is to oversee the therapy and help with any questions or issues that arise during the process. Depending on the local regulations regarding authorized users, they may also need to be present to start the infusion of Lutathera.

An important point is to select an appropriate room for the therapy. It should ideally have an attached bath or at least one in close vicinity. The toilet and surrounding floor should be lined to contain radioactive urine. The room need not be lead-lined, but should only contain one or more patients receiving this same therapy. It can be located within any appropriate areas, such as NM, an oncology infusion area, or Radiation Oncology.

Radiation and release guidelines

The excreted and especially the emitted radiations from this therapy are relatively low, thereby requiring less extreme measures than for some other types of radioisotope therapy such as I-131 for thyroid cancer. Typically, the emitted radiation after administration of Lutathera is 2 mR/h at 1 m. Within 24 h, this has decreased to less than 1 mR/hour at 1 meter. In the United States, this allows for this therapy to be done as an outpatient with the patient returning home if local or staying in a hotel or motel if needed for one night before traveling home if further away. The only need for an overnight stay in the hospital would be if there are any medical complications during the day, or if the patient is unable to manage their urine (i.e., incontinent) in which case there is a high risk for contamination of the home or hotel within the first 24 h.

The patient should be encouraged to exercise good bathroom hygiene and to stay away from children, pregnant women, and crowds for approximately 3 days after the therapy. Hydration should also be encouraged during this time to promote clearance of un-needed radiopharmaceutical.

Response assessment

Similar to confirming progression based on imaging, the clinical trials used conventional imaging (CT and MRI) with RECIST to assess response to PRRT. As such, CT and MRI remain the standard of care (32). On the trial, the response was checked 1 month after the second cycle of therapy. The patient continued on therapy if there was anything but progression at this time point. The response is again assessed after the completion of all four cycles of therapy, at which time the patient goes into long-term follow-up.

As discussed earlier for evaluation of progression, functional imaging (OctreoScan or 68Ga-DOTATATE PET, and even 18F-FDG PET) may have a significant role in the evaluation of response to PRRT especially given that both the imaging and therapy are targeting the same receptor (32). Moreover, this can be combined in the same imaging appointment with PET/CT or PET/MR, respectively. However, the role of functional imaging for response assessment in NET has not yet been evaluated to the same degree that it has been in other malignancies (such as lymphoma). A current roadblock is the limited reimbursement for multiple ^{68}Ga-DOTATATE PET scans per year. Given the additional gamma radiation emitted by Lu-177, another option is to perform gamma-camera and SPECT imaging of ^{177}Lu-DOTATATE immediately after each therapy (Fig. 6.4). This has the added benefit of not requiring any additional radiation for imaging, though the resolution is more limited than a separate ^{68}Ga-DOTATATE PET (33). Once again, however, reimbursement is an issue here. Ultimately, more data are needed to better understand the role of functional imaging in response assessment for this therapy.

Future directions and controversies

While it has been a long road for the clinical approval of Lutathera, there are many future directions for research and optimizing clinical care (34). These include (but are not limited to) improving response assessment, optimizing the number of therapy cycles per patient, consideration of repeat therapy, delivering the therapy intra-arterially instead of intravenously, clarifying the role of Y-90 versus Lu-177, using alpha- instead of beta-emitters, better understanding the sequencing and combination of PRRT with other therapies, using novel peptides to bind SSTRs, and doing personalized dosimetry.

As mentioned earlier, the current standard-of-care for response assessment during and after PRRT is with conventional imaging, which may have significant limitations due to lack of tumor shrinkage or necrosis (32). A large unmet need here is understanding the role of OctreoScan or Ga68-DOTATATE PET for response assessment, especially with the added value of quantitative metrics such as SUV, as well as different combination approaches with CT and MRI (22,35). This may have significant

implications for improving early response assessment, prognosis after therapy, and adjusting the number of cycles of therapy (see in the following section). However, the uptake may change in unexpected ways (i.e., decrease in background organs and increase in metastases) after somatostatin-analog therapy, such that the scan needs to be interpreted in the proper context and with great care (36). Relatedly, blood biomarkers, especially liver enzymes and chromogranin A may transiently rise after the initial cycles of therapy due to radiation inflammation and should not be taken as a progressive disease (37). It should also be noted that 18F-FDG PET, just like in the initial evaluation of the patient, may also have a role in the response assessment of PRRT, especially since 18F-FDG avid disease has a significant negative prognostic value (38).

Most of the larger clinical trials of Lutathera were based on a total of four cycles of therapy. This was (somewhat arbitrarily) chosen to balance the therapeutic benefit with the toxicity. As shown by the results of the NETTER-1 trial, this schedule works quite well for most patients. Having said that, some patients probably don't need all four cycles of therapy, while others could benefit from more cycles of therapy. This will allow for personalized therapy with the potential for decreased toxicity and improved efficacy. As alluded to previously, better ways to assess response to PRRT are needed to fully realize this.

If a patient does respond well to one full course of Lutathera, then it is reasonable to think that the patient may respond well to another course of Lutathera when they subsequently progress. This idea of salvage (repeat) PRRT has been evaluated to some degree by several clinical trials (39). These studies showed that while the PFS is not as long for the second cycle of PRRT as compared to the initial treatment, it is still quite good (presumably similar or longer than other therapeutic options) and safe.

Many patients have a considerable burden of disease, but it is restricted to the liver, as this is a common site for metastatic NET from the bowel. In these patients, it has been advocated to combine the approaches of SIRT and PRRT, by giving Lutathera intra-arterially via the hepatic artery (40). In theory, this will provide higher delivery to the tumor itself (improving efficacy), while reducing the systemic circulation (reducing side effects). This approach has been studied in limited fashion thus far (40).

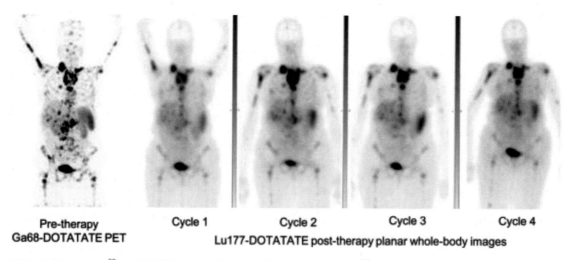

Pre-therapy
Ga68-DOTATATE PET   Cycle 1   Cycle 2   Cycle 3   Cycle 4

Lu177-DOTATATE post-therapy planar whole-body images

FIG 6.4 ● Pre-therapy ^{68}Ga-DOTATATE scan (left), followed by four post-therapy ^{177}Lu-DOTATATE scan images (right) showing distribution of the therapeutic radiopharmaceutical to the same sites of disease seen with the imaging radiopharmaceutical. [68]Ga, Gallium-68.

This approach, while preliminary, shows that the approach can be done successfully. However, they have not yet been done in a comparative manner to systemic PRRT to prove that it is indeed more beneficial. Furthermore, the process is rather complicated, requiring the patient to lay on the interventional radiology table for approximately 4 h, which can be difficult/burdensome to the patient and taxing on the staff.

In the initial phase of PRRT for NET, both Y-90 and Lu-177 were used as the radioisotope. Given the different physical properties described previously, it has been hypothesized (as well as shown in smaller clinical trials) that each may provide different benefits (41). Another approach that has been taken is to give both together or sequentially to take advantage of their respective benefits (12). Principally, Y-90 has a higher energy and thus path length in human tissue. In theory, this would be beneficial for bulkier tumors where the lower energy and shorter path length of Lu-177 would not be able to penetrate. Others argue that as long as there is a viable blood supply to all parts of the bulky tumor, then Lu-177 should be sufficient. Areas without a good blood supply would be prone to necrosis anyway, in which case radiation is not needed. Conversely, the longer path length of Y-90 will also have a greater bystander effect on normal tissues such as the bone marrow and kidneys resulting in higher toxicity, which is generally agreed. It is for these reasons that Lu-177 was chosen as the isotope to move forward for clinical approval. However, the relative benefits of Y-90 versus Lu-177 have not been rigorously studied in a comparative trial so the topic remains open. On a similar note, the use of alpha- instead of these beta-emitters is another area of active research (34).

It has already been mentioned previously that the proper sequencing of PRRT with other available therapies has not been determined yet, and this is a major area of ongoing research (23,42). A related concept to this is the use of combination therapies, such as the use of capecitabine as a radiosensitizer for PRRT (27) or liver-directed therapies in conjunction with system PRRT (42). As the results of these trials (and others yet to be done) become available, we may have a better understanding of proper sequencing and combination therapies. At the current time, this should be discussed in the context of a multidisciplinary conference so that input from multiple experts, especially those familiar with local practices and strengths, can be considered (1).

The SSTR-analogs which are currently used are all agonists for the SSTR. This means they activate the receptor, which ultimately becomes internalized, where the radioisotope is trapped and gives off radiation, which ultimately kills the cells. There has been considerable progress on the next generation of SSTR-analogs which are antagonists to the SSTR. These newer analogs have a higher binding specificity to the SSTR receptor such that even though they do not activate the receptor nor (most likely) get internalized into the cell, they can deliver a higher dose of radiation (43). Several ongoing studies are evaluating these newer analogs (44).

In the beginning, it was mentioned that Lutathera is not specific to the FDA-approved indication of GEP-NETs and it is worth reiterating that in the future, PRRT will likely be extended to many other tumor types. Easily understandable is the treatment of other endocrine malignancies such as lung NETs, and those that are more traditionally treated with I-131 mIBG such as paragangliomas, pheochromocytomas, and medullary thyroid cancer (45). Beyond this, the general concept of PRRT can be extended to other cancers including breast, prostate, gut, pancreas, and brain tumors, that have recently been shown to overexpress several other peptide receptors, such as gastrin-releasing peptide-, neurotensin-, substance P-, glucagon-like peptide 1-, neuropeptide Y-, or corticotropin-releasing factor-receptors. To enable this therapy, a wide range of radiolabeled peptides are being developed for clinical use including newly designed bombesin, neurotensin, substance P, neuropeptide Y, and glucagon-like peptide-1 analogs which offer promise for future PRRT (46).

Lastly, but importantly, is the issue of personalized dosimetry. NETTER-1 and other clinical trials for Lutathera used a fixed dose of 200 mCi (7.4 GBq) of Lu177-DOTATATE per cycle. As can be said for all radioisotope therapies, doing personalized dosimetry would allow for the calculation of an individualized maximum tolerated activity (MTA) which, in theory, should allow for the greatest radiation to the tumors, while limiting toxicity. This has been most well established in thyroid cancer patients with extensive lung or bone metastases, where one wants to give as high a dose as possible without risking pulmonary fibrosis, or severe marrow toxicity. There is even a mandate in Europe to perform individualized dosimetry on all patients. But there are equally others in the community who strongly oppose this approach, especially as a rule for all patients. Many feel that giving a fixed dose works quite well for the vast majority of patients and that there is little added gain by doing personalized dosimetry. This has been borne out in many anecdotal or single-institution experiences but has yet to be studied precisely. Furthermore, it is true that doing dosimetry is a very involved and costly endeavor, which should only be done at a high level. This would preclude many sites from being able to offer these therapies.

Metaiodobenzylguanidine

Aside from somatostatin, the other hormone used for nuclear imaging and therapy of NETs is norepinephrine (or noradrenaline). mIBG (MIBG) or iobenguane is a synthetic analog of guanethidine and is structurally and functionally similar to norepinephrine. Circulating mIBG is thereby taken up in the postganglionic adrenergic neurons (stored in the cytoplasm or secretory granules). Because of this physiology, it is primarily used for neuroblastoma, pheochromocytoma, paraganglioma, and medullary thyroid cancer. Less commonly, it can also be used for other NETs. For imaging, mIBG is typically labeled with Iodine-123. I-123 iobenguane (AdreView, GE Healthcare) was FDA-approved in 2008. For therapy, mIBG is labeled with I-131. I-131 iobenguane (Azedra, Progenics Pharmaceuticals) was FDA-approved in July 2018.

mIBG Imaging

I-123 mIBG imaging (Figs. 6.5–6.9) is relatively straightforward but there are two important points for preparation. Firstly, there are several medications, including some over-the-counter medications, that can interfere with the uptake of the radiopharmaceutical causing a reduction in sensitivity (47). They should be stopped, by the patient's referring physician, for an appropriate amount of time relative to the medication's half-life. Secondly, to decrease the radiation dose to the thyroid, thyroid blockade with either super-saturated potassium iodide (SSKI) drops or potassium iodide pills should be started before the mIBG injection and continued for 2 to 4 days.

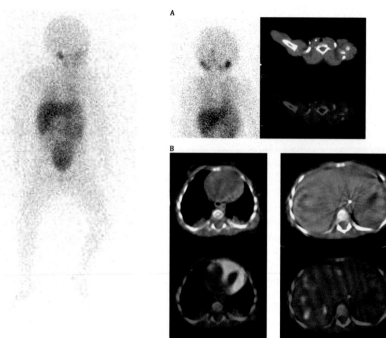

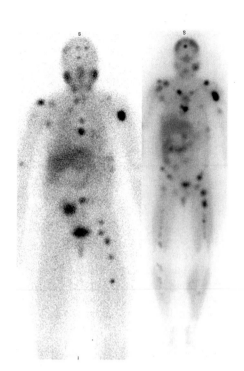

FIG 6.5 ● Normal I-123 mIBG whole-body planar scan in the anterior projection in a pediatric patient being evaluated for neuroblastoma follow-up. Physiologic uptake is seen in the salivary glands, lungs, liver, bowel, and bladder. mIBG, metaiodobenzylguanidine.

FIG 6.6 ● Several examples of physiologic uptake on an I-123 mIBG scan, which should not be confused for abnormal uptake. Panel A shows a planar (left) as well as axial CT and fusion SPECT/CT images (right) of brown fat uptake in the supraclavicular regions. Panel B shows axial CT and fusion SPECT/CT images of uptake in atelectasis (left column), and normal heterogenous uptake in the liver (right column). CT; mIBG, metaiodobenzylguanidine; SPECT.

FIG 6.7 ● Pre-therapy I-123 mIBG scan (left) and post-therapy I-131 mIBG scan (right) in a patient with widely metastatic paraganglioma. The pre-therapy image is used to confirm the uptake and distribution of disease. The post-therapy scan is used to confirm the distribution of the therapeutic radiopharmaceutical to the same areas and to look for additional sites of disease. mIBG, metaiodobenzylguanidine.

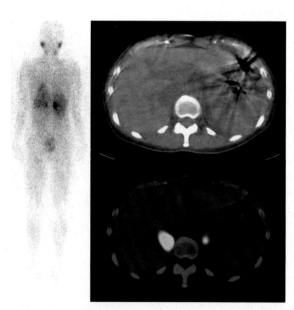

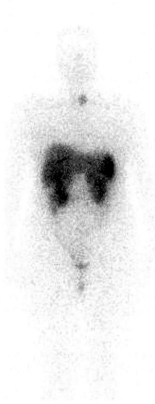

FIG 6.9 ● Abnormal I-123 mIBG whole-body planar scan in the anterior projection in a patient with known medullary thyroid cancer, showing abnormal uptake in the left neck without evidence for metastases. mIBG, metaiodobenzylguanidine.

FIG 6.8 ● I-123 whole-body planar images in the anterior projection (left image) in a patient with suspected pheochromocytoma. There is asymmetrically increased uptake in the right adrenal gland, with physiologic uptake elsewhere. This is better appreciated on the SPECT/CT scan (axial images on the right; low dose CT image on the top, fusion SPECT/CT image on the bottom) showing prominent uptake in the right adrenal gland and mild uptake in the left adrenal gland. This patient subsequently had confirmed pheochromocytoma on the right with compensatory adrenal hyperplasia on the left. CT, computed tomography; SPECT, single photon computed tomography.

Twenty-four hours after the injection of the radiopharmaceutical, a whole-body planar gamma camera image is obtained. At this time, SPECT/CT imaging can also be done as needed. Equivocal findings at this time-point can be further evaluated with 48-h imaging but given the 13.2-h half-life of I-123, counts are limited, and image quality is relatively poor. The applications of mIBG scintigraphy include staging, response assessment, and restaging of patients with disease (48). As a theranostics pair, it is also used to determine eligibility for treatment with I-131 mIBG. To aid in image interpretation, there has been considerable work done on semi-quantitative approaches for mIBG scintigraphy. The two primary ones are the Curie Score, validated through the Children's Oncology Group, and the SIOPEN score, from the International Collaboration for Neuroblastoma Research (49–53). Computer-aided methods have also been developed to automate the process and reduce inter-reader variability (54).

The sensitivity and specificity of mIBG scintigraphy are in the range of 80% to 100% for pheochromocytomas, non-metastatic paragangliomas, and neuroblastoma, but reduced to 50% to 70% for extranodal paragangliomas and medullary thyroid carcinomas. In regard to osseous disease, mIBG is primarily evaluating bone marrow metastases such that full staging of the cortical bone can be completed with a supplementary Tc99m-MDP bone scan. For those tumors that are not mIBG-avid, the next line of imaging would involve either a 68Ga-DOTATATE or 18F-FDG PET depending on whether the pathology shows well-differentiated/low-grade tumor or a poorly differentiated/high-grade tumor, respectively.

mIBG Therapy

The beta and gamma emitting radioisotope, I-131, is attached to mIBG for therapy. I-131 iobenguane (Azedra) was FDA-approved in July 2018 for the treatment of metastatic pheochromocytoma or paragangliomas in patients 12 years of age or older. However, it has been used since the early 1980s in clinical trials for patients with these cancers as well as for those with neuroblastoma and medullary thyroid cancer (55). It is noted again here that PRRT can and has also been used for these same indications, if there is strong SSTR-expression based on imaging, but the data are more limited (21).

Indications and side effects

As described in the European Association of Nuclear Medicine (EANM) procedure guidelines for I-131 mIBG therapy (56), the indications for this treatment include inoperable pheochromocytoma, paraganglioma, or carcinoid tumor, stage III or IV neuroblastoma, and metastatic or recurrent medullary thyroid cancer. The patient also needs to have pre-therapy I-123 or I-131 mIBG scintigraphy to ensure there is sufficient uptake in the sites of metastases to warrant this therapy.

The absolute contraindications for this therapy include a pregnant or breastfeeding patient, life expectancy less than 3 months (except in the case of intractable bone pain), and renal insufficiency requiring dialysis. The relative contraindications include unacceptable medical risk for isolation, unmanageable urinary incontinence, deteriorating renal function (GFR <30 ml/min), progressive hematologic and/or renal toxicity from prior treatment, and myelosuppression (total white cell count $<3 \times 10^9$ per liter and platelets $<100 \times 10^9$ per liter).

The side-effects and toxicity from this therapy can be divided into early and late effects (56). The early effects include temporary nausea and vomiting during the first 2 days after administration and temporary myelosuppression which typically occurs 4–6 weeks post-therapy. Hematological effects are common in children with neuroblastoma after chemotherapy (60%), predominantly as an isolated thrombocytopenia, but are less frequent in adults. But bone marrow depression is likely in patients who have bone marrow involvement at the time of I-131 mIBG therapy and, because of a high whole-body radiation dose, in patients with delayed renal clearance. As with other radio-isotope therapies, there is significantly less hematological toxicity in those patients who have not previously been treated with chemotherapy. Rarely, deterioration of renal function is observed in patients whose kidneys have been compromised by intensive pretreatment with prior nephrotoxic agents. Rarely, in adults with phaeochromocytoma or paraganglioma and children with neuroblastoma, hypertensive crises may be evoked by the release of catecholamines, requiring alpha blockade. In patients with carcinoid, flushing may occur because of the release of serotonin.

Possible long-term effects are those known of I-131 therapy in general, such as hypothyroidism, typically without but sometimes even with adequate thyroid blockade, persistent hematological effects (thrombocytopenia and myelosuppression), and the rare possibility for the induction of leukemia or secondary solid tumors, especially in conjunction with (longstanding) chemotherapy treatment.

Performing the therapy

It was mentioned previously that 177Lu-DOTATATE therapy is significantly more complicated than other therapies such as I-131, Ra-223 dichloride, or Y-90 ibritumomab. Similarly, I-131 mIBG therapy is significantly more complicated than even 1777Lu-DOTATATE therapy. The primary reasons for this are the requirement for pre-therapy dosimetry and the higher radiation dose typically requiring a multi-day hospitalization in an appropriately shielded room.

The primary purpose of pre-therapy whole-body dosimetry is to prevent toxicity. To do this, one must calculate each patient's maximum tolerated dose or activity. Additionally, calculation of the lesion-dose may also be of value. The protocol requires the administration of a small dose of I-131 iobenguane (3–6 mCi) after which three whole-body scans are acquired from day zero through five. Data from those scans can be used in a software program such as OLINDA/EXM to calculate the radiation dose estimates to normal organs and tissues per mCi of administered dose.

The administration of the therapeutic isotope follows within the month and, as mentioned, needs to be done in an appropriate lead-lined hospital room with an en-suite bathroom. Depending on the tumor type, the choice of low-, intermediate-, or high-dose approach, and the results of the pre-therapy dosimetry, the dose of I-131 iobenguane can range from below 100 mCi to greater than 1000 mCi (Azedra is limited to 500 mCi per cycle). As such, different levels of shielding, room lining and preparation, radiation protection, and education for staff and family are needed. The actual administration of the radiopharmaceutical is similar to that for ^{177}Lu-DOTATATE in that one of two techniques can be used: either a two-needle gravity (with or without saline and/or a pump) or a syringe method with a shielded syringe pump. To prevent the short-term side effects of nausea, it is important to provide anti-emetics before and during the therapy. Also similar to ^{177}Lu-DOTATATE, post-therapy imaging is possible due to the beta emissions (Fig. 6.7), typically at the time of discharge from the hospital.

EFFICACY

As stated earlier the indications for I-131 mIBG therapy are relatively broad. As such, the therapy has been utilized in various ways with respect to other therapeutic options, and the results are similarly variable. Some of the approaches are to give it as a monotherapy, to give it over repeated cycles, to give it in combination with another therapy, or to give it up front in newly diagnosed disease as part of induction therapy (57).

Neuroblastoma

Using I-131 mIBG as monotherapy for relapsed or refractory neuroblastoma, the objective response rate is quite wide, in the range of 17% to 66% based on several Phase I and II studies (57). The response rate is higher in patients with fewer prior treatments, a longer time from diagnosis, and older age (58). Because of hematologic toxicity and radiation safety considerations, repeat treatments are typically done at 2- to 3- month intervals. The new approaches to neuroblastoma therapy (NANT) consortium tried the approach of repeated administrations every 14 days, together with autologous hematopoietic cell transplantation (auto-HCT) to ameliorate the hematologic toxicity (59). In this study, patients did not have dose-limiting toxicity, and soft-tissue response (45%) was better than the marrow response (15%).

There have been many studies that look at the combination of I-131 mIBG and other therapeutic options including radiosensitizing chemotherapies, allogeneic stem cell transplantation (allo-HCT) if auto-HCT is not possible, and hyperbaric oxygen (57). Chemotherapies evaluated include cisplatin, cyclophosphamide, etoposide, vincristine, and topotecan/irinotecan, and vorinostat. In some of these studies, the objective response rate was higher (75%) than for I-131 mIBG monotherapy (60). Hyperbaric oxygen can decrease cell proliferation and energy metabolism, and increase lipid peroxidation. These effects may enhance the efficacy of I-131 mIBG. One study showed an OS at 28 months of 32% for a group of patients who received the combination of I-131 mIBG and hyperbaric oxygen therapy, compared to 12% for patients who received I-131 mIBG alone (61). Lastly, several studies have evaluated the role of I-131 mIBG as an up-front, induction therapy in patients with newly diagnosed neuroblastoma, prior to neoadjuvant chemotherapy and/or surgery (57). The results are promising but preliminary and further studies are ongoing.

Pheochromocytoma or paraganglioma

Given the low incidence of pheochromocytomas and paragangliomas, there are limited prospective data with a larger number of patients. Most studies are observational or retrospective with a limited number of patients. Furthermore, the results of these studies are hampered by differences in patient selection, dose, number of treatments, analysis techniques, and follow-up. Despite this relative paucity of data, I-131 mIBG remains an important option for these patients given limited other therapeutic options which include surgery, chemotherapy, tyrosine kinase inhibitors, and liver-directed approaches (62).

However, the limited data does show an objective response with I-131 iobenguane in the range of 20% to 70%, with a 5-year survival rate of 45% to 85% (63,64). Again, the large range is most likely due to the variability in the study design mentioned earlier. One larger prospective Phase II study of 30 patients with either pheochromocytoma or paraganglioma treated with a median dose of 833 mCi of I-131 iobenguane resulted in four patients with complete response, 15 with partial response, one with stable disease, and five with initial response who then progressed (65). This equals an overall response of 67% in this patient group. A more recently published multicenter prospective Phase II trial treated 74 patients with metastatic pheochromocytoma or paraganglioma, with the primary endpoint being at least 50% reduction in baseline antihypertensive medication use lasting at least 6 months (66). Secondary endpoints included objective response, biochemical response, OS, and safety. The results showed 25% met the primary endpoint, and 92% had a partial response or stable disease, 68% had a biochemical response, and the median OS was 36.7 months.

Regarding the toxicity, the most common short-term toxicities include asthenia, nausea, and vomiting (66,67). This may start a few hours after the therapy and last for a week. The incidence is in the range of 4%–16%. The use of antiemetics during this period may help minimize symptoms. The most significant toxicity associated with this therapy is hematologic, primarily thrombocytopenia more than leukopenia and is directly related to dose (62,67). Many if not most patients treated with higher dose (>500 mCi) I-131 mIBG will experience marrow hypoplasia, possibly requiring intervention with platelet transfusions, stimulating factors, epoetin, red blood cells, or peripheral blood stem cell donation (65).

Based on the limited therapeutic options, the published study data, and the manageable toxicity, I-131 iobenguane was FDA-approved for patients 12 years or older with iobenguane scan positive, unresectable, locally advanced or metastatic pheochromocytoma, or paraganglioma who require systemic anticancer therapy (68).

Medullary thyroid cancer

Similar to pheochromocytomas and paragangliomas, there are limited therapeutic options for patients with progressive medullary thyroid cancer aside from surgery, chemotherapy, tyrosine kinase inhibitors, and liver-directed approaches. The data on the use of I-131 mIBG for this application are even more limited but promising.

A case report of a patient with metastatic medullary thyroid cancer treated with 150 mCi of I-131 mIBG showed a durable partial response (69). And in a larger cohort of 13 patients, there were four with partial response, and four with stable disease (70).

CONCLUSION

Radionuclide approaches have a long-standing history for both imaging and therapy of many types of NETs. One approach utilizes somatostatin analogs to investigate the SSTR, and can be utilized broadly across most types of neuroendocrine cells. The FDA-approved radiopharmaceuticals ^{68}Ga-DOTATATE and ^{177}Lu-DOTATATE can be used for imaging and therapy, respectively. Another approach uses a norepinephrine analog to investigate the postganglionic neurons of the sympathetic chain. In this case, the FDA-approved radiopharmaceuticals I-123 mIBG and I-131 mIBG can be used for imaging and therapy, respectively. The data on their utility is very well established for imaging, quite good for ^{177}Lu-DOTATATE therapy for GEP NETs and growing for other indications with both 177Lu-DOTATATE and I-131 mIBG.

References

1. Pavel M, Baudin E, Couvelard A, et al. ENETS consensus guidelines for the management of patients with liver and other distant metastases from neuroendocrine neoplasms of foregut, midgut, hindgut, and unknown primary. *Neuroendocrinology*. 2012;95(2):157–176.
2. Becherer A, Szabo M, Karanikas G, et al. Imaging of advanced neuroendocrine tumors with (18)F-FDOPA PET. *J Nucl Med*. United States. 2004;45(7):1161–1167.
3. Sandostatin LAR® Depot (octreotide acetate for injectable suspension) [package insert]. Novartis Pharmaceuticals Corporation, East Hanover, New Jersey.
4. Enzler T, Fojo T. Long-acting somatostatin analogues in the treatment of unresectable/metastatic neuroendocrine tumors. *Semin Oncol*. 2017;44(2):141–156.
5. Hicks RJ. Use of molecular targeted agents for the diagnosis, staging and therapy of neuroendocrine malignancy. *Cancer Imaging*. 2010;10 Spec no A(1A):S83–S91.
6. Virgolini I, Ambrosini V, Bomanji JB, et al. Procedure guidelines for PET/CT tumour imaging with 68Ga-DOTA-conjugated peptides: 68Ga-DOTA-TOC, 68Ga-DOTA-NOC, 68Ga-DOTA-TATE. *Eur J Nucl Med Mol Imaging*. 2010;37(10):2004–2010.
7. Schuchardt C, Baum RP. Dosimetry in peptide receptor radionuclide therapy (PRRNT): comparative results using Lu-177 DOTA-TATE, DOTA-NOC und DOTA-TOC. *Eur J Nucl Med Mol Imaging*. 2010;37:S244. http://www.embase.com/search/results?subaction=viewrecord&from=export&id=L70975790%5Cnhttp://dx.doi.org/10.1007/s00259-010-1557-3%5Cnhttp://sfx.library.uu.nl/utrecht?sid=EMBASE&issn=16197070&id=doi:10.1007%2Fs00259-010-1557-3&atitle=Dosimetry+in+peptide+r
8. Esser JP, Krenning EP, Teunissen JJM, et al. Comparison of [177Lu-DOTA0,Tyr3]octreotate and [177Lu-DOTA0,Tyr3]octreotide: ehich peptide is preferable for PRRT? *Eur J Nucl Med Mol Imaging*. 2006;33(11):1346–1351.
9. Poeppel TD, Binse I, Petersenn S, et al. 68Ga-DOTATOC Versus 68Ga-DOTATATE PET/CT in functional imaging of neuroendocrine tumors. *J Nucl Med*. 2011;52(12):1864–1870.
10. Velikyan I, Sundin A, Sorensen J, et al. Quantitative and qualitative intrapatient comparison of 68Ga-DOTATOC and 68Ga-DOTATATE: net uptake rate for accurate quantification. *J Nucl Med*. 2014;55(2):204–210.
11. Bodei L, Cremonesi M, Grana CM, et al. Yttrium-labelled peptides for therapy of NET. *Eur J Nucl Med Mol Imaging*. 2012;39 Suppl 1:S93–S102.
12. Kunikowska J, Królicki L, Hubalewska-Dydejczyk A, Mikołajczak R, Sowa-Staszczak A, Pawlak D. Clinical results of radionuclide therapy of neuroendocrine tumours with 90Y-DOTATATE and tandem 90Y/177Lu-DOTATATE: which is a better therapy option? *Eur J Nucl Med Mol Imaging*. 2011;38(10):1788–1797.
13. Kwekkeboom DJ, Bakker WH, Kam BL, et al. Treatment of patients with gastro-entero-pancreatic (GEP) tumours with the novel radiolabelled somatostatin analogue [177Lu-DOTA0,Tyr3]octreotate. *Eur J Nucl Med Mol Imaging*. 2003;30(3):417–422.
14. Teunissen JJM, Kwekkeboom DJ, Krenning EP. Quality of life in patients with gastroenteropancreatic tumors treated with [177Lu-DOTA0,Tyr3]octreotate. *J Clin Oncol*. 2004;22(13):2724–2729.
15. Kwekkeboom DJ, de Herder WW, Kam BL, et al. Treatment with the radiolabeled somatostatin analog [177 Lu-DOTA 0,Tyr3]octreotate: toxicity, efficacy, and survival. *J Clin Oncol*. 2008;26(13):2124–2130.
16. Bodei L, Kidd M, Paganelli G, et al. Long-term tolerability of PRRT in 807 patients with neuroendocrine tumours: the value and limitations of clinical factors. *Eur J Nucl Med Mol Imaging*. 2015;42(1):5–19.
17. Brabander T, Van Der Zwan WA, Teunissen JJM, et al. Long-term efficacy, survival, and safety of [177Lu-DOTA0,Tyr3]octreotate in patients with gastroenteropancreatic and bronchial neuroendocrine tumors. *Clin Cancer Res*. 2017;23(16):4617–4624.
18. Bergsma H, van Lom K, Raaijmakers MHGP, et al. Persistent hematologic dysfunction after peptide receptor radionuclide therapy with 177Lu-DOTATATE: incidence, course, and predicting factors in patients with gastroenteropancreatic neuroendocrine tumors. *J Nucl Med*. 2018;59(3):452–458.
19. Strosberg J, El-Haddad G, Wolin E, et al. Phase 3 trial of 177lu-dotatate for midgut neuroendocrine tumors. *N Engl J Med*. 2017;376(2):125–135.
20. Lutathera® (lutetium Lu177 dotatate) injection [package insert]. Advanced Accelerator Applications, Colleretto Giacosa (TO), Italy. 2018.
21. Bodei L, Mueller-Brand J, Baum RP, et al. The joint IAEA, EANM, and SNMMI practical guidance on peptide receptor radionuclide therapy (PRRNT) in neuroendocrine tumours. *Eur J Nucl Med Mol Imaging*. Germany. 2013;40(5):800–816.
22. Marx M, Winkler C, Lützen U, Zhao Y, Zuhayra M, Henze E. Determination of Tumour-Liver-Ratios (TLR) using Ga-68-DOTATATE PET and grading of patients with Neuroendocrine Tumours (NET) suitable for peptide receptor radionuclide therapy (PRRT). *Eur J Nucl Med Mol Imaging*. 2012;39:S473. http://www.embase.com/search/results?subaction=viewrecord&from=export&id=L70978265%5Cnhttp://dx.doi.org/10.1007/s00259-012-222-x%5Cnhttp://sfx.library.uu.nl/utrecht?sid=EMBASE&issn=16197070&id=doi:10.1007%2Fs00259-012-222-x&atitle=Determination+of+Tumour-
23. Campana D, Capurso G, Partelli S, et al. Radiolabelled somatostatin analogue treatment in gastroenteropancreatic neuroendocrine tumours: factors associated with response and suggestions for therapeutic sequence. *Eur J Nucl Med Mol Imaging*. 2013.
24. Ezziddin S, Opitz M, Attassi M, et al. Impact of the Ki-67 proliferation index on response to peptide receptor radionuclide therapy. *Eur J Nucl Med Mol Imaging*. 2011.
25. Kratochwil C, Stefanova M, Mavriopoulou E, et al. SUV of [68Ga]DOTATOC-PET/CT predicts response probability of PRRT in neuroendocrine tumors. *Mol Imaging Biol*. 2015.
26. Severi S, Nanni O, Bodei L, et al. Role of 18FDG PET/CT in patients treated with 177Lu-DOTATATE for advanced differentiated neuroendocrine tumours. *Eur J Nucl Med Mol Imaging*. 2013.
27. van Essen M, Krenning EP, Kam BL, de Herder WW, van Aken MO, Kwekkeboom DJ. Report on short-term side effects of treatments with 177Lu-octreotate in combination with capecitabine in seven patients with gastroenteropancreatic neuroendocrine tumours. *Eur J Nucl Med Mol Imaging*. 2008.
28. De Keizer B, Van Aken MO, Feelders RA, et al. Hormonal crises following receptor radionuclide therapy with the radiolabeled somatostatin analogue [177Lu-DOTA0,Tyr 3]octreotate. *Eur J Nucl Med Mol Imaging*. 2008.
29. Tapia Rico G, Li M, Pavlakis N, Cehic G, Price TJ. Prevention and management of carcinoid crises in patients with high-risk neuroendocrine tumours undergoing peptide receptor radionuclide therapy (PRRT)_ Literature review and case series from two Australian tertiary medical institutions. 2018;66:1–6.
30. Massimino K, Harrskog O, Pommier S, Pommier R. Octreotide LAR and bolus octreotide are insufficient for preventing intraoperative complications in carcinoid patients. *J Surg Oncol*. 2013;107:842–846.
31. Condron M, Pommier S, Pommier R. Continuous infusion of octreotide combined with perioperative octreotide bolus does not prevent intraoperative carcinoid crisis. *Surgery*. 2016;159(1):358–365.
32. Sundin A, Garske U, Orlefors H. Nuclear imaging of neuroendocrine tumours. *Best Pract Res Clin Endocrinol Metab*. 2007.
33. Sainz-Esteban A, Prasad V, Schuchardt C, Zachert C, Carril JM, Baum RP. Comparison of sequential planar 177Lu-DOTA-TATE dosimetry scans with 68Ga-DOTA-TATE PET/CT images in patients with metastasized neuroendocrine tumours undergoing peptide receptor radionuclide therapy. *Eur J Nucl Med Mol Imaging*. 2012.
34. Bison SM, Konijnenberg MW, Melis M, et al. Peptide receptor radionuclide therapy using radiolabeled somatostatin analogs: focus on future developments. *Clin Transl Imaging*. 2014.
35. Wulfert S, Kratochwil C, Choyke PL, et al. Multimodal imaging for early functional response assessment of 90Y-/177Lu-DOTATOC peptide receptor targeted radiotherapy with DW-MRI and 68Ga-DOTATOC-PET/CT. *Mol Imaging Biol*. 2014.

36. Cherk MH, Kong G, Hicks RJ, Hofman MS. Changes in biodistribution on 68Ga-DOTA-Octreotate PET/CT after long acting somatostatin analogue therapy in neuroendocrine tumour patients may result in pseudoprogression. *Cancer Imaging*. 2018.

37. Brabander T, Van Der Zwan WA, Teunissen JJM, et al. Pitfalls in the response evaluation after peptide receptor radionuclide therapy with [^{177}Lu-DOTA0,Tyr3] octreotate. *Endocr Relat Cancer*. 2017.

38. Nilica B, Waitz D, Stevanovic V, et al. Direct comparison of 68Ga-DOTA-TOC and 18F-FDG PET/CT in the follow-up of patients with neuroendocrine tumour treated with the first full peptide receptor radionuclide therapy cycle. *Eur J Nucl Med Mol Imaging*. 2016.

39. Sabet A, Haslerud T, Pape UF, et al. Outcome and toxicity of salvage therapy with 177Lu-octreotate in patients with metastatic gastroenteropancreatic neuroendocrine tumours. *Eur J Nucl Med Mol Imaging*. 2014.

40. Kratochwil C, Giesel FL, Bruchertseifer F, et al. Dose escalation study of peptide receptor alpha-therapy with arterially administered 213Bi-DOTATOC in GEP-NET patients refractory to beta-emitters. *Eur J Nucl Med Mol Imaging*. 2011;38:S207. http://www.embase.com/search/results?subaction=viewrecord&from=export&id=L70580303%5Cnhttp://dx.doi.org/10.1007/s00259-011-1908-8%5Cnhttp://sfx.library.uu.nl/utrecht?sid=EMBASE&issn=16197070&id=doi:10.1007%2Fs00259-011-1908-8&atitle=Dose+escalation+study+.

41. Gabriel M, Andergassen U, Putzer D, et al. Individualized peptide-related-radionuclide-therapy concept using different radiolabelled somatostatin analogs in advanced cancer patients. *Q J Nucl Med Mol Imaging*. 2010.

42. Van Der Zwan WA, Bodei L, Mueller-Brand J, De Herder WW, Kvols LK, Kwekkeboom DJ. Radionuclide therapy in neuroendocrine tumors. *Eur J Endocrinol*. 2015.

43. Bodei L, Weber WA. Somatostatin receptor imaging of neuroendocrine tumors: from agonists to antagonists. *J Nucl Med*. 2018.

44. Wild D, Fani M, Behe M, et al. First clinical evidence that imaging with somatostatin receptor antagonists is feasible. *J Nucl Med*. 2011.

45. Bomanji JB, Papathanasiou ND. (111)In-DTPA (0)-octreotide (Octreoscan), (131)I-MIBG and other agents for radionuclide therapy of NETs. *Eur J Nucl Med Mol Imaging*. 2012.

46. Reubi JCJC, Ma HR, Krenning EPEP, Mäcke HR, Krenning EPEP. Candidates for peptide receptor radiotherapy today and in the future. *J Nucl Med*. 2005.

47. Bombardieri E, Giammarile F, Aktolun C, et al. 131I/123I-metaiodobenzylguanidine (mIBG) scintigraphy: procedure guidelines for tumour imaging. *Eur J Nucl Med Mol Imaging*. Germany. 2010;37(12):2436–2446.

48. Sharp SE, Trout AT, Weiss BD, Gelfand MJ. MIBG in neuroblastoma diagnostic imaging and therapy. *Radiographics*. United States. 2016;36(1):258–278.

49. Cerny I, Prasek J, Kasparkova H. Superiority of SPECT/CT over planar 123I-mIBG images in neuroblastoma patients with impact on Curie and SIOPEN score values. *Nuklearmedizin*. Germany. 2016;55(4):151–157.

50. Yanik GA, Parisi MT, Shulkin BL, et al. Semiquantitative mIBG scoring as a prognostic indicator in patients with stage 4 neuroblastoma: a report from the Children's oncology group. *J Nucl Med*. United States. 2013;54(4):541–548.

51. Yanik GA, Parisi MT, Naranjo A, et al. Validation of postinduction curie scores in high-risk neuroblastoma: a children's oncology group and SIOPEN group report on SIOPEN/HR-NBL1. *J Nucl Med*. United States. 2018;59(3):502–508.

52. Naranjo A, Parisi MT, Shulkin BL, et al. Comparison of (1)(2)(3)I-metaiodobenzylguanidine (MIBG) and (1)(3)(1)I-MIBG semiquantitative scores in predicting survival in patients with stage 4 neuroblastoma: a report from the Children's Oncology Group. *Pediatr Blood Cancer*. United States. 2011;56(7):1041–1045.

53. Radovic B, Artiko V, Sobic-Saranovic D, et al. Evaluation of the SIOPEN semi-quantitative scoring system in planar simpatico-adrenal MIBG scintigraphy in children with neuroblastoma. *Neoplasma*. Slovakia. 2015;62(3):449–455.

54. Sokol EA, Engelmann R, Kang W, et al. Computer-assisted Curie scoring for metaiodobenzylguanidine (MIBG) scans in patients with neuroblastoma. *Pediatr Blood Cancer*. United States. 2018;65(12):e27417.

55. Kayano D, Kinuya S. Current consensus on I-131 MIBG therapy. *Nucl Med Mol Imaging* (2010). Germany. 2018;52(4):254–265.

56. Giammarile F, Chiti A, Lassmann M, Brans B, Flux G. EANM procedure guidelines for 131I-meta-iodobenzylguanidine (131I-mIBG) therapy. *Eur J Nucl Med Mol Imaging*. Germany. 2008;35(5):1039–1047.

57. Kayano D, Kinuya S. Iodine-131 metaiodobenzylguanidine therapy for neuroblastoma: reports so far and future perspective. *Scientific World J*. United States. 2015;2015:189135.

58. Matthay KK, Yanik G, Messina J, et al. Phase II study on the effect of disease sites, age, and prior therapy on response to iodine-131-metaiodobenzylguanidine therapy in refractory neuroblastoma. *J Clin Oncol*. United States. 2007;25(9):1054–1060.

59. Matthay KK, Quach A, Huberty J, et al. Iodine-131-metaiodobenzylguanidine double infusion with autologous stem-cell rescue for neuroblastoma: a new approaches to neuroblastoma therapy phase I study. *J Clin Oncol*. United States. 2009;27(7):1020–1025.

60. Mastrangelo S, Tornesello A, Diociaiuti L, et al. Treatment of advanced neuroblastoma: feasibility and therapeutic potential of a novel approach combining 131-I-MIBG and multiple drug chemotherapy. *Br J Cancer*. England. 2001;84(4):460–464.

61. Voute PA, van der Kleij AJ, De Kraker J, Hoefnagel CA, Tiel-van Buul MM, Van Gennip H. Clinical experience with radiation enhancement by hyperbaric oxygen in children with recurrent neuroblastoma stage IV. *Eur J Cancer*. England. 1995;31A(4):596–600.

62. Carrasquillo JA, Pandit-Taskar N, Chen CC. I-131 Metaiodobenzylguanidine Therapy of Pheochromocytoma and Paraganglioma. *Semin Nucl Med*. United States. 2016;46(3):203–214.

63. Mukherjee JJ, Kaltsas GA, Islam N, et al. Treatment of metastatic carcinoid tumours, phaeochromocytoma, paraganglioma and medullary carcinoma of the thyroid with (131)I-meta-iodobenzylguanidine [(131)I-mIBG]. *Clin Endocrinol* (Oxf). England. 2001;55(1):47–60.

64. Safford SD, Coleman RE, Gockerman JP, et al. Iodine -131 metaiodobenzylguanidine is an effective treatment for malignant pheochromocytoma and paraganglioma. *Surgery*. United States. 2003;134(6):953–956.

65. Fitzgerald PA, Goldsby RE, Huberty JP, et al. Malignant pheochromocytomas and paragangliomas: a phase II study of therapy with high-dose 131I-metaiodobenzylguanidine (131I-MIBG). *Ann N Y Acad Sci*. United States. 2006;1073:465–490.

66. Pryma DA, Chin BB, Noto RB, et al. Efficacy and safety of high-specific-activity I-131 MIBG therapy in patients with advanced pheochromocytoma or paraganglioma. *J Nucl Med*. United States. 2018.

67. Yoshinaga K, Oriuchi N, Wakabayashi H, et al. Effects and safety of (1)(3)(1)I-metaiodobenzylguanidine (MIBG) radiotherapy in malignant neuroendocrine tumors: results from a multicenter observational registry. *Endocr J*. Japan. 2014;61(12):1171–1180.

68. Azedra® (iobenguane I131) injection [package insert]. Progenics Pharmaceuticals, Inc., New York, NY; 2018.

69. Maiza J-C, Grunenwald S, Otal P, Vezzosi D, Bennet A, Caron P. Use of 131 I-MIBG therapy in MIBG-positive metastatic medullary thyroid carcinoma. *Thyroid*. United States. 2012;22(6):654–655.

70. Castellani MR, Seregni E, Maccauro M, et al. MIBG for diagnosis and therapy of medullary thyroid carcinoma: is there still a role? *Q J Nucl Med Mol Imaging*. Italy. 2008;52(4):430–440.

71. Brabander T, Kwekkeboom DJ, Feelders RA, Brouwers AH, Teunissen JJM. Nuclear medicine imaging of neuroendocrine tumors. *Front Horm Res*. Switzerland. 2015;44:73–87.

CHAPTER SELF-ASSESSMENT QUESTIONS

1. Which of the following is an FDA-approved indication for ^{177}Lu-DOTATATE therapy?

   A. Bronchial carcinoid

   B. Pheochromocytoma

   C. VIPoma

   D. Neuroblastoma

2. Which of the following is the most critical patient-specific factor in choosing ^{177}Lu-DOTATATE therapy versus other therapeutic options?

   A. Grade of NET

   B. Degree of SSTR-expression on imaging

   C. Pathologic subtype of NET

   D. Distribution of disease

3. Which of the following is NOT a known physiologic variant for I-123 mIBG uptake?

   A. Brown fat

   B. Atelectasis

   C. Meningioma

   D. Adrenal glands

4. Which of the following is an FDA-approved indication for I-131 mIBG therapy?

   A. Neuroblastoma

   B. Paraganglioma

   C. Medullary thyroid cancer

   D. Merkel cell carcinoma

Answers to Chapter Self-Assessment Questions

1. C   The FDA approval for Lu177-DOTATATE therapy is for all types of gastro-entero-pancreatic neuroendocrine tumors (NETs) in adults. As an example of a pancreatic NET, VIPoma is the right answer. The others may be treated by this therapy, but they are not FDA-approved indications.

2. B   While all of these are factors in proper patient selection, the clearest link is with the degree of SSTR-expression based on ^{68}Ga-DOTATATE PET (preferably) or an ^{111}In-DTPA-octreotide scan. The others are secondary considerations.

3. C   Mengiomas often express SSTRs and so can be seen on ^{68}Ga-DOTATATE or ^{111}In-DTPA-octreotide scans, but not on I-123 mIBG scans as it is a norepinephrine analog. The others are known reasons for false positives on an I-123 mIBG scan.

4. B   The FDA-approval for I-131 mIBG is for patients 12-years or older with pheochromocytoma or paraganglioma. All of the other answers are examples of tumors that can successfully be treated with this therapy but they are not FDA-approved indications at this time.

Central Nervous System 7

Hossein Jadvar and Patrick M. Colletti

LEARNING OBJECTIVES

1. Describe the major clinical applications of scintigraphy in imaging of the central nervous system.
2. Name the relevant radiotracers and general procedures that are employed in scintigraphic imaging evaluation of cerebrospinal fluid flow, brain death, epilepsy, movement disorders, and brain perfusion reserve in cerebrovascular disease.
3. Create and present parametric brain mapping.

INTRODUCTION

Imaging assessment provides important clues on central nervous system pathology when signs and symptoms suggest an abnormality referable to the brain or spinal cord. Computed tomography (CT) and magnetic resonance imaging (MRI) are mainstay imaging modalities in this clinical setting. However, scintigraphy provides valuable and clinically relevant functional information that complements the findings on anatomic imaging. Various single photon and positron emitting radiopharmaceuticals are available clinically to interrogate the pathophysiology of the central nervous system. This chapter summarizes the major clinical applications of scintigraphy in the imaging assessment of central nervous system including the relevant radiotracers and the imaging techniques.

CLINICAL APPLICATIONS

There are many clinical applications for scintigraphic evaluation of the central nervous system. The essential applications include the following indications, which will be discussed in this chapter briefly. Scintigraphic imaging of dementia and brain tumors is often performed with positron emission tomography and will be presented in Chapter 14.

- Cerebrospinal fluid (CSF) flow (normal pressure hydrocephalus; leak; shunt patency)
- Brain death
- Epilepsy
- Movement disorders
- Cerebrovascular disease
- Dementia

Cerebrospinal fluid flow imaging

CSF is formed by the ventricular choroid plexus as an ultrafiltrate of plasma and absorbed primarily in the arachnoid villi. The total CSF volume is about 120 mL to 150 mL. Scintigraphy provides an effective imaging method to track the CSF flow, which may be hindered in a number of pathological conditions. The major conditions include communicating hydrocephalus, CSF leaks, and assessment of shunt patency.

The most common relevant radiotracer for CSF flow imaging ^{111}In-DTPA, which has a sufficiently long half-life (2.8 days) suited for serial imaging. The radiotracer (~500 uCi) is injected into the subarachnoid space by lumbar puncture. Planar imaging is obtained serially at various intervals (2 h, 24 h, 48 h, and possibly 72 h).

In a normal scan, the activity injected via the lumbar puncture ascends the spinal canal toward the basal cisterns in a few hours (~2–4 h). Delayed images at 24 h will demonstrate further ascent of the activity over bilateral convexities. Presence of significant activity in lateral ventricles is abnormal. If necessary, additional imaging at 48 h and 72 h can be performed to follow the CSF flow if it is relatively slow to reach the convexities.

In communicating (patent foramina of Magendie and Luschka) hydrocephalus (aka. normal pressure hydrocephalus, NPH), anatomic imaging (e.g., CT) demonstrates hydrocephalus without significant cerebral atrophy (1). In rare patients, the classic triad of ataxia, dementia, and urinary incontinence may be seen clinically. Radionuclide cisternogram shows abnormal CSF flow with no transit of the activity over the convexities at 24 h (or longer) with reflux of activity into the enlarged lateral ventricles. The peripheral obstruction to CSF flow is often at the level of temporoparietal lobes (Fig. 7.1)

Localization of CSF leaks (e.g., CSF rhinorrhea or otorrhea) is another major clinical application for radionuclide cisternography. In the more common CSF rhinorrhea, pledgets are placed in the nostrils by otorhinolaryngologist before lumbar puncture injection of the radiotracer. Imaging is performed 1 to 3 h after tracer administration followed by removal of the pledgets at 4 to 6 h, which are then counted for radioactivity in a well counter. Contemporaneous blood sample are obtained and counted to serve as background activity. Pledget/serum activity ratio is calculated. The ratio above a selected value (typically 1.5) is considered abnormal and consistent with CSF leak. It should be noted

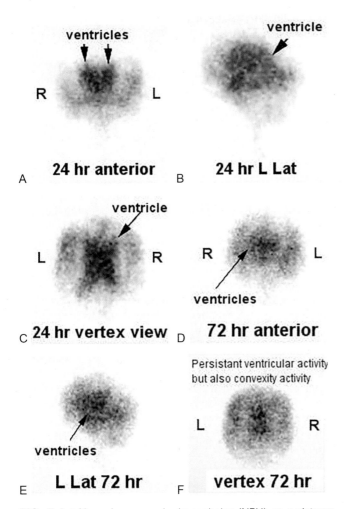

A   **24 hr anterior**   B   **24 hr L Lat**

C   **24 hr vertex view**   D   **72 hr anterior**

Persistant ventricular activity but also convexity activity

E   **L Lat 72 hr**   F   **vertex 72 hr**

FIG. 7.1 ● Normal pressure hydrocephalus (NPH) on a cisternogram with persistent visualization of the ventricles and no cerebral convexity flow. Reprinted with permission from Freeman LM. *Nuclear Medicine Annual 2004*. Philadelphia, PA: Lippincott Williams & Wilkins; 2004.

that there might be no imaging evidence of CSF leak despite abnormal pledget/serum ratio.

Obstruction of ventriculoperitoneal (VP) shunts is a relatively common complication. Scintigraphy can be helpful in localizing the site of obstruction. In this clinical setting, the radiotracer (e.g., ^{111}In-DTPA or ^{99m}Tc-DTPA) is injected in sterile manner into the reservoir followed by serial imaging. It is important to note that while ^{99m}Tc-DTPA is superior to ^{111}In-DTPA as an imaging agent with better counts at lower radiation exposure, ^{99m}Tc-DTPA is not food and drug administration (FDA) approved for potentially intrathecal administration due to the small risk of endotoxins in some forms of this tracer (2). In the normal nonobstructive pattern, diffuse activity reaches the peritoneal cavity in no later than 1 h. Failure in observing peritoneal activity or only focal activity at the distal end of the shunt suggests shunt obstruction. Manual occlusion of the distal limb of the shunt at the time of radiotracer injection can potentially assess the patency of the proximal limb of the shunt system. However, this should be tailored to the clinical situation and the particular CSF shunt system.

Brain death

Brain death is determined by a number of clinical parameters that may include imaging cerebral perfusion scintigraphy (Fig. 7.2). Absence of brain perfusion is compatible with brain death and can be an effective visual tool in aiding difficult discussions about prognosis with patient's family. Local guidelines may be followed for identification and declaration of brain death. Scintigraphic evaluation of cerebral blood flow is accomplished by injecting a radiotracer intravenously followed by dynamic imaging of the head and neck. Blood flow to superficial scalp vessels (external carotid artery territory) may be diminished by an elastic band place over the forehead. However, this maneuver is rarely necessary or performed. Injection of radiotracers that cross the blood–brain barrier and map the cerebral perfusion (e.g., ^{99m}Tc-HMPAO or ^{99m}Tc-ECD) is less dependent on observation of good bolus arrival in the bilateral common carotid arteries or ancillary signs such as the "hot nose" sign. Planar imaging of cerebral perfusion will include anterior–posterior and lateral views.

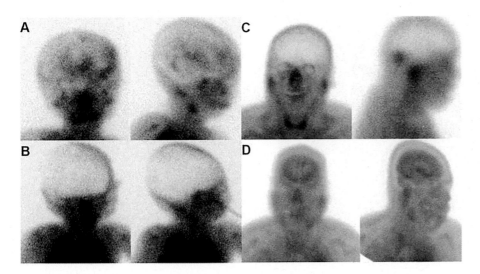

FIG. 7.2 ● Brain death comparison ^{99m}Tc-HMPAO images: **A:** Severe right head trauma post decompression. The entire perfused brain is shifted to the left by hematoma. **B:** Complete absence of brain perfusion: brain death. **C:** Absence of cerebral perfusion with preserved cerebellum. Cerebral death. Note the "Hot Nose" Sign. **D:** Intact cerebral blood flow. The patient was neurologically unresponsive due to a dense midbrain infarction seen on CT. It is unusual for patients receiving brain death studies to survive. All four of these patients were dead within one week of these scans. From Daffner RH. *Clinical Radiology: The Essentials*. 3rd ed. Philadelphia, PA: Wolters Kluwer Health/Lippincott Williams & Wilkins; 2007.

With single photon emission computed tomography (SPECT) imaging, the intracerebral perfusion is clearly depicted without the limitation that may be caused from superficial scalp perfusion. An "empty cranium" is typical for brain death. Occasionally, parts of the brain (e.g., cerebellum in posterior fossa) may show perfusion while there is absence of perfusion in the rest of the brain. Prognosis is poor in this clinical scenario and often repeat brain perfusion scan shows disappearance of the perfusion in entire brain in view of increased intracranial pressure. A practice guideline for brain death scintigraphy has been published (3).

Epilepsy

Clinical workup of epilepsy involves a number of diagnostics procedures including electroencephalography and imaging. In intractable seizures that are not well controlled with medications, localization, and resection of the epileptogenic focus can potentially be curative. MRI is often performed to detect potential morphologic abnormalities (e.g., mesial temporal sclerosis) that may explain the observed seizure activity in correlation with electroencephalography. However, there are occasions that MRI does not depict a specific relevant abnormality. Functional imaging with scintigraphy can be helpful in localization of epileptogenic focus with or without specific MRI abnormality (4,5). Brain perfusion scintigraphy with ^{99m}Tc-HMPAO or ^{99m}Tc-ECD can be performed in the inter-ictal or intra-ictal periods. In inter-ictal period, the brain perfusion SPECT shows hypoperfusion in the region of the brain that may harbor the epileptogenic focus. Such finding can be corroborated with any MRI abnormalities at that location or with intra-ictal brain perfusion SPECT in which the same locus will demonstrate hyperperfusion (Fig. 7.3).

Good quality intra-ictal demands special seizure units in which the patients are monitored actively for seizure activity. When the onset of the seizure activity is observed (clinically and/or with electroencephalography), the previously ready at-hand radiotracer is injected immediately in a previously accessed peripheral vein. The patient is then transferred to nuclear medicine clinic for imaging when the patient is clinically stable. If performed in a timely manner and properly, intra-ictal brain perfusion SPECT is more sensitive in localizing the epileptogenic focus than inter-ictal brain perfusion SPECT.

Movement disorders

Clinical workup of patients with tremor is directed toward differential diagnosis of a variety of etiologies, which lead to different management algorithms. While some patients present with classic sign and symptoms that suggest a particular diagnosis, this is not always the case and uncertainty for an etiology may remain.

^{123}I-Ioflupane (Iodine 123-fluoropropyl (FP)-carbomethoxy-2 beta-(4-iodophenyltropane) or DaTscan with single photon CT is approved for detecting loss of Dopamine transporters (DATs) from presynaptic dopaminergic neuron terminals in the striatum. DaTscan is therefore useful in detecting those conditions that lead to loss of striato-nigral dopamine neurons that occurs in Parkinsonian syndromes (idiopathic Parkinson's disease, multiple system atrophy, progressive supranuclear palsy, corticobasal degeneration) and in dementia with Lewy bodies (6). However, DaTscan is unable to distinguish among these aforementioned conditions, which will require correlation with other relevant clinical information. DaTscan will show preserved striatonigral dopamine neurons in healthy individual, essential tremor,

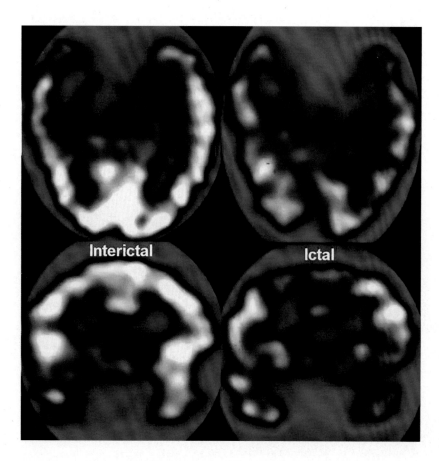

FIG. 7.3 ● This 16-year-old boy had chronic seizures. Interictal ^{99m}Tc-HMPAO axial and coronal SPECT images on the left demonstrate reduced perfusion to the right temporal lobe. Ictal images show increased right temporal activity. Findings are typical for mesial temporal epileptogenic foci.

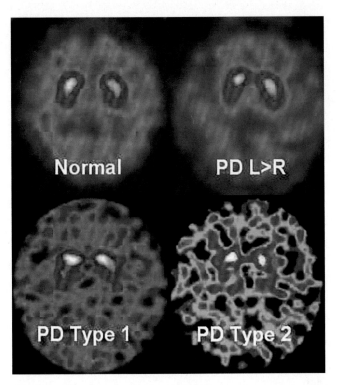

FIG. 7.4 ● ¹²³I-Ioflupane (DaTscan) SPECT scans in a normal patient and in three patients with Parkinsonian syndromes. Asymmetrical putamina loss may be associated with asymmetrical tremor usually more severe on the contralateral side. Severe bilateral loss may be seen in dementia with Lewy body disease.

psychogenic tremor, and drug-induced parkinsonism. Practice guideline for performing DaTscan has been published (7).

Visual interpretation of DaTscan includes the following observations (Fig. 7.4): Normal—symmetric bilateral "comma" shape striata with relatively intense tracer uptake

Grade 1—asymmetrical loss of posterior tail (putamen) in a "comma with full stop" striata

Grade 2—bilateral loss of putamen tails in a "two full stops" striata

Grade 3—near complete loss of both caudate heads and putamen with "fading full stops" appearance

Cerebrovascular disease

CT and MRI are mainstay imaging modalities in patients with suspected or known stroke. A clinically useful scintigraphic technique is related to determining the adequacy of cerebrovascular reserve. This is accomplished with the use of the carbonic anhydrase inhibitor, acetazolamide (Diamox), which leads to vasodilation and increase in cerebral blood flow (8–10). Cerebral perfusion is imaged at baseline and after Diamox administration in separate sessions with SPECT after intravenous injection of ⁹⁹ᵐTc-HMPAO or ⁹⁹ᵐTc-ECD for each scan. The baseline and post-Diamox scans are then compared. The baseline scan often shows preserved (compensated) regional cerebral perfusion. Cerebral regions with perfusion reserve deficit will not respond adequately to Diamox and as such the affected region demonstrates a perfusion deficit in comparison to other brain regions that show Diamox-induced increase in cerebral blood flow (Fig. 7.5). This is in concept similar to blood flow heterogeneity

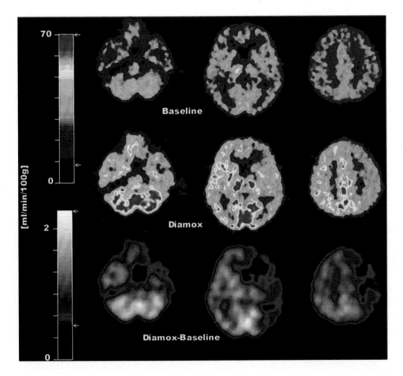

FIG. 7.5 ● Evaluation of cerebrovascular perfusion status in a patient with severe stenosis of the right internal carotid artery. The baseline examination shows a symmetric and normal perfusion. After acetazolamide stimulation, the increase in perfusion is severely decreased in the territory of the right middle cerebral artery, which is also depicted on the difference image at the bottom. Reprinted with permission from von Schulthess GK. *Clinical Molecular Anatomic Imaging: PET, PET/CT and SPECT/CT.* Philadelphia, PA: Lippincott Williams & Wilkins; 2003.

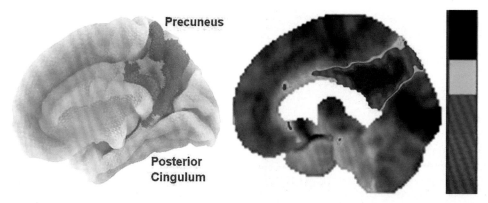

FIG. 7.6 • Posterior Tunnel Schematic and Parametric Imaging example showing reduced metabolism in the cingulate gyrus and precuneus from a patient with Alzheimer disease. The precuneus extends from the marginal branch of the cingulate sulcus to the parieto-occipital sulcus. The cingulate gyrus and pre-cuneus should be identified and analyzed in patients with cognitive impairment. From Brown et al. (12); Sawyer and Kuo (13).

Table 7.1 **CHARACTERISTIC FDG PET FINDINGS IN PATIENTS WITH ALZHEIMER DISEASE, DEMENTIA WITH LEWY BODIES, AND POSTERIOR CORTICAL ATROPHY (13)**

	Brain Region			
Pathology	Precuneus	Post Cingulate	Lateral Occipital	Medial Occipital
Alzheimer	Decreased	Decreased	Preserved	Preserved
Dementia with Lewy Bodies	Decreased	Preserved	Decreased	Preserved
Posterior Cerebral Atrophy	Decreased	Decreased	Decreased	Preserved

"Preserved": relative preservation of activity in a structure compared with an adjacent area of hypometabolism, although activity may not be normal.

Reprinted with permission from Sawyer and Kuo (13).

that is induced by dipyridamole in the coronary bed in myocardial perfusion studies. It is of note that positron emission tomography imaging of brain perfusion (e.g., with ^{15}O-water) may be more sensitive than brain perfusion SPECT in assessing cerebrovascular reserve capacity (11).

Parametric brain SPECT or PET mapping

Voxel-based brain SPECT or PET analysis compares tracer uptake between a patient and normal controls on a voxel-by-voxel basis, highlighting areas of statistically significant differences with color-coded overlays. While brain SPECT with ^{99m}Tc-HMPAO or ^{99m}Tc-ECD is based on relative regional brain perfusion, ^{18}F-FDG PET compares regional brain glucose metabolism. For brain PET parametric analysis, "Cool" blue-based colors indicate areas of FDG hypometabolism while red-based colors represent regional hypermetabolism. As most brain abnormalities are associated with functional loss, blue-based color scales are most useful.

A landmark-based deformation algorithm registers each brain to a standard template. Results are presented as a Z-score color scale: Light blue—2 Standard Deviations (SDs), Dark blue—2.5 SDs, and Purple—3 SDs (12).

For the evaluation of cognitively impaired patients by FDG PET, there is a logical sequence for excluding and including potential diagnoses. One key area to evaluate is the "occipital tunnel" (13). The occipital tunnel is made up of the posterior cingulum and the precuneus (Fig. 7.6). Table 7.1 compares the "occipital tunnel" findings in Alzheimer disease, dementia with Lewy bodies and posterior cerebral atrophy.

The flow chart in Figure 7.7 presents an organized approach to the FDG PET diagnosis of dementia. Example cases of mild cognitive impairment (Fig. 7.8), Alzheimer disease (Fig. 7.9), advanced Alzheimer disease with frontal lobe involvement (Fig. 7.10), vascular dementia (Fig. 7.11), frontal dementia as Pick disease (Fig. 7.12), and dementia with Lewy body disease (Fig. 7.13) are presented. Parametric FDG PET brain mapping may also be helpful in patients with epilepsy as is demonstrated in Figure 7.14.

Positron emission tomography with a variety of brain radiotracers including amyloid and tau markers has also been investigated in these clinical settings. These agents will be discussed in Chapter 14.

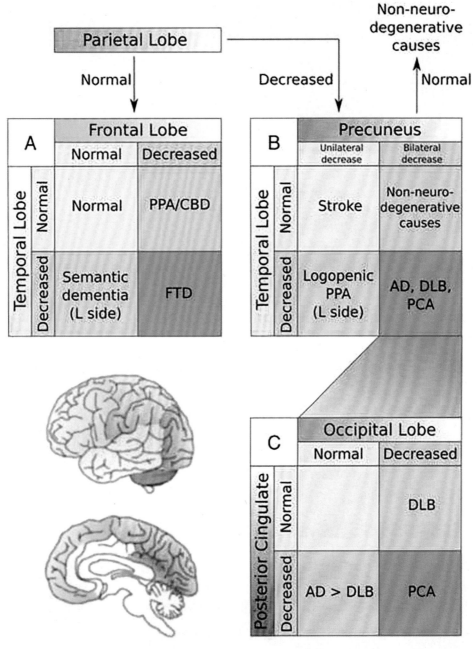

FIG. 7.7 ● This figure displays a "top–down" approach for interpreting FDG PET in patients with dementia. Analysis begins at the parietal lobe. If normal, evaluation of the frontal and temporal lobes follows via *pathway A*. Semantic dementia (SD) is identified with normal frontal and decreased left anterior temporal activity. Normal temporal activity suggests primary progressive aphasia when combined with loss in the left frontal area or corticobasal degeneration when combined with deficits in the frontal lobe, basal ganglia, and primary sensorimotor cortex. Frontotemporal dementia is characterized by decreased frontal and temporal uptake. Alternatively, decreased parietal activity leads to *pathway B*, where the precunei and temporal lobes are evaluated. If the precunei are normal, non-neurodegenerative causes (vascular dementia, depression, drug-induced) should be considered. Vascular insult can also be suggested in the presence of a compromised precuneus if the temporal lobes are preserved. Decreased left temporal activity combined with left precuneal hypometabolism supports a diagnosis of logopenic variant of primary progressive aphasia, a unilateral, left-sided variant of AD. Bilateral decreased uptake in the precuneus in the presence of bilateral temporal hypometabolism suggests Alzheimer disease (AD), dementia with Lewy bodies (DLB), or posterior cortical atrophy (PCA), which can be differentiated according to *pathway C*. Normal occipital activity with posterior cingulate hypometabolism supports AD, although DLB remains possible. Decreased occipital uptake indicates DLB when combined with a relatively preserved posterior cingulate ("cingulate island" sign). Decreased occipital and posterior cingulate activity supports a diagnosis of PCA. Occipital hypometabolism in DLB and PCA can be identified using the "occipital tunnel" sign. Reprinted with permission from Sawyer and Kuo (14).

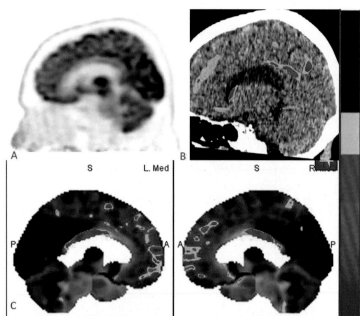

FIG. 7.8 ● 53-year-old man with cognitive decline. There is relatively mild metabolic reduction in the posterior cingulum and precuneus. Mild cognitive impairment may present with memory dysfunction beyond "normal for age" with relatively preservation of other cognitive domains. Up to 12% per year progress to dementia.

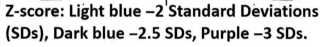

Z-score: Light blue −2 Standard Deviations (SDs), Dark blue −2.5 SDs, Purple −3 SDs.

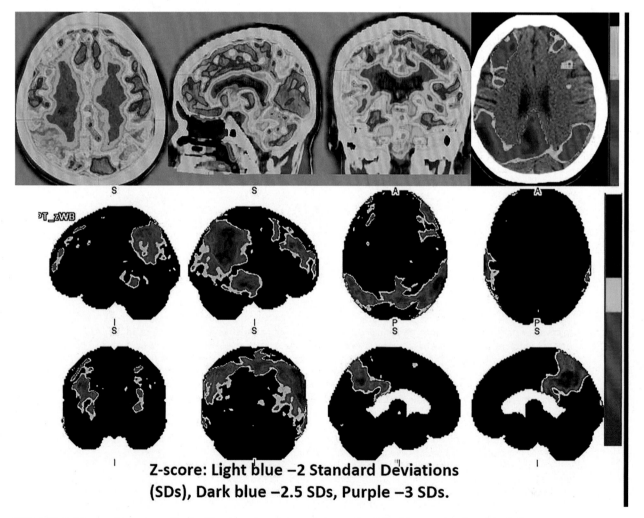

Z-score: Light blue −2 Standard Deviations (SDs), Dark blue −2.5 SDs, Purple −3 SDs.

FIG. 7.9 ● 47-year-old woman with significant memory loss and depression. She has prominent metabolic loss in her posterior cingulum, precuneus, and bilateral parietal–temporal and frontal lobes. Progressive Alzheimer disease.

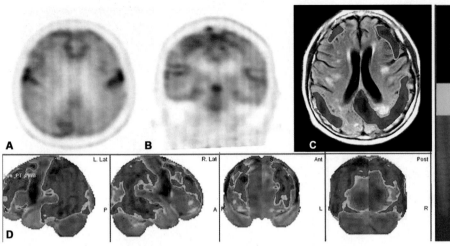

FIG. 7.10 ● An 82-year-old woman with dementia. She has prominent loss of function in her precuneus and parietal, temporal, and frontal lobes with preservation of her motor strip and visual cortex. Progressive Alzheimer disease.

Z-score: Light blue −2 Standard Deviations (SDs), Dark blue −2.5 SDs, Purple −3 SDs.

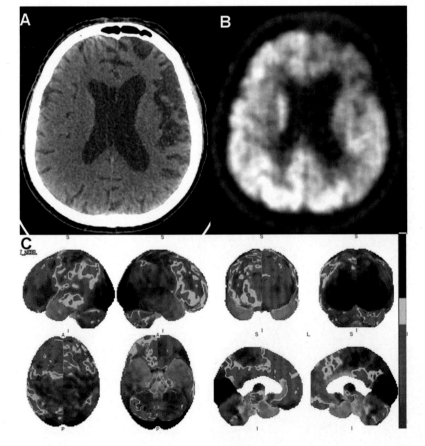

FIG. 7.11 ● A 61-year-old man with dementia, lethargy, and logopenic aphasia: Difficulty retrieving words and word substitutions. Frequently pausing in speech while searching for words. Difficulty repeating phrases or sentences. CT and MR both demonstrate large regions of left frontal and left temporal encephalomalacia associated with significant metabolic dysfunction. The findings are typical of vascular dementia, though functional loss in the left posterior cingulum and precuneus may be either vascular or may be related to a component of Alzheimer disease. Involvement in the left posterior temporal lobe may be associated with logopenic aphasia. Z-score: Light blue—2 Standard Deviations (SDs), Dark blue—2.5 SDs, Purple—3 SDs.

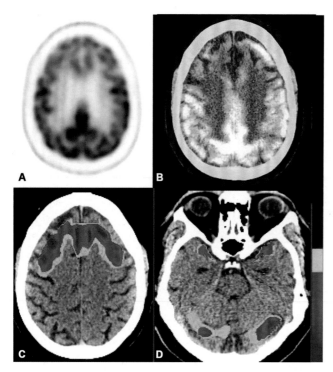

FIG. 7.12 • A 66-year-old man with dementia. He has a history of head trauma. There is CT and metabolic evidence for bilateral frontal loss, right greater than left. Frontal dementia. Z-score: Light blue—2 Standard Deviations (SDs), Dark blue—2.5 SDs, Purple—3 SDs.

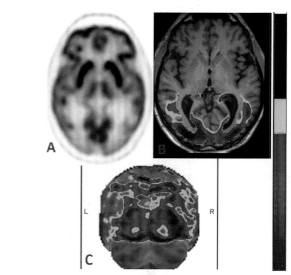

Z-score: Light blue −2 Standard Deviations (SDs), Dark blue −2.5 SDs, Purple −3 SDs.

FIG. 7.13 • A 71-year-old man with cognitive decline. There is specific loss of medial visual cortical dysfunction, typical for dementia with Lewy body disease. A potential confound may occur in patients with significant visual loss.

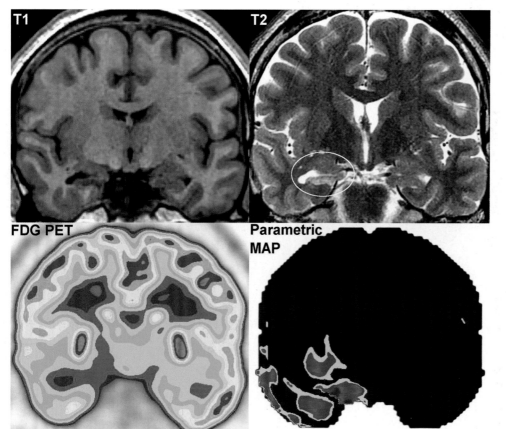

FIG. 7.14 • A 34-year-old man with complex partial seizures. The T1- and T2-weighted coronal MR images demonstrate enlargement of the right choroidal fissure with hippocampal loss and edema (circled). There is associated right mesial temporal functional loss demonstrated on the parametric display, lower right. Right mesial temporal epileptogenic focus. Z-score: Light blue—2 Standard Deviations (SDs), Dark blue—2.5 SDs, Purple—3 SDs.

References

1. Damasceno BP. Neuroimaging in normal pressure hydrocephalus. *Dement Neuropsychol.* 2015;9:350–355.
2. Ponto JA. Special safety considerations in preparation of technetium Tc-99m DTPA for cerebrospinal fluid–related imaging procedures. *J Am Pharm Assoc.* 2008;48:413–416.
3. Donohoe KJ, Agrawal G, Frey KA, et al. SNM practice guideline for brain death scintigraphy 2.0. *J Nucl Med.* 2012;40:198–203.
4. Goffin K, Dedeurwaerdere S, Van Laere K, et al. Neuronuclear assessment of patients with epilepsy. *Semin Nucl Med.* 2008;38:227–239.
5. Van Paesschen W, Dupont P, Sunaert S, et al. The use of SPECT and PET in routine clinical practice in epilepsy. *Curr Opin Neurol.* 2007;20:194–202.
6. Bajaj N, Hauser RA, Grachev ID. Clinical utility of dopamine transporter single photon emission CT (DaT-SPECT) with ^{123}I-ioflupane in diagnosis of parkinsonian syndromes. *J Neurol Neurosurg Psychiatry.* 2013;84:1288–1295.
7. Djang DSW, Janssen MJR, Bohnen N, et al. SNM practice guidelines for dopamine transporter imaging with ^{123}I-Ioflupane SPECT 1.0. *J Nucl Med.* 2012;53:154–163.
8. Kim JS, Moon DH, Kim GE, et al. Acetazolamide stress brain-perfusion SPECT predicts the need for carotid shunting during carotid endarterectomy. *J Nucl Med.* 2000;41:1836–1841.
9. Matsuda H, Higashi S, Kinuya K, et al. SPECT evaluation of brain perfusion reserve by acetazolamide test using 99mTc-HMPAO. *Clin Nucl Med.* 1991;16:572–579.
10. Wong TH, Shagera QA, Ryoo HG, et al. Basal and acetazolamide brain perfusion SPECT in internal carotid artery stenosis. *Nucl Med Mol Imaging.* 2020;54:9–27.
11. Acker G, Lange C, Schatka I, et al. Brain perfusion imaging under acetazolamide challenge for detection of impaired cerebrovascular reserve capacity: positive findings with ^{15}O-water PET in patients with negative ^{99m}Tc-HMPAO SPECT findings. *J Nucl Med.* 2018;59:294–298.
12. Brown RK, Bohnen NI, Wong KK, et al. Brain PET in suspected dementia: patterns of altered FDG metabolism. *Radiographics.* 2014;34:684–701.
13. Sawyer DM, Kuo PH. "Occipital Tunnel" sign on FDG PET for differentiating dementias. *Clin Nucl Med.* 2018;43:e59–e61.
14. Sawyer DM, Kuo PH. Top-down systematic approach to interpretation of FDG-PET for dementia. *Clin Nucl Med.* 2018;43:e212–e214.

CHAPTER SELF-ASSESSMENT QUESTIONS

1. Which statement is FALSE in relation to imaging for brain death?

   A. "Empty cranium" is compatible with brain death.

   B. "Hot nose" sign is necessary for declaration of brain death.

   C. Radiotracers that cross the blood–brain barrier and map the cerebral perfusion can be used.

   D. Observation of only cerebellar perfusion is a poor prognostic sign.

2. DaTscan refers to imaging for which of the following conditions:

   A. Essential tremor

   B. Idiopathic Parkinson's disease

   C. Drug-induced Parkinsonism

   D. Alzheimer disease

3. Diamox in conjunction with scintigraphy may be used for

   A. Localization of the epileptogenic focus

   B. Diagnosis of Parkinson's disease

   C. Brain death

   D. Cerebral perfusion reserve

Answers to Chapter Self-Assessment Questions

1. B "Hot nose" sign is an ancillary finding that can support potential for brain death but is not a necessary sign. Answers A, C, and D are true statements in relation to brain death nuclear imaging.

2. B DaTscan is useful in detecting those conditions that lead to loss of striatonigral dopamine neurons that occurs in Parkinsonian syndromes (idiopathic Parkinson's disease, multiple system atrophy, progressive supranuclear palsy, corticobasal degeneration). DaTscan will show preserved striatonigral dopamine neurons in healthy individual, essential tremor, psychogenic tremor, and drug-induced parkinsonism. DaTscan is not useful for diagnosis of Alzheimer disease.

3. D Cerebral regions with perfusion reserve deficit will not respond adequately to Diamox and as such the affected region demonstrates a perfusion deficit in comparison to other brain regions that show Diamox-induced increase in cerebral blood flow. Diamox is not used in the imaging assessment of brain death, Parkinson's disease, or in localization of epileptogenic focus.

Bone Scintigraphy

8

Hossein Jadvar

LEARNING OBJECTIVES

1. Understand the diagnostic utility of bone scintigraphy in the imaging evaluation of the skeleton in various relevant clinical conditions.
2. Understand the limitations of bone scintigraphy in the imaging evaluation of the skeleton.
3. Discuss non-skeletal imaging utility of bone scintigraphy.

INTRODUCTION

Nuclear medicine has played a major role in the imaging evaluation and treatment of skeletal system. Bone is a crystalline lattice that is comprised of calcium, phosphate, and hydroxyl ions. Bone-seeking radiopharmaceuticals are typically calcium, phosphate, or hydroxyl analogs. The most common radiotracers for imaging are technetium-labeled phosphate analogs including methylene diphosphonate for single-photon planar or single-photon emission computed tomography (SPECT) scintigraphy. Fluorine is a hydroxyl analog and can be used as ^{18}F-sodium fluoride (^{18}F-NaF) with positron emission tomography (PET).

Bone scintigraphy is used for imaging evaluation of infection (e.g., osteomyelitis), noninfectious inflammation (e.g., arthritis), trauma, metabolic bone disease, benign and malignant neoplasms, and specific conditions in children. The scan may include dynamic image data acquisition and involve the whole skeleton or only a specific region of the body. Bone scintigraphy is most effective when correlated with other relevant imaging modalities such as radiography, computed tomography (CT), and magnetic resonance imaging (MRI), which often assists with improving specificity. Procure standards and practice guidelines with either single-photon or positron imaging have been published (1–3).

The uptake of the bone-seeking radiotracers is dependent on blood flow and chemisorption to bone matrix. The skeleton is imaged about 3 h following intravenous administration of the single-photon radiotracer. The delay in imaging improves the target-to-background uptake ratio. With ^{18}F-NaF PET, the tracer uptake is based on chemisorption with an exchange of ^{18}F$^-$ ion for OH$^-$ ion on the surface of the hydroxyapatite matrix of the bone, forming fluoroapatite and migration of the ^{18}F$^-$ ion into the bone crystalline matrix. Due to high first-pass extraction from plasma and rapid renal clearance, imaging with PET can be performed in a shorter time (typically at 45 min to 1 h after intravenous tracer administration) in comparison to ^{99m}Tc-based radiotracers.

NORMAL BIODISTRIBUTION

The normal bone scan shows relatively homogenous tracer distribution in the axial and appendicular skeleton with most activity in the axial skeleton (Fig. 8.1). The calvarial activity may be somewhat patchy. In children, the epiphyseal plates show relatively symmetric and intense tracer accumulation, which diminishes as the child grows into adulthood. There may be increased foci of activity, which may develop with the aging process including degenerative changes (e.g., osteophytosis and arthropathy), and bursitis at tendon insertions. An optimal quality bone scan shows little soft tissue activity with a high bone-to-background activity ratio. Renal and bladder urine activities are reflective of physiologic route of tracer excretion. Unless there are asymmetries due to patient positioning, observed asymmetries in osseous activity may be a sign of abnormality and should be further examined with spot planar imaging, SPECT(/CT), other correlative imaging, and clinical information. The bone-to-background activity ratio (sensitivity) and specificity are generally higher with ^{18}F-NaF PET/CT than planar or whole-body SPECT/CT bone scintigraphy (4).

CLINICAL APPLICATIONS

There is a wide range of clinical applications for bone scintigraphy. These include but are not limited to the following indications:

- Bone pain with normal radiograph.
- Infection (e.g., osteomyelitis vs cellulitis).
- Trauma (e.g., stress fracture, non-accidental injury in children).
- Determination of bone viability.
- Evaluation of prostheses (infection vs loosening).
- Evaluation of metabolic bone disease.
- Staging and treatment monitoring of cancer.

Benign bone lesions

A potential cause for painful bone without a definite radiographic abnormality is osteoid osteoma, which can show high focal activity at the site of the lesion's vascular nidus. Fibrous dysplasia is

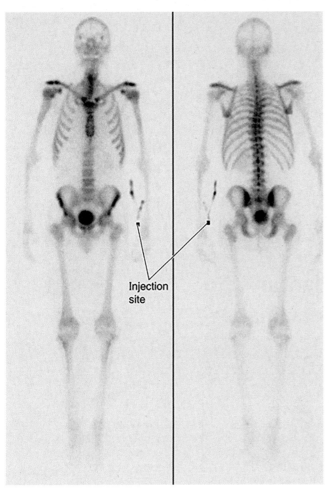

FIG. 8.1 ● Normal bone scan. Reprinted with permission from Dugani S, Alfonsi J, Agur AMR, et al. *Clinical Anatomy Cases: An Integrated Approach with Physical Examination and Medical Imaging.* Philadelphia, PA: Wolters Kluwer; 2016:20–21.

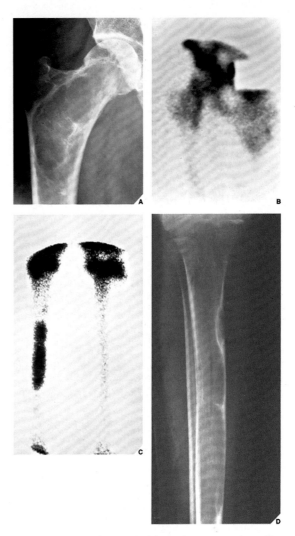

FIG. 8.2 ● Polyostotic fibrous dysplasia. Anteroposterior radiograph (**A**) and bone scan (**B**) of the right hip; bone scan (**C**) and anteroposterior radiograph (**D**) of the right tibia. Reprinted with permission from Greenspan A, Beltran J. *Orthopedic Imaging: A Practical Approach.* 6th ed. Philadelphia, PA: Wolters Kluwer; 2014:770–771.

another benign bone condition that can present as a single lesion or multiple lesions (polyostotic fibrous dysplasia) with typically increase radiotracer accumulation (Fig. 8.2). Correlation with clinical and other imaging information can enhance specificity for differential diagnosis (5).

Infection

The common clinical indications for bone scintigraphy are detection, differentiation (osteomyelitis vs. cellulitis or both), and determination of the extent of infection. Three-phase bone scintigraphy (first phase—flow, second phase—blood pool or tissue, and third phase—delayed or metabolic) can be useful in the differential diagnosis of osteomyelitis and cellulitis. In osteomyelitis, all three phases of bone scintigraphy will be abnormal (hyperperfusion, hyperemia, and hypermetabolic), but in cellulitis, the abnormality is early and compartmentalizes to the soft tissue (Fig. 8.3). Additional imaging with bone marrow scanning and radiolabeled leukocyte scan may be needed for improved specificity (6–8).

Trauma

Bone fractures may be evident on bone scan within 24 h after the injury. However, in the elderly and patients with diminished bone mineral density, increased tracer accumulation

at the site of fracture may be delayed. Non-complicated healing will result in a decline in tracer uptake within a few years. Complicated (e.g., infected) non-healing (e.g., continued trauma) fractures may display high tracer accumulation chronically. Correlative clinical and imaging information can help distinguish pathologic from non-pathologic fractures.

Stress fracture may occur with continued injury at the tendinous insertion of muscles, most often in mid tibia (shin splints) (Fig. 8.4). Bone scintigraphy shows diffuse and/or (multi)focal increased tracer accumulation along the posteromedial aspect of tibia, often with normal radiography (9).

Bone vascularity and viability

Bone scintigraphy can be used to determine blood supply to and viability of bone grafts (e.g., after surgical implantation) and specific sites in the skeleton. Aseptic necrosis is caused by avascular necrosis of bone due to a variety of causes (e.g., trauma and steroids). There is initially decreased tracer activity due to diminished vascularity followed by repair phase, which shows increased activity. Correlation with clinical history and other imaging modalities (particularly MRI) can be helpful for accurate

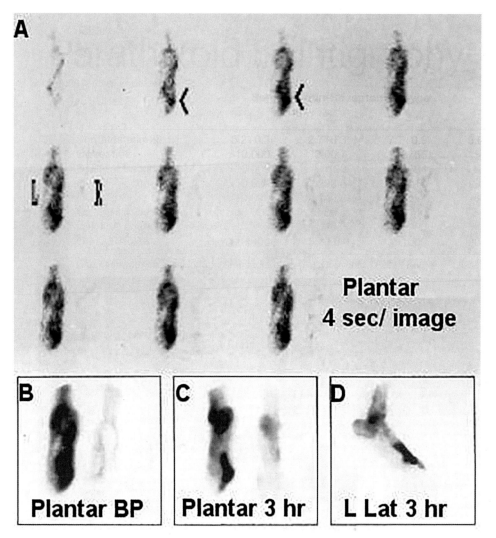

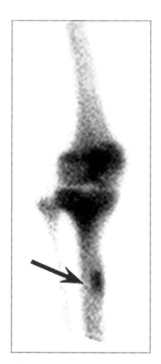

FIG. 8.4 ● Shin splints. A 17-year-old female cross country runner has had tender proximal tibia for 3 months. Plain radiography was negative. Bone scan shows an area of increased uptake in proximal tibia (arrow). Reprinted with permission from Staheli LT. *Fundamentals of Pediatric Orthopedics.* 5th ed. Philadelphia, PA: Wolters Kluwer; 2015:84.

FIG. 8.3 ● First metatarsal osteomyelitis and septic first metatarsal-phalangeal joint. The plantar flow study (**A**) shows increased flow to the left foot and first metatarsal head (arrowheads). The plantar blood pool images (**B**) show diffuse hyperemia in the same areas. The plantar (**C**) and left medial (**D**) views of the static bone scan show intense osteoblastic activity in the entire first metatarsal and the first metatarsal joint region. The asymmetric mildly increased uptake in the left ankle in comparison to the right ankle is due to generalized increased flow (tracer delivery) in the left foot. Reprinted with permission from Brant WE, Helms CA. *Fundamentals of Diagnostic Radiology.* 3rd ed. Philadelphia, PA: Lippincott Williams & Wilkins; 2006:1361–1362.

diagnostic assessment. After radiation therapy, there can be a decline in tracer accumulation in view of diminished vascularity and viable cellularity. Another condition related to vasomotor instability is reflex sympathetic dystrophy syndrome that can be a consequence of a variety of etiologies (e.g., trauma and neurologic abnormality) and associated with pain, swelling, and tenderness. Three-phase bone scintigraphy shows increased perfusion to the affected limb with increased juxtaarticular activity (10–12) (Fig. 8.5).

Prosthesis evaluation

A common clinical request for bone scintigraphy is the discrimination of prosthesis loosening from infection, which requires different clinical management. With regard to hip prosthesis, persistent activity at the caudal tip of prosthesis and the trochanteric region may signal prosthesis loosening (Fig. 8.6). However, in the case of prosthesis infection, there can be generalized hyperactivity around the prosthesis. Bone scintigraphy is also sensitive but nonspecific for differentiating among various conditions that cause painful knee prostheses. If further imaging evaluation is needed, radiolabeled leukocyte scan, ^{68}Ga-citrate scintigraphy, or PET with ^{18}F-fluorodeoxyglucose (^{18}F-FDG) can be contributory (13–17).

Metabolic bone disease

Paget's disease displays relatively intense tracer accumulation in the affected bone that may appear expanded. As the disease transitions from the lytic phase to dense sclerotic phase, the activity increases from a relatively low level to high and then decreases again to near normal activity level (18) (Fig. 8.7).

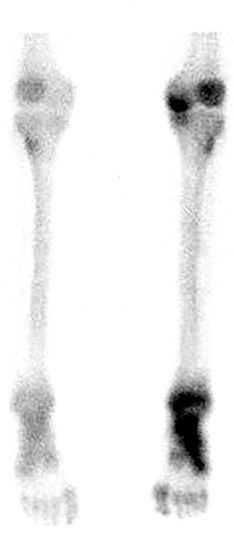

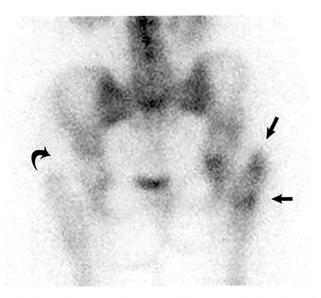

FIG. 8.5 ● Reflex sympathetic dystrophy syndrome. A patient with a 2-year prior left femoral fracture presented with pain and edema in the left lower extremity and increased sensitivity of the skin to pressure and temperature changes. The delayed phase of triple-phase bone scan of both legs shows increased radiotracer uptake in the region of the left knee and left ankle. There was also increased blood flow (first phase) and hyperemia (second phase) on scintigraphy (not shown). Reprinted with permission from Greenspan A, Gershwin ME. *Imaging in Rheumatology: A Clinical Approach*. Philadelphia, PA: Wolters Kluwer; 2017:420–421.

FIG. 8.6 ● Mechanical loosening of hip prosthesis. A patient with bilateral total hip arthroplasties for advanced osteoarthritis reported left hip pain. Bone scan shows focal uptake at the site of femoral component of the left prosthesis only (arrows). There is normal activity surrounding the photopenia of the uncomplicated right total hip arthroplasty (curved arrow). Reprinted with permission from Greenspan A, Gershwin ME. *Imaging in Rheumatology: A Clinical Approach*. Philadelphia, PA: Wolters Kluwer; 2017:50–61.

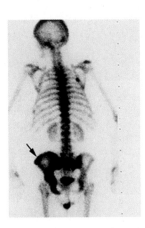

FIG. 8.7 ● Paget's disease. Bone scan (posterior whole body) shows intense activity in an expanded appearance of the entire right hemipelvis (arrow). Reprinted with permission from Yochum TR, Rowe LJ. *Yochum and Rowe's Essentials of Skeletal Radiology*. 3rd ed. Philadelphia, PA: Lippincott Williams & Wilkins; 2004: 665–666.

superscan, diffuse increased activity may be seen in lungs and stomach (19,20).

Renal osteodystrophy is a systemic disorder of bone metabolism due to chronic renal disease, which manifests as abnormalities of calcium, phosphorus, vitamin D, or parathyroid metabolism. These may result in abnormalities of bone mineralization and morphology. Bone scintigraphy typically shows diffuse increase skeletal activity with little or no renal activity (21,22).

Hypertrophic osteoarthropathy is a syndrome characterized by abnormal proliferation of bone and skin in distal extremities. Clinical features include periostosis (subperiosteal new bone formation) of tubular bones, which may be accompanied by pain, and digital clubbing. Hypertrophic osteoarthropathy may be associated with pulmonary disorders (cancer, infections, chronic obstructive disease, and cystic fibrosis), right-to-left cardiac shunts, and less often in other conditions (e.g., Hodgkin lymphoma, sarcoidosis, and cirrhosis). Bone scintigraphy typically demonstrates a symmetric linear increase in tracer accumulation along the diaphyseal and metaphyseal surfaces of long bones (the railroad- or tram-track pattern) (23,24) (Fig. 8.8).

Hyperparathyroidism can also be cause of diffuse increased tracer uptake in the skeleton. In severe cases, "superscan" may be seen with increased activity diffusely in the entire skeleton with little or no renal and bladder activities. There may be particularly increased activity in the skull and facial bones. In advanced cases that are associated with organ calcification, aside from the

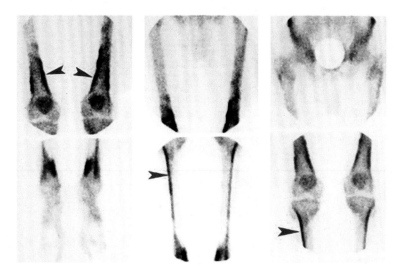

FIG. 8.8 ● Hypertrophic osteoarthropathy. Bone scan in a patient with lung cancer shows increased periosteal uptake in the metaphyses of the lower extremity (arrows). Reprinted with permission from Klein JS, Brant WE, Helms CA, et al. *Brant and Helms' Fundamentals of Diagnostic Radiology*. 5th ed. Philadelphia, PA: Wolters Kluwer; 2018:1636.

Melorheostosis is an uncommon nongenetic developmental sclerosing hyperostosis that typically affects segments of the appendicular skeleton and occasionally occurs in association with another benign generalized sclerosing bone condition, known as osteopoikilosis caused by germline mutations. Surgery may be required for large bone growths, joint impingement syndromes, nerve entrapments, and in remedying limb deformities (25). The characteristic radiographic appearance consists of irregular one-sided cortical hyperostosis resembling melted wax dripping down one side of a candle (26). Bone scan typically shows increased blood flow and uptake in areas involved with increased bone turnover (27).

Erdheim–Chester disease is a rare systemic non-inherited, non-Langerhans cell histiocytosis. It is characterized by xanthomatous or xanthogranulomatous infiltration of tissues by foamy histiocytes, "lipid-laden" macrophages, or histiocytes, surrounded by fibrosis. The disease is typically involved with bilateral metaphyseal and diaphyseal osteosclerosis affecting long bones and sparing epiphyses (28). Bone scan shows symmetric bilateral increased tracer uptake in affected metaphyseal and diaphyseal segments (Fig. 8.9). Other non-osseous classical features on CT scan may include "coated" aorta and "hairy kidney" patterns (29).

Malignant disease

Bone scintigraphy is often used for detection and determination of the extent of metastatic disease involving the bone in patients with primary bone or non-bone neoplasms. Bone scintigraphy is most sensitive for osteoblastic lesions rather than osteolytic lesions. Lesions are typically randomly distributed and often involve axial more than appendicular skeleton (Fig. 8.10). Malignancies that may be associated with primarily osteolytic lesions may be false-negative at least for some lesions and hence may underestimate the extent of osseous metastatic disease (e.g., multiple myeloma, thyroid cancer, and renal cell carcinoma) (30–33).

Bone scintigraphy is often used for staging those cancers that are associated primarily with osteoblastic lesions. The national comprehensive cancer network (NCCN) guidelines should be employed to direct when bone scintigraphy may be most useful for cancer staging. The axial skeleton and pelvis are more commonly involved than the appendicular skeleton. Metastases often present in random distribution although single or few

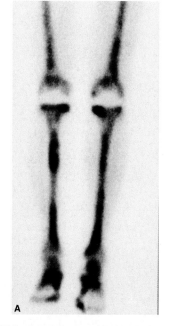

FIG. 8.9 ● Erdheim–Chester disease. Bone scan shows relatively symmetric markedly increased tracer uptake in bilateral femora and tibiae. Reprinted with permission from Peterson JJ. *Berquist's Musculoskeletal Imaging Companion*. 3rd ed. Philadelphia, PA: Wolters Kluwer; 2017:655–656.

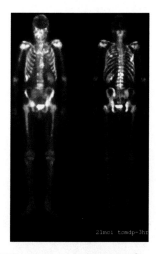

FIG. 8.10 ● Metastatic disease. Anterior and posterior whole-body bone scan shows randomly distributed foci of increased radiotracer uptake in axial and appendicular skeleton.

(oligometastatic) configurations can occur. In patients with heavy burden of osseous metastases, the bone scan is typically associated with diminished soft tissue and renal and bladder urine activities (i.e., superscan) (34). Primary bone malignancy is also typically quite avid for the bone radiotracer. These tumors include, but are not limited to, osteogenic osteosarcoma and Ewing's sarcoma. Osteosarcoma may be associated with reactive soft tissue hyperemia, while Ewing's sarcoma is less often associated with this ancillary finding (35–37).

EXTRA-OSSEOUS UPTAKE

While bone scintigraphy is primarily concerned with the bone conditions, the non-bone tracer uptake can provide clues to many other important clinical conditions. Relatively high soft tissue tracer uptake may be seen with poor radiopharmaceutical preparation (e.g., free pertechnetate accumulating in thyroid and stomach) or renal insufficiency (diminished excretion). Artifactual focal activities may be seen with injection sites, urine contamination, or camera contamination with tracer or urine. Dystrophic calcification, myositis ossificans, tissue infarction, and recent scintigraphy studies are all among many etiologies for extra-osseous bone tracer localization (38–40).

References

1. Bartel TB, Kuruva M, Gnanasegaran G, et al. SNMMI procedure standard for bone scintigraphy 4.0. *J Nucl Med Technol.* 2018;46: 398–404.
2. Segall G, Delbeke D, Stabin MG, et al. SNM practice guideline for sodium ^{18}F-fluoride PET/CT bone scans 1.0. *J Nucl Med.* 2010;51:1813–1820.
3. Van den Wyngaert T, Strobel K, Kampen WU, et al. The EANM practice guidelines for bone scintigraphy. *Eur J Nucl Med Mol Imaging.* 2016;43:1723–1738.
4. Lofgren J, Mortensen J, Rasmussen SH, et al. A prospective study comparing ^{99m}Tc-hydroxyethylene-diphosphonate planar bone scintigraphy and whole-body SPECT/CT with ^{18}F-fluoride PET/CT and ^{18}F-fluoride PET/MRI for diagnosis of bone metastases. *J Nucl Med.* 2017; 58:1778–1785.
5. Van der Wall H, Fogelman I. Scintigraphy of benign bone disease. *Semin Musculoskelet Radiol.* 2007;11:281–300.
6. Palestro CJ. Radionuclide imaging of musculoskeletal infection: a review. *J Nucl Med.* 2016;57:1406–1412.
7. Love C, Palestro CJ. Nuclear imaging of bone infections. *Clin Radiol.* 2016;71:632–646.
8. Palestro CJ. Radionuclide imaging of osteomyelitis. *Semin Nucl Med.* 2015; 45:32–46.
9. Van der Wall H, Lee A, Magee M, et al. Radionuclide bone scintigraphy in sports injuries. *Semin Nucl Med.* 2010; 40:16–30.
10. McDougall IR, Kelling CA. Complications of fractures and their healing. *Semin Nucl Med.* 1988;18:113–125.
11. Lee GW, Weeks PM. The role of bone scintigraphy in diagnosing reflex sympathetic dystrophy. *J Hand Surg Am.* 1995;20:458–463.
12. Agrawal K, Tripathy SK, Sen RK, et al. Nuclear medicine imaging in osteonecrosis of hip: old and current concepts. *World J Orthop.* 2017;8:747–753.
13. Vaz S, Ferreira TC, Salgado L, Paycha F. Bone scan usefulness in patients with painful hip or knee prothesis: 10 situations that can cause pain, other than loosening and infection. *Eur J Orthop Surg Traumatol.* 2017;27:147–156.
14. Verberne SJ, Sonnega RJ, Temmerman OP, et al. What is the accuracy of nuclear imaging in the assessment of periprosthetic knee infection? A meta-analysis. *Clin Ortho Relat Res.* 2017;475:1395–1410.
15. Van der Bruggen W, Hirschmann MT, Strobel K, et al. SPECT/CT in the postoperative painful knee. *Semin Nucl Med.* 2018;48:439–453.
16. Van den Wyngaert T, Paycha F, Strobel K, et al. SPECT/CT in postoperative painful hip arthroplasty. *Semin Nucl Med.* 2018;48:425–438.
17. Zhuang H, yang H, Alavi A. Critical role of 18F-labeled fluorodeoxyglucose PET in the management of patients with arthroplasty. *Radiol Clin North Am.* 2007;45:711–718.
18. Serafini AN. Paget's disease of bone. *Semin Nucl Med.* 1976;6:47–58.
19. Ryan PJ, Fogelman I. Bone scintigraphy in metabolic bone disease. *Semin Nucl Med.* 1997;27:291–305.
20. Hain SF, Fogelman I. Nuclear medicine studies in metabolic bone disease. *Semin Musculoskelet Radiol.* 2002;6:323–329.
21. De Graaf P, Schicht IM, Pauwels EK, et al. Bone scintigraphy in renal osteodystrophy. *J Nucl Med.* 1978;19:1289–1296.
22. Ambrosoni P, Olaizola I, Heuguerot C, et al. The role of imaging techniques in the study of renal osteodystrophy. *Am J Med Sci.* 2000;320:90–95.
23. Yap FY, Skalski MR, Patel DB, et al. Hypertrophic osteoarthropathy: clinical and imaging features. *Radiographics.* 2017;37:157–195.
24. Kaur H, Muhleman M, Balon HR. Hypertrophic osteoarthropathy on bone scintigraphy. *J Nucl Med Technol.* 2018;46:147–148.
25. Wordsworth P, Chan M. Melorheostosis and osteopoikilosis: a review of clinical features and pathogenesis. *Calcif Tissue Int.* 2019;104:530–543.
26. Greenspan A, Azouz EM. Bone dysplasia series. Melorheostosis: review and update. *Can Assoc Radiol J.* 1999;50:324–330.
27. Janousek J, Preston DF, Martin NL, Robinson RG. Bone scan in melorheostosis. *J Nucl Med.* 1976;17:1106–1108.
28. Haroche J, Amaud L, Cohen-Aubart F, et al. Erdheim–Chester disease. *Curr Rheumatol Rep.* 2014; 16:412.
29. Moulis G, Sailer L, Bonneville F, Wagner T. Imaging in Erdheim–Chester disease: classic features and new insights. *Clin Exp Rheumatol.* 2014;32:410–414.
30. Vaz S, Usmani S, Gnanasegaran G, van den Wyngaert T. Molecular imaging of bone metastases using bone targeted tracers. *Q J Nucl Med Mol Imaging.* 2019;63:112–128.
31. Yang HL, Liu T, Wang XM, et al. Diagnosis of bone metastases: a meta-analysis comparing 18FDG PET, CT, MRI and bone scintigraphy. *Eur Radiol.* 2011;21:2604–2617.
32. Liu T, Wang S, Liu H, et al. Detection of vertebral metastases: a meta-analysis comparing MRI, CT, PET, BS, and BS with SPECT. *J Cancer Res Clin Oncol.* 2017;143:457–465.
33. Dasgeb B, Muligan MH, Kim CK. The current status of bone scintigraphy in malignant diseases. *Semin Musculoskelet Radiol.* 2007;11:301–311.
34. Manohar PR, Rather TA, Khan SH, Malik D. Skeletal metastases presenting as superscan on technetium 99m methylene diphosphonate whole body bone scintigraphy in different type of cancers: a 5-year retro-prospective study. *World J Nucl Med.* 2017;16:39–44.
35. Picci P. Osteosarcoma (osteogenic sarcoma). *Orphanet J Rare Dis.* 2007;2:6.
36. Cummings JE, Elzey JA, Heck RK. Imaging of bone sarcomas. *J Natl Compr Canc Netw.* 2007;5:438–447.
37. Focacci C, Lattanzi R, Ideluca ML, Campioni P. Nuclear medicine in primary bone tumors. *Eur J Radiol.* 1998;27 Suppl 1:S123–S131.
38. Gentili A, Miron SD, Bellon EM. Nonosseous accumulation of bone-seeking radiopharmaceuticals. *Radiographics.* 1990;10:871–881.
39. Loutfi I, Collier BD, Mohammed AM. Nonosseus abnormalities on bone scans. *J Nucl Med Technol.* 2003;31:149–153.
40. Zuckier LS, Freeman LM. Nonosseous, nonurologic uptake on bone scintigraphy: atlas and analysis. Semin Nucl Med. 2010;40:242–256.

CHAPTER SELF-ASSESSMENT QUESTIONS

1. Which of the following is not a typical indication for bone scintigraphy?
   A. Staging and treatment monitoring of cancer
   B. Infection
   C. Paget's disease
   D. Crohn's disease

2. All of the following can be a potential condition for extra-osseous tracer uptake on a bone scan except:
   A. Poor radiopharmaceutical preparation
   B. Tissue infraction
   C. Myositis ossificans
   D. Melorheostosis

3. Which statement regarding "superscan" pattern is incorrect:
   A. Can be seen with hyperparathyroidism
   B. Is typically associated with little or no renal and bladder activities
   C. Is associated with oligometastatic disease
   D. Is commonly demonstrated with high bone tumor burden

Answers to Chapter Self-Assessment Questions

1. **D** Staging and treatment monitoring of cancer, infection, and Paget's disease are all common indications for bone scintigraphy. Crohn's disease, which is an inflammatory bowel disease, is not an indication for bone scanning.

2. **D** Poor radiopharmaceutical preparation may result in free pertechnetate that can accumulate in thyroid and stomach. Both myositis ossificans and tissue infraction, which may be associated with dystrophic calcification, can demonstrate bone tracer uptake. Bone scan typically shows increased blood flow and uptake in areas involved with increased bone turnover in melorheostosis, which is a developmental sclerosing hyperostosis condition involving the appendicular skeleton.

3. **C** "Superscan" pattern on bone scan may be seen with hyperparathyroidism and with high bone tumor burden, often associated with low renal and bladder activities. Oligometastatic disease refers to only few (typically <5) tumor sites.

Infection and Inflammation

9

Søren Hess and Abass Alavi

LEARNING OBJECTIVES

1. Describe the basics of radionuclide imaging in infection and inflammation.
2. Compare pros and cons of imaging modalities in selected indications within the domain of infectious and inflammatory diseases.

INTRODUCTION

Radionuclide imaging has played a major role in the diagnostic workup of suspected infection and inflammation in the past almost 50 years since the incidental discovery that ^{67}Ga-citrate accumulated in inflammatory tissue while investigating its use in Hodgkin lymphoma—the exact mechanism is still not fully understood, but ^{67}Ga-citrate is taken up by transferrin and other iron-carriers ion and the ^{67}Ga-citrate-complexes accumulate at sites of inflammation by a combination of hyperperfusion, increased vascular permeability, and direct binding to leucocytes or bacterial siderophores. Although ^{67}Ga-citrate scintigraphy displayed good sensitivity for both acute and chronic inflammation, specificity was lacking due to widespread physiologic tracer distribution throughout the body for several days after tracer administration, which necessitated delaying imaging for as much as 72 to 96 h. Furthermore, ^{67}Ga has an unfavorable long half-life and high energy gamma photons leading to a relatively high radiation burden. The next generation infection scintigraphy based on labeled white blood cells (WBC) was introduced in 1976 with ^{111}In-oxine, 10 years later with ^{99m}Tc-HMPAO, and later ^{18}F-fluorodeoxyglucose-positron emission tomography (FDG-PET) was applied to infection and inflammation (1,2).

With increasing availability, FDG-PET/CT has been applied in most common inflammatory and infectious indications. While ^{67}Ga-citrate SPECT/CT remains an effective method for demonstrating spinal infection and active pneumonitis and nephritis and chronic infections, it is no longer considered the radionuclide gold standard for infection and inflammation. The usual clinical choices in infection imaging is now limited to WBC scintigraphy or FDG-PET/CT.

It has become apparent that the diagnostic value of FDG-PET/CT is at least comparable to WBC scintigraphy in most clinical settings. FDG-PET/CT is performed within 1 h with a contemporaneous CT, all without the task of collecting, labeling, and risk of reinjecting the patient's blood, or waiting 24 to 48 h for the final results. Thus, FDG-PET/CT should be considered the modality of choice for most indications—this chapter outlines the most common use of radionuclide imaging in infectious and inflammatory diseases (Table 9.1).

Basic principles of imaging labeled white blood cell scintigraphy

Two inherently different agents are available for ex-vivo labeling of WBC, ^{111}In-oxine, and ^{99m}Tc-HMPAO. Both are based on ex-vivo labeling of autologous WBC. After withdrawal of whole blood, red blood cells are sedimented and plasma is centrifuged to segregate the leucocytes, primarily neutrophils, which in turn are labeled and reinjected into the patient. ^{111}In-oxine is lipid soluble and readily diffuses across the cellular membrane and forms stable binds to cytoplasmic components, whereas ^{99m}Tc-HMPAO is lipophilic. Isotope half-life and radiation dose is lower with ^{99m}Tc-labeled HMPAO compared to ^{111}In-oxine, and the decay energy and image quality is also more favorable with the former than the latter (1).

Regardless of labeling method, interpretation is based on uptake patterns over time, that is, within about an hour after injection leucocytes migrate to sites of infection as a result of chemotaxis and most reports use increased uptake on sequential scans to define a positive WBC scintigraphy, whereas stable or decreasing uptake is not considered indicative of infection (3–5). However, several caveats and pitfalls need to be acknowledged; first of all, the rate of accumulation depends on several factors including the site (e.g., faster in vascular tissue and slower in bone due to compromised blood flow), type of pathogen, virulence, and extent (i.e., more or less chemotactic signals to accumulate leucocytes) (3). Secondly, the bio-distribution of the labeled cells is important, as both ^{111}In-oxine-labeled and ^{99m}Tc-HMPAO-labeled WBC accumulate in the lungs rapidly after injection and subsequently lung activity clear after 3 to 4 h. Labeled WBCs also accumulate in the liver, spleen, and bone marrow as part of the reticuloendothelial system where they are retained. However, because of differences in labeling attributes, over time, ^{99m}Tc elutes the cells and is excreted in urine and stool, thus radioactivity from ^{99m}Tc-HMPAO-labeled WBC is visible in the entire urinary and gastrointestinal system, for example, kidneys, bladder, gall bladder and especially colon, which limits the usage in suspected inflammation in these organs (1,4). Thus, specific imaging protocols should be employed depending on the clinical challenge, for example, early–late phase images in suspected

Table 9.1 **OVERVIEW OF SELECTED COMMON INDICATIONS WITH POTENTIAL DIAGNOSTIC VALUE OF RADIONUCLIDE MODALITIES IN INFECTIOUS AND INFLAMMATORY DISEASES—NUMBERS ARE FURTHER EXPLAINED AND QUALIFIED IN THE TEXT**

Indications	WBC scintigraphy		FDG-PET/CT	
	Sensitivity	Specificity	Sensitivity	Specificity
Fever of unknown origin	33%	83%	83%–98%	58%–86%
Bacteremia/metastatic infection	-	-	46%–74%[§]	-
Febrile neutropenia	-	-	-	-
Large vessel vasculitis	-	-	80%–90%	89%–98%
Osteomyelitis	100%[*]	89%–97[*]	86%–94%[*]	76%–100%[*]
	11%–38%[**]	-	88%–100%[**]	93%–95%[**]
Spondylodiscitis	63%–84%	55%–100%	95%–97%	88%–90%
Prosthetic joint infection	83%–89%	84%–93%	86%–88%[$]	88%–93%[$]
			70%–72%[□]	80%–84%[□]
Vascular graft infection	82%–100%	85%–100%	>90%	61%–83%
Endocarditis	64%–86%	97%–100%	61%–81%	85%–88%
Cardiac device infections	~85%	~90%	93%–96%[#]	97%–98%[#]
			65%–76%[##]	83%–88%[##]

[§] Detection rate of infectious foci or metastatic infection.

[*]/[**] Peripheral/axial osteomyelitis.

[$]/[□] Hip/knee prostheses.

[#]/[##] Pocket/lead infections.

From Doroudinia and Tavakoli (81).

abdominal infection, especially if ^{99m}Tc-HMPAO is used, delayed images in suspected bone or prosthetic joint infection, or completely refraining from using labeled WBC if infection in the spine is suggested (5).

Basic principles of imaging FDG

As a glucose analogue, FDG in many respects imitates the distribution and cellular uptake of glucose throughout the body. A multitude of clinical settings are characterized by increased glucose uptake, most prominently exploited by FDG-PET/CT in imaging malignancies; it is well-known that cancer cells adhere to the so-called Warburg effect, that is, their metabolism is based on glucose consumption rather than the more energy-efficient oxidative phosphorylation even under aerobic conditions, so the net effect is a generally increased glucose metabolism through upregulation of GLUT. Inflammatory cells also utilize glucose; in fact, the increased uptake of FDG in inflammatory cells was initially dismissed as a nuisance leading to false-positive findings in patients suspected of malignant disease, but already in the early days of FDG-PET, it became clear that the effect was not specific to cancer (6,7). One of the first to present FDG-PET used directly in the diagnostic workup of infection was Tahara et al., who presented two case reports of abdominal abscesses with clearly increased FDG-uptake compared to adjacent soft tissue, both visually and semi-quantitatively (8). Subsequent preclinical pathophysiologic studies established that GLUT were not only upregulated in cancer cells but also by immune-mediated cytokine release in inflammatory settings; autoradiography showed increased expression of GLUT in the activated granulocytes that dominate early phases of inflammation in artificially induced septic inflammation, and in the macrophages that dominate more

chronic stages of inflammation in artificial aseptic turpentine-induced inflammation (9,10). Thus, the potential use in inflammatory diseases was slowly recognized, but FDG did not become a serious contender in inflammation imaging until the recently increased availability in the past two decades.

Patient preparation before FDG-PET/CT in infection and inflammation imaging generally follows the same principles as for tumor imaging, that is, fasting for at least 4 to 6 h prior to injection to ensure optimum blood glucose levels of <150 mg/dL (8.3 mmol/L) (11,12). It seems though that the effect of relative hyperglycemia is less pronounced on inflammatory cells compared to cancer cells; several studies including meta-analysis of large populations suggest limited effect as long as blood glucose is kept below 200 mg/dL (11.1 mmol/L), and chronic hyperglycemia has less impact than acute hyperglycemia or hyperinsulinemia (13–15). On the other hand, prolonged fasting for up to 12 to 18 h preceded by low-carb-high-fat dietary restraints are important measures to shift the physiologically predominant glucose-driven metabolism of the heart toward free fatty acids to suppress physiologic FDG uptake sufficiently to assess suspected cardiac inflammation and infections (16).

Some medication may generally interfere with interpretation of FDG-PET/CT, for example, metformin should be discontinued for 48 to 72 h prior to the scan if pathology in the bowel is suspected, and this is also the case in infection and inflammation. More specifically, the mainstay treatment strategy of several noninfectious inflammatory disorders includes corticosteroids and the impact on sensitivity may be significant as it has been shown in large vessel vasculitis; sensitivity of visual as well as semi-quantitative assessment was not affected after 3 days but was significantly reduced after 10 days' treatment; thus, imaging in suspected inflammatory disease should be performed before or shortly after treatment is instituted, and otherwise discontinuation should be considered (17).

Clinical imaging strategies in selected clinical settings

Radionuclide imaging is employed in a multitude of clinical settings of infectious and inflammatory diseases, and it is beyond the scope of this chapter to present an exhaustive review. In the following sections, we present some overall considerations regarding the most common or well-established indication in systemic diseases as well as focal/local organ specific affection. Generally, WBC scintigraphy is of little use in the initial diagnostic workup of suspected systemic inflammation; FDG-PET/CT provides a better solution on most accounts. On the other hand, some WBC scintigraphy is still considered routine examination or even the modality of choice in several local infections, for example, suspected prosthetic infection.

One of the issues that is often broad forth is the relatively non-specificity of FDG compared to labeled WBC, but it is important to remember that the migration of leucocytes is also governed by relatively nonspecific chemotactic signaling, adhesion molecules, and diapedesis. These are specific markers of leucocytic infiltration rather than infection per se[2]. There may also be differences between bacterial strains. A scintigraphic study of WBC distribution and uptake in a rabbit model also showed considerable differences between induced gram-positive and gram-negative osteomyelitis in femur and vertebra. Pathologic WBC uptake was seen in 88% of gram-positive animals (both femur and vertebra) but only in 13% of gram-negative animals (both femur and vertebra), and the authors speculated that circulating anti-chemotactic factors secreted by gram-negative bacteria could account for the lack of WBC accumulation (18).

In a study of 132 patients with suspected infection who underwent WBC scintigraphy, 62 were considered positive for infection, and 30% had positive WBC scintigraphy. They found WBC scintigraphy overall clinically useful in 48% of patients but with variations according to indications; WBC scintigraphy was most helpful in osteomyelitis (70%) or vascular graft infections (67%), and least helpful in fever of unknown origin (FUO, 34%) (19). Nonetheless, however interesting such studies are, obviously the choice of modality in clinical practice is guided very little by such post-hoc analyses in the setting of infectious and inflammatory disorders because of the often nonspecific presentation.

Systemic infection and inflammation

A major and relatively well-established indication for FDG-PET/CT is FUO, a challenging clinical condition first defined by Petersdorf et al. in 1961 as unclear diagnosis despite relevant workup in patients with fever admitted for prolonged periods. Today, the definition has been revised slightly to fit contemporary outpatient-based healthcare. Although final diagnoses may be divided into overarching groups of infection (20%–40%), noninfectious inflammation (10%–30%), cancer (20%–30%), and miscellaneous (10%–20%), most patients present with relatively few, nonspecific symptoms and diagnostic clues, and as many as one third of patients remain without a firm final diagnosis despite extensive diagnostic workup (20–22). Before the FDG-PET/CT era, ^{67}Ga-citrate and WBC scintigraphy were used with the formerly considered gold standard. Currently, FDG-PET/CT offers a faster, more sensitive, and more patient convenient whole-body assessment with less radiation exposure and less expense in many settings. In the case of FUO, the relative non-specificity of FDG is an advantage in a highly heterogeneous patient population with more than 200 differential diagnoses. Positive scans may point the clinicians toward potential sites of disease regardless of the underlying etiology (Figs. 9.1 and 9.2), whereas negative scans generally exclude treatable focal disease and harbor good prognoses (23,24). On the downside, the non-specificity also gives rise to a significant proportion of false-positive findings that may lead to unnecessary diagnostic procedures. As for ^{67}Ga-citrate and WBC scintigraphy, ^{67}Ga-citrate is as nonspecific as FDG, while labeled WBCs may be more specific for septic inflammation and to some extent aseptic inflammation, but with less sensitivity. Labeled WBCs may also accumulate in some malignancies. This is underlined in a recent meta-analysis with sensitivities and specificities for FDG-PET/CT, FDG-PET, ^{67}Ga-citrate, and WBC scintigraphy that strongly favor FDG-PET/CT, that is, 86% and 52%, 76% and 50%, 60% and 63%, and 33% and 83%, respectively, with an overall diagnostic yield of 58%, 44%, 35%, and 20%, respectively (25).

Several other meta-analyses also support the use of FDG-PET/CT in FUO with pooled sensitivities and specificities of 83% to 98% and 58% to 86%, respectively (26–28), although several caveats pertain to the underlying literature; most are retrospective, definitions of FUO is highly variable, populations are relatively small, final diagnoses was not reached in varying proportions, and some older studies use stand-alone PET only. Also, due to the heterogeneous etiologies, sensitivity and specificity may not be the best outcome measures, so most studies instead report on the proportion of patients in whom FDG-PET/CT was considered helpful in the diagnostic process, which ranged from 26% to 92% depending on patient population and selection. It is also important to realize that in many of the studies FDG-PET/CT was performed late in the diagnostic process and many cases could be considered the most challenging ones where a diagnosis had not yet been reached by other modalities (29). Accordingly, several factors may influence diagnostic yield, including inflammatory markers. Prior studies have shown a positive correlation between increased CRP and ESR and positive scans, and generally FDG-PET/CT should not be performed in patients with normal inflammatory markers (30,31).

A different but also serious systemic infectious condition is bloodstream infection. Prognosis and treatment strategy depend on whether the bacteremia is uncomplicated or complicated, that is, with metastatic foci (for instance prosthetic material or spondylodiscitis). Mortality is higher in complicated bacteremia. To ensure sufficient eradication, treatment is usually required for several weeks longer than in uncomplicated cases. Consequently, it is imperative to locate any metastatic foci to ascertain patient prognosis and facilitate a proper treatment strategy. Achieving this may be a challenge since half the patients present without any signs or symptoms related to infectious foci (32). One of the only large prospective studies on this topic demonstrated significant differences between two groups of patients with bacteremia, one who underwent FDG-PET/CT during workup, and a matched historic control group undergoing workup without FDG-PET/CT. Metastatic foci were found in significantly more cases than controls (67.8% vs. 35.7%), and relapse rate and mortality was significantly lower in cases than in controls (i.e., 2.6% vs. 7.4%, and 19.1% vs. 32.2%, respectively) (33,34). Similar to FUO, definitions are different in various studies; some studies report the number of metastatic foci, others the detection rate for infectious foci, but semantics aside the rates of detection of metastatic infectious foci are comparable, that is, 46% to 74% (33–39). Some

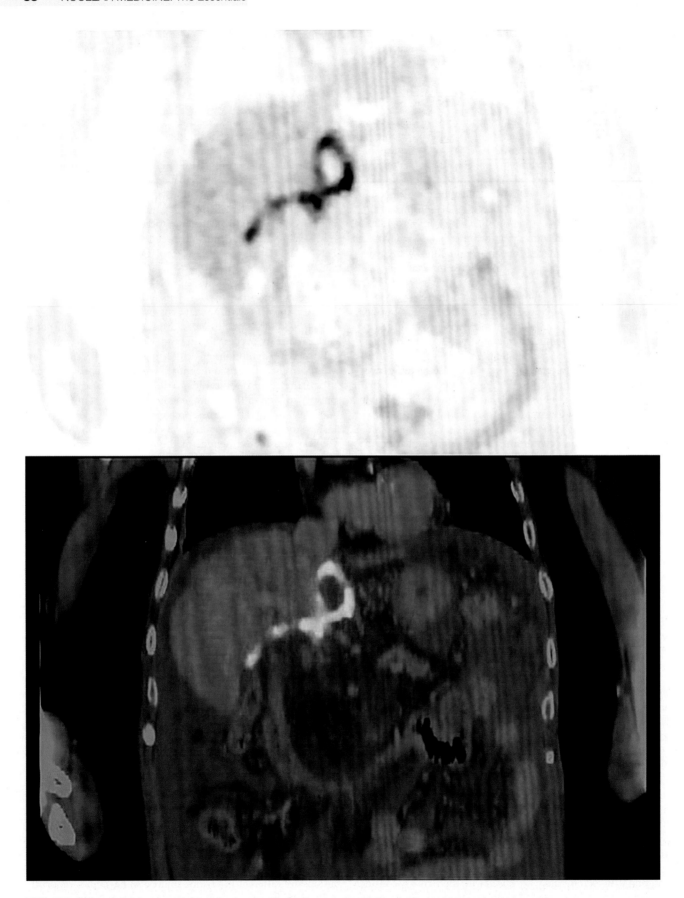

FIG. 9.1 ● Fever of unknown origin; patient presenting with general malaise, prolonged fever of unknown origin, and nonspecific abdominal discomfort. Initial chest x-ray was negative and abdominal ultrasonography was equivocal. FDG-PET/CT showed marked FDG-uptake in the circumference of a liver abscess with a fistula to the gall gladder bed.

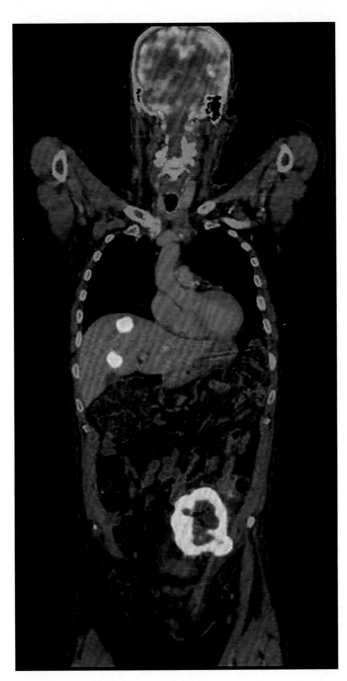

FIG. 9.2 ● Fever of unknown origin; patient presenting with general malaise and prolonged fever of unknown origin. FDG-PET/CT showed high FDG-uptake in the circumference of sigmoidal process and several focal liver lesions. Biopsy confirmed a highly metabolically active disseminated neuroendocrine tumor of the sigmoid with liver metastases.

mainstay treatment strategy includes broad-spectrum antibiotic, but febrile neutropenia is only caused by infection in 30% to 50% cases. To improve patient outcome, but to avoid overtreatment, potential side effects, and microbial resistance, it is equally important to find and to exclude infectious foci (41). WBC scintigraphy is logically inappropriate in febrile neutropenia. FDG-PET/CT generally performs favorably in case–control diagnostic studies with versus without FDG-PET/CT. Thus in febrile neutropenia, FDG-PET/CT offers a higher detection rate and a high degree of clinical impact including changes in treatment strategy (42–44). Nonetheless, a more recent study showed more equivocal results with only moderate sensitivity, only limited impact on diagnosis and treatment, and no apparent advantage over CT (45). Thus, results remain equivocal and most studies are small and methodologically weak with poorly defined reference standards primarily based on hematological malignancies while almost devoid of results from solid tumors. At first glance and from a strictly pathophysiologic point of view, FDG should perhaps not be the tracer of choice in febrile neutropenia for the same reason as WBC are not; sensitivity could be hampered as the prerequisite of the method is believed to be FDG uptake in the activated neutrophils, but the uptake in macrophages and granulation tissue as seen in the aforementioned autoradiography studies. Alternatively, nonspecific FDG uptake in underlying malignant cells and metastases may confound the search for infection. Fortunately, because of the increased use of FDG-PET/CT as part of the routine workup in cancers, baseline scans are often available for comparison, limiting issues with sensitivity and specificity (29).

Large vessel vasculitis is a chronic autoimmune inflammatory condition of aorta and its main branches with or without involvement of cranial arteries. Symptoms are often nonspecific, and diagnosis may therefore be difficult. Treatment is imperative to avoid serious complications like blindness, but the required high doses of glucocorticoids are associated with side effects. Hitherto, the diagnosis has been based on nonspecific and subjective clinical criteria, and temporal artery biopsy considered the gold standard, but false-negative findings are common (46). Besides, cranial involvement is only present in a proportion of patients and biopsy is not readily performed from larger arteries. Currently, large vessel vasculitis is divided in those with primary whole-body disease and these with predominantly cranial affection (47). FDG-PET/CT is considered most adept in whole-body affected patients with meta-analyses consistently reporting sensitivities and specificities of 80% to 90% and 89% to 98%, respectively (48,49). Cranial vessels, though, were not considered accessible to PET imaging due to resolution issues related to the small caliber of temporal arteries and the close proximity to the high physiologic FDG activity in the brain (46). However, a recent retrospective case–control study established the possibility to detect cranial artery inflammation with high sensitivity and specificity (i.e., 82% and 100%, respectively) (50) and these results were recently confirmed in a prospective, double-blinded study (51).

Localized or organ specific infection and inflammation

Bone-related infections are an important healthcare issue. The number of patients with joint prostheses are increasing and most bone infections require antibiotic therapy for prolonged time periods. The diagnosis may be challenging as symptoms and findings mimic noninfectious conditions like degeneration or prosthetic loosening, and metallic artifacts from implanted hardware reduce image quality. Consequently, controversies remain regarding the

studies have found direct clinical impact of FDG-PET/CT on patient management such as changes in treatment in 47% to 74% of cases (35–37), and in one series relapse rates and mortality was similar in patients with uncomplicated bacteremia compared to a group with bacteremia with high risk of metastatic spread, but negative echocardiography and FDG-PET/CT who were treated with antibiotics for the same duration (40).

A subset of systemic infection in the interface between FUO and bacteremia is febrile neutropenia encountered in cancer patients during therapy. As it is a potentially lethal condition, the imaging modality of choice in various settings. In acute osteomyelitis, MRI is the modality of choice with limited added value of radionuclide imaging, but in more chronic, low-grade osteomyelitis, radionuclide imaging may be more helpful. In peripheral osteomyelitis, WBC scintigraphy and SPECT/CT have performed better than FDG-PET/CT, that is, sensitivity and specificity of 100% and 89% to 97%, respectively, versus 86% to 94% and 76% to 100%, respectively. In the axial skeleton, however, there is no role for WBC SPECT/CT as sensitivities are reported as low as 11% to 38%, whereas FDG-PET/CT has demonstrated consistently high values, that is, 88% to 100% sensitivity and 73% to 95% specificity. Two older meta-analyses found FDG-PET superior to comparative methods with sensitivities and specificities of 92% to 96% and 91% to 92% (FDG-PET or FDG-PET/CT), 74% and 88% (WBC scintigraphy), 78% and 84% (combined bone scintigraphy and WBC scintigraphy), and 84% and 60% (MRI). Importantly, similar results were found regardless of spinal metal implants with sensitivity, specificity, and accuracy around 90% (52–56).

An important subgroup of osteomyelitis is infectious spondylodiscitis, which may be either primary hematogenous (e.g., in metastatic bacteremia, Fig. 9.3) or secondary to spine surgery. MRI has been considered the modality of choice, but structural imaging may be hampered by nonspecific morphologic changes, artifacts from metallic implants, or limited sensitivity in the early phases. As mentioned earlier, WBC scintigraphy has very limited sensitivity in the axial skeleton, including spondylodiscitis, with reported sensitivities of 63% to 84% and highly variable specificities of 55% to 100% (54). Several meta-analyses have reported consistently high diagnostic values for FDG-PET/CT, that is, sensitivities and specificities of 95% to 97% and 88% to 90%, respectively, with no discernible negative effect from spinal implants and other potential confounders, compared to 76% to 85% and 62% to 66%, respectively, for MRI (57–59). Furthermore, as mentioned earlier, there are significant differences in diagnostic performance related to different time points; a recent comparative study found overall diagnostic values for MRI and FDG-PET/CT comparable to the meta-analyses (i.e., 67% and 84% versus 96% and 95%), but interestingly, the accuracy of MRI was only 58% within the first 2 weeks after symptoms and 82% in later phases, whereas the diagnostic performance of FDG-PET/CT was unrelated to timing of the scan relative to symptom start (60).

An important subset of localized infections are those related to various implanted prosthetic material, and the diagnoses may be even more challenging due to the inherent artifacts that such exogenous material may induce—thus, although the individual clinical entities are different, they also share some common features.

Although prosthetic joint infections only occur in <5%, the challenge to healthcare is considerable due to the increasing number of inserted prostheses; generally, one third occurs early (within 3 months), one third delayed (within 1 year), and one third late (more than a year after insertion). Early and delayed infections are a direct consequence of microorganisms introduced during surgery, while late infections are usually caused by hematogenous spread from another focal point in bacteremia. The diagnosis may be challenging with nonspecific symptoms and findings; pain are present in most patients, whereas the presence of fever is highly variable (5%–40%), and the usual inflammatory markers like redness and swelling that are usually present in acute infection are rarely found in the often more chronic low-grade infections of prosthetic joints. Inflammatory markers like erythrocyte sedimentation rate or c-reactive protein are usually elevated, but may also be so physiologically for prolonged periods following

surgery. Plain radiography are insensitive and nonspecific, CT as well as MRI are hampered by metallic artifacts, and the reference standard joint aspiration may be specific (92%–100%) but with highly variable sensitivity (28%–92%). Thus, radionuclide imaging plays a key role, but the modality of choice remains controversial. Many consider WBC scintigraphy the modality of choice, preferably enhanced with SPECT/CT and combined with bone marrow scintigraphy. Bone marrow scintigraphy is added to increase specificity by differentiating leukocyte accumulation in periprosthetic-infected tissue from physiologic activity in aberrant bone marrow displaced during insertion of the prosthesis; several studies have presented consistent sensitivities, specificities, and accuracy of 83% to 89%, 84% to 93%, and 89%, respectively (54,61). FDG-PET/CT is usually considered less specific, especially in the early post-operative phase; for instance, increased FDG uptake was seen in 100% of sternotomy scars 3 months after surgery and activity remained 1 year post-surgery in 40%. Similarly, nonspecific periprosthetic uptake was seen around 80% of non-symptomatic hip arthroplasties and activity was still present 5 years after insertion in 71%. In contrast, a rat study showed that only septic inoculated surgical incisions were positive on WBC scintigraphy, whereas physiologic wound healing was negative, but several older studies found varying degrees of leukocyte accumulation around more than half of hip arthroplasties several years after insertion (61). In an attempt to better specificity, several interpretation criteria for FDG-PET/CT have been proposed in suspected prosthetic joint infection as uptake patterns are probably more important than intensity. Regardless of interpretation criteria, several meta-analyses on FDG-PET/CT in suspected prosthetic joint infections have demonstrated overall diagnostic values almost comparable to WBC scintigraphy with better performance in hip prostheses than knee prostheses, that is, pooled sensitivities and specificities of 86% to 88% and 88% to 93%, respectively, in hip prostheses, and 70% to 72% and 80% to 84%, respectively, in knee prostheses (62,63). Interestingly, a prospective comparison reported significantly better sensitivity for FDG-PET/CT compared to WBC scintigraphy; that is, sensitivity, specificity, positive predictive value, and negative predictive values of FDG-PET in hip prostheses were 82%, 93%, 79%, and 94%, respectively. Corresponding values for knee prostheses were 95%, 88%, 69%, and 98%, respectively. Sensitivity, specificity, positive predictive value, and negative predictive values of combined WBC scintigraphy/bone marrow imaging in hip prostheses yielded 39%, 96%, 71%, and 85%, respectively, whereas the values for knee prostheses were 33%, 89%, 25%, and 92%, respectively (64).

Vascular graft infections are relatively rare (incidence <5%) but dreaded due to mortality as high as 25% to 88%; early and correct diagnosis is important to avoid under-treatment with fatal consequences and over-treatment with unnecessary high-risk surgery or prolonged antibiotics. However, it is a clinically challenging diagnosis with nonspecific symptoms, and it is seldom possible to obtain biopsy verification. CT has been the imaging modality of choice, because it can visualize characteristic morphologic features of vascular graft infections, for example, peri-graft soft tissue, fluid, or gas, but sensitivity and specificity is only moderate, especially in low-grade infections, that is, one meta-analysis found pooled sensitivity and specificity of only 67% and 63%, respectively. Thus, FDG-PET/CT has been suggested to increase sensitivity and specificity, and generally speaking, it has been successful regarding sensitivity, whereas results are more equivocal regarding specificity.

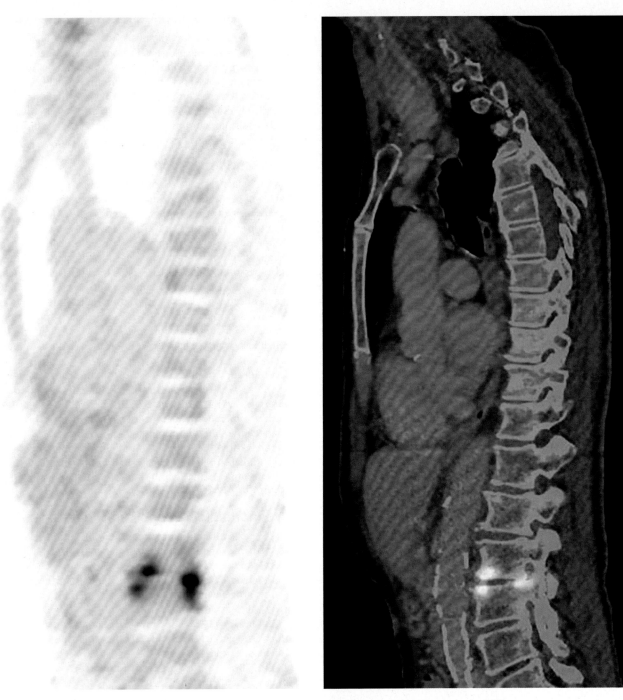

FIG. 9.3 ● Bacteremia; patient presenting with fever, back pain, and ***Staphylococcus aureus*** bacteremia. MRI was not performed due to claustrophobia, and FDG-PET/CT showed marked FDG uptake around the vertebral disc between L2/L3 with an intra-foraminal phlegmonous component consistent with spondylodiscitis.

This is due to the physiological immune response to synthetic graft materials resulting in common mild-to-moderate diffuse FDG-uptake along the prosthesis. This inflammation may linger for several years or even decades and be misread as low-grade FDG avid infection, especially if there are nonuniformities between various graft materials (65). Furthermore, comparison between studies is difficult because there is currently no consensus on interpretation criteria, for example, visual or semi-quantitative assessment, but sensitivity is generally high whereas specificity is lower. According to three recent meta-analyses, it is possible to achieve sensitivities

>90% depending on interpretation criteria but with generally lower specificities ranging 61% to 83% (65–67).

Due to the somewhat disappointing specificity of FDG-PET/CT, WBC scintigraphy (especially when enhanced with SPECT/CT) is still considered by some to be the radionuclide reference standard with several newer studies reporting impressive results; overall sensitivities (82%–100%) are generally comparable to those of FDG-PET/CT albeit with overall better specificity (85%–100%) (54,68,69). One of the recent meta-analyses also compared FDG-PET/CT to WBC SPECT/CT and found overall better accuracy of the latter, but they still suggested FDG-PET/

CT as first-line imaging due to its more widespread accessibility and more simple performance (67).

Infectious endocarditis (IE) comprises several subsets with different challenges, for example, native-valve endocarditis (NVE), prosthetic-valve endocarditis (PVE), and implanted cardiac device-infections (ICDI), and regardless of subtype, initial presentation is diverse and relatively nonspecific. Initial diagnostic evaluation is usually based on modified Duke criteria and echocardiography, both with good sensitivity in native endocarditis, but more limited values in PVE (due to artifacts), early in the disease course, or in patients with already initiated antibiotic treatment. Thus, alternative imaging is in high demand, and FDG-PET/CT has been investigated, but as mentioned earlier, imaging the heart with FDG requires sufficient patient preparation, may give false-positive results in the immediate post-operative course, and false-negative results in patients heavily pretreated with antibiotics. Initial reports, including meta-analyses, found only moderate overall pooled sensitivities and specificities, that is, 61% to 81% and 85% to 88%, respectively, presumably because NVE and PVE were included alike and because preparatory measures like prolonged fasting was not routinely applied, but generally the diagnostic performance improved when only PVE was considered (62,70). This was underlined in a recent study that compared NVE and PVE and found sensitivity of 22% and 90%, respectively, with comparable specificity (70).

Controversy remains regarding the role of WBC scintigraphy versus FDG-PET/CT in IE, but recent results point toward comparable diagnostic values with dedicated SPECT/CT protocols in PVE. In a head-to-head comparison in 39 patients with PVE, FDG-PET/CT displayed higher sensitivity (93% vs. 64%), WBC SPECT/CT higher specificity (100% vs. 71%) with discrepant findings in 31% of patients (5 false-negatives with WBC, 6 false-positive with FDG)—the latter cases were all imaged within the first 2 months post-surgery (71). In a head-to-head comparison regarding extra-cardiac foci in 55 patients, FDG-PET/CT found significantly more than WBC-SPECT/CT (91 vs. 37) and the clinical utility of the former was considered significantly better (72). However, the meta-analysis from Juneau et al. found overall comparable results for both modalities, that is, sensitivity and specificity of 81% and 85%, respectively, for FDG-PET/CT, and sensitivity and specificity of 86% and 97%, respectively, for WBC scintigraphy, and they concluded that both are useful (73). The same is currently the case for ICDI; recent studies including meta-analyses have found comparable results for FDG-PET/CT and WBC-SPECT/CT, that is, sensitivities and specificities around 85% and 90%, respectively (62,74). For FDG-PET/CT, there was significant differences in subgroup analyses of pocket infections (93%–96% sensitivity and 97%–98% specificity) versus lead electrode infections (65%–76% sensitivity and 83%–88% specificity), and also better sensitivity in patients with sufficient preparation (i.e., overall pooled sensitivity of 92%).

Thus, generally speaking, the clinical setting, local availability, and patient considerations should guide the choice—WBC protocols employ imaging up till 24 hours post-injection, whereas FDG-PET/CT requires prolonged patient preparation but faster results. FDG-PET/CT should be reserved for PVE, and caution should be advised in the immediate post-operative period and in patients heavily pretreated with antibiotics; both conditions seem to affect WBC SPECT/CT to a lesser extent. In suspected extra-cardiac foci, FDG-PET/CT probably performs better, and the same is probably the case in ICDI, especially with pocket infections.

A multitude of other indications have also been investigated with FDG-PET/CT for diagnosis, response evaluation, recurrence detection, and prognostication, albeit less established in clinical practice or with more controversial or equivocal results in the literature; that is, results are interesting, usually scientifically sound, and with promising potential, but more data are needed to more firmly establish FDG-PET/CT in these settings that include tuberculosis, human immunodeficiency virus, sarcoidosis, IBD, psoriasis, and venous thromboembolism (75,76).

Novel and future aspects

As a consequence of the relative non-specificity of FDG and WBC much work has been put into developing the modalities toward higher specificity or to find new methods altogether. Several technical improvement of PET/CT has been suggested, for example, multiple-time-point imaging to improve differentiation between malignant and inflammatory cells, and more advanced quantification based on global disease assessment instead of the flawed semi-quantitative standard uptake value-based values, but neither has been widely implemented in clinical practice (77). On the hardware front, hybrid PET/MR is obviously interesting with its aptitude for soft-tissue imaging, but the availability is still very limited and available literature on infection and inflammation is sparse (78).

A multitude of novel tracers for both gamma camera imaging and PET/CT has been introduced and developed for direct bacterial imaging with tracers aimed at more or less specific cellular or membrane features of singular bacterial strains, for instance radiolabeled antibiotics. Although results are interesting and mostly scientifically sound, the obstacles are not negligible, studies are highly variable, and only very few have been translated into human studies and that without much success (79,80).

Nuclear medicine aspects of COVID-19

On December 31, 2019, a pneumonia of unknown cause was detected in Wuhan, in Hubei province, China, and was first reported to the WHO.

On January 10, 2020, WHO issued a tool for the detection of the novel coronavirus developed with reference to other coronaviruses, such as SARS and MERS.

On January 11–12, China made genome sequencing of novel coronavirus publicly available, for other countries to develop specific diagnostic kits.

On January 13, the first case of novel coronavirus outside of China was confirmed in Thailand.

On January 23, the members of the International Health Regulations Emergency Committee decided that at that time the outbreak of novel coronavirus (2019-nCoV) did not constitute a Public Health Emergency of International Concern (PHEIC), even though Human-to-human transmission was reported to occur, with a preliminary R0 estimate of 1.4–2.5 and that of confirmed cases, 25% were reported to be severe.

Only one week later, on January 30, the second meeting of the Committee agreed that the outbreak met the criteria for a PHEIC and WHO eventually declared the 2019-nCoV outbreak a PHEIC.

On February 11, novel coronavirus disease was named COVID-19.

On February 17, WHO has outlined planning considerations for organizers of mass gatherings, in light of the COVID-19 outbreak, and has issued advice on how to detect and take care of ill travelers, who are suspected COVID-19 cases at Points of Entry—international airports, seaports, and ground crossings.

By February 21, according to WHO, the window of opportunity to contain the outbreak was "narrowing" world widely and WHO itself and countries separately were engaged in large-scale preparedness activities.

By that time, through massive worldwide campaigns, individuals and businesses were instructed on how to protect themselves and others from the virus.

Despite worldwide preparation, on March 2, WHO recognized shortages of personal protective equipment, endangering health workers worldwide.

To meet rising global demand, WHO estimated that industry should increase manufacturing of personal protective equipment by 40%. Frontline health responders around the world would need at least 89 million masks, 30 million gowns, 1.6 million goggles, 76 million gloves and 2.9 million liters of hand sanitizer every month.

On March 11, WHO characterizes COVID-19 as a pandemic.

By July 1, 2020, there were over 10 million worldwide cases of CoVID-19 with over 5 million recovered and over 500,000 worldwide COVID deaths.

While there is no primary role for nuclear medicine in the diagnosis or treatment of COVID-19, a number of patients with incidental COVID-19 have undergone nuclear medicine or PET examinations (81–100). The diagnosis of COVID-19 has most often been first suspected based on CT lung findings; bilateral peripheral ground-glass consolidative pulmonary opacities (Figure 9.4). Most often these were asymptomatic, as patients with apparent signs and symptoms of COVID are generally diverted from the nuclear medicine scanning environment (101–104).

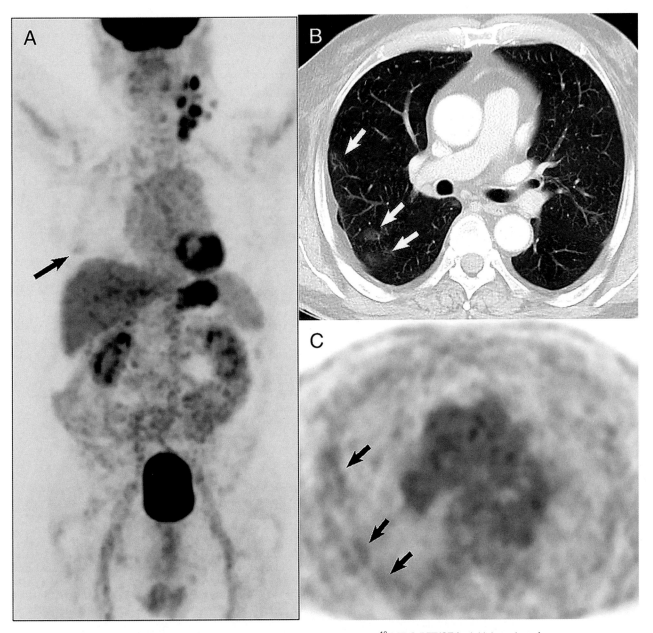

FIG. 9.4 ● This 70-year-old asymptomatic man from La Rioja, Spain, underwent ¹⁸F-FDG PET/CT for initial staging of Hodgkin lymphoma. His diagnostic workup included contrast-enhanced CT, followed by 18F-FDG PET/CT, with both examinations reported together. He had no clinical evidence for COVID-19 infection including no known risk contacts.

(Continued)

FIG. 9.4 ● (Continued) MIP images (A) showed bilateral cervical lymphadenopathy with abnormal ^{18}F-FDG uptake, predominantly in the left side (SUVmax, 9.0). The right lower lung (arrow, A) had ill-defined low-grade activity (SUVmax, 2.4). On CT (B), there were bilateral tree-in-bud opacities and several peripheral and subpleural ground-glass opacities (GGO), predominantly in the right lung (arrows). These showed mild activity on axial PET (arrows, C). GGOs have been reported as a primary CT findings in COVID-19, whereas pleural effusions and the tree-in-bud sign are atypical in COVID-19, possibly related to complications (pleural effusions) or superadded bacterial infection (tree-in-bud sign). Although the patient was asymptomatic, with no fever or cough, his CT findings were typical for COVID-19. The same day as the PET/CT, a reverse transcriptase-polymerase chain reaction (RT-PCR) test had negative results for COVID-19 virus. Given the high clinical suspicion for COVID-19, the patient was immediately isolated, and a repeat RT-PCR at 72 hours was positive for COVID-19. Repeat laboratory tests showed high IL-6 (4.4 pg/mL) and ferritin (1433 ng/mL), with normal D-dimer (<200 µg/L), lymphocytes, and LDH (127 units/L). Reprinted with permission from Boulvard Chollet et al. (100).

References

1. Salmanoglu E, Kim S, Thakur ML. Currently Available radiopharmaceuticals for imaging infection and the Holy Grail. *Semin Nucl Med.* 2018;48(2):86–99.
2. Boerman OC, Rennen H, Oyen WJ, Corstens FH. Radiopharmaceuticals to image infection and inflammation. *Semin Nucl Med.* 2001;31(4):286–295.
3. Signore A, Jamar F, Israel O, Buscombe J, Martin-Comin J, Lazzeri E. Clinical indications, image acquisition and data interpretation for white blood cells and anti-granulocyte monoclonal antibody scintigraphy: an EANM procedural guideline. *Eur J Nucl Med Mol Imaging.* 2018;45(10):1816–1831.
4. Ady J, Fong Y. Imaging for infection: from visualization of inflammation to visualization of microbes. *Surg Infect.* 2014;15(6):700–707.
5. Glaudemans AW, Israel O, Slart RH. Pitfalls and limitations of radionuclide and hybrid imaging in infection and inflammation. *Semin Nucl Med.* 2015;45(6):500–512.
6. Larson SM. Cancer or inflammation? A Holy Grail for nuclear medicine. *J Nucl Med.* 1994;35(10):1653–1655.
7. Strauss LG. Fluorine-18 deoxyglucose and false-positive results: a major problem in the diagnostics of oncological patients. *Eur J Nucl Med.* 1996;23(10):1409–1415.
8. Tahara T, Ichiya Y, Kuwabara Y, et al. High [18F]-fluorodeoxyglucose uptake in abdominal abscesses: a PET study. *J Comput Assist Tomogr.* 1989;13(5):829–831.
9. Sugawara Y, Gutowski TD, Fisher SJ, Brown RS, Wahl RL. Uptake of positron emission tomography tracers in experimental bacterial infections: a comparative biodistribution study of radiolabeled FDG, thymidine, L-methionine, 67Ga-citrate, and 125I-HSA. *Eur J Nucl Med.* 1999;26(4):333–341.
10. Yamada S, Kubota K, Kubota R, Ido T, Tamahashi N. High accumulation of fluorine-18-fluorodeoxyglucose in turpentine-induced inflammatory tissue. *J Nucl Med.* 1995;36(7):1301–1306.
11. Jamar F, Buscombe J, Chiti A, et al. EANM/SNMMI guideline for 18F-FDG use in inflammation and infection. *J Nucl Med.* 2013;54(4):647–658.
12. Boellaard R, Delgado-Bolton R, Oyen WJ, et al. FDG PET/CT: EANM procedure guidelines for tumour imaging: version 2.0. *Eur J Nucl Med Mol Imaging.* 2015;42(2):328–354.
13. Zhao S, Kuge Y, Tsukamoto E, et al. Effects of insulin and glucose loading on FDG uptake in experimental malignant tumours and inflammatory lesions. *Eur J Nucl Med.* 2001;28(6):730–735.
14. Zhuang HM, Cortes-Blanco A, Pourdehnad M, et al. Do high glucose levels have differential effect on FDG uptake in inflammatory and malignant disorders? *Nucl Med Commun.* 2001;22(10):1123–1128.
15. Rabkin Z, Israel O, Keidar Z. Do hyperglycemia and diabetes affect the incidence of false-negative 18F-FDG PET/CT studies in patients evaluated for infection or inflammation and cancer? A Comparative analysis. *J Nucl Med.* 2010;51(7):1015–1020.
16. Osborne MT, Hulten EA, Murthy VL, et al. Patient preparation for cardiac fluorine-18 fluorodeoxyglucose positron emission tomography imaging of inflammation. *J Nucl Cardiol.* 2017;24(1):86–99.
17. Nielsen BD, Gormsen LC, Hansen IT, Keller KK, Therkildsen P, Hauge EM. Three days of high-dose glucocorticoid treatment attenuates large-vessel 18F-FDG uptake in large-vessel giant cell arteritis but with a limited impact on diagnostic accuracy. *Eur J Nucl Med Mol Imaging.* 2018;45(7):1119–1128.
18. Elgazzar AH, Dannoon S, Sarikaya I, Farghali M, Junaid TA. Scintigraphic patterns of indium-111 oxine-labeled white blood cell imaging of gram-negative versus gram-positive vertebral osteomyelitis. *Med Princ Pract.* 2017;26(5):415–420.
19. Lewis SS, Cox GM, Stout JE. Clinical utility of indium 111-labeled white blood cell scintigraphy for evaluation of suspected infection. *Open Forum Infect Dis.* 2014;1(2):ofu089.
20. Mulders-Manders C, Simon A, Bleeker-Rovers C. Fever of unknown origin. *Clin Med (Lond).* 2015;15(3):280–284.
21. Petersdorf RG, Beeson PB. Fever of unexplained origin: report on 100 cases. *Medicine.* 1961;40:1–30.
22. Palestro CJ, Love C. Nuclear medicine imaging in fever of unknown origin: the new paradigm. *Curr Pharm Des.* 2018;24(7):814–820.
23. Besson FL, Chaumet-Riffaud P, Playe M, et al. Contribution of (18)F-FDG PET in the diagnostic assessment of fever of unknown origin (FUO): a stratification-based meta-analysis. *Eur J Nucl Med Mol Imaging.* 2016;43(10):1887–1895.
24. Takeuchi M, Nihashi T, Gafter-Gvili A, et al. Association of 18F-FDG PET or PET/CT results with spontaneous remission in classic fever of unknown origin: A systematic review and meta-analysis. *Medicine.* 2018;97(43):e12909.
25. Takeuchi M, Dahabreh IJ, Nihashi T, Iwata M, Varghese GM, Terasawa T. Nuclear imaging for classic fever of unknown origin: meta-analysis. *J Nucl Med.* 2016;57(12):1913–1919.
26. Dong MJ, Zhao K, Liu ZF, Wang GL, Yang SY, Zhou GJ. A meta-analysis of the value of fluorodeoxyglucose-PET/PET-CT in the evaluation of fever of unknown origin. *Eur J Radiol.* 2011;80(3):834–844.
27. Hao R, Yuan L, Kan Y, Li C, Yang J. Diagnostic performance of 18F-FDG PET/CT in patients with fever of unknown origin: a meta-analysis. *Nucl Med Commun.* 2013;34(7):682–688.
28. Kan Y, Wang W, Liu J, Yang J, Wang Z. Contribution of 18F-FDG PET/CT in a case-mix of fever of unknown origin and inflammation of unknown origin: a meta-analysis. *Acta Radiol.* 2019;60(6):716–725.
29. Hess S. FDG-PET/CT in fever of unknown origin, bacteremia, and febrile neutropenia. *PET Clin.* 2020;15(2):(in press).
30. Balink H, Veeger NJ, Bennink RJ, et al. The predictive value of C-reactive protein and erythrocyte sedimentation rate for 18F-FDG PET/CT outcome in patients with fever and inflammation of unknown origin. *Nucl Med Commun.* 2015;36(6):604–609.
31. Bleeker-Rovers CP, Vos FJ, Mudde AH, et al. A prospective multi-centre study of the value of FDG-PET as part of a structured diagnostic protocol in patients with fever of unknown origin. *Eur J Nucl Med Mol Imaging.* 2007;34(5):694–703.
32. Kouijzer IJ, Vos FJ, Bleeker-Rovers CP, Oyen WJ. Clinical application of FDG-PET/CT in metastatic infections. *Q J Nucl Med Mol Imaging.* 2017;61(2):232–246.
33. Vos FJ, Bleeker-Rovers CP, Sturm PD, et al. 18F-FDG PET/CT for detection of metastatic infection in gram-positive bacteremia. *J Nucl Med.* 2010;51(8):1234–1240.

34. Vos FJ, Kullberg BJ, Sturm PD, et al. Metastatic infectious disease and clinical outcome in Staphylococcus aureus and Streptococcus species bacteremia. *Medicine.* 2012;91(2):86–94.

35. Berrevoets MAH, Kouijzer IJE, Aarntzen E, et al. (18)F-FDG PET/CT optimizes treatment in staphylococcus aureus bacteremia and is associated with reduced mortality. *J Nucl Med.* 2017;58(9):1504–1510.

36. Tsai HY, Lee MH, Wan CH, Yang LY, Yen TC, Tseng JR. C-reactive protein levels can predict positive (18)F-FDG PET/CT findings that lead to management changes in patients with bacteremia. *J Microbiol Immunol Infect.* 2018;51(6):839–846.

37. Brondserud MB, Pedersen C, Rosenvinge FS, Hoilund-Carlsen PF, Hess S. Clinical value of FDG-PET/CT in bacteremia of unknown origin with catalase-negative gram-positive cocci or Staphylococcus aureus. *Eur J Nucl Med Mol Imaging.* 2019;46(6):1351–1358.

38. Pijl JP, Glaudemans A, Slart R, Yakar D, Wouthuyzen-Bakker M, Kwee TC. FDG-PET/CT for detecting an infection focus in patients with bloodstream infection: factors affecting diagnostic yield. *Clin Nucl Med.* 2019;44(2):99–106.

39. Yildiz H, Reychler G, Rodriguez-Villalobos H, et al. Mortality in patients with high risk Staphylococcus aureus bacteremia undergoing or not PET-CT: a single center experience. *J Infect Chemother.* 2019;25(11):880–885.

40. Berrevoets MAH, Kouijzer IJE, Slieker K, et al. (18)F-FDG-PET/CT-guided treatment duration in patients with high-risk Staphylococcus aureus bacteremia: a proof of principle. *J Nucl Med.* 2019;60(7):998–1002.

41. Vos FJ, Donnelly JP, Oyen WJG, Kullberg BJ, Bleeker-Rovers CP, Blijlevens NMA. 18F-FDG PET/CT for diagnosing infectious complications in patients with severe neutropenia after intensive chemotherapy for haematological malignancy or stem cell transplantation. *Eur J Nucl Med Mol Imaging.* 2012;39(1):120–128.

42. Koh KC, Slavin MA, Thursky KA, et al. Impact of fluorine-18 fluorodeoxyglucose positron emission tomography on diagnosis and antimicrobial utilization in patients with high-risk febrile neutropenia. *Leuk Lymphoma.* 2012;53(10):1889–1895.

43. Guy SD, Tramontana AR, Worth LJ, et al. Use of FDG PET/CT for investigation of febrile neutropenia: evaluation in high-risk cancer patients. *Eur J Nucl Med Mol Imaging.* 2012;39(8):1348–1355.

44. Gafter-Gvili A, Paul M, Bernstine H, et al. The role of (1)(8)F-FDG PET/CT for the diagnosis of infections in patients with hematological malignancies and persistent febrile neutropenia. *Leuk Res.* 2013;37(9):1057–1062.

45. Camus V, Edet-Sanson A, Bubenheim M, et al. (1)(8)F-FDG-PET/CT imaging in patients with febrile neutropenia and haematological malignancies. *Anticancer Res.* 2015;35(5):2999–3005.

46. Gholami S, Fardin S, Houshmand S, Hansson SH, Alavi A, Hess S. Applications of FDG-PET/CT in assessment of vascular infection and inflammation. *Cur Mol Imaging (Discontinued).* 2014;3(3):230–239.

47. Nielsen BD, Gormsen LC. 18F-FDG PET/CT in the diagnosis and monitoring of giant cell arteritis. *PET Clin.* 2020;15(2):(in press).

48. Besson FL, Parienti JJ, Bienvenu B, et al. Diagnostic performance of (1)(8)F-fluorodeoxyglucose positron emission tomography in giant cell arteritis: a systematic review and meta-analysis. *Eur J Nuc Med Mol Imaging.* 2011;38(9):1764–1772.

49. Soussan M, Nicolas P, Schramm C, et al. Management of large-vessel vasculitis with FDG-PET: a systematic literature review and meta-analysis. *Medicine.* 2015;94(14):e622.

50. Nielsen BD, Hansen IT, Kramer S, et al. Simple dichotomous assessment of cranial artery inflammation by conventional 18F-FDG PET/CT shows high accuracy for the diagnosis of giant cell arteritis: a case-control study. *Eur J Nucl Med Mol Imaging.* 2019;46(1):184–193.

51. Sammel AM, Hsiao E, Schembri G, et al. Diagnostic accuracy of positron emission tomography/computed tomography of the head, neck, and chest for giant cell arteritis: a prospective, double-blind, cross-sectional study. *Arthritis Rheumatol.* 2019;71(8):1319–1328.

52. Termaat MF, Raijmakers PG, Scholten HJ, Bakker FC, Patka P, Haarman HJ. The accuracy of diagnostic imaging for the assessment of chronic osteomyelitis: a systematic review and meta-analysis. *J Bone Jt Surg Am.* 2005;87(11):2464–2471.

53. Kwee TC, Basu S, Alavi A. Should the nuclear medicine community continue to underestimate the potential of 18F-FDG PET/CT with present generation scanners for the diagnosis of prosthetic joint infection? *Nucl Med Commun.* 2015;36(7):756–757.

54. Sollini M, Lauri C, Boni R, Lazzeri E, Erba PA, Signore A. Current status of molecular imaging in infections. *Curr Pharm Des.* 2018;24(7):754–771.

55. Govaert GA, FF IJ, McNally M, McNally E, Reininga IH, Glaudemans AW. Accuracy of diagnostic imaging modalities for peripheral post-traumatic osteomyelitis - a systematic review of the recent literature. *Eur J Nucl Med Mol Imaging.* 2017;44(8):1393–1407.

56. Wang GL, Zhao K, Liu ZF, Dong MJ, Yang SY. A meta-analysis of fluorodeoxyglucose-positron emission tomography versus scintigraphy in the evaluation of suspected osteomyelitis. *Nucl Med Commun.* 2011;32(12):1134–1142.

57. Prodromou ML, Ziakas PD, Poulou LS, Karsaliakos P, Thanos L, Mylonakis E. FDG PET is a robust tool for the diagnosis of spondylodiscitis: a meta-analysis of diagnostic data. *Clin Nucl Med.* 2014;39(4):330–335.

58. Yin Y, Liu X, Yang X, Guo J, Wang Q, Chen L. Diagnostic value of FDG-PET versus magnetic resonance imaging for detecting spondylitis: a systematic review and meta-analysis. *Spine J.* 2018;18(12):2323–2332.

59. Kim SJ, Pak K, Kim K, Lee JS. Comparing the diagnostic accuracies of F-18 fluorodeoxyglucose positron emission tomography and magnetic resonance imaging for the detection of spondylodiscitis: a meta-analysis. *Spine.* 2019;44(7):E414–e422.

60. Smids C, Kouijzer IJ, Vos FJ, et al. A comparison of the diagnostic value of MRI and (18)F-FDG PET/CT in suspected spondylodiscitis. *Infection.* 2017;45(1):41–49.

61. Palestro CJ, Love C. Role of nuclear medicine for diagnosing infection of recently implanted lower extremity arthroplasties. *Semin Nucl Med.* 2017;47(6):630–638.

62. Treglia G. Diagnostic performance of (18)F-FDG PET/CT in infectious and inflammatory diseases according to published meta-analyses. *Contrast Media Mol Imaging.* 2019;2019:3018349.

63. Kwee TC, Kwee RM, Alavi A. FDG-PET for diagnosing prosthetic joint infection: systematic review and metaanalysis. *Eur J Nucl Med Mol Imaging.* 2008;35(11):2122–2132.

64. Basu S, Kwee TC, Saboury B, et al. FDG PET for diagnosing infection in hip and knee prostheses: prospective study in 221 prostheses and subgroup comparison with combined (111)In-labeled leukocyte/(99m)Tc-sulfur colloid bone marrow imaging in 88 prostheses. *Clin Nucl Med.* 2014;39(7):609–615.

65. Sunde SK, Beske T, Gerke O, Clausen LL, Hess S. FDG-PET/CT as a diagnostic tool in vascular graft infection: a systematic review and meta-analysis. *Clin Trans Imaging.* 2019;7(4):255–265.

66. Rojoa D, Kontopodis N, Antoniou SA, Ioannou CV, Antoniou GA. 18F-FDG PET in the diagnosis of vascular prosthetic graft infection: a diagnostic test accuracy meta-analysis. *Eur J Vasc Endovasc Surg.* 2019;57(2):292–301.

67. Reinders Folmer EI, Von Meijenfeldt GCI, Van der Laan MJ, et al. Diagnostic imaging in vascular graft infection: a systematic review and meta-analysis. *Eur J Vasc Endovasc Surg.* 2018;56(5):719–729.

68. Erba PA, Leo G, Sollini M, et al. Radiolabelled leucocyte scintigraphy versus conventional radiological imaging for the management of late, low-grade vascular prosthesis infections. *Eur J Nucl Med Mol Imaging.* 2014;41(2):357–368.

69. Puges M, Berard X, Ruiz JB, et al. Retrospective study comparing WBC scan and (18)F-FDG PET/CT in patients with suspected prosthetic vascular graft infection. *Eur J Vasc Endovasc Surg.* 2019;57(6):876–884.

70. de Camargo RA, Bitencourt MS, Meneghetti JC, et al. The role of 18F-FDG-PET/CT in the Diagnosis of left-sided Endocarditis: native vs. prosthetic valves endocarditis. *Clin Infect Dis.* 2020;70(4): 583–594.

71. Rouzet F, Chequer R, Benali K, et al. Respective performance of 18F-FDG PET and radiolabeled leukocyte scintigraphy for the diagnosis of prosthetic valve endocarditis. *J Nucl Med.* 2014;55(12):1980–1985.

72. Lauridsen TK, Iversen KK, Ihlemann N, et al. Clinical utility of (18) F-FDG positron emission tomography/computed tomography scan vs. (99m)Tc-HMPAO white blood cell single-photon emission computed tomography in extra-cardiac work-up of infective endocarditis. *Int J Cardiovasc Imaging.* 2017;33(5):751–760.

73. Juneau D, Golfam M, Hazra S, et al. Molecular Imaging for the diagnosis of infective endocarditis: A systematic literature review and meta-analysis. *Int J Cardiol.* 2018;253:183–188.

74. Holcman K, Malecka B, Rubis P, et al. The role of 99mTc-HMPAO-labelled white blood cell scintigraphy in the diagnosis of cardiac device-related infective endocarditis. *Eur Heart J Cardiovasc Imaging.* 2020;21(9):1022–1030.

75. Alavi A, Hess S, Werner TJ, Hoilund-Carlsen PF. An update on the unparalleled impact of FDG-PET imaging on the day-to-day practice of medicine with emphasis on management of infectious/inflammatory disorders. *Eur J Nucl Med Mol Imaging.* 2020;47(1):18–27.

76. Hess S, Blomberg BA, Zhu HJ, Hoilund-Carlsen PF, Alavi A. The pivotal role of FDG-PET/CT in modern medicine. *Acad Radiol.* 2014;21(2):232–249.

77. Hess S, Blomberg BA, Rakheja R, et al. A brief overview of novel approaches to FDG PET imaging and quantification. *Clin Transl Imaging.* 2014;2:11.

78. Sollini M, Berchiolli R, Kirienko M, et al. PET/MRI in infection and inflammation. *Semin Nucl Med.* 2018;48(3):225–241.

79. Auletta S, Galli F, Lauri C, Martinelli D, Santino I, Signore A. Imaging bacteria with radiolabelled quinolones, cephalosporins and siderophores for imaging infection: a systematic review. *Clin Transl Imaging.* 2016;4:229–252.

80. Auletta S, Varani M, Horvat R, Galli F, Signore A, Hess S. PET radiopharmaceuticals for specific bacteria imaging: a systematic review. *J Clin Med.* 2019;8(2):197.

81. Doroudinia A, Tavakoli M. A case of coronavirus infection incidentally found on FDG PET/CT scan. *Clin Nucl Med.* 2020;45: e303–e304

82. Liu C, Zhou J, Xia L, et al. 18F-FDG PET/CT and serial chest CT findings in a COVID-19 patient with dynamic clinical characteristics in different period. *Clin Nucl Med.* 2020;45:495–496.

83. Playe M, Siavellis J, MD, Braun T, Soussan M. FDG PET/CT in a patient with mantle cell lymphoma and COVID-19: typical findings. *Clin Nucl Med.* 2020;45:e305–e306.

84. Prabhu M, Raju S, Chakraborty D, et al. Spectrum of 18F-FDG uptake in bilateral lung parenchymal diseases on PET/ CT. *Clin Nucl Med.* 2020;45:e15–e19.

85. Sinha P, Sinha S, Schleh E, Schlehr JM. COVID-19: incidental diagnosis by 18F-FDG PET/CT. *Clin Nucl Med.* 2020;00:00–00.

86. Artigas C, Lemort M, Mestrez F, et al. COVID-19 pneumonia mimicking immunotherapy-induced pneumonitis on 18F-FDG PET/ CT in a patient under treatment with nivolumab. *Clin Nucl Med.* 2020;00:00–00.

87. Goetz C, Fassbender TF, Meyer PT. Lung scintigraphy imaging features in a young patient with COVID-19. *Clin Nucl Med.* 2020;00: 00–0.0

88. Qin C, Liu F, Yen TC, et al. 18F-FDG PET/CT findings of COVID-19: a series of four highly suspected cases. *Eur J Nucl Med Mol Imaging.* 2020;47(5):1281–1286.

89. Xu X, Yu C, Qu J, et al. Imaging and clinical features of patients with 2019 novel coronavirus SARS-CoV-2. *Eur J Nucl Med Mol Imaging.* 2020;47:1275–1280.

90. Albano D, Bertagna F, Bertolia M, et al. Incidental findings suggestive of COVID-19 in asymptomatic patients undergoing nuclear medicine procedures in a high prevalence region. *J Nucl Med.* 2020;61(5): 632–636.

91. Zou S, Zhu X. FDG PET/CT of COVID-19. *Radiology.* 2020;296(2): E118.

92. Huang HL, Allie R, Gnanasegaran G, et al. COVID-19—nuclear medicine departments, be prepared! *Nucl Med Commun.* 2020;41: 297–299.

93. Paez D, Gnanasegaran G, Fanti S, et al. COVID-19 pandemic: guidance for nuclear medicine departments. *Eur J Nucl Med Mol Imaging.* 2020.

94. Notghi A, Pandit M, O'Brien J, et al. COVID-19: Guidance for infection prevention and control in nuclear medicine. *BNMS.* 2020:12. https://cdn.ymaws.com/www.bnms.org.uk/resource/resmgr/news_&_press_office/news/26-03-2020_nuclear_medicine_.pdf. Accessed 18 April, 2020.

95. Deng Y, Lei L, Chen Y, et al. The potential added value of FDG PET/CT for COVID-19 pneumonia. *Eur J Nucl Med Mol Imaging.* 2020.

96. Joob B, Wiwanitkit V. 18F-FDG PET/CT and COVID-19. *Eur J Nucl Med Mol Imaging.* 2020.

97. Lutje S, Marinova M, Kutting D, et al. Nuclear medicine in SARS-CoV-2 pandemia: 18F-FDG-PET/CT to visualize COVID-19. *Nuklearmedizin.* 2020.

98. Polverari G, Arena V, Ceci F, et al. 18F-FDG uptake in asymptomatic SARS-CoV-2 (COVID-19) patient, referred to PET/CT for Non-Small Cells Lung Cancer restaging. *J Thorac Oncol.* 2020. doi:10.1016/j.jtho.2020.03.022

99. Kirienko M, Padovano B, Serafini G, et al. CT, [18F]FDG-PET/CT and clinical findings before and during early COVID-19 onset in a patient affected by vascular tumour. *Eur J Nucl Med Mol Imaging.* 2020 Apr 25:1–2. [Epub ahead of print].

100. Boulvard Chollet XLE, Romero Robles LG, Garrastachu P, et al. 18F-FDG PET/CT in Hodgkin Lymphoma with unsuspected COVID-19. *Clin Nucl Med.* 2020;45(8):652–653.

101. Czernin J, Fanti S, Meyer PT, et al. Imaging clinic operations in the times of COVID-19: strategies, precautions and experiences. *J Nucl Med.* 2020 Apr 1:jnumed.120.245738.

102. Skali H, Murthy VL, Al-Mallah MH, et al. Guidance and best practices for nuclear cardiology laboratories during the coronavirus disease 2019 (COVID-19) pandemic: an information statement from ASNC and SNMMI. *Zenodo.* 2020:13. http://doi.org/10.5281/zenodo.3738020. Accessed Apr 16, 2020.

103. Tulchinsky M, Fotos JS, Slonimsky E. Incidental CT findings suspicious for Covid-19 associated pneumonia on nuclear medicine exams: recognition and management plan. *Clin Nucl Med.* 2020;45:531–533.

104. Lu Y, Zhu X, Yan SX, Lan X. Emerging attack and management strategies for nuclear medicine in responding to COVID-19—ACNM member experience and advice. *Clin Nucl Med.* 2020;45:534–535.

CHAPTER SELF-ASSESSMENT QUESTIONS

1. This 35-year-old man has fever shortness of breath and cough. What is the most likely diagnosis?

   A. Chronic Bronchitis

   B. Cystic Fibrosis

   C. Mounier-Kuhn syndrome

   D. Relapsing polychondritis

2. This 82-year-old man has renal failure and difficulty voiding and abdominal pain. What is the most likely diagnosis?

   A. Carcinoid

   B. Crohn's disease

   C. IgG4 disease

   D. Lymphoma

   E. Sarcoidosis

   F. Tuberculosis

3. This 23-year-old woman has fever and malaise. What is her most likely diagnosis?

   A. ASVD

   B. Giant cell

   C. PAN

   D. Takayasu

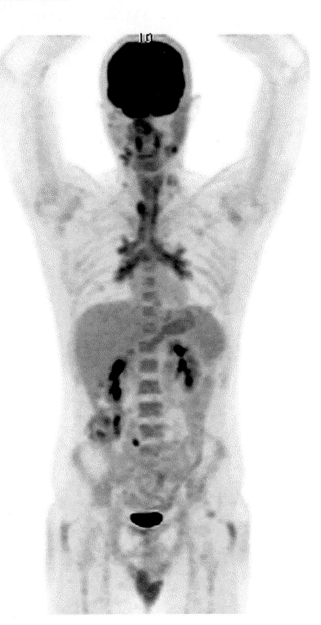

Answers to Chapter Self-Assessment Questions

1. The abnormal finding is increased central bronchotracheal activity, SUVmax = 13.8. This activity is much greater than expected for chronic bronchitis (A), cystic fibrosis (B) or Mounier-Kuhn Syndrome (C). The prominent central bronchotracheal activity is typical for relapsing polychondritis (D).

2. The abnormal findings are increased bilateral hilar, renal, pancreatic, aortoiliac, and pancreatic activity. Carcinoid (A), Crohn's disease (B), Lymphoma (D), Sarcoidosis (E), and Tuberculosis (F) would not be expected to have all of these findings. The correct answer is IgG4 disease (C). Adenopathy and pancreatic involvement are common. Nephritis, prostatitis, and vasculitis may all occur. Chronic pancreatitis with biliary obstruction was a recurrent problem in this patient.

3. There is increased aortic, brachial cephalic, and iliac arterial activity. ASVD (A) and Giant cell arteritis (B) would be most unusual in this 23-year-old woman. PAN would be expected to involve smaller arteries than is demonstrated in this patient. Thus, the correct answer is Takayasu.

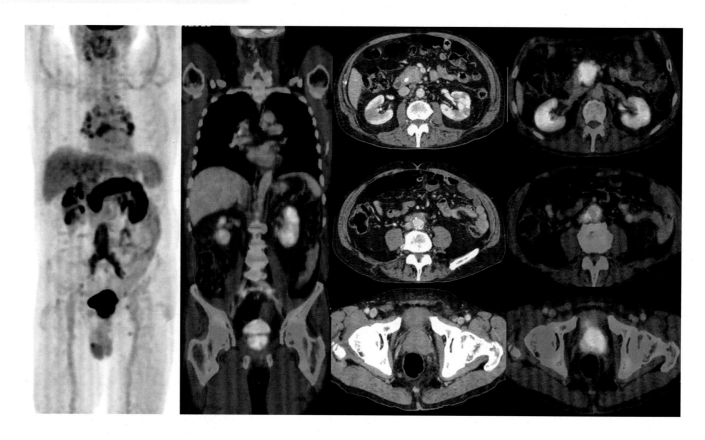

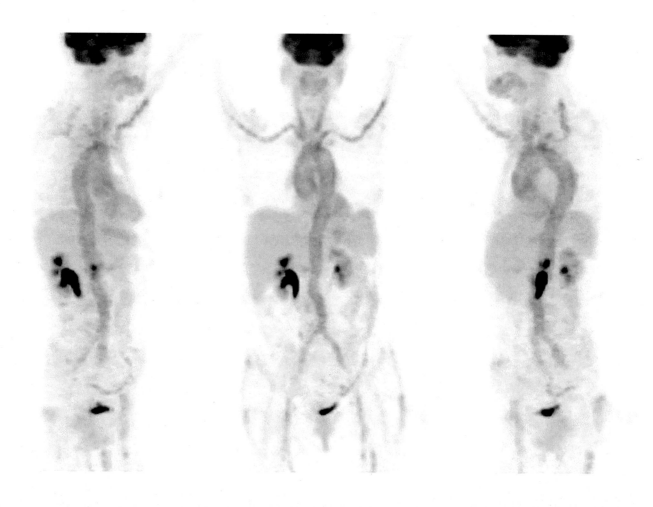

Cardiovascular Nuclear Medicine

10

Patrick M. Colletti

LEARNING OBJECTIVES

1. Determine myocardial function with gated blood pool imaging.
2. Interpret myocardial volumes and ejection fraction with myocardial perfusion single photon emission computed tomography (SPECT).
3. Select the optimal myocardial perfusion agent based on required performance.
4. Select the appropriate myocardial stress method based on patient presentation.
5. Interpret and report myocardial perfusion SPECT exams.
6. Apply nuclear medicine techniques to evaluate myocardial viability.
7. Select the optimal method for the diagnosis of cardiovascular infection.
8. Select and optimize methods for the diagnosis of myocardial sarcoidosis.
9. Diagnosis and interpret pyrophosphate myocardial SPECT in suspected myocardial amyloidosis.

MYOCARDIAL FUNCTION

Myocardial function is examined with gated blood pool imaging and myocardial perfusion imaging. Gated blood pool imaging, also known as "MUGA," for "multiple gated acquisition" is a quantitative technique performed most commonly when reliable and reproducible left ventricle ejection fractions are required, typically to evaluate and follow patients treated with cardiotoxic drugs (1).

The blood pool is labeled with technetium-99m (Table 10.1) either with a modified in vivo or more reliably with an in vitro technique. Both methods use the reducing agent stannous pyrophosphate to deliver stannous ion to red cell where ^{99m}Tc-pertechnetate will later bind to hemoglobin.

Upon tagging of the blood pool, sequential electrocardiogram (ECG)-gated images are then acquired in anterior, left anterior oblique (LAO), and lateral views. The best LAO view is selected for separation of the ventricles. Caudal–cephalic tilting may help in separating the left ventricle from the left atrium. The end-diastolic frame is acquired at the "R" wave and the R-R cycle is divided into 24 frames with an R-R tolerance window set at between 10% and 20% (1).

The left ventricular ejection fraction is calculated as

$$LVEF = \{[ED - ES]/[ED - Bk]\} \times 100\%$$

where
LVEF = Left ventricular ejection fraction,
ED = End-diastolic counts,
ES = End-systolic counts,
Bk = Background counts.

The placement of the three region of interests (ROIs) is important, as misplacement results in erroneous ejection fraction calculations (Fig. 10.1).

Figure 10.2 shows adriamycin cardiotoxicity in a 55-year-old woman with breast cancer presenting with shortness of breath; end-diastolic frames in red, end-systolic frames in green, background in yellow.

Top row: initial examination prior to chemotherapy; LVEF = 60% at 65 bpm.

Bottom row: follow-up exam upon completion of chemotherapy; LVEF = 30% at 93 bpm. Note the visually dilated end-systolic frame.

Myocardial function can also be reliably quantitated with gated myocardial perfusion SPECT or positron emission tomography (PET) imaging. In fact, the myocardial volumes measured at SPECT and PET are similar to those measured with cardiac magnetic resonance (MR) (2). A significant advantage for SPECT and PET is the ease with which these volumes are determined after simply locating the myocardium and allowing the computer to rapidly present the results for end-diastolic volume, end-systolic volume, left ventricular ejection fraction, and myocardial mass.

Table 10.2 presents some typical cardiac volumes with their calculated LVEFs and cardiac outputs for a given heart rate. We can see that the LVEF is a global measure of left ventricular health and the simple measurement of LVEF is strongly associated with cardiac outcomes. The normal LVEF is on the order of 65% with a range of between 50% and 80%. LVEFs measured for smaller hearts may be falsely elevated by MUGA or by gated

Table 10.1 **RBC LABELING TECHNIQUES**

Labeling Technique	Advantages	Disadvantages
In vivo	Simple and rapid No risk of blood handling	Incomplete labeling with higher background activity More sensitive to confounding drugs
In vivo/in vitro	Faster than in vitro labeling	Labeling efficient less than in vitro Some handling of blood
In vitro	Highest labeling efficiency and stability	Risk of blood handling Patient blood identification errors Requires more technical expertise More expensive, more time consuming

RBC, red blood cell(s).

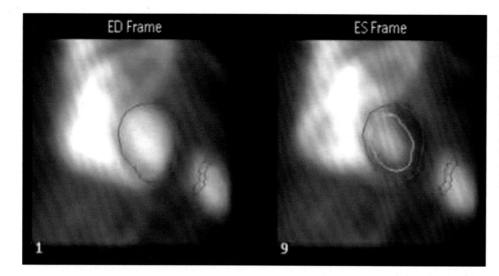

FIG. 10.1 ● **Background ROI placed over the spleen.** Misplacement of the background ROI over the spleen results in a falsely high measurement subtracted from the denominator results on a low denominator and therefore a falsely high ejection fraction. The LVEF calculated in this case was 90%. Repeat with a correctly placed background between the spleen and the LV results in the correct LVEF = 60%.

LVEF, left ventricular ejection fraction; ROI, region of interest.

Table 10.2 **MYOCARDIAL VOLUME ANALYSIS**

Condition	EDV (mL)	ESV (mL)	Stroke Volume (mL)	Ejection Fraction (%)	Cardiac Output (L/min)
Normal	150	50	100	67%	6L at 60 bpm
Dilated Cardiomyopathy	300	200	100	33%	6L at 60 bpm
Acute MI	150	100	50	33%	3L at 60 bpm 6L at 120 bpm
Chronic MI	300	200	100	33%	6L at 60 bpm
Aortic Insufficiency	300	100	200 (100 + 100 R)	67% (with 50% RF)	6L + 6L at 60 bpm
Papillary Muscle Rupture	150	50	100 (50 + 50 R)	67% (with 50% RF)	3L + 3L at 60 bpm 6L + 6L at 120 bpm
Papillary Muscle Rupture + AMI	150	100	50 (25 + 25 R)	33% (with 50% RF)	3L + 3L at 120 bpm

AMI, acute myocardial infarction; bpm, beats per minute; EDV, end-diastolic volume; ESV, end-systolic volume; MI, myocardial infarction; R, regurgitation; RF, regurgitation fraction (%).

myocardial perfusion SPECT as the small end-systolic lumen may be obscured by blur from the myocardial walls. Thus, we typically report all very high LVEFs as >80%.

Myocardial perfusion

Myocardial perfusion is typically performed with the intravenous administration of ^{99m}Tc tetrofosmin or ^{99m}Tc sestamibi during treadmill or post-coronary vasodilator regadenoson and at rest. SPECT imaging is then acquired, and images are reconstructed in the short axis, vertical long axis, and horizontal long axis (3). Relative regional myocardial perfusion can then be evaluated visually and with computer analysis.

The characteristics of myocardial perfusion imaging radiopharmaceuticals (4,5) are summarized in Table 10.3.

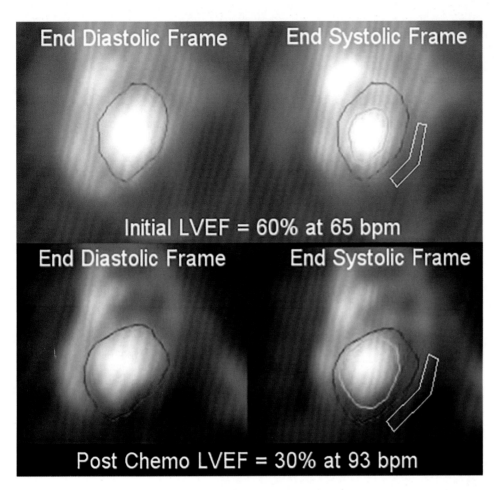

Initial LVEF = 60% at 65 bpm

Post Chemo LVEF = 30% at 93 bpm

FIG. 10.2 ● **is an example of results in a patient with LVEF of 60% at baseline dropping to 30% due to adriamycin cardiotoxicity.**

LVEF, left ventricular ejection fraction.

Table 10.3 **MYOCARDIAL PERFUSION AGENTS**

Agent	Half-life	Energy (keV)	Extraction (%)	Dose (mCi)	Radiation (mSv)
[201]Tl-chloride	73.1 h	68–80, 135, 167	85	3	7
[99m]Tc sestamibi	6 h	140	65	10–30	5
[99m]Tc tetrofosmin	6 h	140	54	10–30	5
[82]Rb-chloride	75 s	511	65	40	2.8
[13]N-ammonia	9.6 min	511	80	40	8
[18]F-flurpiridaz*	109 min	511	94	14	6.4

*Investigational radiopharmaceutical.

While ideally patients are stressed on a treadmill, many patients are unable to exercise adequately for myocardial perfusion scintigraphy. Most commonly, patients are challenged with hyperemic agents like dipyridamole, adenosine, or regadenoson, or by the β1-adrenoceptor stimulator dobutamine. Myocardial pharmacologic agents are summarized in Table 10.4.

As most gamma camera myocardial perfusion SPECT requires on the order of 10 minutes per acquisition or 6 minutes for a half acquisition exam, it is clear that data are not acquired rapidly enough to estimate absolute myocardial blood flow in mL/min/g of myocardium. Myocardial perfusion PET may be acquired in rapid list mode such that temporal resolution of between 0.2 and 10 seconds per data point may be achieved (4,5). Interestingly, rapid dynamic SPECT imaging with cadmium zinc telluride (CZT) crystal technology may achieve temporal resolution of 3 seconds with

the ability to quantitate myocardial blood flow with ^{99m}Tc sestamibi or ^{99m}Tc tetrofosmin (6).

In current practice, myocardial perfusion SPECT is interpreted visually, with or without computer-assisted interpretation. Relative activity from each myocardial region is compared to all of the other myocardial regions. Convincing defects seen only on the post-stress images are interpreted as myocardial ischemia, while regional defects noted at both rest and stress are either infarction, hibernating myocardium, or attenuation artifact. Causes for false-positive and false-negative myocardial perfusion SPECT are listed in Table 10.5.

Absence of stress-induced myocardial perfusion SPECT defects is typically noted in patients without significant coronary artery stenosis. Patients with dilated cardiomyopathy typically demonstrate a dilated left ventricle with reduced left ventricular

Table 10.4 **MYOCARDIAL PHARMACOLOGIC STRESS AGENTS**

Agent	Role	Administration
Adenosine	Hyperemic agent	140 mcg/kg/min IV over 6 min
Dipyridamole	Hyperemic agent	0.142 mg/kg/min IV over 4 min
Regadenoson	Hyperemic A2A adenosine receptor agonist	5 mL (0.4 mg) IV Push
Dobutamine	β1-Adrenoceptor stimulator	5–40 mg/kg/min IV in 3-min stages
Nitroglycerin	Coronary vasodilator viability agent	0.4 mg sublingually or 1 spray
Aminophylline	Reverses hyperemic agent effects	100 mg IV over 30–60 s

Table 10.5 **CAUSES OF MYOCARDIAL PERFUSION SPECT ERRORS**

False Positive	False Negative
Abdominal attenuation: inferior in men	"Roll off" due to low tracer extraction
Breast attenuation: anterior and lateral in women	"Balanced" triple vessel disease
Motion blur	Inadequate stress
Abdominal activity distorts myocardial SPECT	Caffeine reduces hyperemic response

SPECT, single photon emission computed tomography.

ejection fraction. Patients with elevated left atrial pressures and prolonged pulmonary transit times may also demonstrate increased lung as in Figure 10.3.

Coronary artery ischemia presents on myocardial perfusion single photon emission computed tomography (SPECT) as stress-induced defects that normalize at rest. Stress-induced defects may be associated with stress-induced wall motion abnormalities and regional dilatation as in Figures 10.4 and 10.5. Figure 10.5 also demonstrates how multivessel coronary artery disease may present as a single defect in the most severely affected region as these techniques demonstrate relative perfusion, not absolute perfusion in mL/min/g of myocardium. One may be suspicious of multivessel disease in Figure 10.5 only because of the relative stress-induced left ventricular dilatation visibly noted.

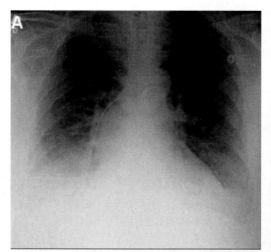
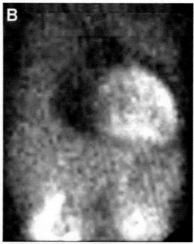
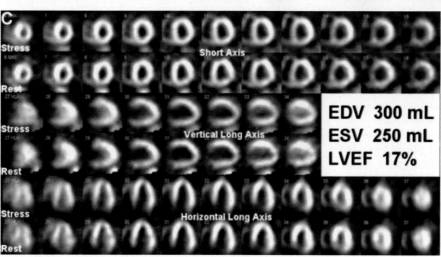

EDV 300 mL
ESV 250 mL
LVEF 17%

FIG. 10.3 ● **Shortness of breath in a 62-year-old man with dilated cardiomyopathy.** Bedside sitting AP chest radiography **(A)** demonstrates cardiomegaly, bilateral effusions, and upper lobe venous dilatation. Raw projection post-regadenoson ^{99m}Tc-tetrofosmin image **(B)** demonstrates marked bilateral lung retention typical for prolonged pulmonary transit time and elevated left atrial pressure. Myocardial perfusion SPECT **(C)** demonstrates a dilated left ventricle without perfusion defects. The left ventricle is markedly dilated with an end-diastolic volume of 300 mL and a very low 17% left ventricular ejection fraction.

AP, anterior-posterior; EDV, end-diastolic volume; ESV, end-systolic volume; LVEF, left ventricular ejection fraction; SPECT, single photon emission computed tomography.

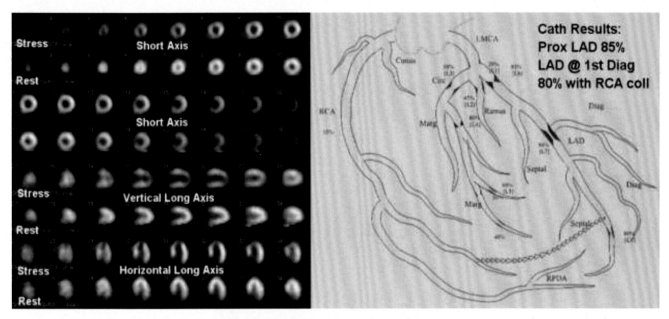

FIG. 10.4 ● **Apical septal ischemia in a 52-year-old man with 85% stenosis of the proximal LAD and 80% mid-LAD stenosis at the first diagonal branch.** Myocardial perfusion SPECT (**left**) demonstrates a large regadenoson stress-induced apical septal defect with associated dilatation. A map of the results of his coronary angiography (**right**) shows two significant LAD lesions with collateral vessels from his normal right coronary artery.

LAD, left anterior descending; RDC, right coronary artery; SPECT, single photon emission computed tomography.

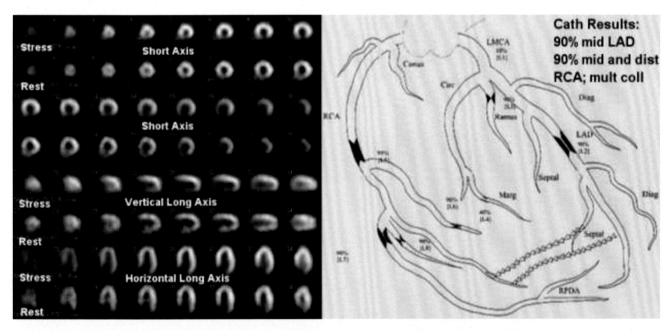

FIG. 10.5 ● **Inferior ischemia in a 58-year-old man with severe multivessel disease and right coronary occlusions with multiple collateral vessels.** Myocardial perfusion SPECT (**left**) demonstrates a large regadenoson stress-induced inferior wall defect with associated dilatation. A map of the results of his coronary angiography (**right**) shows multiple significant lesions with right coronary artery occlusion and multiple collateral vessels limited by 90% occlusion of his mid left anterior descending coronary artery.

LAD, left anterior descending; RCA, right coronary artery; SPECT, single photon emission computed tomography.

MYOCARDIAL VIABILITY

Why is viability important? Revascularization of viable myocardium improves quality of life, while revascularization of nonviable myocardium increases risk and potentially misallocates vascular resources such as the left internal mammillary artery that may more effectively be applied elsewhere.

Wall motion and thickening, uptake of any myocardial perfusion agent, or uptake of flurodeoxyglucose (FDG) are all evidence for myocardial viability. Evidence for nonviability includes delayed contrast enhancement with gadolinium- and iodine-based extracellular agents and absence of FDG activity. Myocardial thinning to less than 5 mm is also typical for nonviability.

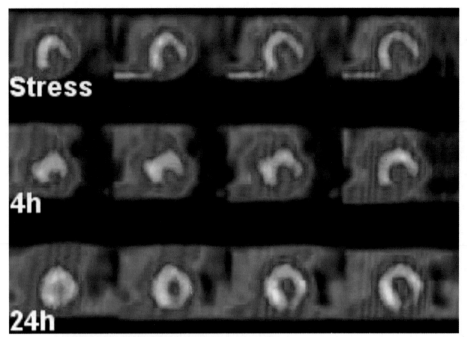

FIG. 10.6 ● **Thallium 24-hour study demonstrates viability.** This 60-year-old man presented with chest pain and shortness of breath. Regadenoson short axis images demonstrated a large inferior wall defect with transient dilatation. The apparent luminal volume is reduced on the 4-hour exam with reduction in the inferior defect but with a large seemingly fixed inferior defect typical for infarction with surrounding ischemia. By 24 hours, the residual defect is now minimal, demonstrating near total inferior wall viability. Coronary angiography demonstrated 85% RCA stenosis.

RCA, right coronary artery.

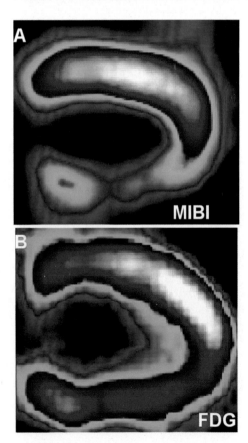

FIG. 10.7 ● **FDG demonstrates a large area of inferior wall viability.** This 61-year-old woman with hypertension and hyperlipidemia presented with shortness of breath and chest pain. Cardiac catheterization demonstrated significant triple vessel coronary stenosis and inferior akinesia. The MIBI vertical long-axis regadenoson stress (not shown) and rest **(A)** image demonstrated a large fixed inferior wall defect without wall motion. ^{18}F-FDG vertical long-axis imaging after insulin and glucose loading demonstrated inferior wall viability **(B)**. Hibernating myocardium.

FDG, flurodeoxyglucose; MIBI, sestamibi.

While dobutamine echocardiography and delayed contrast-enhanced cardiac MR are effective methods for evaluating myocardial viability, nuclear methods may be very effect. Evidence of myocardial perfusion by thallium, sestamibi, tetrofosmin, rubidium, or ammonia excludes the need for further viability analysis.

201-Thallium can be quite effective in demonstrating myocardial viability. Stress-induced or resting perfusion defects noted initially may fill in at 4 or 24 hours as thallium washes out of the normally perfused areas and appears to increase in more poorly perfused areas including hibernating myocardium (Fig. 10.6). This process may be enhanced with administration of the coronary artery dilator nitroglycerin administered as 0.4 mg sublingually or 1 spray.

[18]F-fluorodeoxyglucose PET is an appropriate agent for myocardial viability evaluation, as the ischemic or hibernating myocardium selectively metabolizes glucose , as compared to the normal myocardium which selectively metabolizes fatty acids (Fig. 10.7). Insulin is required for myocardial glucose metabolism, so control of insulin is important when myocardial FDG uptake is desirable, as in myocardial viability analysis (7,8), or when myocardial FDG is undesirable, as in routine cancer imaging, or especially when the myocardium is to be analyzed for tumor or sarcoid lesions (9). Alternatively, low-dose heparin may have lipolytic activity capable of markedly lowering fatty acids, driving the myocardium to selectively metabolize glucose as a preparation for FDG myocardial viability imaging (10). Tables 10.6 and 10.7 compare the available methods for evaluating myocardial viability.

INFECTIVE, INFLAMMATORY, AND DEPOSITION-RELATED CONDITIONS

While the metastatic infections resulting from endocarditis and septic emboli are readily detected with ^{111}In-white blood cell(s) (WBCs) (11) or ^{18}F-FDG PET/CT (12–15), the causal valvular vegetations are more difficult to detect (Fig. 10.8).

The addition of SPECT/CT to ^{111}In-WBC exams may be helpful although the routine availability of flurodeoxyglucose positron emission tomography/ computed tomography (FDG PET/CT) may

Table 10.6 PATIENT PREPARATION FOR ^{18}F-FDG MYOCARDIAL PET

Viability Studies (7,8)		Sarcoidosis (9)	
6-h fast followed by glucose loading plus insulin		*High-fat, low-carb diet 3 d before FDG-PET/CT*	
Fasting BG < 250 mg/dL	Oral glucose loading (25–100 g orally)	Permitted foods	Poultry, fish, and meat; eggs; non-sweet butter; non-
Fasting BG > 250 mg/dL	Glucose not necessary		processed cheese; animal and vegetable oil;
BG at 45–90 min after glucose loading:	Suggested insulin dose		Non-starchy vegetables; water or coffee or tea without milk or sugar
130–140 mg/dL	1U regular insulin		
140–160 mg/dL	2U regular insulin	Prohibited foods	Sugar, sugar substitutes, pastas, bread, rice, cereal, starchy
160–180 mg/dL	3U regular insulin		vegetables, fruits, milk, candy or
180–200 mg/dL	5U regular insulin		gum, barbeque or salad sauce, alcohol in any form
>200 mg/dL	Reassess patient; Consider scanning after 5U regular insulin*	At least 4 h prior to FDG administration	Fried chicken or bacon; omelet with 4 eggs; at least 2 spoons of olive oil; water or black coffee

*It may be advantageous to delay scanning to 60–90 min in patient with diabetes.
BG, blood glucose; CT, computed tomography; FDG, flurodeoxyglucose; PET, positron emission tomography.

Table 10.7 MYOCARDIAL VIABILITY STUDIES

Method	Advantages	Disadvantages
Dobutamine echo	Shows viability and function (30 min)	Dobutamine risk Less helpful with DCM
24-h thallium	Also evaluate ischemia	Low sensitivity 24-h delay
FDG PET	Metabolic viability (2 h)	Less available; need insulin-glucose clamp
Delayed CE-MRI	Available, rapid (20 min), easy to visualize	Displays nonviability Difficult with cardiac devices
Delayed CE-CT	Available, rapid (20 min), easy to visualize	Displays nonviability Contrast agent, radiation

CE, contrast enhanced; CT, computed tomography; DCM, dilated cardiomyopathy; FDG, flurodeoxyglucose; MRI, magnetic resonance imaging; PET, positron emission tomography.

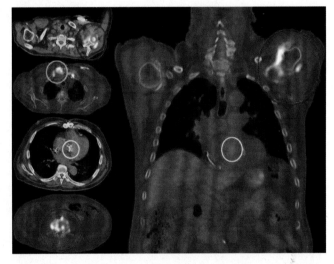

FIG. 10.8 ● *Staphylococcus aureus* bioprosthetic aortic valve endocarditis with sepsis and multiple infections in a 62-year-old man. ^{18}F-FDG PET/CT demonstrates symptomatic pyogenic infections of the left shoulder (red circles), right sternoclavicular joint (green circle), and L3–L4 disk space (blue circle) with SUVmax ranging from 16 to 23. There is relatively lower activity SUVmax = 6 in the prosthetic aortic valve (yellow circles), which was positive for vegetations by transesophageal echocardiography.

CT, computed tomography; FDG, flurodeoxyglucose; MIBI, sestamibi; PET, positron emission tomography.

be advantageous. Ideally, patients evaluated with FDG PET/CT for cardiac infections should be prepped for their exam in a manner as similar as possible to preparation for cancer or myocardial sarcoidosis (low-carb, high-fat diet) (9), as normal myocardial FDG metabolism confounds evaluation of infection and inflammation.

Myocardial sarcoidosis is associated with difficult to manage ventricular arrhythmias including multifocal ventricular tachycardia and ventricular fibrillation. Patients with myocardial sarcoidosis are often treated with implantable cardioverter defibrillato (ICDs), immunosuppressive therapy, and chronic corticosteroid coverage. The presence of ICDs makes cardiac MRI impractical for most patients with myocardial sarcoidosis. In addition, cardiac MR may be difficult to interpret due to the heterogenous distribution of the condition, especially if the patient has an arrhythmia. Thus, ^{18}F-FDG PET/CT has become more popular for diagnosing and following the activity of the myocardial lesions of sarcoidosis

(16–18). Proper patient preparation with a low-carb, high-fat diet is essential for satisfactory FDG PET/CT exams (Table 10.6). Typical patient FDG PET/CT examinations for myocardial sarcoid are demonstrated in Figures 10.9 and 10.10.

Myocardial amyloidosis is caused by amyloid deposits related to misfolded light chain (AL) or transthyretin (TTR) proteins. Patients with myocardial TTR amyloidosis may present with heart failure. Myocardial amyloid deposition associated with wild-type TTR may cause a restrictive cardiomyopathy. TTR

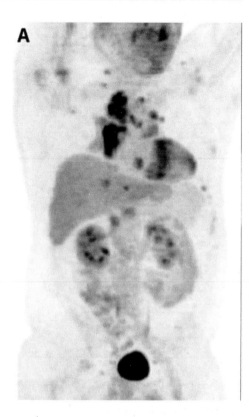

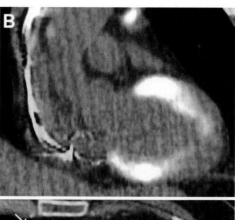

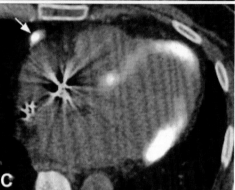

FIG. 10.9 ● **Widespread sarcoidosis with myocardial involvement.** This 52-year-old man received an ICD 8 years prior for ventricular arrhythmias related to known myocardial sarcoidosis with nodal involvement. He was initially treated with methotrexate and has been on chronic corticosteroid therapy. RAO MIP FDG PET CT **(A)** demonstrates hypermetabolic thoracic lymph nodes (SUVmax 15.0 in a subcarinal lymph node), abdominal lymph nodes (SUVmax 5.5 in a peripancreatic lymph node), and pelvic lymph nodes. The MIP image and coronal **(B)** and axial **(C)** FDG PET images demonstrate patchy hypermetabolism within the left ventricular myocardium involving the lateral wall (SUVmax 10.0), interventricular septum (Max SUV 6.5), superior wall (max SUV 9.7), inferior wall (max SUV 9.0), and apex (Max SUV 6.5), typical for active myocardial sarcoidosis. Arrow in C denotes a hyperactive right paracardiac node, SUVmax = 8.

CT, computed tomography; FDG, flurodeoxyglucose; ICD, implantable cardioverter defibrillato; PET, positron emission tomography.

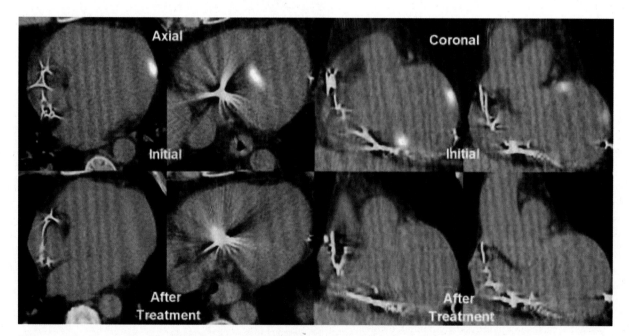

FIG. 10.10 ● **Myocardial sarcoidosis before and after treatment.** This 56-year-old man initially presented with a high-grade AV block with non-sustained ventricular tachycardia and recurrent PVCs. He had an ICD placed and active cardiac sarcoidosis was initially confirmed by focal FDG hypermetabolic myocardial lesions, SUVmax = 7, upper-row axial, and coronal images. Myocardial lesions are no longer seen on repeat FDG PET/CT after treatment initially with methotrexate followed by chronic corticosteroids, lower-row axial, and coronal images.

CT, computed tomography; FDG, flurodeoxyglucose; ICD, implantable cardioverter defibrillato; PET, positron emission tomography.

cardiomyopathy is seen in up to 3% of older Black men. This is most commonly seen in men over the age of 70. Interestingly, autopsies of men over the age of 80 typically demonstrate TTR-derived amyloid deposits. Heart failure likely requires enough amyloid has to cause measurable myocardial wall thickening (19,20).

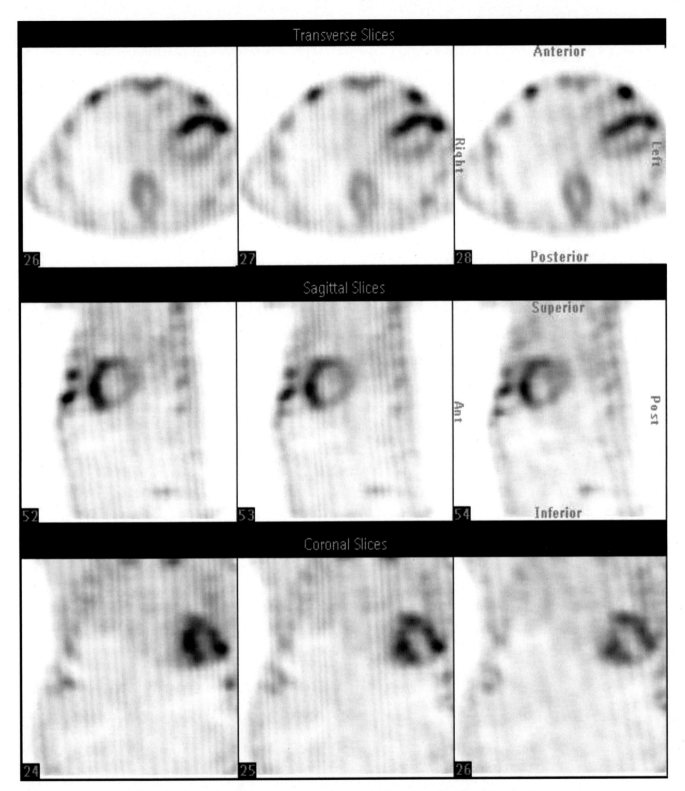

FIG. 10.11 ● **This 48-year-old man has shortness of breath due to transthyretin amyloid cardiomyopathy.** Axial, sagittal, and coronal ^{99m}Tc-pyrophosphate SPECT images clearly demonstrate Grades 2 to 3 myocardial activity typical for transthyretin amyloid cardiomyopathy.

SPECT, single photon emission computed tomography.

No special preparation for amyloid scanning. A dose of 10 to 20 mCi of ^{99m}Tc-pyrophosphate is administered intravenously and imaging is performed at 1 to 3 hours with SPECT or SPECT/CT equipment. Images may be visually graded on a 0 to 3 scale where Grade 0 has no myocardial activity, Grade 1 has myocardial activity less than ribs, Grade 2 has myocardial activity equal to ribs, and Grade 3 has myocardial activity greater than rib activity. Grades 2 and 3 are considered positive (Fig. 10.11) (20,21).

References

1. Hesse B, Lindhardt TB, Acampa W, et al. EANM/ESC guidelines for radionuclide imaging of cardiac function. *Eur J Nucl Med Mol Imaging*. 2008;35:851.

2. Berman DS, Germano G. The clinical value of assessing left ventricular function from gated SPECT perfusion studies. *Rev Port Cardiol*. 2000;(Suppl. 1):131–137.

3. Henzlova JM, Cerqueira MD, Hansen CL, Taillefer R, Yao SS. ASNC imaging guidelines for nuclear cardiology procedures stress protocols and tracers. *J Nucl Cardiol*. 2009;16:331–344.

4. Maddahi J, Packard RRS. Cardiac PET perfusion tracers: current status and future directions. *Semin Nucl Med*. 2014 Sep;44(5):333–343.

5. Packard RR, Huang SC, Dahlbom M, Czernin J, Maddahi J. Absolute quantitation of myocardial blood flow in human subjects with or without myocardial ischemia using dynamic flurpiridaz F 18 PET. *J Nucl Med*. 2014;55:1438–1444.

6. Agostini D, Roule V, Nganoa C, Roth N, Baavour R, Parienti JJ, et al. First validation of myocardial flow reserve assessed by dynamic 99mTc-sestamibi CZT-SPECT camera: head to head comparison with 15O-water PET and fractional flow reserve in patients with suspected coronary artery disease. The WATERDAY study. *Eur J Nucl Med Mol Imaging*. 2018;45:1079–1090.

7. Dilsizian V, Bacharach SL, Beanlands RS, et al. Imaging guidelines for nuclear cardiology procedures: PET myocardial perfusion and metabolism clinical imaging. *J Nucl Cardiol*. 2009;16:651.

8. https://www.professionalradiology.com/media/documents/Cardiac%20Pet.pdf. Accessed January, 15, 2020.

9. Lu Y, Grant C, Xie K, et al. Suppression of myocardial 18F-FDG uptake through prolonged high-fat, high-protein, and very-low-carbohydrate diet before FDG-PET/CT for evaluation of patients with suspected cardiac sarcoidosis. *Clin Nucl Med*. 2017;42:88–94.

10. Asmal AC, Leary WP, Thandroyen F, et al. A dose-response study for the anticoagulant and lipolytic activities of heparin in normal subjects. *Br J Clin Pharmacol*. 1979;7:531–533.

11. Erba PA, Conti U, Lazzeri E, et al. Added value of 99mTc-HMPAO-labeled leukocyte SPECT/CT in the characterization and management of patients with infectious endocarditis. *J Nucl Med*. 2012;53:1235–1243.

12. Amraoui S, Tlili G, Sohal M, et al. Contribution of PET imaging to the diagnosis of septic embolism in patients with pacing lead endocarditis. *JACC Cardiovasc Imaging*. 2016;9:283–290.

13. Calais J, Touati A, Grail N, et al. Diagnostic impact of 18F-fluorodeoxyglucose positron emission tomography/computed tomography and while blood cell SPECT/computed tomography in patients with suspected cardiac implantable electronic device chronic infection. *Cir Cardiovasc Imaging*. 2019;12:e007188.

14. Chen W, Sajadi MM, Dilsizian V. Merits of FDG PET/CT and functional molecular imaging over anatomic imaging with echocardiography and CT angiography for the diagnosis of cardiac device infections. *JACC Cardiovasc Imaging*. 2018;11:1679–1691.

15. Mahmood M, Kendi AT, Ajmal S, et al. Meta-analysis of 18F-FDG PET/CT in the diagnosis of infective endocarditis. *J Nucl Cardiol*. 2019;26:922–935.

16. Youssef G, Leung E, Mylonas I, et al. The use of 18F-FDG PET in the diagnosis of cardiac sarcoidosis: a systematic review and meta-analysis including the Ontario experience. *J Nucl Med*. 2012;53:241–248.

17. Schatka I, Bengel FM. Advanced imaging of cardiac sarcoidosis. *J Nucl Med*. 2014;55:99–106.

18. Ohira H, Tsujino I, Ishimaru S, et al. Myocardial imaging with 18F-fluoro-2-deoxyglucose positron emission tomography and magnetic resonance imaging in sarcoidosis. *Eur J Nucl Med Mol Imaging*. 2008;35:933–941.

19. Ruberg FL, Berk JL. Transthyretin (TTR) cardiac amyloidosis. *Circulation*. 2012;126:1286–300.

20. https://www.asnc.org/Files/Practice%20Resources/Practice%20Points/ASNC%20Practice%20Point-99mTechnetiumPyrophosphateImaging2016.pdf. Accessed January 16, 2020.

21. Falk RH, Quarta CC, Dorbala S. How to image cardiac amyloidosis. *Circ Cardiovasc Imaging*. 2014;7:552–562.

CHAPTER SELF-ASSESSMENT QUESTIONS

1. What is the most common cause for a false-positive myocardial perfusion SPECT study?

   A. Attenuation

   B. Inadequate stress

   C. Motion

   D. Tracer "roll-off"

2. What is the most common cause for a false-negative myocardial perfusion SPECT study?

   A. Attenuation

   B. Inadequate stress

   C. Motion

   D. Tracer "roll-off"

Answers to Chapter Self-Assessment Questions

1. A Attenuation. Foe Tc-99m, 4.6 cm of tissue will reduce transmitted counts by 50%. Prone imaging can be very helpful in reducing attenuation artifact from abdominal tissue as is more commonly seen in men. Properly performed attenuation correction as, for example, with SPECT/CT can be extremely helpful for reducing artifacts from abdominal or breast attenuation. Motion artifact can occasionally cause false-positive exams. Inadequate stress and roll-off are causes for false-negative exams.

2. D Tracer "roll-off" is the most common cause for false-negative exams. Roll-off is caused by incomplete first-pass myocardial extraction. Table 10.1 compares the available myocardial perfusion agents. The popular SPECT agent 99mTc tetrofosmin has a low extraction rate of 54% compared with Ti-201 with an 85% extraction fraction.

Inadequate stress (B) can also cause false-negative exams. This usually does not occur because stress lab personnel can readily convert an inadequate treadmill stress to a regadenoson exam where coronary blood flow is increased by up to 5 times the baseline perfusion.

Attenuation (A) and motion (C) typically are associated with false-positive exams.

Pulmonary Scintigraphy

11

Søren Hess

LEARNING OBJECTIVES

1. Summarize the basic challenges in the diagnosis of pulmonary embolism (PE).
2. Describe basic imaging strategies in PE.
3. Perform and interpret ventilation–perfusion pulmonary scintigraphy (V/Q scan).
4. Apply V/Q scanning for non-PE problem-solving.

INTRODUCTION

Acute pulmonary embolism (PE) is a common, ubiquitous, and potentially life-threatening condition. Overall annual occurrence is estimated to be 300,000 to 700,000 in the United States and Europe with annual incidence rates of 75 to 269/100,000 increasing with age to 700/100,000 in patients above age 70. With increasing age demographics, incidences are expected to rise and physicians in virtually every field of clinical medicine will have to care for patients with suspected PE, not only in settings classically associated with high incidences such as emergency departments with a reported incidence of 1/400, but also in patients with chronic medical or psychiatric conditions. Effective anticoagulant treatment is available to reduce morbidity and mortality but is itself associated with potentially dangerous side effects such as bleeding. Thus, accurate diagnosis is imperative to institute correct and timely treatment but also to limit the number of patients subjected to the risks of anticoagulation. However, PE is a notoriously difficult clinical diagnosis due to nonspecific signs and symptoms, and imaging is usually necessary to confirm or exclude the diagnosis. This chapter outlines the basic features of radionuclide ventilation–perfusion pulmonary scintigraphy (V/Q scan) (1,2).

CLINICAL ASPECTS OF PULMONARY EMBOLISM

Basic work on thrombus and embolus including clinical definitions date back to the mid-nineteenth century and German pathologist and polyhistor Rudolph Virchow: a thrombus is a clot forming in the vasculature, and an embolus is a fragment dislodged from a thrombus and transported by the blood stream to another location where it lodges. Although PE is commonly referred to as a blood clot in the lung, the initial fragment may also arise from fat, air, amniotic fluid, or even cement from joint prostheses or vertebroplasty. Nonetheless, PE most commonly arises from deep venous thromboses (DVT) in the lower extremity and there is a close connection between lower extremity DVT and PE, which are together termed venous thromboembolism (VTE). Nearly 50% of proximal DVT progress to PE, and lower

extremity DVT, can be found in most cases of PE, whereas non-symptomatic or silent PE is seen in 40% of DVT (3,4).

The pathophysiologic basis for DVT begins with the so-called Virchow's triad, which describe the three overarching risk factors for DVT: stasis (e.g., immobilization from long-haul travel or bed rest), endothelial damage (e.g., surgery or indwelling catheters), and hypercoagulability (e.g., hereditary disorders, or secondary to pregnancy, disease, or medication). While the factors described by Virchow's triad may increase the risk of DVT formation, addressing these risk factors, for example, moving about during flights to reduce risk of VTE may be preventative. It is important, though, that risk increases with increasing risk factors present. For example, the risk of DVT from long-haul flights remains low for the average traveler without additional risk factors (3,5).

While history and physical exam are important to ascertain the presence of potential risk factors, signs and symptoms are usually nonspecific (Table 11.1). In symptomatic patients, acute onset dyspnea, chest pain, syncope, and hemoptysis are often present alone or in combination—but these symptoms are also present alone or in combination in many patients presenting to the emergency department (ED) without PE. The same is the case with clinical findings. While heart rate, blood pressure, arterial oxygen saturation, and respiratory frequency should be recorded in patients with acute cardiopulmonary symptoms, no firm differences in physiological signs are found between patients with or without PE (6).

EKG and chest radiographs are also important examinations, primarily for differential diagnoses. Several so-called specific PE-associated findings are described, for example, S1Q3T3-pattern on EKG (S-wave in lead I, Q-wave in lead III, and inverted T-wave in lead III), and Westermark's sign on chest radiography (focal oligemia). Both signs are in fact nonspecific, the S1Q3T3-pattern is a general sign of right heart strain more than PE specifically, and neither sign is present in more than about 10% of cases (3,6).

In order to improve the selection of patients for further testing, clinical prediction scores have been developed, for example, Well's score, which based on several disposing factors, symptoms, and signs stratifies patients according to clinical probability for

Table 11.1 **PROPORTION OF SELECTED SYMPTOMS, SIGNS, AND BASIC DIAGNOSTIC RESULTS IN PATIENTS WITH AND WITHOUT PULMONARY EMBOLISM (BASED ON REFERENCE [6])**

	PE	Non-PE
Symptoms		
Dyspnea	50%–78%	29%–50%
Chest pain	39%–44%	28%–30%
Syncope	6%–26%	6%–13%
Hemoptysis	8%–9%	4%–5%
Signs		
Tachycardia	24%	23%
Hypotension	3%	2%
ECG		
Right heart strain	50%	12%
S1Q3T3	12%	–
Chest X-ray		
Pleural effusion	23%	–
Oligemia	8%	–

PE, that is, low (~10%), intermediate (~30%), or high (~65%), respectively, or dichotomized as "PE likely" (~30%) or "PE unlikely" (~12%). In conjunction with d-dimer, a fibrin degradation product that is increased in VTE, but also in many nonembolic conditions, clinical scores may guide whether more advanced diagnostic imaging is warranted or not. This has become increasingly important as the actual confirmation rate of PE in patients undergoing diagnostic workup has decreased significantly over the past decades, according to some reports as much as from 50% to 5%, which suggests a significant overutilization of advanced diagnostic procedures (5).

OVERALL IMAGING STRATEGIES IN PULMONARY EMBOLISM

The clinical diagnosis of PE remains difficult (6), and according to current international literature, including a recent guideline and a meta-analysis from our own group, controversies remain regarding the diagnostic modality of choice in patients with suspected PE (5,7–11).

Over the years, several imaging modalities have been employed in the diagnostic workup of suspected PE, that is, catheter-based pulmonary angiography, magnetic resonance imaging, V/Q scan, computer tomography angiography (CTA), and positron emission tomography (8,12–14). In recent years, the choice has been narrowed to CTA and V/Q scan—both have a place in suspected PE, but with different advantages and shortcomings, and controversies remain regarding first-line imaging (8).

CTA is available around the clock at most hospitals, offering rapid direct evidence for PE or alternative important diagnoses. CTA may not disclose smaller, peripheral PEs, which may be associated with chronic pulmonary hypertension. The radiation dose to breast tissue may be a consideration in younger females (15), and contrast media is administered with the risk of allergic

reactions and it may be relatively contraindicated in patients with renal impairment (7–9).

On the other hand, with V/Q scan, the radiation burden may be less and no contrast media is employed, but there may be limited access to scintigraphy and radiopharmaceuticals in some settings. Ventilation or aerosol studies can be a challenge with patients in respiratory distress (7). Previously, V/Q scan was characterized by a substantial number of nondiagnostic studies, and it offered no alternative diagnoses (7,15–17). Recent developments in 3D-imaging and fusion with low-dose CT have ameliorated this (7,8,18).

PRACTICAL ASPECTS OF V/Q SCAN

The basic principles of V/Q scan have remained virtually unchanged for more than 50 years and are as the name implies based on combined assessment of perfusion and ventilation.

Pulmonary perfusion is assessed by intravenously injected radiolabeled microparticles (i.e., ^{99m}Tc-labeled macroaggregated albumin; ^{99m}Tc-MAA). The usual adult receives 200,000 to 500,000 particles that comprise an administered patient dose of 100 to 200 MBq mix uniformly with venous blood and distribute uniformly throughout the pulmonary vasculature before they lodge in the precapillary arterioles because the particles are larger (10–90 μm) than the vessel diameter (<15 μm). Tracer distribution is subsequently registered by the gamma camera, but if the vasculature is blocked by an embolus, particles will not reach the vessels distal to it. Thus, obstructed regions remains devoid of radioactivity and appears as photopenic perfusion defects in the scintigraphic images with a wedge-shaped appearance as a consequence of the segmental anatomy of the lungs (19). It seems counterintuitive to essentially induce multiple micro emboli, but due to the vastness of pulmonary vasculature, the particles only transiently block less than 0.1% of the capillary bed. They are subsequently hydrolyzed to smaller particles and phagocytized with a biologic half-life of 3 to 4 h. The dose should be reduced in pregnant women and children, and the number of particles reduced should be reduced to 50,000 to 100,000 in patients with suspected of right-to-left shunt (to minimize the risk of systemic emboli) or pulmonary hypertension (to reduce the risk of severe pulmonary deterioration as the particles lodge more centrally due to reduced lumen) (20), while infants and children typically are prescribed 10,000 to 50,000 particles.

Perfusion images are usually supplemented with an assessment of the ventilation to improve specificity and help differentiate primary perfusion defects caused by PE from perfusion defects due to hypoxic vasoconstriction secondary to impaired ventilation. Ventilation images are based on inhalation of radiolabeled gas (^{133}Xenon or ^{81m}Krypton) or aerosol (^{99m}Tc-labeled DTPA or ^{99m}Tc-labeled Technegas®) that distributes throughout ventilated areas of the lungs.

The gaseous ^{81m}Kr with a 13s physical half-life has to be breathed continuously by mask; most patients with respiration impairment can accommodate this, and because it has different gamma energy (190 keV) than ^{99m}Tc-MAA (140 keV), the entire examination can be performed as a simultaneous dual-isotope examination. However, with the short half-lives of ^{81m}Kr and its mother isotope ^{81}Rubidium, generator lifetime is equally short, it is no longer available in the United States, where ^{133}Xe is the available radioactive gas for ventilation exams.

^{133}Xe has an energy of 80 keV, so thus, ideally xenon ventilation studies are performed prior to ^{99m}Tc-MAA perfusion exams. Because 133Xe has a 5-day physical half-life, it has a long shelf life and it is used to evaluate single breath (vital capacity), 2-min rebreathing (total lung volume equilibrium), and sequential 20-s washout images are performed to demonstrate air trapping. As the normal lung washout biological half-life is 20 s, the apparent residual lung activity should normally reduce by 50% on each sequential image. The short biological half-life of ^{133}Xe dominates in reducing the radiation exposure associated with the 5-day physical half-life of ^{133}Xe.

Recent shortages and associated price rises for ^{133}Xe have led to use of alternative airspace imaging with radioaerosols. As ^{99m}Tc is more widely available, radioaerosol ^{99m}Tc-DTPA has replaced ^{133}Xe in many practices. Aerosols are not as uniformly distributed as radioactive gasses and they may be retained in central airway mucus in patients with obstructive lung disease. Especially if the relatively deep inhalations required for uniform, distribution may not be achievable in all patients (19,21). In Europe and Australia, ^{99m}Tc-Technegas® with its more gas-like ultrafine particles is replacing radioaerosol ^{99m}Tc-DTPA, with more reliable pulmonary distribution.

In the early days of V/Q scanning, planar images in 4 to 8 projection were the mainstay. However, planar images may not visualize all segments of the lungs sufficiently as photopenic areas may be obscured by radioactivity in adjacent segments, especially in the basal medial segments of the right lower lobe. Thus, in recent years, single photon emission computed tomography (SPECT) or hybrid SPECT/CT has become much more widespread, and a recent meta-analysis clearly found SPECT and SPECT/CT to be equivalent to, or even better than CTA, but comparative literature is sparse. Also, somewhat longer acquisition times may be to lengthier than patients with respiratory impairment can accommodate (7,8).

INTERPRETATION OF V/Q SCINTIGRAPHY—PULMONARY EMBOLISM OR NO PULMONARY EMBOLISM

The Achilles heel of V/Q scan has always been the interpretation criteria, and over the years several have been introduced, revised, or revoked again. In the early days of planar images, a simplistic approach based on the abovementioned basic assumptions were used, that is, wedge-shaped segmental perfusion defects in areas with preserved ventilation ("mismatch") signified PE, whereas areas with decreased perfusion AND ventilation ("match") did not. However, with this approach, sensitivity and specificity were only around 80%, and consequently 20% were misdiagnosed, which is not negligible in a disease that may be deadly both with treatment and as a direct consequence of treatment (7,13). In 1990, the pivotal multicenter prospective investigation of pulmonary embolism diagnosis (PIOPED) study introduced a more elaborate interpretation scheme with much more advanced and somewhat complicated criteria based on various parameters beyond mere match/mismatch, for example, number, size, and shape of perfusion defects (Table 11.2a). Results were now reported in a probabilistic manner, that is, scans were divided into normal scans or positive scans with high, intermediate, low, or very low probability of PE. When scans were considered conclusive and diagnostic (i.e., high probability scans and very low probability or normal scans), taken together, they displayed high sensitivity and specificity (>95%). However, only about half of the scans fell into either categories; the remainder (intermediate probability and low probability) were considered

nondiagnostic with overall 30% risk of PE but highly dependent on pretest probability. To referring physicians, vague V/Q became a nuisance. To overcome this, the PIOPED criteria were revised several times, but the nondiagnostic rate remained relatively high (7,22). Attempts were also made to improve diagnostic efficacy using planar perfusion-only images; the so-called prospective investigative study of acute pulmonary embolism diagnosis (PISA-PED) study managed to achieve relatively high sensitivity and specificity (>90%), but the prerequisite was interpretation of chest X-rays by very experienced readers, and the results were not readily reproducible (7,23). The uncertainties of planar images with high nondiagnostic rates helped to pave the way for CTA when spiral CT was introduced in the early 1990s: It offered several advantages over V/Q scan, primarily much more dichotomous classification of patients as either positive or negative for PE and clinically relevant differential diagnoses, but also a more simple, faster examination, and more widespread availability around the clock. On the downsides were the use of contrast media and radiation dose to certain critical organs. Furthermore, it is worth noticing that the initial enthusiastic reports of spiral CT with sensitivities and specificities of 90%–100% were based on assessment of central vessels only—as soon as subsegmental branched were included, sensitivity dropped dramatically to ~50% (7,8,13). Although technological advancements have improved this in later years, the overall sensitivity of CTA (80%–85%) remains inferior to state-of-the-art V/Q SPECT/CT (98%) with comparable specificity (95%) and nondiagnostic rates (1%–5%) (8). The improvements of V/Q SPECT/CT is not only based on the obvious advances in technology but also on implementation of novel interpretation criteria, which are paradoxically based on the much more simplistic dichotomous match/mismatch pattern of the past (Table 11.2b and Fig. 11.1)—these criteria yield the highest sensitivities and specificities (>95%) with a nondiagnostic rate of 1%–3%. This is at least comparable to CTA, and it is important to remember that CTA is relatively contraindicated in a significant proportion of patients, for example, as many as 25% is excluded from clinical studies due to impaired renal function (7,8). Another benchmark for the modality of choice is the ability to provide relevant differential diagnoses, and state-of-the-art V/Q SPECT/CT now provide just as many non-thrombotic ones as CTA, for example, pneumonia, chronic obstructive pulmonary disease (COPD), and tumors (4).

As mentioned, CTA may miss smaller, peripheral PE, but controversy remains regarding the clinical importance of subsegmental PE—some advocate they foretell future events of potentially larger PE, others that they simply represent an important physiologic filter function of the lung for small emboli. Generally, patients with single subsegmental PE without underlying cardiopulmonary disease may be managed conservatively, whereas antithrombotic intervention may be considered in patients with reduced cardiopulmonary reserve or persistent risk factors of PE (4).

Some clinical conditions may cause false-positive mismatch, for example, central lung tumors that compress the soft vessels but to a lesser extent the harder bronchi, or vasculitis causing obstructive luminal inflammation. However, a central lung tumor will often be visible with SPECT/CT, and pulmonary vasculitides are relatively rare conditions. When both tracers are ^{99m}Tc based, the necessary higher activity of the perfusion tracer results in better count statistics, and perfusion defects (for instance at interlobar fissures) may therefore be more clearly outlined than the more blurred ventilation images although they are matched. This may cause false-positive interpretation, but again the CT-part

Table 11.2a THE NEWEST (REVISED) PIOPED CRITERIA (BASED ON REFERENCE [15])

High probability

- ≥2 large (>75% of a segment) segmental perfusion defects without corresponding ventilation or roentgenographic abnormalities or substantially larger than either matching ventilation or chest roentgenogram abnormalities
- ≥2 moderate segmental (≥25% and ≤75% of a segment) perfusion defects without matching ventilation or chest roentgenogram abnormalities and 1 large mismatched segmental defect
- ≥4 moderate segmental perfusion defects without ventilation or chest roentgenogram abnormalities

Intermediate probability (indeterminate)

- Not falling into normal, very-low-, low-, or high-probability categories
- Borderline high or borderline low
- Difficult to categorize as low or high
- Single moderate mismatched segmental perfusion defect with normal chest roentgenogram

Low probability

- Nonsegmental perfusion defects (e.g., very small effusion causing blunting of the costophrenic angle, cardiomegaly, enlarged aorta, hila, and mediastinum, and elevated diaphragm)
- Large or moderate segmental perfusion defects involving no more than 4 segments in 1 lung and no more than 3 segments in 1 lung region with matching ventilation defects either equal to or larger in size and chest roentgenogram either normal or with abnormalities substantially smaller than perfusion defects

Very low probability

- ≤3 small segmental perfusion defects with a normal chest roentgenogram.
- Nonsegmental perfusion abnormalities. These are enlargement of the heart or hilum, elevated hemidiaphragm, linear atelectasis, or costophrenic angle effusion with no other perfusion defects in either lung.
- Perfusion defect smaller than corresponding radiographic lesion.
- >2 matched V/Q defects with regionally normal chest radiograph and some areas of normal perfusion elsewhere in the lungs.
- 1 to 3 small segmental perfusion defects (<25% of a segment).
- Solitary triple matched defect (defined as a matched V/Q defect with associated matching chest radiographic opacity) in the middle or upper lung zone confined to a single segment.
- Stripe sign, which consists of a stripe of perfused lung tissue between a perfusion defect and the adjacent pleural surface (best seen on a tangential view).
- Pleural effusion equal to one third or more of the pleural cavity with no other perfusion defect in either lung.

Normal

- No perfusion defects present.
- Perfusion outlines exactly the shape of the lungs as seen on the chest roentgenogram. (Hilar and aortic impressions may be seen, chest roentgenogram and/or ventilation study may be abnormal.)

Table 11.2b THE NEWEST DICHOTOMOUS INTERPRETATION CRITERIA FOR SPECT AND SPECT/CT RECOMMENDED BY EANM (BASED ON REFERENCE [4])

Pulmonary embolism

- V/Q mismatch of at least one segment or two subsegments in keeping with the pulmonary vascular anatomy (wedge-shaped defects with the base projecting to the lung periphery

No pulmonary embolism

- Normal perfusion pattern in keeping with the anatomic boundaries of the lung
- Matched or reversed-mismatched V/Q defects of any size, shape, or number in the absence of mismatch
- Mismatch that does not follow a lobar, segmental, or subsegmental pattern

Nondiagnostic for pulmonary embolism

- Widespread V/Q abnormalities not typical of specific disease

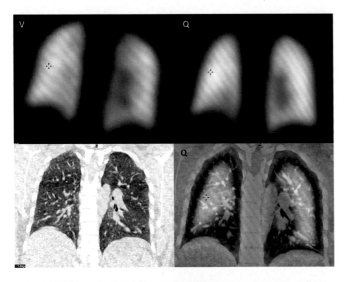

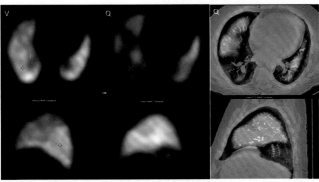

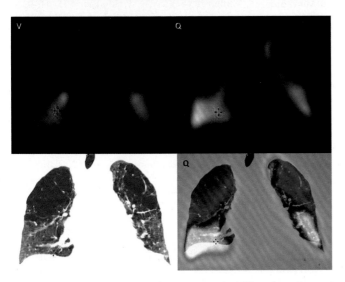

FIG. 11.1 ● Classical V/Q patterns. **A:** Normal V/Q pattern; coronal ventilation (upper left) and perfusion (upper right), low-dose CT (lower left), and hybrid perfusion SPECT/CT (lower right). **B:** Mismatched V/Q pattern; transaxial and sagittal ventilation (left column), perfusion (middle column), and hybrid perfusion SPECT/CT (right column) show wedge-shaped segmental mismatched perfusion defects typical for PE. **C:** Matched and reversed-mismatched V/Q pattern; coronal ventilation (upper left) and perfusion (upper right), low-dose CT (lower left), and hybrid perfusion SPECT/CT (lower right) show tracer distribution and morphology typical for well-known bullous COPD and no PE.

may help, and such defects most likely have a non-segmental presentation not signifying PE (4,7).

Suspected recurrence in patients with previous clots on V/Q scans may pose a challenge. Although the clot resolution rate is generally high with complete normalization of perfusion within months after the incident, in some patients unresolved perfusion defects remain. As recurrence is reported to have predilection for sites of previous clots, it may be difficult to conclude if clots are old or new. Generally, older unresolved or only partly resolved clots present with non-segmental perfusion defects with varying ventilatory match. To facilitate recurrence assessment follow-up, V/Q scan after 6 to 12 months or at cessation of therapy may be considered to provide a novel baseline in patients with irreversible or persistent risk factors of VTE (7).

Unresolved PE may also progress to chronic PE, a less common condition with the potential to develop further into chronic thromboembolic pulmonary hypertension (CTEPH), which may in turn lead to right heart failure, arrhythmias, and ultimately death. V/Q scan has significantly better sensitivity than CTA in diagnosing the peripheral PEs of CTEPH, that is, 97% versus 50%, and there is generally poor agreement between the two modalities, albeit CTA and right heart catheterization are important in the further management after the diagnosis has been established (4).

NON-PULMONARY EMBOLISM USE

Various distribution patterns seen on V/Q scan but not indicative of PE may contribute in non-PE conditions, for instance, COPD is often characterized by varying degrees of uneven ventilation and reverse mismatch, albeit similar patterns may also be encountered in pneumonia. Non-segmental, antigravitational perfusion patterns, for example, increased perfusion in anterior lung segments with the patient in the supine position, may indicate left heart failure, and it may cause false-positive mismatch as ventilation is less affected. Although these uses may have potential clinical relevance, they are generally less well established and not widely implemented compared to PE diagnostics (4).

In other clinical settings, the methodology is used directly to assess a specific condition different from PE, for example, right-to-left shunt. Caution is advised in suspected right-to-left shunts due to a risk of systemic emboli from the injected particles. However, the particles may in fact be used to assess and quantify such a shunt. The size of the macro-aggregated particles suits the gauge of the precapillary vessels so they lodge almost exclusively before entering the systemic circuit, but in case of an anatomic right-to-left shunt (e.g., persistent foramen ovale), particles may bypass pulmonary trapping. Similarly, in physiologic right-to-left shunt (e.g., hepatopulmonary syndrome), the diameter of the vessels is dilated through mechanisms that are not fully understood but allow the particles to pass through to the systemic vessels. An undiagnosed shunt may be suspected if tracer uptake is visually detected outside the pulmonary vasculature, for example, in the kidneys, which are typically included in the scan field. If a shunt is otherwise suspected or diagnosed, ^{99m}Tc-MAA is the most common method available to quantify it based on tracer distribution (i.e., the fraction of injected activity relative to whole-body dose located in either the brain or the kidneys, which may have prognostic implications) (24). Quantification of perfusion is also used to estimate post-therapeutic lung function in patients scheduled for tumor resection or volume-reducing interventions like endo-bronchial valves or bulla resection (25).

Whereas the abovementioned non-PE indications take advantage of the perfusion tracer, measurement of mucociliary clearance is based on inhalation of the nebulized ventilation aerosol ^{99m}Tc-labeled colloids; the cilia and the mechanism of mucociliary clearance is part of a bronchial defense strategy to reduce inflammation or impact from inhaled noxious particles. Thus, if cilia function is compromised inflammation ensues, as is seen in cilia dyskinesia. This rarely used technique is especially adept in ruling out primary cilia dyskinesia, but only very few centers in the world employ this test and only in select patients (26,27).

TAKE HOME POINTS

- Symptoms of PE are nonspecific, and the clinical diagnosis is notoriously difficult.
- Basic workup in PE includes arterial blood gas analysis, ECG, chest X-ray, and d-dimer but findings are nonspecific and primarily serve to establish differential diagnosis.

- Clinical prediction scores like Wells score may help to decide whether advanced diagnostic imaging is warranted in suspected PE.
- V/Q scan is a valid method in suspected PE and with SPECT or SPECT/CT is comparable to CTA.
- Reporting should be dichotomized as "PE present" or "PE not present" and only few percent should be characterized as "non-diagnostic" in a trinary manner.
- If imaging results are discordant with clinical probability, further testing is recommended.
- A normal V/Q scan excludes PE.
- A positive V/Q scan and high clinical likelihood confirms PE.
- Follow-up scans should be considered in patients with persistent risk factors.
- Non-PE indications include right-to-left shunt, pre-operative assessment of pulmonary function, and measurements of mucociliary clearance.

References

1. Konstantinides SV, Barco S, Lankcit M, Meyer G. Management of pulmonary embolism: an update. *J Am Coll Cardiol*. 2016;67(8):976–990.
2. Serhal M, Barnes GD. Venous thromboembolism: a clinician update. *Vasc Med (London, England)*. 2019;24(2):122–131.
3. Dalen JE. Pulmonary embolism: what have we learned since Virchow? Natural history, pathophysiology, and diagnosis. *Chest*. 2002;122(4):1440–1456.
4. Bajc M, Schumichen C, Gruning T, et al. EANM guideline for ventilation/perfusion single-photon emission computed tomography (SPECT) for diagnosis of pulmonary embolism and beyond. *Eur J Nucl Med Mol Imaging*. 2019;46(12):2429–2451.
5. Konstantinides SV, Meyer G, Becattini C, et al. 2019 ESC Guidelines for the diagnosis and management of acute pulmonary embolism developed in collaboration with the European Respiratory Society (ERS). *Eur Heart J*. 2019;41(4):543–603.
6. Madsen PH, Hess S. Symptomatology, clinical presentation and basic work up in patients with suspected pulmonary embolism. *Adv Exp Med Biol*. 2017;906:33–48.
7. Hess S, Madsen PH. Radionuclide diagnosis of pulmonary embolism. *Adv Exp Med Biol*. 2017;906:49–65.
8. Hess S, Frary EC, Gerke O, Madsen PH. State-of-the-Art imaging in pulmonary embolism: ventilation/perfusion single-photon emission computed tomography versus computed tomography angiography - controversies, results, and recommendations from a systematic review. *Semin Thromb Hemost*. 2016;42(8):833–845.
9. Mortensen J, Gutte H. SPECT/CT and pulmonary embolism. *Eur J Nucl Med Mol Imaging*. 2014;41 Suppl 1:S81–S90.
10. Roach PJ, Schembri GP, Bailey DL. V/Q scanning using SPECT and SPECT/CT. *J Nucl Med*. 2013;54(9):1588–1596.
11. Laurence IJ, Redman SL, Corrigan AJ, Graham RN. V/Q SPECT imaging of acute pulmonary embolus - a practical perspective. *Clin Radiol*. 2012;67(10):941–948.
12. Madsen PH, Hess S, Jorgensen HB, Hoilund-Carlsen PF. [Diagnostic imaging in acute pulmonary embolism in Denmark. A survey]. *Ugeskrift for laeger*. 2005;167(41):3875–3877.
13. Hess S, Madsen PH, Jorgensen HB, Hoilund-Carlsen PF. [Diagnostic imaging in acute pulmonary embolism. The use of spiral computed tomography, lung scintigraphy and echocardiography]. *Ugeskrift for laeger*. 2005;167(41):3870–3875.

14. Hess S, Madsen PL, Iversen ED, et al. Efficacy of FDG PET/CT imaging for venous thromboembolic disorders: preliminary results from a prospective, observational pilot study. *Clin Nucl Med*. 2015;40(1):e23–e26.
15. Freeman LM, Stein EG, Sprayregen S, Chamarthy M, Haramati LB. The current and continuing important role of ventilation-perfusion scintigraphy in evaluating patients with suspected pulmonary embolism. *Semin Nucl Med*. 2008;38(6):432–440.
16. Marmolin ES, Moller L, Johansen A, Madsen PH, Hess S. [Therapeutic consequences of lung scintigraphy in patients with intermediate probability of pulmonary embolism]. *Ugeskrift for laeger*. 2009;171(19):1594–1597.
17. Siegel A, Holtzman SR, Bettmann MA, Black WC. Clinicians' perceptions of the value of ventilation-perfusion scans. *Clin Nucl Med*. 2004;29(7):419–425.
18. Alis J, Latson LA Jr., Haramati LB, Shmukler A. Navigating the Pulmonary perfusion map: dual-energy computed tomography in acute pulmonary embolism. *J Comput Assist Tomogr*. 2018;42(6):840–849.
19. Bajc M, Neilly JB, Miniati M, et al. EANM guidelines for ventilation/perfusion scintigraphy: Part 1. Pulmonary imaging with ventilation/perfusion single photon emission tomography. *Eur J Nucl Med Mol Imaging*. 2009;36(8):1356–1370.
20. Ciofetta G, Piepsz A, Roca I, et al. Guidelines for lung scintigraphy in children. *Eur J Nucl Med Mol Imaging*. 2007;34(9):1518–1526.
21. Bajc M, Neilly B, Miniati M, Mortensen J, Jonson B. Methodology for ventilation/perfusion SPECT. *Semin Nucl Med*. 2010;40(6):415–425.
22. Value of the ventilation/perfusion scan in acute pulmonary embolism. Results of the prospective investigation of pulmonary embolism diagnosis (PIOPED). *JAMA*. 1990;263(20):2753–2759.
23. Miniati M, Pistolesi M, Marini C, et al. Value of perfusion lung scan in the diagnosis of pulmonary embolism: results of the Prospective Investigative Study of Acute Pulmonary Embolism Diagnosis (PISA-PED). *Am J Respir Crit Care Med*. 1996;154(5):1387–1393.
24. Madsen PH, Hess S, Madsen HD. A case of unexplained hypoxemia. *Respir Care*. 2012;57(11):1963–1966.
25. Mortensen J, Berg RMG. Lung scintigraphy in COPD. *Semin Nucl Med*. 2019;49(1):16–21.
26. Munkholm M, Mortensen J. Mucociliary clearance: pathophysiological aspects. *Clin Physiol Funct Imaging*. 2014;34(3):171–177.
27. Munkholm M, Nielsen KG, Mortensen J. Clinical value of measurement of pulmonary radioaerosol mucociliary clearance in the work up of primary ciliary dyskinesia. *EJNMMI Res*. 2015;5(1):118.

CHAPTER SELF-ASSESSMENT QUESTIONS

1. What is the most likely explanation for these findings?

   A. Abscesses

   B. Bulli

   C. Emboli

   D. Metastasis

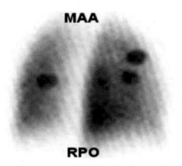

2. What scintigraphic finding is demonstrated?

   A. Fissure sign

   B. Hampton hump

   C. Rim sign

   D. Stripe sign

   E. Westermarck sign

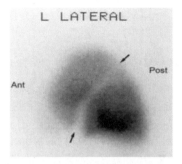

3. What scintigraphic finding is demonstrated?

   A. Fissure sign

   B. Hampton hump

   C. Rim sign

   D. Stripe sign

   E. Westermarck sign

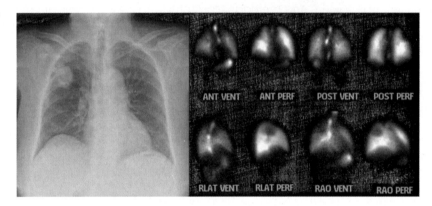

Answers to Chapter Self-Assessment Questions

1. Abscesses (A), bulli (B) and metastases (D) are most commonly photopenic defects. In this case, the correct answer is emboli (C). This has been reported with many radiopharmaceuticals, especially when blood is inadvertently mixed with the tracer and radioactive clots form in the tracer syringe and are injected into the patient and trapped in the lungs.

2. This is the "fissure sign" (A). The fissure sign is most typically seen with pleural effusion. The other choices are incorrect. "Hampton Hump" (B) is a pleural-based opacity radiographic sign of pulmonary infarction. The "rim sign" (C) is a hepatobiliary scintigraphic sign of gangrenous cholecystitis. The "stripe sign" (D) is a perfusion scan sign of perfusion peripheral to a perfusion defect. This is not a sign of PE. "Westermarck sign" (E) is a radiographic region of lucent lung with reduced vessel density as a sign of PE.

3. This is an example of a triple-matched perfusion, ventilation, and radiographic abnormality. This is usually not PE if it is seen in the upper or mid-lung. The specific sign presented here is the "stripe sign" (D) of perfusion seen peripheral to a perfusion defect. This is also not a sign of PE. This triple-matched region demonstrated non-small cell lung cancer on bronchoscopic biopsy.

Gastrointestinal & Hepatobiliary Scintigraphy

12

James Connelly, Jan Fjeld, and Mona-Elisabeth Revheim

LEARNING OBJECTIVES

1. Describe methods to investigate gastrointestinal (GI) function in different parts of the GI tract.
2. List commonly used gastrointestinal and hepatobiliary track tracers.
3. Describe methods to investigate specific types of GI pathology including salivary gland diseases, gastro-esophageal reflux, Meckel's diverticulum, GI bleed, protein loss enteropathy, biliary acid recirculation.
4. List different ways hepatobiliary scintigraphy can be used to image different clinical indications.
5. Describe tracers and methods to identify and image different aspects of liver and splenic tissue.

GASTROINTESTINAL FUNCTIONAL STUDIES

Gastrointestinal symptoms can be diffuse, nonspecific, and difficult to pinpoint due to the length and motile mature of the gastrointestinal tract and correlation between the different regions. Nuclear medicine provides a relatively physiological approach to image all or part of the gastrointestinal tract during consumption of a meal and its progress through the esophagus, stomach, small-bowel, colon, and excretion. Usually, the investigation is truncated to the part of the GI tract most affected, with gastric emptying being the most frequently performed investigation. However, it is worth remembering that regional motility is dependent on both input and output, so some representation of this should be included in the imaging study. There is close relationship with radiological and endoscopic techniques. Whereas nuclear medicine does not provide the anatomical detail of the other methods, it provides a complementary overview and slow dynamic imaging methods that are not really practical with X-ray, compute tomography (CT) or even magnetic resonance (MR).

GASTRIC EMPTYING SCINTIGRAPHY

Abnormal gastric emptying may be a consequence of various diseases, leading to either too slow or too fast emptying rate. Symptoms and signs indicating gastric emptying problems are difficult to interpret, and the problem is frequently psychologic. Therefore, objective method for assessment of gastric emptying is a necessity. With a radiolabeled meal and dynamic scintigraphy, it is easy to assess gastric emptying.

The emptying rate is highly dependent on the meal. Therefore, standardized meals must be used, and reference intervals for these meals must be established (1). Moreover, there is a relatively broad biologic variation in gastric emptying rate, which leads to wide reference intervals also when standardized meals are used (2). For a person with an emptying rate close to the center of the normal reference interval for a specific meal, a relatively large deviation from the normal rate is necessary to avoid a false-negative result.

Nuclear medicine test methods with solid food are considered the gold standard for measuring gastrointestinal emptying, but emptying studies with liquids are also of interest, especially in small children and patients fed through various types of tubes. The examination can be modified into a double isotope method with a mixture of differentially labeled solid food and liquid, for example, ^{111}In-DTPA in water that is drunk with the solid test meal labeled with ^{99m}Tc-DTPA. The usefulness of this, however, seems limited.

Delayed emptying is seen with mechanical hindrances in the pylorus (cancer or ulcer with stenosis), diabetes mellitus with autonomic neuropathy, hypothyroidism, after a vagotomy, in collagen diseases, amyloidosis, uremia, anorexia, and depression, as well as idiopathic. Aberrant rapid emptying may be seen after gastric surgery, in patients with Zollinger–Ellison syndrome, carcinoid syndrome, duodenal ulcers, hyperthyroidism, and diabetes in the early phase.

SCINTIGRAPHIC PRINCIPLE

Radioactivity, most often a ^{99m}Tc-labeled radiopharmaceutical, is added to a standardized meal (3). The radiopharmaceutical added must be of a kind that is not absorbed from the gastrointestinal tract, and it must follow the test meal within the gastrointestinal tract. Examples are ^{99m}Tc-labeled sulfur colloid or DTPA. After intake of the test meal, the gastric emptying rate is measured by dynamic scintigraphy from time of intake and for the next 60 or 90 min, and sometimes for a longer period if the emptying is slow.

Indications

- Unexplained dyspepsia
- To detect or exclude gastroparesis, most often in patients with type 1 diabetes and autonomic neuropathy

- Verify dumping syndrome
- Detection of gastroesophageal reflux

Following up previously detected motility disorders Contraindication, special precautions, side effects

- There are no special contraindications. Side effects are not described. Breastfeeding can continue without interruption.

GENERAL STUDY PROTOCOL

The patients are instructed to fast without food and drinks for at least 4 h, preferably 8-h fast overnight. To be scheduled for investigation, the next morning is most convenient in combination with an overnight fast.

Diabetics should postpone their morning insulin until after the test meal. Early morning doses of drugs that affect the stomach's emptying should, if possible, be brought along and taken immediately after the investigation. Opiates, calcium blockers, anticholinergics, antidepressants, levodopa, histamine H2-antagonists, proton pump inhibitors, and antacids with aluminum tend to slow down the emptying rate. Erythromycin, metoclopramide, and cisapride increase the emptying rate.

Body mass index (BMI), age, and a history of smoking are of marginal significance to gastric emptying. However, emptying will depend on the volume of the meal and its composition, if the meal is solid or a liquid, and whether the person is standing, sitting or lying down. Hence, one must therefore strive for identical testing conditions, including standardization of the composition of test meals. A variety of standard meals are used. Eggs and bread are frequently used. With egg meals, only the egg white may be used. The yolk has a high content of fat and calories, and both these factors may reduce the emptying rate. Egg white from two eggs scrambled in the microwave oven and put between two halves of a slice of white bread is used by these authors for adult patients. The ^{99m}Tc-sulfur colloid is added to the egg white before the heating procedure.

Individual adaptation of meal volumes or composition in relation to allergies or other illnesses, or administration routes, should be evaluated by a physician for best possible administration. Children, dependent on age, drink 150 mL of cow's milk or other liquid nutrition, or solid food as for adults, in reduced amount. For tube-fed patients, the tube position in the stomach must be verified. The intake phase should be finished within maximum 10 min.

Camera recording should start immediately after the meal has been finished. Dynamic registration is performed over the abdominal area:

- Simultaneously, front and rear imaging, with a two-headed camera and calculating the decay-corrected geometric average.
- In addition to the stomach, the lower part of the esophagus, and the duodenum and the upper part of the small intestine, must be in the field of view.
- Time: approx. 90 min (5400 s), typically 90 s per image.

For very restless children, one can take static images at regular intervals (approximately every 10 min). If the only camera available has one detector, the left anterior oblique (LAO) projection is preferable to anterior (ANT) projection. It may be appropriate to follow up with more images throughout the day. Static images should be taken in 256 × 256 format every 10 min or so.

It is important with some anatomical landmarks on these scintigrams with very little anatomy except for the gastrointestinal tract, for example by marking right shoulder.

INTERPRETATION AND REPORTING

After ingestion, solid food will remain for some time in the stomach. In this lag period or plateau phase, peristalsis prepares the food for emptying to the duodenum. Then an exponential fall in radioactive gastric content following a solid meal is observed. Men, and women after menopause, have a somewhat faster gastric emptying than premenopausal women. But this gender difference is small, and separate reference ranges are not necessary. The difference in emptying between the different patients groups is frequently due to a different length of the initial plateau phase.

Compared with solid food, the liquid test meals are poorer at discriminating between normal and pathological emptying. Different liquids may also differ in their emptying rate. The emptying immediately after intake, with no plateau phase, and there is no significant difference between genders. In adults, the normal half-life is 10 to 60 min. In children, there seems to be a particularly large difference in emptying patterns depending on the volume of milk ingested and methodology in general. Breast milk and water are emptied exponentially, as with liquid test meals in adults, while test meals of cow's milk or infant formula often have long plateaus. Rectilinear fall with an immediate start can also be seen. Generally applicable reference values for children are lacking.

If gastrointestinal emptying examinations are carried out consistently, the emptying parameters will be reasonably well reproduced with a variation coefficient of about 15%. Patient movement bringing the stomach completely or partly outside the region of interest (ROI) is a source of error, which can be corrected and can easily be observed if the scintigrams are displayed dynamically in connection with processing. The overlap between gastric ROI and small intestine activity is another source of error.

As many practices are performing 4-h gastric emptying studies, it is useful to remember the *upper limit of normal at two standard deviations above the mean forgastric retention* as: (1 h: 90%; 2 h: 60%; 3 h: 30%; 4 h: 10%)

GASTROESOPHAGEAL REFLUX AND PULMONARY ASPIRATION

The two main problems with gastrointestinal reflux are esophagitis and pulmonary aspiration. Like in gastrointestinal emptying, dynamic scintigraphy is also well suited for monitoring if an ingested meal takes a retrograde course from the stomach into the esophagus, and further into the lungs.

Pulmonary aspiration might happen in situations with reduced consciousness after trauma or anesthesia or due to a reduced gag reflex. However, the cases suitable for scintigraphic investigation are those with a confirmed gastroesophageal reflux, and suspected to have a lung problem caused by aspiration of acidic ventricular content. Most patients with this problem are children (4).

Various investigations outside the nuclear medicine field are applied on patients suspected of having a gastric reflux problem. An X-ray examination using contrast of the upper gastrointestinal tract can detect underlying abnormalities in the esophagus, stomach, and duodenum, as well as demonstrating esophageal motility. A Meckel's scintigraphy can detect Barrett's esophagus with ectopic epithelium. Endoscopy and an esophagus biopsy can be used to detect esophagitis. The gold standard for reflux detection is 24 h of pH measurement in the esophagus. A fall in acidity below pH 4 for more than 4% in a 24-h period is considered pathological.

Scintigraphic examinations of gastroesophageal reflux are not invasive and produce a very low radiation dose. Sensitivity to detection of reflux is highest with patients in supine position, and equivalent to the sensitivity of pH measurement in the esophagus. The method's main limitation is that the examination period is necessarily short. It is not possible to monitor the patient throughout the whole day and night. Nevertheless, scintigraphy is probably the most effective method available for detecting pulmonary aspiration (5).

Scintigraphic principle

A ^{99m}Tc-labeled radiopharmaceutical that is not absorbed from the GI-tract is added to a test meal. After intake of the test meal, gastric emptying is measured by dynamic scintigraphy, with lungs and upper part of the abdomen within the camera field of view. Hence, gastric emptying, reflux to the esophagus and aspiration will be revealed.

Indications

- Confirmation of gastroesophageal reflux
- Clarify if lungs problems are due to aspiration of gastric content

Contraindications

- There are no special contraindications. Side effects are not described. Breast feeding can continue without interruption.

General study protocol

The investigation should start in the morning, after the patient has eaten breakfast. Hospitalized patients are studied with juice or milk (at least 150 mL). Children are given 10 mL of juice, milk, or a nutrition liquid with 10 MBq ^{99m}Tc-DTPA, followed by as much as possible of the nonradioactive juice/milk/nutrition. Infants should have a feeding bottle with milk or other kind of nutrition that they are usually fed with. Adults are given 75 mL of fluid with 10 MBq ^{99m}Tc-sulfur colloid and then 75 mL fluid without radioactivity. The patient should sit on a chair with the camera posteriorly over the thorax. Dynamic registration is performed for a total time of typically 60 s, 1 s per image. Then, after drinking, the patient lays down on their back for a dynamic registration posteriorly over the thorax, typically for a total of 2700 s (45 min), 30 s per image.

It is important to add an anatomic landmark to the images to know where the radioactive test meal is located within the gastrointestinal tract. The patient can eat and drink normally after the examination. If the indication for the examination is reflux into the lungs, an extra static image in front and back view of the thorax is appropriate later the same day, and the next morning as well. By following the ROI of the stomach and esophagus during a recording period of approximately 45 min, a time activity curve will give indication whether reflux is present or not. The static images will also add valuable information.

Interpretation and reporting

Almost all children have gastroesophageal reflux the first weeks of life. Some show symptoms, but the symptoms usually disappear when a child reaches 12 months of age. Persistent reflux can cause eating discomfort and "failure to thrive," and can also cause respiratory symptoms, including aspiration pneumonia and asthma. The normal transit period through the esophagus is 6 to 15 s. Any reflux is graded according to duration and proximal extent. Short-term gastroesophageal reflux into the lower part of the esophagus is not to be regarded as abnormal, but detectable pulmonary aspiration is clearly pathological.

No sign of focal activity in the lungs on late scintigrams does not exclude aspiration because the patient may have coughed up aspirate or insufficient amount of activity was left in the stomach during reflux and aspiration. Further imaging has no value when the stomach is completely empty. Scintigraphy cannot replace an X-ray contrast examination when the representation of anatomical details is of interest or necessary.

SMALL BOWEL AND COLON TRANSIT STUDIES

Small and large bowel investigations are performed as a modified continuation of gastric emptying studies(6). Intestinal transit studies have been around for a while but frequently done in a multitude of different ways. To promote more standardized practice, a joint guideline was issued by the society of nuclear medicine and molecular imaging (SNMMI) and European Association of Nuclear Medicine (EANM) in 2013 (7).

Indications

- Suspected gastroparesis
- Dyspepsia
- Irritable bowel syndrome
- Chronic constipation, chronic diarrhea
- Chronic idiopathic intestinal pseudo-obstruction
- Scleroderma
- Celiac disease
- Malabsorption syndromes

Procedure

Preparation for intestinal transit is the same as for gastric emptying (which is the starting point for the investigation):

- Note food allergies/intolerances
- Fast overnight or a minimum of 8 h
- Review medication in advance and discontinue medications that influence motility at least 48 to 72 h in advance (medications that slow transit such as opioids and anticholinergics and prokinetic medications, e.g., erythromycin, laxatives) unless this is an assessment intended to be on ongoing or subsequent treatment.
- Diabetic patients should aim to be euglycemic.
- Normal diet 2 days before and during the 4 to 6 days of a colon study.

Protocols

The following procedures are recommended:

Two tracers, ^{99m}Tc and ^{111}In; ^{67}Ga is an alternative to indium but infrequently used.

Options of either (A) whole-gut transit (including gastric emptying, small bowel and colon transit), (B) small bowel transit (without the colonic section), or (C) colon transit study. The main difference between the methods is option B stops after 24 h, options A and C involve imaging up to 72 h or longer.

The two tracers allow two protocols for each option, either as a single or as a dual isotope method. In all protocols, the small bowel and colonic study is done with a labeled water phase (^{111}In-DTPA, unless single-phase small-bowel transit only, for which ^{99m}Tc-DTPA can be used) and with a solid phase that may be labeled with ^{99m}Tc-DTPA. In practice, this means 300 mL of labeled water and a standard meal (and for solid gastric emptying: egg white omelet, 2 slices white bread, 30 g strawberry jam,

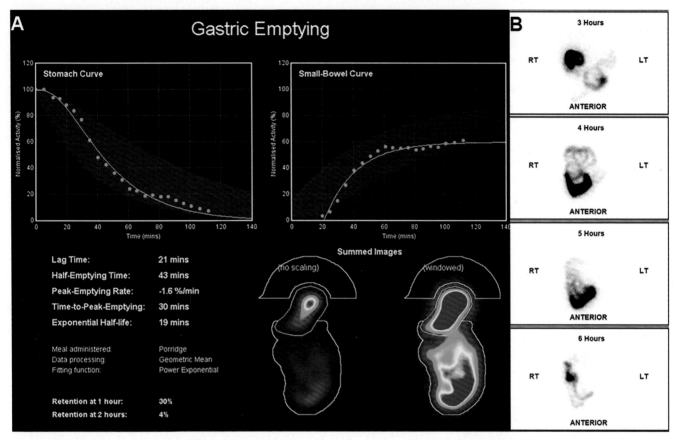

FIG. 12.1 ● Gastric emptying and small bowel transit in a patient following a ^{99m}Tc-labeled solid meal. (A) Analysis showing curves derived for regions of interest over the stomach and small bowel for the first 2 h using a dynamic imaging protocol. (B) Hourly images mapping the progression of tracer through the small bowel and into the terminal ileum at 5 h and cecum at 6 h.

120 mL water). There is one exception. For colon transit, an enteric-coated capsule containing ^{111}In-activated charcoal particles that dissolves in the small bowel and delivers a bolus of activity in the terminal ileum have been established, however, the capsule is not generally available.

The general imaging procedure is based on the whole-gut transit study.

- Large field of view, medium energy collimator for ^{111}In $\pm ^{99m}$Tc, 128 × 128 matrix.
- A cobalt positioning marker on the iliac crest for anatomical reference.
- Anterior and posterior images for 1 min at hourly intervals for 6 h for both ^{111}In-DTPA or ^{99m}Tc-DTPA liquid phase methods.
- If there is a ^{99m}Tc-labeled solid phase, then the gastric emptying imaging protocol is used initially up to 4 h.
- Further images for 4 min at 24, 48, and 72 (and more if necessary) h for ^{111}In. If ^{99m}Tc-DTPA is used for small bowel transit, then only additional imaging is performed up to 24 h.
- Correction is made for isotope decay.

Image analysis

Small bowel transit starts as a gastric emptying investigation then maps the progress of tracer through the small bowel until it reaches the terminal ileum and transfers into the cecum, typically within 6 h of the meal.

An example of a gastric emptying study together with a small bowel uptake curve over 2 h is shown in Figure 12.1A followed by hourly imaging up to 6 h in Figure 12.1B. The images show normal emptying and progression through the small bowel. A quantitative measure of the small bowel is the small bowel transit index at 6 h that measures the total counts in the terminal ileum and colon divided by the average total abdominal counts on the 2 to 5 h images. Geometric mean decay counts are used. Table 12.1 shows reference values for studies based on the guideline protocol.

Potential errors in assessment can arise in identifying the terminal ileum and cecum. The terminal ileum has a reservoir role so transfer to the colon occurs at a different rate, and an image at 24 h is a useful check to see if there is normal transfer to the cecum and that a more proximal hold up has not been misinterpreted as the terminal ileum. Slow transit to the cecum may also be secondary to delayed colonic transit

Table 12.1	**REFERENCE VALUES FOR SMALL BOWEL AND COLON TRANSIT TIMES (FROM [7])**
Small bowel transit index at 6 h	>50%
Colon emptying at 24 h	>14%
48 h	>41%
72 h	>67%
Rapid colonic transit	>40%

Colon transit assessment ideally follows a bolus of activity from the cecum to excretion and is the motivation for a capsule method where the tracer is released in the terminal ileum. The capsule method is not generally available so the protocol begins with combined standard meal and ^{111}In-DTPA water and follows hourly and then daily imaging as previously described. Analysis is based on measuring geometric mean counts in segments of the colon, corrected for decay and normalized to the initial total abdominal counts. Typically, five or seven segments are defined. Counts in each segment can be given as percentage of the total or as a geometric center value, calculated by multiplying the fraction of the total counts in a segment by a weighting factor according to how distal the segment is in the colon and summing over all segments. Figure 12.2 shows analysis of a normal colonic transit case.

There are three main abnormal patterns of slow colonic transit. Generalized slow transit is typically characterized by delayed progression with widespread retention of tracer involving multiple segments. A case is shown in Figure 12.3A. Colonic inertia is rather characterized by delayed accumulation of tracer before the splenic flexure. Functional outlet obstruction is where there is accumulation of tracer in the rectosigmoid region but without proportionate excretion. Figure 12.3B shows a case of rectosigmoidal delay, although relatively normal total colonic transit. By

using standardized protocols, reference values can provide useful guidance. These protocols and reference values should either be defined carefully locally or follow established guidelines.

There are potential a plethora of factors that can affect bowel transit including medication, past surgery, lesions, and age. Transit studies form part of a panel of procedures and investigations to identify the underlying cause and provide only one piece of the usually much larger diagnostic jigsaw associated with bowel pathology.

SALIVARY GLAND FUNCTION

The salivary glands consist of three pairs of exocrine glands. The largest are the parotid glands located immediately posterior to the mandibular ramus with a duct that extends forward and opens into the mouth in the mid buccal region. The second largest are the submandibular glands that are placed medially to the posterior lower edge of the mandibular. The ducts from these glands extend anteriorly to exit through sublingual caruncles either side of the frenulum. Finally, the sublingual glands are located anteriorly submucosally in the floor of the mouth and also drain either side of the frenulum.

Salivary gland scintigraphy was established as a method in the 1970s. There are a number of different protocols described

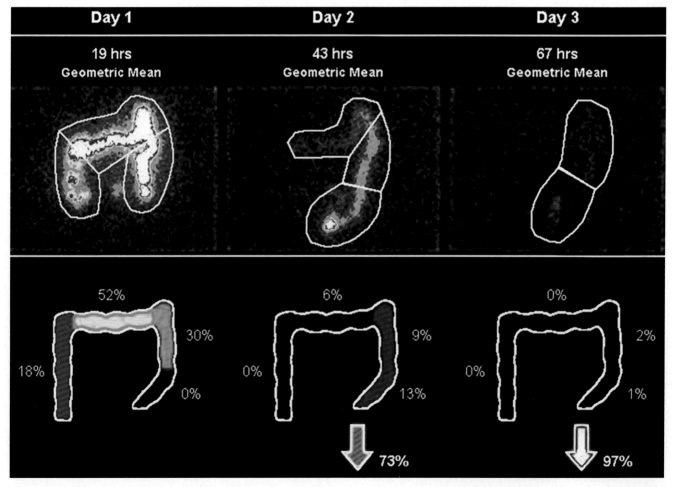

FIG. 12.2 ● Colonic transit study using ^{111}In-DTPA demonstrating segmental analysis (ascending, transverse, descending, rectosigmoid, and excretion segments) showing percentages of total activity in each segment. Normal transit.

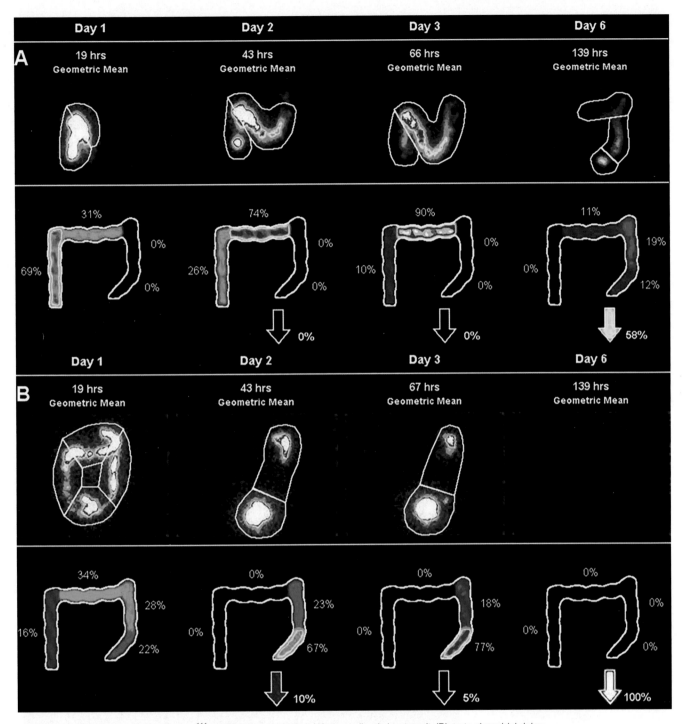

FIG. 12.3 ● Colonic transit study using ^{111}In-DTPA demonstrating (A) generalized slow transit, (B) recto sigmoidal delay.

in the literature. Most are aimed at semi-quantitation of function to evaluate the degree of xerostomia (dryness of the mouth) (8).

A dynamic scan following intravenous injection of ^{99m}Tc pertechnetate allows uptake of tracer into the salivary glands to be followed. Uptake is assumed to be proportional to glandular function. To assess excretion, lemon juice is given toward the end of the registration to stimulate salivary glands to empty. This also allows the drainage conditions to be evaluated.

Indications

- Sjøgren's syndrome to estimate grade of xerostomia grade
- Infectious (viral/bacterial) sialadenitis
- Saliva stone or suspected obstructed salivary gland for some other reason
- Grading of radiation damage (radioiodine induced or due to external radiation therapy)
- Unexplained dry mouth

Contraindications

- Allergic reaction has been described, but is extremely rare
- Check that the patient has not had recent X-ray contrast, iodine supplements, perchlorate thyroid protection (last 24 h) or is on medication that have dry mouth as a significant side effect.

- It is not usually necessary to do this investigation during pregnancy or while breastfeeding. The European Nuclear Medicine Guide (9) suggests breastfeeding must be interrupted for 12 h and pumped milk during that time should be discarded.

PROTOCOL

Gamma Camera with Low Energy, High-Resolution Collimator (LEHR)

- The patient should fast for an hour before the test.
- The patient is placed under the camera with the head in a headrest and as far back as possible. 185–370 MBq ^{99m}Tc pertechnetate is given intravenously.
- Dynamic registration in AP position, zoom × 2, 128 × 128 format, 20 s per image for 50 min. The patient is asked not to swallow unnecessarily during the examination.
- After 40 min, the patient is given 2 mL of concentrated lemon juice using a plastic pipette to ensure minimal head movement. The patient holds the lemon juice in the mouth 15 to 20 s before swallowing. Imaging continues for a further 10 min.
- Effective dose 4.7 mSv/370 MBq. The colon and thyroid gland receive the highest equivalent dose.

- The images are processed by defining five oval regions of interest placed over the oral cavity and the four major salivary glands, respectively, as well as two smaller background regions temporally and sub mentally, respectively, near the parotid and submandibular glands, as shown in the Figure 12.4. Time activity curves are produced for each gland.
- Parameters such as the ejection fraction post lemon juice stimulation, visual appearance scores, uptake curve parameters, and excretion time intervals can be measured and used as objective measures of xerostomia and to follow progression over time.

Applications

Salivary gland scintigraphy is almost always used in conjunction with radiological techniques and frequently after biopsy, so the diagnosis is known. It primarily provides a means to assess function.

Normal uptake and secretion are demonstrated in Figures 12.4A and 12.4B. Figures 12.4C and 12.4D show a patient with xerostomia after treatment for thyroid carcinoma and subsequent metastatic recurrence with two courses of radioactive iodine. There is virtually no tracer uptake in the parotid glands, which were atrophied on CT and ultrasound. There is also significantly

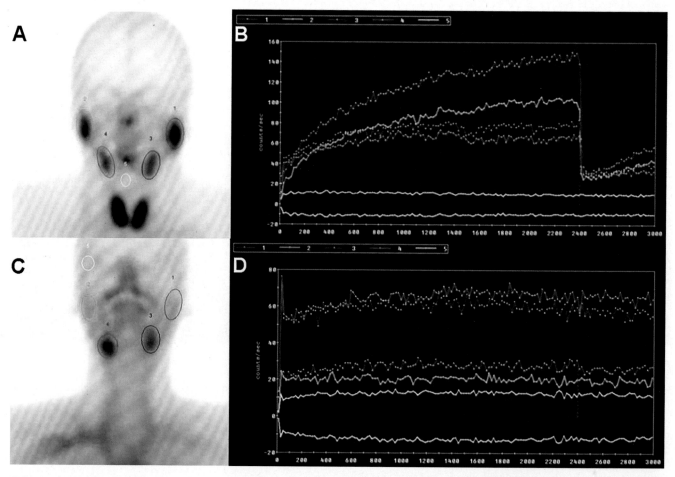

FIG. 12.4 ● Salivary gland scintigraphy. Normal uptake is shown in A and B. (A) Summed uptake of all images defining regions of interest (ROI) over the parotid glands (region 1 and 2 red/green), over the salivary glands (ROI 3 & 4 blue/purple) and background (ROI 5, white). (B) Time activity curves for each ROI. Lemon juice is given after 2400 s (vertical red dotted line). C & D show a patient treated for thyroid carcinoma with postradiation xerostomia and are processed as in A & B. There is considerable reduced tracer uptake by the glands, virtually negligible in the parotid glands, and no significant excretion stimulated by lemon juice.

reduced uptake in the submandibular glands with no response to lemon juice stimulation. Studies suggest that the parotid gland is more susceptible to radiation damage, that subjective dry mouth symptoms are more strongly associated with submandibular gland dysfunction and that there is a dose-response relationship between radiation dose and salivary dysfunction parameters.

Oral cavity activity parameters are also useful to discriminate between normal and patients with different stages of Sjøgren's syndrome (8).

The largest source of error arises from inconsistency in the instillation of lemon juice. Less significant is competitive inhibition of the tracer by other sources of iodide, for example, X-ray contrast, food supplements, or similar anions such as perchlorate used in other nuclear medicine investigations to block or protect the thyroid.

MECKEL'S SCINTIGRAPHY

Meckel's diverticulum is a congenital diverticulum in the ileum, with an incidence of 2%. Most people go through life without any problems related to it, not even knowing that they were born with this anatomic variation, and only 25% to 40% of them will experience symptoms from this diverticulum localized 50 to 100 cm from the ileocecal valve. As 25% of the diverticula contain heterotopic gastric mucosa, this congenital defect may be the origin of a gastrointestinal bleed. This is most common in childhood, and most frequently before the age of 5 years. Less frequently, a Meckel's diverticulum may also lead to complications like diverticulitis, obstruction, or perforation. These complications are more common in adult patients. It is very seldom that patients presenting with Meckel-related complications are over the age of 40.

Scintigraphic principle

In addition to the thyroid and salivary glands, ^{99m}Tc-pertechnetate is concentrated in gastric mucosa cells, and the goal of scintigraphy is to look for ectopic gastric mucosa, i.e., not the bleeding per se. The typical patient is an otherwise healthy child suspected of intestinal bleeding before the age of 5 years, most often less than 2 years. Within this relatively rare group of children with a gastrointestinal bleed a Meckel's diverticulum with ectopic gastric mucosa is a frequent explanation for the situation.

Table 12.2 **PREPARATION FOR A MECKEL SCAN**

Adults and Children

H2 receptor blocker the day before arrival
H2 receptor blocker same morning
Fasting increases sensitivity, but is not mandatory
X-ray contrast media from previous investigations in the gastrointestinal system may attenuate gamma radiation

Indications

- Patients with gastrointestinal bleeding suspected of having ectopic gastric mucosa as the focus for the bleeding.

General study protocol

The H2 receptor antagonist is administered to stabilize and increase the retention of ^{99m}Tc-pertechnetate in topic as well as ectopic gastric mucosa. This increases the sensitivity by increasing the intensity of the uptake in the Meckel's diverticulum and reducing the possibility that intestinal content of ^{99m}Tc-pertechnetate released from gastric mucosa to intestine is misinterpreted as Meckel's diverticulum, Table 12.2 (10,11).

With the patient in position on the camera, ^{99m}Tc-pertechnetate (3 MBq/kg bw) is administered IV in a peripheral vein usually in the antecubital region. Dynamic registration in two different dynamic series:
- 5 s/frame during the first of minute planar acquisition.
- 1 min/frame planar acquisition for the next 60 min.

The purpose of the angiographic dynamic images acquired during the first minute is to reveal vascular malformations that otherwise can be mistaken for ectopic mucosa. The second series is designed to reveal a Meckel's diverticulum, where the uptake often is at its maximum after 20 min. If no focus is seen on the planar images within 60 min, further imaging has no value.

If a Meckel's diverticulum is suspected from the planar images, SPECT/CT may add value to the investigation by more precise localization.

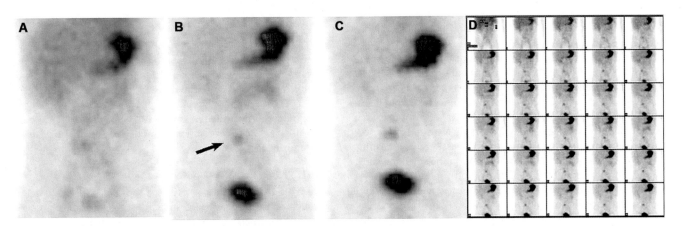

FIG. 12.5 ● Meckel's scintigraphy. Nine-year-old patient with intermittent abdominal pain. Blood per rectum, proctoscopy, and colonoscopy were negative. The scintigrams show focal uptake in the right and lower quadrant of the abdomen already 8–10 min after injection of ^{99m}Tc-pertechnetate consistent with ectopic gastric epithelium in a Meckel's diverticulum (A). The activity increases and persists through the whole 60 min (B & C) acquisition.

Interpretation and reporting

A focal uptake in the terminal part of the ileum is interpreted as a Meckel's diverticulum with ectopic gastric mucosa.

In children with gastrointestinal bleeding in their medical history, sensitivity, specificity, and diagnostic accuracy in detecting ectopic epithelium are 85%, 95%, and 90%, respectively. It is easy to overlook this condition when a diverticulum is located in the pelvis in contact with the bladder unless bladder evacuation and supplementary SPECT are performed. There must also be a certain volume of ectopic epithelium for the scintigraphic detection to be successful. Sensitivity is significantly lower in adults, down to 60%, and diagnostic accuracy is below 50%. Adults rather develop diverticulitis, mechanical ileus, and perforation.

When a Meckel's diverticulum with ectopic gastric mucosa has been confirmed (Fig. 12.5), further investigations, most often endoscopy, may be carried out to confirm bleeding from the area.

Radioactive gastric juice that has passed into the small intestine and urinary tract activity may be mistaken for a Meckel's diverticulum. More frequently false-positives are caused by bowel diseases that need surgical intervention, such as intestinal tumors, arteriovenous malformations, inflammations, invagination, or mechanical ileus for other reasons. The uptake dynamics in these conditions will differ, however, from the uptake in ectopic epithelium. The false-positives typically have highest uptake, i.e., a vascular blush, immediately after the injection. True positives, i.e., gastric mucosa, are seldom visualized before after 20 min after the IV injection. Gastrointestinal duplication is a rare anomaly that can be misinterpreted as Meckel's diverticulum.

In the thorax, neurenteric cysts and Barrett's esophagus will show uptake of ^{99m}Tc-pertechnetate. If the patient has been examined for gastrointestinal bleeding in advance using an in vivo or in vivo/in vitro labeling technique, intravenously injected ^{99m}Tc-pertechnetate will for several days and even weeks after the bleeding examination label the erythrocytes rather than concentrate in the gastric mucosa. However, this is not a problem with pure in vitro erythrocyte labeling.

BILIARY ACID RECIRCULATION

Bile acids are derived from cholesterol, and are either synthetized in the liver (primary bile acids), or produced by bacteria in the colon (secondary bile acids). Bile acids are necessary for digestion, and for absorption of fat and the fat-soluble vitamins. Bile acids are made water soluble by conjugation with the amino acids taurine or glycine in the liver. Sodium and potassium salts of these conjugates form bile salts.

There is an enterohepatic circulation of bile acids. They are secreted from the liver to the intestine, and absorbed by a specific cell membrane transport system in the ileum, bringing bile from the intestinal lumen to the blood. Reduction in this uptake from ileum to the blood is the topic of this section. A variety of gastrointestinal diseases may affect the bile acid uptake mechanism and give a secondary biliary acid malabsorption. These diseases include Crohn's disease, celiac disease, bacterial overgrowth in the small intestine, a variety of other small bowel diseases, and pancreatic diseases. Sometimes, no disease other than the biliary acid malabsorption is found, a condition known as primary biliary acid malabsorption.

Scintigraphic principle

^{75}Se-HomoCholicAcid Taurine (^{75}Se-HCAT) is a synthetic bile acid. After oral intake, about 95% of the preparation is absorbed, mainly in the ileum, and follows the enterohepatic cycle. Normal

Table 12.3 **75-SE-HOMOCHOLICACID TAURINE RETENTION**	
Retention after 7 days:	
>15%:	Normal
10%–15%:	Mild malabsorption
5%–10%:	Moderate malabsorption
<5%:	Serious malabsorption

biologic half-life (for about 97% of the injected activity) is 2.6 days or more, i.e., 15% or more is retained after 7 days (Table 12.3).

Indications

- Evaluation of bile acid malabsorption
- Evaluation of the ileum function in inflammatory intestinal diseases
- Quantification of loss from the bile acid pool
- Study of other factors affecting the enterohepatic cycle

General study protocol

Cholesterol binders must be stopped from 24 h before the appointment, and throughout the 7 days investigation period. No anti-diarrhea medication from the day before and, if possible, throughout the 7 days period.

Day 1: The patient swallows a capsule with 370 MBq ^{75}Se-HCAT together with a glass of water. After 2 h, the initial body content of HCAT is measured by counting with a gamma camera without the collimator. Five minutes counting time. Anterior and posterior camera position over the abdomen. Background counting without the patient in the camera room. Remove radioactive sources of any kind from the room and ensure effective shielding against other radioactive sources in nearby rooms.

Day 7: Repeat counting procedure from day 1. Ensure exactly reproducible camera position and distance between camera and the body on days 1 and 7 measurements. Calculate percent retained radioactivity after 7 days. Use geometric mean of AP and PA counts, adjusted for background and decay.

Applying 15% retention as a lower normal limit gives a specificity of 99%, while 8% retention as upper limit for pathology gives a specificity of 97% (12).

PROTEIN-LOSING ENTEROPATHY

Plasma protein loss to the intestinal lumen lowers the plasma protein level, leading to low osmotic pressure and edema problems. Protein loss may be the dominating problem, such as the seldom disease primary lymphangiectasia, or other types of lymphangiectasia. The protein loss may also be connected with intestinal diseases where protein loss is moderate and is one of many other consequences of the disease.

Scintigraphic principle

Measuring ^{111}In-chloride in feces is a sensitive method to detect pathological elevated gastrointestinal protein loss, and the excreted amount specified as a percentage of the injected dose is a good semi-quantitative measurement for assessing the amount of protein leakage. For daily feces collection and blood sampling during the entire collection period, a leak can be quantitated in milliliter of plasma per day by relating the amount excreted in the feces to the average plasma concentration for the previous day, and then calculate the mean value for several days of measurements.

Gastrointestinal protein loss involves exuding of plasma, and a radiolabeled high-molecular plasma protein that is not reabsorbed after leakage into the gastrointestinal tract can be used to measure protein loss. The precursor of the current method was the injection of ^{51}Cr-chloride. Due to the gamma energy of ^{51}Cr (320 keV) and the fact that over 90% of the photons are internally converted, ^{51}Cr is not suited to scintigraphy. The current methods are based on plasma protein labeling with ^{111}In-chloride. ^{111}In-ions are trivalent and behave like trivalent iron. If not completely saturated with iron, transferrin will have binding capacity for indium ions, and can be labeled with ^{111}In by incubating citrate plasma with ^{111}In-chloride. The iron transporter transferrin has a molecular weight close to the quantitatively dominating plasma protein albumin, and will model this molecule in a situation with plasma protein loss. Hence, in patients with gastrointestinal protein loss, there will also be an increased excretion of ^{111}In-transferrin. Free ^{111}In after digestion of the ^{111}In-transferrin in the intestinal tract will not be reabsorbed. ^{111}In has characteristics that allow scintigraphic visualization of protein leakage. The physical half-life is 2.8 days, which allows quantitation in feces from several days of collection.

The transition from other radionuclides to ^{111}In-chloride as a routine method started in the beginning of the 1990s (13). ^{111}In-chloride was originally produced for in vitro labeling of antibodies for in vivo use. Accordingly, a citrated plasma sample is incubated with the ^{111}In-chloride in vitro before injection. Citrate binds ^{111}In in a negative complex that prevents precipitation, but because the indium-ions affinity to transferrin is much higher than its affinity to citrate, and trivalent ^{111}In-ions will bind to the unsaturated transferrin in the plasma sample. Any possible excess of ^{111}In-citrate are removed using anion exchangers.

After IV injection of the autologous plasma containing radiolabeled transferrin, the loss of plasma proteins can be followed scintigraphically and by radioactivity counting. Two different methods for quantification are available: Collection and counting in feces, or by whole body counting. Whole body counting requires exclusion of any non-enteropathy protein lowering mechanism, primarily proteinuria (14).

Indications

- Detection and quantification of pathological gastrointestinal protein loss
- Localization of the leakage point
- Follow-up of disease activity in patients with stomach/intestinal illnesses with known pathological gastrointestinal protein loss.

General study protocol

The patient should not take iron supplements the last 24 h before the investigation, as transferrin binding sites may be saturated with iron; no other patient preparation.

A blood sample is taken for determination of plasma levels of iron and transferrin, and transferrin saturation is calculated. The blood sample for radiolabeling is then mixed with ^{111}In-chloride. Assessment of the labeling efficiency is performed using an anion exchange column that elutes uncharged proteins while anions, including any citrate-bound indium, are attached to the column.

The patient is injected with the ^{111}In-labeled plasma, and image acquisitions are done with the gamma camera in anterior position over the abdomen. As mentioned in the introduction, there are two alternative procedures for localization and quantification of gastrointestinal protein loss: (1). collection and counting of feces combined with imaging to localize the intestinal

leaking spot; (2). whole body counting combined with imaging to localize the leaking spot.

1. Collection of feces combined with imaging
   All feces must be collected for 5 days. It is important to note that feces collection must be complete. Anterior and posterior scintigraphy of the abdominal and pelvic region to localize the leakage spot starts immediately after the injection on day 1, typically 10 min acquisition periods starting 5, 30, 60, 120, 180, 240, and 360 min after the injection. Depending on the result from the planar images, SPECT/CT may be helpful. The patient attends for a final image on day 2 and for delivery of the collected feces on day 5.
2. Whole body counting combined with imaging
   Anterior and posterior scintigraphy of the abdominal and pelvic region to localize the leakage spot starts immediately after the injection, same procedure as described earlier for the imaging combined with feces collection. Whole body counting is performed with an uncollimated gamma camera, with distance of about 4 m between patient and camera. Acquisition time 5 min, and correction, is made for background. The whole body counting is repeated on day 2 after the imaging procedure and thereafter more whole body counts on day 4 and 5.

Interpretation and reporting

Normally, transferrin is not fully saturated with iron and the labeling efficacy is at least 80%, typically 90%. If the patient has ingested ferrous preparations in the last 24 h before the injection, the labeling might be poor.

On the scintigram, uptake in the bone marrow is normal. Moreover, leakage into the bowel might happen, but seldom within the first 6 h. Occasionally, the colon is visualized as a normal phenomenon after 24 h. Kidney and bladder activity is normally not visualized. Normal half-life in plasma is 15 to 20 h.

In conditions with increased gastrointestinal protein loss, the leakage is visible after 3 to 4 h. Scintigrams acquired approximately 6 h after labeled plasma injection tend to best locate the leakage. It is important to keep in mind that the initial leakage of plasma into the GI-tract is moving with the intestinal content. If the gastrointestinal protein loss is only slightly increased, the method can fail to localize the leakage point. Only major leaks are located with reasonable certainty. Leakage into the stomach is difficult to visualize because it can be challenging to separating the radioactivity of the stomach from blood pool activity in the liver and spleen.

A gastrointestinal protein loss into the 5 days' feces collection exceeding 1.2% is defined as pathologic. Fecal excretion from 1.2% to 2.5% is described as slightly elevated, from 2.4% to 4% as moderately elevated, and over 4% clearly elevated gastrointestinal protein loss. A loss of 15% or higher is rare. When whole body counting is applied, the normal loss measured on day 5, that is, after 96 h, has been measured to 1.8% ± 1.3% (15).

GASTROINTESTINAL BLEEDING SCINTIGRAPHY

Bleeding into the gastrointestinal tract is a common medical problem. Most of the cases are diagnosed by upper endoscopy, or proctoscopy and colonoscopy. However, when the origin of the bleeding is situated in the small intestine or the upper part of the colon, conventional endoscopic localization may be difficult. Scintigraphic localization is then an option, based on extravascular leakage of an intravascular radioactive tracer. Alternatively, radiological angiography is a more precise method for localization of the bleeding, but active bleeding during the radiologic contrast injection is a prerequisite, and the blood flow must be at least 1 mL/min. Wireless capsule endoscopy where the patient swallows a capsule with a radio transmitter that takes pictures frequently while it passes the digestive tract is also an option. Intestinal peristalsis moves the capsule along the digestive tract and the entire tract becomes available for consideration. Double balloon enteroscopy is another option.

Scintigraphic principle

Autologous erythrocytes are labeled *in vitro* with ^{99m}Tc-pertechnetate. Leakage of circulating radiolabeled erythrocytes into the stomach or intestines indicates bleeding.

Pure *in vivo* labeling of erythrocytes must be avoided. Poor erythrocyte labeling and high level of free ^{99m}Tc-pertechnetate will give scintigrams with poor contrast, ample urine activities and ^{99m}Tc absorption in the thyroid, salivary glands, and stomach. Uptake in the salivary glands and stomach leads to release of radioactivity into the gastrointestinal tract. Even after an in vitro labeling procedure with a labeling efficacy of 98%, radioactivity can occasionally be seen in the colon after 24 h due to free ^{99m}Tc-pertechnetate.

Gastrointestinal bleeding is often intermittent. Information about time of the last bleeding is important information in the interpretation of the images. In contrast to the alternative methods, a scintigraphy procedure can be prolonged as long as the gamma camera count rate is high enough. With ^{99m}Tc-labeled erythrocytes, the patient can be followed with extra scintigrams for about 24 h, sometimes 30 h.

- IndicationsLocate non-life-threatening but transfusion-dependent gastrointestinal bleeding when the site of the bleeding cannot be located by endoscopy.
- Occult bleeding cannot be detected.

General study protocol

No preparation is required, but it is an advantage if the patient's stomach is not filled with food. Erythrocyte labeling may be reduced if the patient has received an intravenous injection of X-ray contrast media within the last 24 h. Moreover, residual X-ray contrast media in the gastrointestinal tract after a previous radiologic procedure can shield radioactivity in the intestines (16). The pulse and blood pressure should be measured upon arrival to ensure that the patient is not hypotensive. Since the examination involves injection of autologous erythrocytes handled in vitro, it is especially important to avoid reinjection of labeled blood products into the wrong patient. Sodium perchlorate is administered to reduce the pertechnetate uptake in the thyroid, and salivary glands and gastric mucosa.

A sample of 2 mL of blood is drawn, and erythrocytes are labeled. Reinjection of erythrocytes should be done within 30 min after finishing the labeling. Immediately, upon reinjection of labeled erythrocytes, a two-phase dynamic scintigraphy with frame mode recording of the abdomen can be acquired, preferably simultaneous anterior and posterior imaging with a double-headed camera:

- First phase 3 s/acquisition for 60 s.
- Second phase 120 s/acquisition for 60 min.
- If these two procedures do not provide positive findings, continue repeating at short (approx. 10 min.) dynamic series after 2, 3, 4, and 6 h, and possibly static images the next morning.

It may improve the localization to do a SPECT/CT. Minimum dose for children are 90 MBq. If it is difficult to draw blood, an in vivo labeling can be a solution.

Poor labeling effect can occasionally be a problem. Some medications have this effect, such as cyclosporine, nifedipine, verapamil, apresoline, propranolol, and digoxin. Cephalosporin cefotaxime can also interfere in manner similar to the antineoplastic agents etoposide and idarubicin. Other neoplastic agents such as doxorubicin, 5-fluorouracil, cyclophosphamide, vincristine, and cisplatin do not interfere.

Interpretation and reporting

Some ^{99m}Tc will be released from the erythrocytes and the bladder will always be visualized, while the intensity in the urinary tract and the kidneys are usually on a level that corresponds to intravascular activity. Progressive activity outside the bloodstream and the urinary tract indicates bleeding. The activity will follow the gut content and progress distally in the gastrointestinal tract (Fig. 12.6). It is essential that the imaging results are examined in CINE mode.

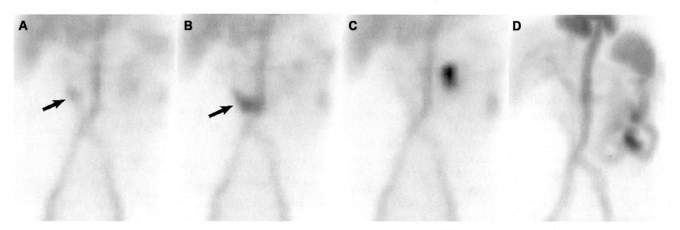

FIG. 12.6 ● Gastrointestinal bleeding scintigraphy. Middle-aged man s/p liver transplant due to liver cirrhosis secondary to hepatitis C presented with postoperative melena and anemia. Gastroduodenoscopy was negative. Immediately following injection of radiolabeled erythrocytes, a 2-phase dynamic scan of the abdomen was acquired. Focal activity was seen 31 min later at the right side of the aorta (A), moving initially toward the right side, (B) and then to the left side of the abdomen (C). Serial scintigrams 120 s/acquisition for 60 min (D). Based on location and the movement pattern of the activity, the focus of bleeding was (and later confirmed), to be in the descending duodenum.

Table 12.4 **COMMON HEPATOBILIARY AND SPLENIC SCINTIGRAPHIC INVESTIGATIONS**

	Investigation	Tracer	Mechanism	Alternative methods
Liver and biliary function	Cholescintigraphy	^{99m}Tc IDA derivatives	Bilirubin like clearance and excretion	MRCP or with biliary specific contrast, ERCP
Liver function		^{99m}Tc-GSA	Uptake by hepatocytes	CT or MR volumetry
Liver cavernous hemangioma,	Red blood cell liver scan	^{99m}Tc-labeled red blood cells	Visualizing vascularity and relative flow	MR, CT, ultrasound
Liver, spleen, bone marrow reticuloendothelial function	Colloid liver-spleen scan	^{99m}Tc colloid	Uptake by Kupfer cells in the liver, macrophages in spleen and marrow	MR
Splenunculi, splenosis	Denatured red blood cell scan	^{99m}Tc-labeled red blood cells	Macrophage uptake in splenic red pulp	MR

IDA, iminodiacetic acid; GSA, galactosyl human serum albumin; ERCP, endoscopic retrograde cholangiopancreatography; MRCP, magnetic resonance cholangiopancreatography.

The advantage of this scintigraphic method is the possibility to detect intermittent bleeding. Occult bleeding cannot be detected, and 5 mL of blood is the absolute smallest quantity that can be detected. However, this presupposes that the blood volume is not diluted. Active peristalsis in the small intestine tends to dilute the intraluminal blood volume and reduce the count rate. As a rule of thumb, for detection of a bleed, the flow should be at least 0.3 mL/min, corresponding to a transfusion need of about 450 mL blood per 24 h. However, bleeding rates of one third of this may occasionally be detected. Sensitivity and specificity for detection of transfusion-dependent bleeding is approximately 90%.

Localization of the bleeding focus is more difficult than detection of the bleeding per se. It takes time before the bleeding target to background ratio is high enough. Bleeding can be located incorrectly and distal to its origin, especially if the focus is located in the small intestine. In the colon, where the movement of intestinal content is slower, localization is easier. However, retrograde movement of the blood can occur, and then the bleeding focus is incorrectly localized proximal to the starting point. A prerequisite for reasonably correct localization of the origin of the gastrointestinal bleeding is that the images are viewed in cine mode. Vascular structures like mesenteric varices, corpora cavernosa penis, and urinary tract activity, such as in the pelvis of a transplanted kidney, should not be misinterpreted as gastrointestinal bleeding.

Hepatobiliary and splenic scintigraphy

Hepatobiliary imaging has undergone many changes since cholescintigraphy was first done in the 1960s. Many investigations from the time before CT and ultrasound such as assessment of cirrhosis have become of historical interest. However, the underlying nuclear medicine principle of imaging function, combined with SPECT and positron emission tomography (PET), means that the original techniques are finding their place in ever more refined imaging techniques that combine radiological anatomy with nuclear medicine function.

There are a number of strategies for investigating the liver, and commonly used tracers are listed in Table 12.4 together with mechanisms. The predominant imaging method, cholescintigraphy, is based around tracer uptake by the liver and excretion through the biliary system into the duodenum. This allows visualization of kinetics of uptake in liver parenchyma and allows a proxy assessment of liver function. Following the excretion process provides a tool to assess biliary and extrahepatic atresia, obstruction, cholecystitis, and post hepatic and biliary surgery.

CHOLESCINTIGRAPHY

The precursor of liver and biliary tract scintigraphy was the ^{131}I rose Bengal test. This test was based on radiolabeling the fluorescent dye rose Bengal that has a long history of use in microscopy and some clinical uses. After intravenous injection, the plasma clearance of ^{131}I-rose Bengal was used as a liver function test, liver activity time curves were assessed, and percentage of the injected dose excreted in feces measured. Subsequently, ^{99m}Tc-labeled radiopharmaceuticals have been developed that are also rapidly absorbed into the hepatocytes and excreted via the bile that allow dynamic imaging of the liver parenchyma, biliary ducts, gallbladder, and bile excretion to the small intestine. Since the 1990s, ^{99m}Tc-labeled hepatobiliary iminodiacetic acid (HIDA) derivatives have been available. Trimethyl-bromo-iminodiacetate (Mebrofenin) is commonly used due to higher hepatic extraction and performance in patients with hepatic dysfunction. The tracer is rapidly extracted from the blood almost exclusively by hepatocytes using a mechanism similar to other organic amines. It is not significantly metabolized or conjugated and is rapidly excreted (clearance half-life is under 20 min). Normally about 98% is excreted unchanged via the bile. As such, HIDA derivatives can be used to assess liver function and biliary excretion in an analogous dynamic way to MAG3 and renal function (17).

^{99m}Tc-HIDA scintigraphy can be supplemented with several pharmacological interventions. Analogues of the gastrointestinal hormone, cholecystokinin (CCK), stimulate liver and bile secretion, gallbladder contraction, and relaxation of the sphincter of Oddi. Sincalide (CCK-8) is a synthetic octapeptide that consists of the 8 amino acids at the C-terminus of CCK. The half-life of CCK-8 in the blood is approx. 2.5 min so is given with as an infusion or a slow bolus. An alternative to CCK-8 is a fatty meal such as 300 mL of whole milk. Although intuitively this method is more physiological, it is less reproducible and reference data have a wider normal range. Morphine causes contraction of the Sphincter of Oddi, reduces excretion of bile to the duodenum, increases biliary duct pressure, and is used to stimulate gallbladder filling. It has a half-life of 2.5 h. Phenobarbital induces microsomal liver enzymes and increases bilirubin conjugation and excretion as well as increasing bile flow. It is typically given in investigations to diagnose biliary atresia in neonates.

Radiopharmaceuticals

Current radiotracers are based on ^{99m}Tc-labeled iminodiacetic acid analogues. The most common are ^{99m}Tc-bromotriethyl IDA (mebrofenin) and ^{99m}Tc diisopropyl IDA (disofenin or DISIDA). The European Nuclear Medicine Guide (9) recommends adult activities between 111 and 185 MBq. Higher activities are suggested in patients with hyperbilirubinemia. Pediatric activities are adjusted according to weight, for example, using the EANM pediatric dose calculator, down to a minimum of 20 MBq. The effective dose for ^{99m}Tc-HIDA is 16 microSv/MBq, or 1.8 to 3.0 mSv. The large intestine receives the highest dose, followed by the gallbladder depending on the patient's individual physiology.

Indications

- Upper right quadrant pain variants/functional bile pain syndromes with normal radiological findings-biliary dyskinesia
- Measurement of gallbladder ejection fraction (GBEF) in chronic cholecystitis/gallbladder dyskinesia (chronic, stone-free gallbladder disease)
- Postsurgical complications including suspected bile leakage or obstruction post-traumatic or postoperative (liver transplantation, biliary tract surgery, Kasai procedure)
- Post-cholecystectomy syndrome/sphincter of Oddi dysfunction
- Enterogastric reflux and afferent loop syndrome. Biliary reflux to the esophagus after gastrectomy
- Congenital biliary system anomalies; biliary atresia, choledochal cysts
- Evaluation of liver transplants
- Functional liver evaluation before liver resection
- Cholecystitis

Contraindications

- Very high plasma bilirubin (e.g., above 600 mmol/L) indicates a high degree of hepatocellular injury so that liver uptake and bile excretion are poorly visualized, and the dynamics of the investigation are altered.
- CCK-8 is contraindicated in patients who have previously had severe side effects or who have known intestinal obstruction.
- Rapid intravenous injection of significantly higher doses than 20 ng Sincalide per kg body weight commonly causes abdominal discomfort (transient colic pain and nausea). Ideally, CCK-8 is delivered over a 1-h infusion.

General study protocol

Patient preparation
To ensure the gallbladder is not contracted in patients under investigation for biliary dyskinesia, fasting for between 2 and 6 h

is required. If filling of the gallbladder is not an important point, fasting is not necessary, for example in biliary atresia.

Technique

- Dynamic planar imaging of the liver and biliary system using a large field of view gamma camera with a low energy general purpose collimator.
- Short frames (e.g., 1–2 s frames) at time of injection, for 60 s to observe the blood pool phase. Then 1 min frames for 60–90 min.
- If the gallbladder is not visualized at 60 min, right lateral and left anterior oblique views can be useful to distinguish possible gallbladder uptake from the liver.

With the normal hepatobiliary scintigram (Fig. 12.7), liver activity maximizes within 12 min, with a normal liver activity T1/2 of less than 20 min. Bile dusts visualize at 5 to 20 min and the gallbladder fills from 10 to 40 min. Activity is seen in the duodenum and small bowel after 15 to 60 min if gallbladder present or less than 10 min post-cholecystectomy.

Hepatobiliary scintigraphy sources of errors (18) include the following:

- Activity in the duodenum, renal pelvis or enlarged cystic duct that may be mistaken for gallbladder activity.
- Lack of visualization of the biliary tract should be interpreted with caution in all patients with bilirubin concentrations over 300 mmol/L.
- Lack of visualization may also be due to short fasting (<2–4 h), too long fasting (> 24 h), high-grade choledochal obstruction, or severe intercurrent disease.
- Morphine and related preparations can cause spasm of sphincter Oddi and give a pattern as in choledochal obstruction.
- Diaper activity (possibly with skin contamination) may be interpreted as bowel activity.

Postprandial epigastric pain

Scintigraphy has been based around demonstrating lack of gallbladder filling on a standard protocol and absent filling on delayed imaging or following morphine, to induce increased biliary duct pressure. Although scintigraphy has very high sensitivity (97%) and specificity (94%), acute cholecystitis investigation has been essentially replaced by ultrasound, which can visualize gallstones and signs of inflammation in a fraction of the time taken for scintigraphy or magnetic resonance cholangiopancreatography (MRCP).

In patients with biliary type pain without gallstones or signs of inflammation on ultrasound or findings on other investigation, cholescintigraphy is useful to assess gallbladder function. Both filling and emptying of the gallbladder are useful assessments. Normally, within the first hour postinjection, there is rapid blood pool clearance and liver uptake and excretion, biliary drainage with gallbladder filling, and tracer transfer to the small bowel. If the gallbladder is not visualized after 60 min, an injection of morphine IV (0.04 mg/kg) can be given slowly over 2 to 3 min, which is intended to increase the tone in the sphincter of Oddi, increase biliary pressure, and facilitate gallbladder filling. If the tracer is already washed out to the small bowel, a new tracer injection should be given before the morphine. Continue imaging for another 30 min. Non-visualization of gallbladder after this maneuver is compatible acute cholecystitis.

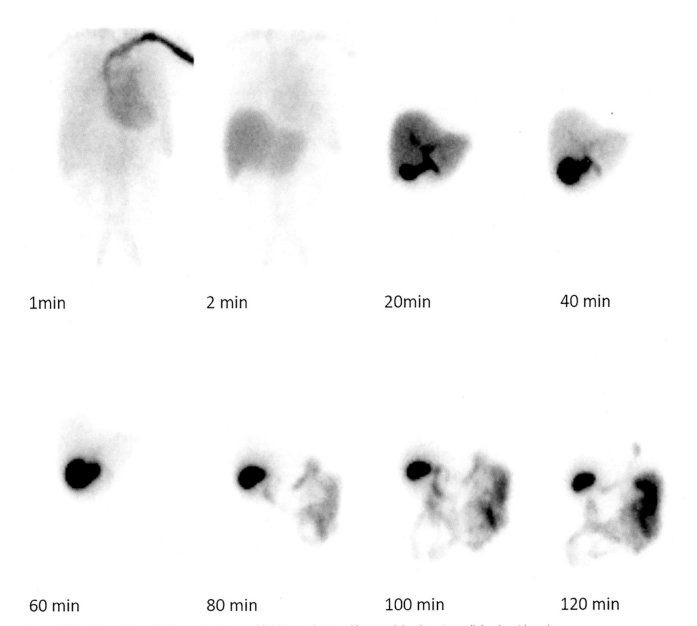

1min   2 min   20min   40 min

60 min   80 min   100 min   120 min

FIG. 12.7 ● Normal hepatobiliary scintigraphy. Middle-aged man with unexplained postprandial epigastric pain for several years accompanied with occasional nausea, bloating, and pallid stools. The first 60 min demonstrate a normal study with filling of the gallbladder. The second 60 min demonstrate gallbladder emptying during CCK infusion. The GBEF is 65%.

Gallbladder emptying can be assessed using CCK to stimulate gallbladder contraction. An GBEF of less than 38% is considered abnormal and compatible with chronic cholecystitis and/or biliary dyskinesia. Normal value is typically greater than 50% (75% ± 20%). Various protocols for CCK administration are described with infusions ranging from 3 to 60 min although the 60 min protocol is best validated. Figure 12.7 demonstrates a case measuring the GBEF. The first 60 min follows the standard protocol. Then CCK intravenous infusion (0.02 mcg/kg over 60 min) is given. The GBEF is calculated from the gallbladder ROI as the counts at 60-min post-CCK infusion counts divided by the pre-CCK infusion counts.

Postsurgical complications

The time frame of nuclear medicine investigations over minutes to hours can be advantageous when one is looking for complications of surgery. Nuclear medicine investigation of early complications such as bleeding and vascular problems has largely been supplanted by radiological investigations. The exception is where the issue is intermittent or low volume and there are multiple potential sites of complication. An example is biliary leakage after complex surgery such as liver transplantation or small bowel reconstruction after gastric or pancreatic surgery.

Cholescintigraphy can be helpful in problem solving of late surgical complications that may be related to biliary excretion and drainage. Stent patency and effect on function can be evaluated. Persistent post cholecystectomy colic in the absence of radiological findings can be investigated. Guidelines suggest the use of a CCK infusion 10 min before and during a standard cholescintigraphy investigation in patients with suspected sphincter of Oddi dysfunction. Cholescintigraphy may also be helpful

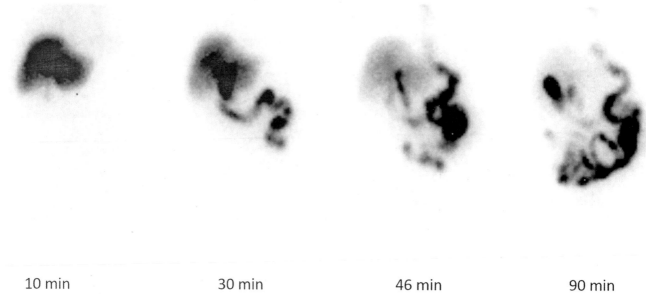

| 10 min | 30 min | 46 min | 90 min |

FIG. 12.8 ● Patient with biliary reflux after gastric bypass surgery. The hepatobiliary scan images show normal liver uptake and biliary excretion to the jejunal anastomosis. For the first 45 min, there is anterograde biliary flow into the small bowel. After 45 min, there is retrograde biliary reflux to the gastric pouch and into the esophagus that persists to the end of the scan.

in cases of postsurgical recurrent gastric or esophageal biliary reflux (Fig. 12.8). In these cases CCK infusion, delayed imaging and SPECT-CT may all be useful tools to demonstrate the problem.

Biliary atresia

This is a rare disease that presents in newborn infants characterized by narrow, blocked, or absent bile ducts. The incidence varies with ethnicity, between 1:5000 and 1:15000. Prompt diagnosis is required as surgical treatment, such as the Kasai procedure (hepatoportoenterostomy), can delay liver failure and the need

for liver transplantation. The infant presents with neonatal jaundice, and the aim of investigation is to differentiate atresia from other causes of neonatal jaundice.

Phenobarbital given 5 mg/kg for 5 days before the investigation increases bilirubin conjugation and excretion as well as increasing bile flow. The infant does not need to be fasted. Tracer uptake in the small bowel rules out atresia but delayed or no transfer of tracer to the small bowel is not specific for atresia. Delayed planar imaging up to 24 h is done if no tracer transfer to the small bowel is seen. Figure 12.9 shows an example of patent common bile duct in a jaundiced infant without biliary atresia.

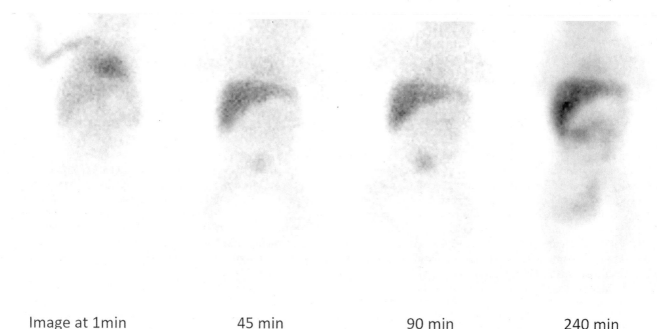

| Image at 1min | 45 min | 90 min | 240 min |

FIG. 12.9 ● Hepatobiliary scintigraphy to investigate conjugated hyperbilirubinemia in a neonatal infant. Images show rapid tracer uptake in the liver but very slow biliary excretion and transfer of tracer to the small bowel, which is only seen on the 4-h delayed image. Transfer of tracer to the small bowel rules out biliary atresia.

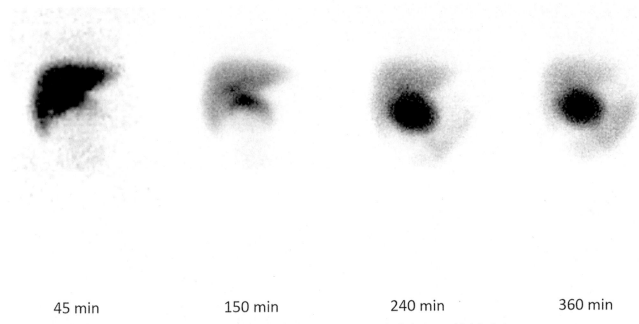

| 45 min | 150 min | 240 min | 360 min |

FIG. 12.10 ● Cholescintigraphy imaging of a patient with Todani type 4a choledochal cysts, which includes a large cyst in the proximal common bile duct that overlaps the cystic duct as well as a central intrahepatic cyst. The slow clearance of tracer from the liver suggests a degree of biliary obstruction.

Choledochal cysts

Choledochal cysts are rare (fewer than 1/150,000 births) and are more prevalent in Asia and in females (3:1). The cysts are classified according to the Todani system based on number and position of cysts. Most cases are diagnosed during childhood although can also be diagnosed later. Management is predominantly surgical excision although one type (Todani type 3) with a cyst at the distal end of the common bile duct may be treated by endoscopic retrograde cholangiopancreatography (ERCP). Choledochal cysts increase the risk for cholangiocarcinoma, even after excision and regular follow-up is necessary. Figure 12.10 shows an example of a Todani Type 4A choledochal cyst.

Liver function and surgical planning pre-liver resection

The liver has both a capacity for regeneration and a relative functional over capacity in healthy people. This makes liver resection, to treat both primary liver tumors and metastases, a procedure with limited morbidity and mortality, although a reliable assessment of the capacity of the postsurgical liver remnant to maintain function is required. There are a number of established methods to assess liver function including blood tests and clinical scoring systems, such as the Child–Pugh–Turcotte score. Liver volumetry using CT or MR provides a method to assess the fractional liver remnant but assumes a linear proportionality between volume and function. Studies have shown that liver resection in normal liver is safe when there is a remaining volume of 25% to 30%. In diseased liver, the threshold rises to 40% although this is an empirical value with many caveats. Ideally, methods with a spatially distributed measure of function that can be imaged would be a way to combine both approaches and potentially provide a more reliable and individualized assessment of remnant liver function.

Methods have been developed using a number of radiotracers listed in Table 12.1. Mebrofenin is the most generally available and

there are a number of methods in the literature describing protocols, quantitative assessment, and threshold functional values based on them. Table 12.4 outlines a method developed in Amsterdam (19). A quantitative method for the assessment of liver function has been developed in Amsterdam (19). After a standard patient preparation, using a SPECT-CT camera with LEHR collimator, dynamic hepatic uptake of mebrofenin is measured in 38 frames of 10 s/frame, in anterior and posterior planar projections. SPECT-CT is performed immediately after the dynamic phase for 60 frames at 8 s/frame along with low-dose CT (e.g., 20 mA, 110 kV) without breath-hold. A dynamic excretion phase is acquired for 20 frames at 60 s/frame, 128 matrix, in anterior and posterior projections.

Mebrofenin uptake rate (MUR) is calculated from the dynamic series, first calculating the geometric mean for each frame, then time activity curves for liver, blood pool (left ventricle and aortic root), and total field of view and finally fitting the curves to an appropriate kinetic model. The MUR is calculated as percentage of total administered mebrofenin accumulated in the liver per minute (%/min) and normalized to body surface area (%/min/m^2). MUR is used as a measure of global liver function. Functional methods can be used to assess function and plan interventions such as portal vein embolization and associating liver partition and portal vein ligation for staged hepatectomy (ALPPS) that aim to stimulate lobar hypertrophy before resection.

Figure 12.11 shows an example of a patient undergoing right portal vein embolization before right hemihepatectomy for metastases. There is significant left lobe hypertrophy in the space of weeks and the left lobar function, measured as the normalized MUR, rises from 1.0% to 2.7%/min/m^2. Studies in the literature suggest that a value of 2.7%/min/m^2 is a conservative lower limit for future remnant liver (FRL) function in patients undergoing liver resection for biliary tumors. The variability of this threshold depending on disease type has yet to be established.

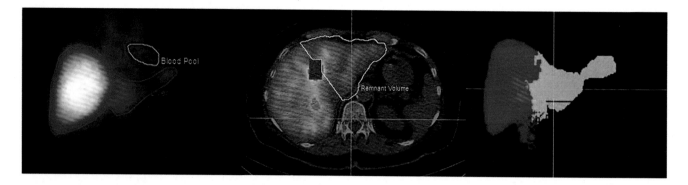

Pre intervention dynamic scan   ROIs Left and right liver segmentation   Predicted FRL

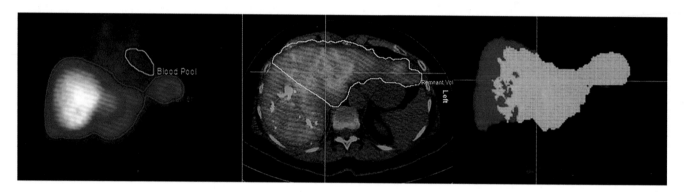

Post intervention dynamic scan ROI Left and right liver segmentation   Predicted FRL

FIG. 12.11 • Planning scintigraphic scans of the liver pre and post right portal vein embolization before right hemihepatectomy for metastases. (A) Example planar image early in the dynamic scan with regions of interest to calculate mebrofenin uptake rate. (B) Left liver lobe region of interest, with the central biliary duct masked out. (C) Segmented liver. (D) Early dynamic scan image post right portal vein embolization. (E) Hybrid image showing embolization material in the right lobe. F) Segmented liver showing hypertrophy of the left lobe and reduction of the right lobe. FRL = future remnant liver.

LIVER ASSESSMENT BEFORE SELECTIVE INTERNAL RADIATION THERAPY

This treatment employs embolization with small ^{90}Y-labeled beads (microspheres) that emit beta particles and result in localized radiotherapy. There are two main indications:

• Treatment of unresectable primary liver tumors or various types of liver metastases
• Neoadjuvant treatment of tumors before resection or liver transplantation

The tumors derive their circulation from the hepatic arterial supply, so treatment is achieved by selectively catheterizing the lobar or segmental artery supplying the tumor region. The tumor typically has high blood flow and the particles largely accumulate in the vascular regions of the tumor. Normal liver parenchyma largely derives its blood supply from the portal vein, has relatively low arterial demand, and receives only a minor fraction of the treatment dose. There is a risk that the tumor creates an arteriovenous shunt so that some of the dose bypasses the tumor into the hepatic vein and this should be assessed before SIRT is given. This is done as part of the planning angiography workup where once the catheter position for treatment has been planned, and

an injection of ^{99m}Tc macroaggregated albumin (MAA) is given. Angiography is also employed to assess and avoid or embolize any small arteries connecting the hepatic and gastroduodenal circulation, which can also be assessed on the ^{99m}Tc-MAA scan. The patient is then imaged immediately after angiography using planar imaging of thorax and abdomen and possibly also SPECT/CT to establish more accurate distribution of tracer in the liver and lungs. The systemic shunt from the liver to the lungs is calculated as the proportion of the total activity in the lungs. Too high a dose of particles shunting into the lungs runs the risk of radiation pneumonitis and ultimately pulmonary fibrosis. Guidelines suggest reductions in administered microsphere dose for shunts between 10% and 20%. Therapy is contraindicated for a shunt over 20%. Figure 12.12 shows a patient with a large hepatocellular carcinoma with a hepato-systemic shunt of 11%.

Other applications

It is worth mentioning that ^{99m}Tc colloid has had past utility in assessing liver cirrhosis as well as localizing lesions such as hepatic adenoma, focal nodular hyperplasia, carcinoma, and metastases. Other than as an alternative method to assess functional reserve liver, ^{99m}Tc colloid scintigraphy has almost entirely been replaced by radiological techniques. Blood pool imaging using ^{99m}Tc red

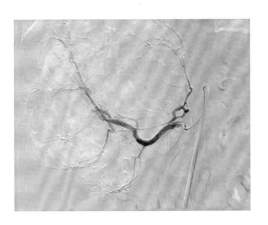
A

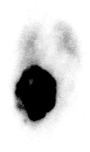
B

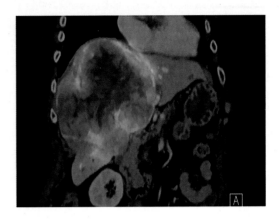
C

FIG. 12.12 • SIRT treatment of a patient with a large hepatocellular carcinoma. **A:** Angiogram of the tumor during workup showing the position of the catheter for treatment. **B:** Planar scintigraphy following injection of ^{99m}Tc-MAA from the catheter. The majority of the tracer is in the tumor but there is an 11% shunt to the lungs. **C:** ^{90}Y PET-CT of the tumor posttreatment showing predominantly peripheral distribution of tracer in the centrally necrotic tumor. ^{90}Y may be scanned either with Bremsstrahlung imaging or as ^{90}Zr PET. The ^{90}Y dose is reduced depending on the degree of lung shunting. Lung shunt fraction (LSF) less than 10% requires no dose reduction. LSF between 10% and 15% as in this patient requires a 20% dose reduction. LSF between 15% and 20% requires a 40% dose reduction. LSF greater than 20% usually makes ^{90}Y SIRT inappropriate unless the shunt can be located and occluded.

blood cells to visualize cavernous hemangioma, where decreased perfusion and increased blood pool uptake is seen, is occasionally still done instead of MRI.

A recent publication on quantitative PET of liver functions by Keiding et al. (20) looked at the use of dynamic PET to assess function. With the high spatial and time resolution afforded by PET, parameters relating to various kinetic compartment models can be measured. ^{18}F-fluoro-D-galactose (^{18}F-FDGal) is almost exclusively metabolized in hepatocytes and provides a measure of hepatic carbohydrate metabolism. They show that SUV measured on a static scan at 10 to 20 min postinjection correlates linearly with the metabolic clearance rate and can replace quantification from a dynamic scan. This provides the PET equivalent of the liver function assessment using mebrofenin cholescintigraphy, as described earlier, for preoperatively estimating metabolic future remnant liver.

The most commonly available PET tracer, ^{18}F-FDG, has more complex kinetics due to competitive metabolism with glucose. However, there are a number of studies investigating the use of ^{18}F-FDG to measure effects of insulin and drugs on the liver as well as the effect of disease such as nonalcoholic fatty liver disease on glucose metabolism. PET also provides a potentially useful tool for measuring bile acid secretion (e.g., ^{11}C-CSar), lipid metabolism (e.g., ^{11}C-palmitate), and amino acid metabolism (e.g., ^{11}C-methionine).

SPLENIC SCINTIGRAPHY

The spleen has hematological, lymphatic, and reticuloendothelial/mononuclear phagocyte system functions. Typically used radiotracers include the following:

- ^{99m}Tc-labeled heat-denatured red blood cells (HDRBC)
- ^{99m}Tc-labeled sulfur colloid or phytate
- ^{99m}Tc-labeled while blood cells

There are a number of studies demonstrating that the HDRBC method is more sensitive than sulfur colloid in imaging spleen. About 90% of heat-denatured RBCs localize to the spleen compared with 5% to 10% of colloid tracer where the majority is taken up in the liver. Colloid does, however, have the advantage of not requiring blood handling, which necessitates more involved procedures and quality control.

Heat-denatured erythrocytes have altered shape and become more spherical and less flexible, so they are stopped in the splenic capillary bed. The denatured erythrocytes are sequestered and disposed of by the spleen. As a result, the radioactive tracer localizes to splenic tissue and this provides a means to identify the spleen and any other splenic tissue. Images are taken 1 to 2 h after reinjection of labeled blood (21). A radiolabeled white blood cell or leucocyte scan has the advantage of being a well-established technique for infection, but the preparation is more involved than for HDRBC.

Indications

- Accessory spleens, or splenunculi, are a common finding, frequently arising as developmental variants and usually local to the spleen and often easily identified.
- More widespread dispersal of splenic tissue, splenosis, can be seen after trauma or surgery and can be more difficult to distinguish from other possible lesions.
- An increasingly common indication is ruling out splenic tissue as the cause for a hypervascular lesion in the pancreas.
- Assessing functional hyposplenism and asplenia, for example, in sickle cell disease or amyloidosis.

Protocol

In the denatured erythrocyte method (9), a modification of the general RBC radiolabeling method is used with the additional step of a gentle heat-denaturing step before reinjection.

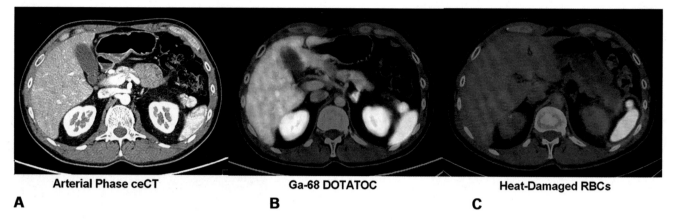

Arterial Phase ceCT   **Ga-68 DOTATOC**   **Heat-Damaged RBCs**

A   **B**   **C**

FIG. 12.13 ● Splenic scintigraphy. Patient with lesion in the tip of the pancreatic tail that (A) is hypervascular on the arterial CT, (B) is 68 Ga DOTATOC positive, and (C) shows strong heat-denatured erythrocyte uptake on scintigraphy consistent with splenic tissue

- The patient does not need any specific preparation.
- Preparing erythrocytes with stannous pyrophosphate either *in vitro* or *in vivo*, for example using a commercial pyrophosphate kit, and administering an intravenous injection of ca 4 mg stannous chloride/12 mg sodium pyrophosphate and waiting 30 min.
- Treating 6 mL of heparinized blood with 75 MBq ^{99m}Tc pertechnetate.
- Incubating the labeled blood in a thermally stabilized water bath at 49°C to 50°C for 35 min.
- Checking for aggregates (thick blood film under the microscope).
- Reinjecting the blood sample.
- Imaging after 60 to 90 min. EANM guidelines suggest planar imaging followed by SPECT/CT of the abdomen and/or other areas in question. If the indication is characterization of known lesions rather than extent, then proceeding straight to SPECT/CT may be most productive.

The aim is to obtain as high-resolution images as possible as lesions are often small and in close proximity to the high uptake within the spleen (use LEHR collimator, iterative reconstruction).

An example is shown in Figure 12.13 where there is a hypervascular and somatostatin receptor tracer positive lesion in the pancreatic tail. Other radiological techniques have been unable to differentiate whether this lesion is ectopic splenic tissue or a well-differentiated neuroendocrine tumor.

One would expect high diagnostic efficiency for detection of ectopic splenic tissue; however, there are examples where cytologically verified splenic tissue has been scintigraphically negative. Given that scintigraphy can also be used to assess functional hyposplenism, it is possible that some ectopic splenic tissue has impaired function due to its location. Other sources of error include deficient preparation, variation in the thermal denaturation temperature, small size of lesion, and high nearby background activity.

ACKNOWLEDGMENT

The authors thank Dr Alp Notghi for providing the small bowel and colonic transit cases.

References

1. Knight LC, Kantor S, Doma S, Parkman HP, Maurer AH. Egg labeling methods for gastric emptying scintigraphy are not equivalent in producing a stable solid meal. *J Nucl Med.* 2007;48(11):1897–1900.
2. Hunt JN, Stubbs DF. The volume and energy content of meals as determinants of gastric emptying. *J Physiol.* 1975;245(1):209–225.
3. Donohoe KJ, Maurer AH, Ziessman HA, Urbain JL, Royal HD, Martin-Comin J, et al. Procedure guideline for adult solid-meal gastric-emptying study 3.0. *J Nucl Med Technol.* 2009;37(3):196–200.
4. Bar-Sever Z. Scintigraphic evaluation of gastroesophageal reflux and pulmonary aspiration in children. *Semin Nucl Med.* 2017;47(3):275–285.
5. Falk GL, Beattie J, Ing A, Falk SE, Magee M, Burton L, et al. Scintigraphy in laryngopharyngeal and gastroesophageal reflux disease: a definitive diagnostic test? *World J Gastroenterol.* 2015;21(12):3619–3627.
6. Maurer AH, Camilleri M, Donohoe K, Knight LC, Madsen JL, Mariani G, et al. The SNMMI and EANM practice guideline for small-bowel and colon transit 1.0. *J Nucl Med.* 2013;54(11):2004–2013.
7. Solnes LB, Sheikhbahaei S, Ziessman HA. Nuclear scintigraphy in practice: gastrointestinal motility. *AJR Am J Roentgenol.* 2018;211(2):260–266.
8. Aung W, Murata Y, Ishida R, Takahashi Y, Okada N, Shibuya H. Study of quantitative oral radioactivity in salivary gland scintigraphy and determination of the clinical stage of Sjogren's syndrome. *J Nucl Med.* 2001;42(1):38–43.
9. Hustinx R, Muylle K. European Nuclear Medicine Guide. European Association of Nuclear Medicine. 2018. https://www.eanm.org/publicpress/european-nuclear-medicine-guide/(accessed July 18, 2021)
10. Spottswood SE, Pfluger T, Bartold SP, Brandon D, Burchell N, Delbeke D, et al. SNMMI and EANM practice guideline for meckel diverticulum scintigraphy 2.0. *J Nucl Med Technol.* 2014;42(3):163–169.
11. ACR–SPR Practice parameter for the performance of gastrointestinal scintigraphy. 2020. https://www.acr.org/-/media/ACR/Files/Practice-Parameters/GI-Scint.pdf (accessed 7/18/2021)
12. Merrick MV, Eastwood MA, Ford MJ. Is bile acid malabsorption underdiagnosed? An evaluation of accuracy of diagnosis by measurement of SeHCAT retention. *Br Med J.* 1985;290(6469):665–668.
13. Aburano T, Yokoyama K, Kinuya S, Takayama T, Tonami N, Hisada K, et al. Indium-111 transferrin imaging for the diagnosis of protein-losing enteropathy. *Clin Nucl Med.* 1989;14(9):681–685.
14. Simonsen JA, Braad PE, Veje A, Gerke O, Schaffalitzky De Muckadell OB, Hoilund-Carlsen PF. (111)Indium-transferrin for localization and

quantification of gastrointestinal protein loss. *Scand J Gastroenterol.* 2009;44(10):1191–1197.

15. de Kaski MC, Peters AM, Bradley D, Hodgson HJ. Detection and quantification of protein-losing enteropathy with indium-111 transferrin. *Eur J Nucl Med.* 1996;23(5):530–533.

16. Dam HQ, Brandon DC, Grantham VV, Hilson AJ, Howarth DM, Maurer AH, et al. The SNMMI procedure standard/EANM practice guideline for gastrointestinal bleeding scintigraphy 2.0. *J Nucl Med Techno*l. 2014;42(4):308–317.

17. Tulchinsky M, Ciak BW, Delbeke D, Hilson A, Holes-Lewis KA, Stabin MG, et al. SNM practice guideline for hepatobiliary scintigraphy 4.0. *J Nucl Med Technol.* 2010;38(4):210–218.

18. Low CS, Ahmed H, Notghi A. Pitfalls and limitations of radionuclide hepatobiliary and gastrointestinal system imaging. *Semin Nucl Med.* 2015;45(6):513–529.

19. Rassam F, Olthof PB, Richardson H, van Gulik TM, Bennink RJ. Practical guidelines for the use of technetium-99m mebrofenin hepatobiliary scintigraphy in the quantitative assessment of liver function. *Nucl Med Commun.* 2019;4(40):297–307.

20. Keiding S, Sorensen M, Frisch K, Gormsen LC, Munk OL. Quantitative PET of liver functions. *Am J Nucl Med Mol Imaging.* 2018;8(2):73–85.

21. Armas R, Thakur ML, Gottschalk A. A simple method of spleen imaging with 99mTc-labeled erythrocytes. *Radiology.* 1979;132(1):215–216.

CHAPTER SELF-ASSESSMENT QUESTIONS

1. A patient is examined with salivary gland scintigraphy. The scan shows mildly reduced uptake and excretion in both parotid and submandibular glands but in addition, asymmetrically reduced uptake in the parotid glands, substantially lower in the right parotid gland.

   Which of the following explain the results?

   A. Radiotherapy for tonsillar cancer

   B. Salivary stone

   C. Lupus

   D. Tolterodine, taken for bladder instability

2. The images from a radiolabeled leukocyte SPECT-CT and contrast CT are from a patient with several lesions above and below the diaphragm. What is the most likely explanation for the findings?

   A. Metastatic pancreatic NET

   B. Hemangiomas

   C. Functional hyposplenism

   D. Traumatic splenosis

Answers to Chapter Self-Assessment Questions

1. A. Choice A is the most likely cause, either the result of recent treatment and a subacute response, or the long-term effect of a significant dose of radiation to the nearby right tonsil, typically performed with 60–70 Gy. Salivary stones (B) are often symptomatic, most frequently in the submandibular gland ducts. Acute cases are investigated by radiography, CT, or ultrasound. The chronic effects may result in inflammation, atrophy, and dry mouth. About 14% to 18% of patients with Lupus (C) also have Sjøgren's syndrome, which is typically bilateral. Tolterodine (D) is a nonselective antimuscarinic that is used to treat urinary urgency and incontinence. Dry mouth is a common side effect. The effect may differ between submandibular and parotid glands reflecting their slightly different physiological roles. Both answers C and D demonstrate largely symmetrical diminished salivary gland activity.

2. D. Spleen is missing but there are high focal areas of activity, which are compatible with likely post-traumatic splenosis as the explanation for the imaging findings. The patient had a history of splenic trauma, splenectomy, and was investigated for extent of splenosis. Radiolabeled leukocyte scan is not suitable for imaging evaluation of neuroendocrine tumors. Hemangiomas may show mild uptake with radiolabeled leukocyte scan but the preferred radiotracer for assessing hemangiomas is radiolabeled RBCs. Functional hyposplenism showed reduced radiolabeled leukocyte uptake.

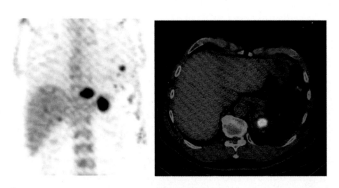

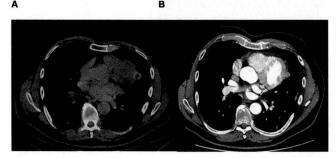

A   B

C   D

Renal Scintigraphy

13

Hossein Jadvar

LEARNING OBJECTIVES

1. Recognize various radiotracers employed in renal scintigraphy.

2. Name a number of renal diseases that may be evaluated effectively with scintigraphy.

3. Describe the utility and limitations of positron emission tomography with ^{18}F-flurodeoxyglucose in the imaging evaluation of renal cell carcinoma.

Scintigraphy offers imaging-based diagnostic information on renal structure and function. Many single-photon radiotracers have long been in routine clinical use in renal scintigraphy. They are tailored to provide physiological information complementing the primarily structural-based imaging modalities, such as ultrasonography, computed tomography (CT), and magnetic resonance imaging (MRI). With the rapid expansion of positron emission tomography (PET), and more recently hybrid structural–functional imaging systems such as PET/CT, additional unprecedented opportunities have developed for quantitative imaging evaluation of renal diseases in both clinical and research arenas. In this chapter, we review the unique contribution of scintigraphy, including PET, in the imaging evaluation of renal structure and function. We first launch with a brief discussion of the common radiopharmaceuticals used in renal scintigraphy. Following a review of the normal patterns, we focus on various disease processes in which scintigraphy has been particularly contributory.

RADIOPHARMACEUTICALS

Technetium-99m diethylenetriaminepentaacetic acid

Technetium-99m diethylenetriaminepentaacetic acid (^{99m}Tc-DTPA) is the common agent for assessing glomerular filtration rate (GFR). The ideal agent for measuring GFR is cleared only by glomerular filtration and is not secreted or reabsorbed. ^{99m}Tc-DTPA satisfies the first requirement but has variable degrees of protein binding which deviate its kinetics from the ideal agent such as inulin. For a 20 mCi (740 MBq) dose, the radiation exposures to the kidneys and urinary bladder are 1.8 and 2.3 rads, respectively (1).

Iodine-131 orthoiodohippurate

The mechanism of iodine-131 orthoiodohippurate (^{131}I-OIH) renal clearance is about 20% by GFR and 80% by tubular secretion. ^{131}I-OIH is an acceptable alternative to

para-aminohippuric acid (PAH) for determining renal plasma flow although its clearance is 15% lower than that of PAH. PAH is not entirely cleared by the kidneys with about 10% of arterial PAH remaining in the renal venous blood. Therefore, ^{131}I-OIH measures *effective* renal plasma flow (ERPF). The tubular extraction efficiency of ^{131}I-OIH is 90% and there is no hepatobiliary excretion. OIH may also be labeled with ^{123}I that not only provides equivalent urinary kinetics as that for ^{131}I label but also offers improved image quality due to typically larger administered dose in view of its more favorable radiation exposure. For a 300-uCi (11 MBq) dose of ^{131}I-OIH, the radiation exposures to the kidneys and urinary bladder are 0.02 and 1.4 rads, respectively. Few drops of nonradioactive iodine (e.g., saturated solution of potassium iodide) orally minimize the thyroid uptake of free ^{131}I (1).

Technetium-99m mercaptoacetyltriglycine

Technetium-99m mercaptoacetyltriglycine (^{99m}Tc-MAG3) has similar properties to OIH but has significant advantages of better image quality and less radiation exposure. The tubular extraction fraction of MAG3 is lower than OIH at about 60% to 70%. There is also about 3% hepatobiliary excretion which increases with renal insufficiency. Despite these features, however, MAG3 is a common agent used in the scintigraphic evaluation of renal function. For a 10-mCi (370 MBq) dose, the radiation exposures to the kidneys and urinary bladder are 0.15 and 4.4 rads, respectively (1).

Technetium-99m dimercaptosuccinic acid

Technetium-99m dimercaptosuccinic acid (^{99m}Tc-DMSA) localizes to renal cortex at high concentration and has slow urinary excretion rate. About 50% of the injected dose accumulates in the renal cortex at 1 h. The tracer is bound to the renal proximal tubular cells. Because of the high retention of DMSA in the renal cortex, it has become useful for the imaging of renal parenchyma. For a 6-mCi (11 MBq) dose, the radiation exposures to the kidneys and urinary balder are 3.78 and 0.42 rads, respectively (1).

Fluorine-18 fluorodeoxyglucose

Fluorodeoxyglucose (FDG) is the most common positron-labeled radiotracer in PET. ^{18}F-labeled deoxyglucose is a modified form of glucose in which the hydroxyl group in the 2-position is replaced by the ^{18}F positron emitter. FDG accumulates in cells in proportion to glucose metabolism. Cell membrane glucose transporters facilitate the transport of glucose and FDG across the cell membrane. Both glucose and FDG are phosphorylated in the 6-position by the hexokinase. The conversion of glucose-6-phosphate or FDG-6-phosphate back to glucose or FDG, respectively, is affected by the enzyme phosphatase. In most tissues, including cancer, there is little phosphatase activity. FDG-6-phosphate cannot undergo further conversions and, therefore, is trapped in the cell. FDG is excreted in the urine. The typical FDG dose is 0.144 mCi/kg (minimum 1 mCi and maximum 20 mCi). The urinary bladder wall receives the highest radiation dose from FDG (2,3). The radiation dose depends on the excretion rate, the varying size of the bladder, the bladder volume at the time of FDG administration, and an estimated bladder time–activity curve. For a typical 15 mCi FDG dose and voiding at 1 h after tracer injection, the average estimated absorbed radiation dose to the adult bladder wall is 3.3 rads (0.22 rads/mCi) (4). The doses to other organs are between 0.75 and 1.28 rads (0.050–0.085 rads/mCi) for an average organ dose of 1.0 rad (4).

NORMAL RENAL FUNCTION

GFR and ERPF may be assessed using dynamic quantitative nuclear imaging techniques. The GFR quantifies the amount of filtrate formed per minute (normal: 125 mL/min in adults). Only 20% of renal plasma flow is filtered through the semi-permeable membrane of the glomerulus. The filtrate is protein-free and nearly completely reabsorbed in the tubules. Filtration is maintained over a range of arterial pressures with autoregulation. The ideal agent for the determination of GFR is inulin which is only filtered but is neither secreted nor reabsorbed (1,5).

^{99m}Tc-DTPA is often employed to demonstrate renal perfusion and assess glomerular filtration, although 5% to 10% of injected DTPA is protein-bound and 5% remains in the kidneys at 4 h. A typical imaging protocol includes posterior 5-s flow images for 1 min followed by 1 min per frame images for 20 min. The GFR may be obtained using the Gates method that employs images of renal uptake during the second through third minute after DTPA administration. Regions of interest (ROIs) are drawn over the kidneys and background activity correction is applied. A standard dose is counted by the gamma camera for normalization. Depth photon attenuation correction is made based on a formula relating body weight and height. A split GFR can be obtained for each kidney which is not possible with the creatinine clearance method (1,5).

The ERPF (normal: 585 mL/min in adults) can be obtained by using OIH and MAG3 imaging (6). However, OIH has been largely replaced by MAG3 because of MAG3's better imaging characteristics and dosimetry (due to radiolabeling with ^{99m}Tc). At present, MAG3 is the renal imaging agent of choice primarily because of the combined renal clearance of MAG3 by both filtration and tubular extraction which leads to the ability for obtaining relatively high-quality images even in patients with impaired renal function. The imaging protocol includes posterior 1-s images for 60 s (flow study) followed by 1-min images for 5 min and then 5-min images for 30 min. The relative tubular function may be obtained by drawing renal ROIs corrected for background activity. A renogram is constructed to depict the renal tracer uptake over time. The first portion of the renogram has a sharp upslope occurring in about 6 s following peak aortic activity (Phase I) representing perfusion followed by the extension to the peak value representing both renal perfusion and early renal clearance (Phase II). The next phase (Phase III) is downsloping and represents excretion. Normal perfusion of the kidneys is symmetric (50% ± 5%). The renogram peak occurs at about 2 to 3 min (vs. 3–5 min with DTPA) in normal adults and by 30 min, more than 70% of tracer is cleared and present in the urinary bladder (Fig. 13.1) (1,5).

Renal cortical structure can be imaged with DMSA which correlates strongly with differential glomerular filtration and differential renal blood flow. Imaging is started 90 to 120 min after tracer administration, although images can be obtained at up to 4 h. Planar images are obtained in the anterior, posterior, left anterior (LAO)/right anterior (RAO), and right posterior oblique (RPO)/left posterior oblique (LPO) projections. Single-photon emission CT (SPECT) is also often obtained. A normal scan shows evenly distributed renal cortical uptake. Normal variations include dromedary hump (splenic impression on the left kidney), fetal lobulation, horseshoe kidney, crossed fused ectopia, and hypertrophied column of Bertin. The renal images also allow accurate assessment of the relative renal size, position, axis, and presence of cortical infarct (Fig. 13.2) (1,5).

CLINICAL APPLICATIONS

Renal failure

In renal failure, glomerular and tubular dysfunctions are reflected by abnormal renal scans and renograms. Renal uptake of MAG3 is prolonged with tubular tracer stasis and little or no excretion. It has been shown that in patients with acute renal failure, the demonstration of MAG3 renal activity more than hepatic activity at 1 to 3 min indicates likely recovery while when renal uptake is less than the hepatic uptake, dialysis may be needed (7). In chronic renal failure, there is diminished renal perfusion, cortical tracer extraction, and excretion. However, this imaging pattern is nonspecific and needs to be interpreted in the clinical context (1).

Renal infection

Acute pyelonephritis is associated with fever, flank pain, leukocytosis, and pyuria. Radiolabeled leukocyte (e.g., ^{111}In-WBC) and ^{67}Ga-citrate scans can help identify acute pyelonephritis. However, these methods have the drawbacks of extended imaging time (more than 24 h) and higher radiation exposure. Cortical imaging with DMSA is highly sensitive for detecting acute

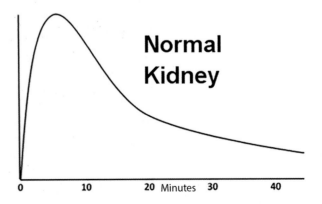

FIG. 13.1 ● Normal ^{99m}Tc-MAG3 renogram. ^{99m}Tc-MAG3, Technetium-99m mercaptoacetyltriglycine.

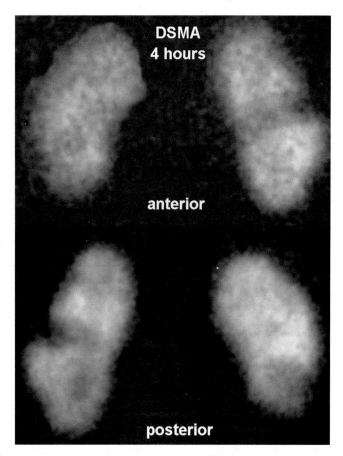

FIG. 13.2 ● Anterior and posterior planar ^{99m}Tc-DMSA scintigraphy obtained 4 h after radiotracer administration showed small (upper lateral) and larger (mid-lateral) peripheral cortical defects in left kidney compatible with renal infarcts. SPECT (not shown) may be used for improved definition of the extent of renal cortical defects. ^{99m}Tc-DMSA, Technetium-99m dimercaptosuccinic acid; SPECT, single-photon emission computed tomograpy.

pyelonephritis in the appropriate clinical setting (8). Acute pyelonephritis demonstrates segmental regions of decreased tracer uptake in oval, round, or wedge pattern. There may also be diffuse generalized decrease in renal uptake which in association with normal or slightly enlarged kidney is suspicious for an acute infectious process. The pathophysiologic basis for decline in DMSA cortical uptake in infection is related to diminished tracer delivery to the infected area and to direct infectious injury to the tubular cells compromising their function and tracer uptake. A wedge-shaped cortical defect with regional decrease in renal size is compatible with post-infectious scarring. Renal infarcts may also have a similar appearance (1,5).

Renal obstructive disease

A frequent clinical request is to evaluate for obstructive uropathy. Although the Whitaker test remains the standard for the determination of obstruction, diuretic renography is a much less invasive procedure and is an excellent test to evaluate for obstructive uropathy. In general, it is recommended that the patient be well hydrated. In children and adults with noncompliant bladder, catheterization of the bladder may be used to ensure drainage and reduce back pressure in the urinary system. MAG3 scintigraphy is often employed. Furosemide (Lasix) is administered intravenously (1 mg/kg; higher dose in cases of renal insufficiency) when the renal pelvis and ureter are maximally distended (9). This may occur in as early as 10–15 min and as late as 30–40 min after tracer administration. ROIs are drawn around each renal pelvis with the background regions as crescent shapes lateral to each kidney. Following furosemide administration, rapid emptying of the collecting system with a subsequent steep decline in the renogram curve is compatible with dilatation without obstruction. Obstruction can be excluded if the clearance half time ($T_{1/2}$) of the renal pelvic emptying is less than 10 min. A curve that reaches a plateau or continues to rise after administration of furosemide is an obstructive pattern with a clearance $T_{1/2}$ of greater than 20 min (Fig. 13.3). A slow downslope after furosemide may

FIG. 13.3 ● Abnormal ^{99m}Tc-MAG3 renogram following furosemide administration demonstrating left hydronephrosis and diminished left urinary clearance kinetics caused by ureteropelvic junction obstruction. ^{99m}Tc-MAG3, Technetium-99m mercaptoacetyltriglycine.

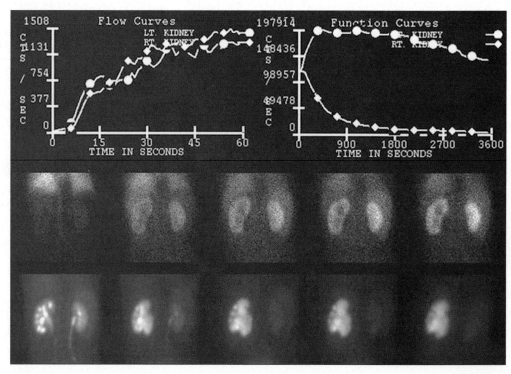

indicate partial obstruction. An apparent poor response to furosemide may also be seen in severe pelvic dilatation (reservoir effect). Other pitfalls include poor injection technique of either the diuretic or the radiotracer, impaired renal function, and dehydration in which delayed tracer transit and excretion may not be overcome by the effect of a diuretic. Kidneys in neonates (<1 month in age) may be too immature to respond to furosemide and are not suitable candidates for diuretic renal scintigraphy (1,5).

Renovascular disease

Angiotensin-converting enzyme (ACE) inhibition prevents the conversion of angiotensin I to angiotensin II. In renal artery stenosis, angiotensin II constricts the efferent arterioles as a compensatory mechanism to maintain GFR despite diminished afferent renal blood flow. Therefore, ACE inhibition in renal artery stenosis reduces GFR by interfering with the compensatory mechanism.

Before the study, the patient should be well hydrated. ACE inhibitors should be discontinued (captopril for 2 days; enalapril or lisinopril for 4–5 days), since otherwise diagnostic sensitivity of the study may be reduced. Diuretics should be discontinued preferably for 1 week. Dehydration resulting from diuretics may potentiate the effect of captopril and contribute to hypotension. Captopril (25–50 mg) crushed and dissolved in 250 mL water is administered orally followed by blood pressure monitoring every 15 min for 1 h. Alternatively, enalaprilat (40 µg/kg up to 2.5 mg) is administered intravenously over 3 to 5 min. A baseline scan can be performed before captopril renography (1-day protocol) or the next day, only if captopril study is abnormal (2-day protocol).

The affected kidney in renovascular hypertension (RVH) often has a renogram curve with reduced initial slope, a delayed time to peak activity, prolonged cortical retention, and a slow downslope following peak. These findings are due to slowed renal tracer transit owing to increased solute and water retention in response to ACE inhibition. Reduced urine flow causes delayed and decreased tracer washout into the collecting system in ^{99m}Tc-MAG3 and ^{131}I-OIH studies. ^{99m}Tc-DTPA demonstrates reduced uptake on the affected side (10).

Consensus reports regarding methods and interpretation of ACE renography elaborate on a scoring system of renogram curves (11–13). It has been recommended that high (>90%), intermediate (10%–90%), and low (<10%) probability categories be applied to captopril renography based on change of renogram curve score between baseline and post-captopril renograms. Among quantitative measurements, relative renal function, the time to peak activity, and the ratio of 20-min renal activity to peak activity (20/peak) are used more commonly than other parameters. For MAG3 renal scintigraphy, a 10% change in relative renal function, peak activity increase of 2 min or more, and a parenchymal increase in 20 per peak post captopril by 0.15 represent a high probability of RVH (14).

Captopril renography has a sensitivity of 80% to 95% and a specificity of 50% to 94% for the detection of RVH (10). With bilateral renovascular stenosis, the detection of stenosis by captopril-stimulated renography may be more complicated (10). It is more the exception than the rule for bilateral renovascular stenosis to have symmetric findings on captopril renography. Studies in canine models with bilateral renal artery stenosis demonstrated that captopril produced striking changes in the time-activity curve of each kidney, which are even more pronounced in the more severely stenotic kidney (10).

Renal transplant assessment

Renal transplantation is a common procedure in the United States. Patients with end-stage renal disease who receive successful transplants have a higher quality of life than those who are treated with chronic dialysis. There are several complications associated with renal transplantation. These include vascular compromise (arterial or venous thrombosis), lymphocele formation, urinary extravasation, acute tubular necrosis (ATN), drug toxicity, and organ rejection. Scintigraphy provides important imaging information about these potential complications which can then prompt corrective intervention (15).

The earliest complication may be hyperacute rejection which is often apparent immediately after transplantation and is due to preformed cytotoxic antibodies. Other early complications may include sudden urine output decline and acute urinary obstruction. Scintigraphy with DTPA or MAG3 shows an absence of perfusion and function with complete renal artery or vein thrombosis. A sensitive but nonspecific finding for acute rejection is when there is >20% decline in the ratio of renal activity to aortic activity (16).

Renal scintigraphy performed few days after the transplantation often shows intact perfusion but delayed and decreased tracer excretion and some cortical tracer retention. This is typically due to ATN and is more common with cadaveric grafts than with living-related grafts (Fig. 13.4). If both perfusion and function continue to decline, then rejection is considered. However, ATN, obstruction, drug (cyclosporine) toxicity, and rejection can have a relatively similar scintigraphic appearance. The differential diagnosis should be considered in the clinical context and the interval since transplantation, although two or more of these conditions may coexist. In a study, a non-ascending second phase of MAG3 renogram curve was predictive of graft dysfunction. However, patients with ATN were not

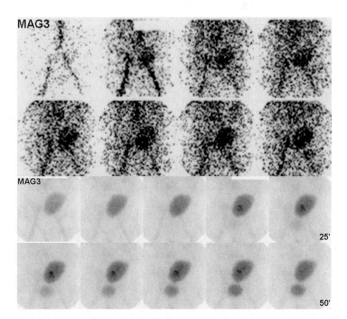

FIG. 13.4 • Anterior planar renal ^{99m}Tc-MAG3 image shows a functioning left pelvic renal transplant. The mild cortical retention of ^{99m}Tc-MAG3 is related to mild ATN. Note the progressive accumulation of excreted urine in the urinary bladder. 25' and 50' are denote 25 and 50 minutes (from the time of radiotracer administration), respectively; ATN, acute tubular necrosis; ^{99m}Tc-MAG3, Technetium-99m mercaptoacetyltriglycine.

significantly more likely to have a non-ascending curve than those with acute rejection. An ascending curve was nonspecific and could be seen in both normally and poorly functioning grafts (17).

Urine extravasation may be noted on the renal scan as a collection of excreted radiotracer outside of the transplant and the urinary bladder. Small urine leaks and impaired renal transplant function make the identification of a leak difficult on scintigraphy. However, a cold defect that becomes warmer with time on the sequential images usually represents a urinoma or a urinary leak. If the activity declines with voiding, then the finding is likely a urinoma. A chronic photopenic defect may represent a hematoma and/or a lymphocele (18). For assessing potential obstructive disease, scintigraphy with diuretic may be considered as discussed earlier.

RENAL CANCER

Renal cell carcinoma (RCC) arises from the renal tubular epithelium and accounts for the majority of adult kidney tumors. The tumor is angioinvasive and is associated with widespread hematogenous and lymphatic metastases especially to the lung, liver, lymph nodes, bone, and brain. Metastases are present in about 50% of patients at initial presentation. Radical nephrectomy is the main treatment for the early stages of the disease, although palliative nephrectomy may also be performed in advanced disease with intractable bleeding. Solitary metastasis may also be resected. RCC responds poorly to chemotherapy. Radiation therapy for RCC is used for palliation of metastatic sites, specifically, bone and brain. Immunotherapy with biologic response modifiers, such as interleukin-2 and interferon-alpha, and more recently with checkpoint inhibitors has the most impact on the treatment of metastatic disease (19). The 5-year survival may be as high as 80% to 90% for the early stages of the disease while advanced disease carries a poor prognosis (20).

Preliminary studies of PET imaging of RCC have revealed a promising role in the evaluation of indeterminate renal masses, in pre-operative staging and assessment of tumor burden, in detection of osseous and non-osseous metastases, in restaging after therapy, and in the determination of the effect of imaging findings on clinical management (21–26). However, few other PET studies have demonstrated less enthusiastic results and no advantage over standard imaging methods (27–29).

A relatively high false-negative rate of 23% has been reported with FDG PET in the preoperative staging of RCC when compared to histological analysis of surgical specimens. In a recent study, PET exhibited a sensitivity of 60% (vs. 91.7% for CT) and specificity of 100% (vs. 100% for CT) for primary RCC tumors. For retroperitoneal lymph node metastases and/or renal bed recurrence, PET was 75.0% sensitive (vs. 92.6% for CT) and 100.0% specific (vs. 98.1% CT). PET had a sensitivity of 75.0% (vs. 91.1% for chest CT) and a specificity of 97.1% (vs. 73.1% for chest CT) for pulmonary metastases. PET had a sensitivity of 77.3% and specificity of 100.0% for bone metastases, compared to 93.8% and 87.2% for combined CT and bone scan (30). For restaging RCC, a sensitivity of 87% and a specificity of 100% have been reported (31). A comparative investigation of bone scan and FDG PET for detecting osseous metastases in RCC revealed sensitivity and specificity of 77.5% and 59.6% for bone scan and 100% and 100% for PET, respectively (26). Another report revealed a negative predictive value of 33% and a positive

predictive value of 94% for restaging RCC (22). Other studies have reported high accuracy in characterizing indeterminate renal masses with a mean tumor-to-kidney uptake ratio of 3.0 for malignancy (21).

These mixed observations are probably related to the heterogeneous expression of glucose transporter-1 (GLUT-1) in RCC, which may not correlate with the tumor grade or extent (32,33). A negative study may not exclude disease while a positive study is highly suspicious for malignancy. If the tumor is FDG avid, then PET can be a reasonable imaging modality for follow-up after treatment and surveillance (Fig. 13.5). Moreover, it has been shown that FDG PET can alter clinical management in up to 40% of patients with suspicious locally recurrent and metastatic renal cancer (24).

The diagnostic accuracy of FDG PET appears not to be improved by semi-quantitative image analysis, which is probably due to the fundamental variability of glucometabolism in RCC (29). In one study, the maximum and average standardized uptake values (SUVs) for FDG-positive, primary renal malignant tumors were 7.9 ± 4.9 and 6.0 ± 3.6, respectively. The maximum and average SUVs of metastatic renal masses were 6.1 ± 3.4 and 4.7 ± 2.8, respectively. There was no significant difference in maximum and average SUVs between primary and metastatic renal masses (34). Since FDG is excreted in the urine, the intense urine activity may confound lesion detection in and near the renal bed. Intravenous administration of furosemide has been proposed to improve urine clearance from the renal collecting system although the exact benefit of such intervention in improving lesion detection remains undefined.

Other PET tracers (e.g., ^{11}C-acetate, ^{18}F-fluoromisonidazole, radiolabeled prostate-specific membrane antigen agents) have been investigated in the imaging evaluation of patients with RCC but further studies are needed to establish the exact role of these and other non-FDG tracers in this clinical setting (35–37). Moreover, despite several studies supporting the diagnostic synergism of the combined PET/CT or PET/MRI imaging systems, their impact on patient outcome will need further investigations (38–40).

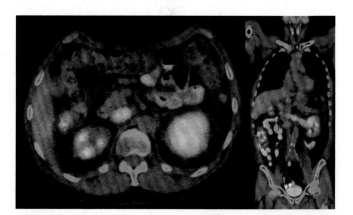

FIG. 13.5 ● Renal cell carcinoma. Fused axial (left panel) and coronal (right panel) FDG PET/CT images show a hypermetabolic left renal mass with the extension of the hypermetabolism along the course of the left renal vein to IVC compatible with left renal tumor with associated left renal vein and IVC tumor thrombus. CT, computed tomography; FDG, fluorodeoxyglucose; IVC, inferior vena cava; PET, positron emission tomography.

References

1. Perlman SB, Bushnell DL, Barnes WE. Genitourinary System. In: Wilson MA editor. *Textbook of nuclear medicine*. Lippincott-Raven Publishers: Philadelphia; 1998. p. 117–136.
2. Mejia AA, Nakamura T, Masatoshi I, et al. Estimation of absorbed doses in humans due to intravenous administration of fluorine-18-fluorodeoxyglucose in PET studies. *J Nucl Med*. 1991;32:699–706.
3. Hays MT, Watson EE, Thomas SR, et al. MIRD dose estimate report No. 19: radiation absorbed dose estimates from 18F-FDG. *J Nucl Med*. 2002;43:210–214.
4. Jones SC, Alavi A, Christman D, et al. The radiation dosimetry of 2[F-18]fluoro-2-deoxy-D-glucose in man. *J Nucl Med*. 1982;23:613–617.
5. Kuni CC, duCret RP. Genitourinary system. In: *Manual of nuclear medicine imaging*. Thieme Medical Publishers: New York; 1997. p. 106–128.
6. Bagni B, Portaluppi F, Montanari L, et al. ^{99m}Tc-MAG3 versus ^{131}I-orthoiodohippurate in the routine determination of effective renal plasma flow. *J Nucl Med Allied Sci*. 1990;34:67–70.
7. Lin EC, Gellens ME, Goodgold HM. Prognostic value of renal scintigraphy with Tc-99m MAG3 in patients with acute renal failure. *J Nucl Med*. 1995;36:232P–233P.
8. Bjorgvinsson E, Majd M, Eggli KD. Diagnosis of acute pyelonephritis in children: comparison of sonography and ^{99m}Tc-DMSA scintigraphy. *AJR Am J Roentgenol*. 1991;157:539–543.
9. Saremi F, Jadvar H, Siegel M. Pharmacologic interventions in nuclear radiology: indications, imaging protocols, and clinical results. *Radiographics*. 2002;22:477–490.
10. Nally JV Jr, Black HR. State-of-the-art review: captopril renography-pathophysiological considerations and clinical observations. *Semin Nucl Med*. 1992;22:85–97.
11. Taylor A, Nally J, Aurell M, et al. Consensus report on ACE inhibitor renography for detecting renovascular hypertension. Radionuclides in Nephrourology Group. Consensus Group on ACEI Renography. *J Nucl Med*. 1996;37:1876–1882.
12. Taylor AT Jr, Fletcher JW, Nally JV Jr, et al. Procedure guideline for diagnosis of renovascular hypertension. Society of Nuclear Medicine. *J Nucl Med*. 1998;39:1297–1302.
13. Nally JV Jr, Chen C, Fine E, et al. Diagnostic criteria of renovascular hypertension with captopril renography: a consensus statement. *Am J Hypertens*. 1991;4:749S–752S.
14. Fine EJ. Interventions in renal scintigraphy. *Semin Nucl Med*. 1999;29:128–145.
15. Dubovsky EV, Russell CD, Erbas B. Radionuclide evaluation of renal transplants. *Semin Nucl Med*. 1995;25(1):49–59.
16. Dunagin P, Alijani M, Atkins F, et al. Application of the kidney to aortic blood flow index to renal transplants. *Clin Nucl Med*. 1983;8:360–364.
17. Lin E, Alavi A. Significance of early tubular extraction in the first minute of Tc-99m MAG3 renal transplant scintigraphy. *Clin Nucl Med*. 1998;23:217–222.
18. Fortenbery EJ, Blue PW, Van Nostrand D, et al. Lymphocele: the spectrum of scintigraphic findings in lymphoceles associated with renal transplant. *J Nucl Med*. 1990;31:1627–1631.
19. Bedke J, Stuhler V, Stenzi A, Brehmer B. Immunotherapy for kidney cancer: status quo and the future. *Curr Opin Urol*. 2018;28:8–14.
20. Frank IN, Graham Jr S, Nabors WL. Urologic and male genital cancers. In: Holleb AI, Fink DJ, Murphy GP editors. *Clinical Oncology*. American Cancer Society; 1991. p. 272–274.
21. Goldberg MA, Mayo-Smith WW, Papanicolaou N, et al. FDG PET characterization of renal masses: preliminary experience. *Clin Radiol*. 1997;52:510–515.
22. Jadvar H, Kherbache HM, Pinski JK, Conti PS. Diagnostic role of [F-18]-FDG positron emission tomography in restaging renal cell carcinoma. *Clin Nephrol*. 2003;60:395–400.
23. Mankoff DA, Thompson JA, Gold P, et al. Identification of interleukin-2-induced complete response in metastatic renal cell carcinoma by FDG PET despite radiographic evidence suggesting persistent tumor. *AJR Am J Roentgenol*. 1997;169:1049–1050.
24. Ramdave S, Thomas GW, Berlangieri SU, et al. Clinical role of F-18 fluorodeoxyglucose positron emission tomography for detection and management of renal cell carcinoma. *J Urol*. 2001;166:825–830.
25. Wahl RL, Harney J, Hutchins G, Grossman HB. Imaging of renal cancer using positron emission tomography with 2-deoxy-2-(^{18}F)-fluoro-D-glucose: pilot animal and human studies. *J Urol*. 1991;146(6):1470–1474.
26. Wu HC, Yen RF, Shen YY, et al. Comparing whole body 18F-2-deoxyglucose positron emission tomography and technetium-99m methylene diphosphate bone scan to detect bone metastases in patients with renal cell carcinomas - a preliminary report. *J Cancer Res Clin Oncol*. 2002;128:503–506.
27. Majhail NS, Urbain JL, Albani JM, et al. F-18 fluorodeoxyglucose positron emission tomography in the evaluation of distant metastases from renal cell carcinoma. *J Clin Oncol*. 2003;21:3995–4000.
28. Seto E, Segall GM, Terris MK. Positron emission tomography detection of osseous metastases of renal cell carcinoma not identified on bone scan. *Urology*. 2000;55:286.
29. Zhuang H, Duarte PS, Pourdehand M, et al. Standardized uptake value as an unreliable index of renal disease on fluorodeoxyglucose PET Imaging. *Clin Nucl Med*. 2000;25:358–360.
30. Kang DE, White RL Jr, Zuger JH, et al. Clinical use of fluorodeoxyglucose F 18 positron emission tomography for detection of renal cell carcinoma. *J Urol*. 2004;171(5):1806–1809.
31. Safaei A, Figlin R, Hoh CK, et al. The usefulness of F-18 deoxyglucose whole-body positron emission tomography (PET) for re-staging of renal cell cancer. *Clin Nephrol*. 2002;57:56–62.
32. Miyakita H, Tokunaga M, Onda H, et al. Significance of 18F-fluorodeoxyglucose positron emission tomography (FDG-PET) for detection of renal cell carcinoma and immunohistochemical glucose transporter 1 (GLUT-1) expression in the cancer. *Int J Urol*. 2002;9:15–18.
33. Nagase Y, Takata K, Moriyama N, et al. Immunohistochemical localization of glucose transporters in human renal cell carcinoma. *J Urol*. 1995;153(3 Pt 1):798–801.
34. Kumar R, Chauhan A, Lakhani P, Xiu Y, Zhuang H, Alavi A. 2-Deoxy-2-[F-18]fluoro-D-glucose-positron emission tomography in characterization of solid renal masses. *Mol Imaging Biol*. 2005;7(6):431–439.
35. Lawrentschuk N, Poon AM, Foo SS, et al. Assessing regional hypoxia in human renal tumors using 18F-fluoromisonidazole positron emission tomography. *BJU Int*. 2005;96:540–546.
36. Shreve P, Chiao PC, Humes HD, et al. Carbon-11-acetate PET imaging in renal disease. *J Nucl Med*. 1995;36:1595–1601.
37. Ahn T, Roberts MJ, Abduljabar A, et al. A review of prostate-specific membrane antigen (PSMA) positron emission tomography in renal cell carcinoma (RCC). *Mol Imaging Biol*. 2019;21:799–807.
38. Ma H, Shen G, Liu B, et al. Diagnostic performance of 18F-FDG PET or PET/CT in restaging renal cell carcinoma: a systematic review and meta-analysis. *Nucl Med Commun*. 2017;38:156–163.
39. Liu Y. The place of FDG PET/CT in renal cell carcinoma: value and limitations. *Front Oncol*. 2016;6:201.
40. Kelly-Morland C, Rudman S, Nathan P, et al. Evaluation of treatment response and resistance in metastatic renal cell cancer (mRCC) using integrated ^{18}F-fluorodeoxyglucose (18F-FDG) positron emission tomography/magnetic resonance imaging (PET/MRI); the REMAP study. *BMC Cancer*. 2017;17:392.

CHAPTER SELF-ASSESSMENT QUESTIONS

1. Which of the following radiotracers is best suited for the imaging assessment of renal infarct

   A. FDG

   B. ^{11}C-acetate

   C. ^{99m}Tc-DMSA

   D. ^{99m}Tc-DTPA

2. Which statement below regarding RCC is correct

   A. There is a heterogenous expression of glucose transporter-1 in RCC

   B. FDG PET has absolutely no role in the imaging evaluation of RCC

   C. Diagnostic accuracy of FDG PET is improved by semi-quantitative image analysis

   D. Lack of FDG excretion in urine is advantageous in FDG PET imaging of RCC

Answers to Chapter Self-Assessment Questions

1. C ^{99m}Tc-DMSA, localizes to renal cortex at high concentration. While the other radiotracers mentioned may also reveal renal infarct by the relative decline of activity in the infarcted renal cortex, they are not the primary radiotracer for specific scintigraphic imaging valuation of renal infarction.

2. A While FDG PET is useful in the imaging evaluation of RCC in specific clinical situations, the heterogeneity of results may be fundamentally due to the heterogeneous expression of glucose transporter-1 in RCC. Studies have suggested that, in general, the diagnostic accuracy of FDG PET is not improved by semi-quantitative image analysis. FDG is excreted in urine.

Positron Emission Tomography (PET), PET/CT, and PET/MRI

14

Farshad Moradi and Andrei H. Iagaru

LEARNING OBJECTIVES

1. Describe the major clinical applications of fluorodeoxyglucose (FDG) positron emission tomography (PET)/CT.

2. Name several PET radiotracers and their common utility in PET scintigraphy.

3. Describe clinical conditions in which PET/MRI may provide advantage over PET/CT.

INTRODUCTION

Radiopharmaceuticals and instrumentation

Positron emission tomography radionuclides in clinical and investigational human use

Fluorine-18 (F-18) is a positron emitter and currently the most commonly used radionuclide in PET. The relatively low energy resulting in short range of the emitted positron leads to superior image quality compared to most other positron emitters. The 109-min half-life of F-18 is suitable for majority of clinical applications and allows for accumulation of radiopharmaceuticals in target structures and washout of background activity before significant decay. F-18 is produced in a cyclotron and can be distributed to imaging facilities up to several hours away from the cyclotron and radiochemistry unit.

N-13 (used as NH_3 for imaging myocardial perfusion) and C-11 (which is extensively used for research applications due to favorable chemistry for organic compounds) produce positrons with higher energies than that of F-18 although the effect on image quality for human applications is not significant. However, the shorter half-lives of 10 and 20 min, respectively, require the producing cyclotron to be in the immediate vicinity of imaging centers, limiting the availability of these radiotracers for widespread clinical use.

Rb-82 and O-15 (which are used for evaluation for myocardial or brain perfusion) emit high-energy positrons (which results in degraded image resolution blur due to longer positron path) and have very short half-lives (1.27–2 min), requiring a generator or cyclotron to be on-site.

Positron-emitting radiometals such as Ga-68 are in increasing clinical use because of the applicability in labeling both small compounds and macromolecules. Ga-68 is most commonly available from a $^{68}Ge/^{68}Ga$ generator system (1), although successful efforts to implement cyclotron production have been reported recently. The images suffer an image penalty when compared to F-18 due to higher positron energy and complex scatter.

Radiometals with longer half-lives are particularly useful for tagging monoclonal antibodies and allowing imaging over multiple days. The slow decay, however, limits the amount of administered activity in human due to concerns about radiation. Some radiometals are not pure positron emitters and produce gamma rays that can interfere (directly or indirectly) with the coincidence detection in PET cameras, blurring the image and producing quantification errors (2). Some radiometals (e.g., Y-90) (3) primarily emit high-energy beta-particles (i.e., electron) that are useful for internal radiation therapy (RT) but produce some positrons that allow imaging their biodistribution using PET. Table 14.1 is a summary list of major clinically relevant PET radionuclides (Table 14.1).

Positron emission tomography scanners design

PET scanners use a 360° array of detectors to collect pairs of photons emitted by a positron-emitting radionuclide interacting with an electron. Detector rings are stacked together resulting in an axial field of view of 15 to 26 cm. Longer axial field of view systems covering the entire torso or entire length of body have been recently introduced (6,7). Allowing coincidence detection between different detector rings (3D mode acquisition) significantly increases the sensitivity of the PET camera compared to older versions using 2D mode in which thin lead or tungsten septa are used to eliminate photons originating outside of the plane of each detector ring in order to avoid saturating the detectors. Elimination of collimators and geometric efficiency of ring detectors result in exquisite sensitivity that is orders of magnitude higher than single photon emission computed tomography (SPECT) or other molecular imaging techniques in clinical use.

Annihilation of each positron during the interaction with an electron results in two simultaneous photons moving in opposite directions (with a small deviation from 180° due to preservation of momentum of the original particles). If both photons are detected, the source can be localized to the line connecting the locations of corresponding scintillation events. Depending on how far the source is from each detector, there may be a short

Table 14.1 PHYSICAL PROPERTIES AND CHARACTERISTICS OF RADIONUCLIDES USED IN PET FOR HUMAN CLINICAL AND INVESTIGATIONAL APPLICATIONS (2,4,5)

Radionuclide	Half life	β+ decay (alternative)	Range, mean (max), mm	Production	Examples
F-18	110 min	97% (EC)	0.7 (2.6)	Cyclotron	^{18}F-FDG, ^{18}F-FACBC ^{18}F-NaF, ^{18}F-DCFPyL
Ga-68	68 min	88.9%# (EC)	3.6 (10.3)	Ge68/Ga68 generator	^{68}Ga-DOTATATE, ^{68}Ga-DOTATOC, ^{68}Ga-DOTANOC, ^{68}Ga-PSMA-11
N-13	10 min	100%	1.7 (5.6)	Cyclotron	^{13}N-NH3
C-11	20.4 min	99.8% (EC)	1.3 (4.5)	Cyclotron	^{11}C-acetate
O-15	2 min	99.9% (EC)	3 (9)	Cyclotron	^{15}O-H$_2$O
Rb-82	1.27 min	95.5%# (EC)	7.5 (18.6)	Sr82/Rb82 generator	Rubidium chloride
Cu-64	12.7 h	17.9% (39% β-, 45% EC, 0.5% γ)	0.7 (2.9)	Cyclotron	^{64}Cu-ATSM
Zr-89	3.3 days	23% (EC)	1.3 (3.8)	Cyclotron	^{89}Zr-trastuzumab
I-124	4.2 days	12.7%# (EC)	3.4 (11.7)	Cyclotron	^{124}I
Y-90	64 h	0## (99.98% β-)	1 (3)	90Sr/90Y generator	SIR-Spheres®, TheraSphere®

#Complex decay schemes with coincident gamma emission.

##Pair production (0.0032%)

time difference between scintillation events (less than 3 ns for a 70-cm ring diameter), a fact that time-of-flight cameras use to further pinpoint the source along the line of response. Increased time window in systems with lower temporal resolution (typically 6–12 ns) increases the chance of coincidentally registering photons from unrelated annihilation events, degrading image quality. Conversely, newer scanners with improved timing resolution have improved image quality.

The high energy of coincident photons (511 keV) requires the use of scintillating crystals with high effective Z and high density to maintain good detection efficiency (stopping power) and reduce thickness. Thicker crystals affect image quality by reducing spatial, temporal, and energy resolutions, and can increase cost. The commonly employed crystals include bismuth germanium oxide (BGO), lutetium oxyorthosilicate (LSO), and lutetium–yttrium oxyorthosilicate (LYSO). The light output is less than that of sodium iodide (NaI) (i.e., lower-energy resolution and less efficient scatter rejection). BGO has the highest stopping power (efficiency) but the light output (corresponding to energy resolution) and temporal resolution are lower than other crystals. LSO and LYSO crystals used in time-of-flight cameras have rapid decay times minimizing the dead time (enabling higher count rates than BGO particularly in 3D mode) and provide a temporal resolution of <1 ns (translating to a 30-cm bracket along the line of response). With optimization of electronics for time-of-flight PET, modern systems have a timing resolution of 500 ps or better (8) (symbol or vice versa 400 ps using silicon photomultipliers based detectors PET [9]). Timing information improves image quality and higher signal to noise ratio particularly for larger patients as temporal resolution of the system increases (10).

Scintillating crystals are either coupled to photomultiplier tubes, or to solid-state single-photon-sensitive devices (silicon photomultipliers or avalanche photodiodes) that unlike photomultiplier tubes can operate in the presence of strong external magnetic fields (as in PET/MRI). The photomultiplier output is amplified and is digitized and read out. State-of-the-art systems improve signal to noise by directly converting photons into a digital signal.

Image reconstruction

The lines of response determined by each pair of coincidentally detected photons are organized into projections. Projections within a plane (as in 2D mode) construct a sinogram that can be back projected to reconstruct an image (generally after correcting for oversampling by applying a filter, i.e., filtered back projection). The image can be refined by an iterative expectation maximization (EM) algorithm, implemented for computational efficiency by dividing the data into ordered sets (OSEM). Bayesian methods try to further improve the quality of the reconstructed image by taking advantage of knowledge of the image (e.g., non-negative tracer concentration and only small variations between neighboring voxels). Regularized Bayesian reconstruction methods have better contrast recovery for small structures and better tissue uniformity compared to OSEM (11).

In addition to correcting for random events and scatter events, the reconstruction should also account for the attenuation of photons primarily due to Compton's scatter, which is proportional to the density of the absorber. PET is more sensitive than SPECT to attenuation artifact (even accounting for lower absorption of 511-keV photons compared to typical gamma emitters) since a coincidence would not be registered if either photon produced in the decay of positron is attenuated. Attenuation can be measured directly using a germanium rod source (which adds significantly to the scan time and is no longer used in current clinical scanners), or from CT (which is very quick although the measured attenuation may be different given lower photon energies due to photoelectric effect particularly when metal or CT contrast material is present). Respiratory misregistration or motion can introduce artifacts.

MR data cannot be directly used for attenuation correction, but attenuation map must be estimated based on known attenuation factors of different tissue types such as fat- or soft tissue (12). Time-of-flight information can be used to estimate attenuation and can be used in conjunction with MR-derived attenuation maps to correct for body parts outside of the MR field of view or deviations in attenuation due to metallic implants, internal air, or dense bones that are poorly visualized and characterized on MR sequences (13).

Hybrid imaging: PET/CT

Integrated PET systems are a combination of a PET and a CT or MRI system with a single, conjoined patient handling system (bed) that allows acquisition of co-registered functional and anatomical information with the patient in the same position for both modalities.

Images are acquired using PET and CT scanners in tandem. The CT provides detailed anatomical and structural information that guides interpretation of PET, improving sensitivity and specificity of findings particularly in areas of heterogenous physiologic uptake such as bowel in FDG PET or degenerative spine in sodium fluoride (NaF) PET. CT images are additionally used to create attenuation correction maps. To minimize the additional radiation from the CT component, the X-ray tube current is reduced (low-mA, 60–100 mAs). A high tube voltage (typically 120 or 140 kVp) is preferred to reduce the photoelectric effect. The use of intravenous or oral contrast material in certain applications improves delineation of lesions and normal anatomy, but in most instances the benefit from administration of contrast is limited and presence of contrast may introduce small quantification errors. If needed, additional dedicated contrast-enhanced CT studies or 4D respiratory-correlated CT for RT planning may be performed in the same session.

To minimize motion and registration artifacts in the chest and upper abdomen, the patients should be instructed to breath-hold at normal end expiration during CT. In large patients, artifacts related to truncation (part of body outside of CT beam) may be seen. PET/CT is usually well tolerated and requires shorter scan time compared to legacy PET scanners or PET/MRI systems. Claustrophobic patients or patients who have difficulty staying still may benefit from sedation.

PET/MRI

PET and MRI are both clinically utilized as functional imaging modalities. Features such as transverse relation (depicted on T2-weighted images), restricted diffusion, or enhancement can be used to identify and characterize various pathologies such as cancer or inflammation, and these features may be complementary to specific information that can be measured using PET such as metabolism or somatostatin receptor (SSTR) expression. MRI can provide excellent anatomical and structural details and soft-tissue contrast that assist in interpretation of PET imaging. PET/MRI systems can be used in scenarios that neither PET or MRI is by themselves sufficient to address diagnostic information needed for clinical decision-making without requiring two separate exams, particularly in applications that high-fidelity registration is desired, or as in pediatric population, eliminating CT to minimize radiation is a priority.

The conventional PET hardware uses photomultiplier tubes which are susceptible to high magnetic fields permanently present in an MRI environment. The advent of silicon-based systems allowed simultaneous acquisition of PET and MRI, and with optimization of MRI- or PET-based attenuation correction algorithms, the resulting images appear similar in diagnostic quality to PET/CT systems with comparable detectors and acceptable acquisition time. In skull to thigh or whole-body acquisition, time per bed station is typically limited by the MRI portion of the study. The exam duration is typically longer than a comparable PET/CT exam, providing higher counts for PET images for the same amount of administered activity. Alternatively, the administered activity can be reduced to minimize radiation while obtaining similar quality to PET/CT.

A primary drawback of MRI is evaluation of lung parenchyma and pulmonary nodules. Gradient-echo-based sequences such as diffusion-weighted echoplanar images (DWI) or Dixon-based sequences are particularly susceptible to magnetic field differences between air and tissue. Sub-centimeter pulmonary nodules therefore may be missed particularly in breath-hold T1-weighted images. T2-weighted images with respiratory triggering improve sensitivity for pulmonary nodules (60% sensitivity) but require longer acquisition (3–5 min) (14). Diagnostic accuracies of ~80% are reported using ultra-short or zero echo time sequences (15). A dedicated chest CT is often needed when focal uptake in the lung on PET is not well visualized on MRI or if pulmonary imaging with CT is standard of care for staging/restaging.

Patient comfort is affected by smaller bore size, acoustic noise, side-effects of MRI such as heat and peripheral nerve stimulation, and longer duration of study. Claustrophobic patients may require sedation or anesthesia. Exam in pediatric patients may require general anesthesia.

Quantification

Reconstructed images are corrected for attenuation, scatter and random events, and decay of radionuclide. Corrected images reflect the amount of radioactivity (radiopharmaceutical and its radioactive metabolites) during acquisition time window per volume calibrated to a specific time. The resulting raw activity values (often expressed in kBq/mL) depend on the amount of administered radioactivity and several other factors, and these values are not directly clinically useful. Comparing raw activity within a volume of interest with a reasonable reference value can provide meaningful information about the distribution of radiotracer at the time of PET acquisition. Reference values are either derived from the PET images (e.g., activity in mediastina blood pool or liver) or estimated from administered radioactivity and expected volume of distribution.

Physiological activity in specific structure(s) can be used as reference for visual or qualitative scoring. For example, blood pool and liver parenchyma are used for assessment of response in lymphoma using FDG PET (Deauville or Lugano 5-point scale), whereas liver is used for selecting patients with well-differentiated neuroendocrine tumors prior to peptide receptor radionuclide therapy (PRRT) (Krenning score), and cerebellar white matter can be used for evaluation of cortical plaque burden with amyloid PET.

A commonly used semi-quantitative measure, standardized uptake value (SUV), uses uniform distribution of radiotracer throughout the body (i.e., dose divided by body weight) as the reference value for normalization of activity:

SUV = measured activity/(administer dose/body weight)

For example, 100 MBq FDG administered to a 100-kg patient is consistent with 1 MBq/kg (or 1 kBq/g) if distributed uniformly throughput the body. In this case, a measured activity of 2 kBq/g can be expressed as SUV of 2 g/mL. Variants of SUV such as SUV$_{lbm}$ and SUV$_{bsa}$ replace body weight with lean body mass or body surface area, respectively, which may better reflect the actual volume of distribution of FDG or other radiotracers. SUVs regardless of normalization method can vary significantly between sessions and between different scanners. When scan protocols are kept similar, a decrease of 25% or an increase of 33% in SUV generally indicate an actual change. With meticulous control of physiologic and scan parameters the variability can be reduced to as low as 10% (16).

Most practices report the highest activity in the region of the lesion (SUV$_{max}$). SUV$_{max}$ reduces partial volume effects in areas of heterogeneity and necrosis and at the boundaries of lesion, and in contrast to several other measures such as lesion size, volume, and average activity (SUV$_{mean}$), it does not depend on how the operator delineates the lesion.

The volume of the lesion on PET can be automatically estimated by thresholding and inclusion of nearby voxels at a certain fraction of the SUV$_{max}$ (typically 40%–42%) or a fixed number (e.g., 2.5 g/mL for FDG PET) (17). For FDG PET, the term *metabolic tumor volume* (MTV) is used, and summed activity of all voxels within the lesion (using the same threshold for segmentation) is termed *total lesion glycolysis* (TLG). SUV$_{peak}$ is a variation of SUV$_{max}$ that." Modify to : 'SUV$_{peak}$ is a variation of SUV$_{max}$ that, instead of using the single voxel of maximum activity, measures activity within a prespecified region (i.e., 1-cm^3 sphere) centered at the maximum voxel location. PET Response Criteria in Solid Tumors (PERCIST 1.0) uses SUV$_{peak}$ and normalization based on lean body mass instead of body weight.

Dynamic PET (acquiring images at multiple time intervals) enables visualization of radiotracer kinetics in vivo (18). PET images are superpositions of activities of radiotracer and its radioactive metabolites in different compartments such as blood, and extracellular and intracellular moieties. Kinetic models describing how activities in each compartment evolve over time depending on other compartments can detangle the underlying signals and derive quantitative measurements of specific physiologic parameters such as metabolic rate of glucose. The information content of the PET data is inadequate to support complex and sophisticated models. Continuous or multiple-time point arterial plasma sampling may be needed to measure the input function. Simplified models or tools such as multiple-time graphical analysis technique (19) are generally used to measure desired kinetic or physiologic parameters and can provide more robust estimates than complex models that are close to the actual values.

Radiation

The effective radiation to the patient is primarily determined by the administered radioactivity, biodistribution, and effective half-life. Many PET radiopharmaceuticals in clinical use including FDG have high urinary clearance, and hydration and frequent voiding can reduce overall radiation and specifically radiation to the bladder wall. CT contributes to the radiation to the patient. However, radiation exposure associated with FDG PET/CT carried out with a low-dose CT scan can be well below that of a diagnostic multiphase contrast-enhanced CT scan.

In obese patients, increased attenuation and scatter affect image quality. Adjusting acquisition time based on body mass index (BMI) or patient weight may be needed and for LSO and LYSO detectors can result in better image quality compared to increasing the administered dose.

PET/MRI eliminates radiation from CT and enables reduction of administered radioactivity due to longer MRI acquisition time.

Positron emission tomography radiopharmaceuticals

PET can image and quantify biological processes at the cellular and subcellular level by using radioactive ligands and chemicals that target specific molecular mechanisms such as cell membrane transporters, peptide receptors, enzymes, or antigens. A few commonly used tracers are discussed in detail.

FDG

FDG is a glucose analogue that is taken up by living normal or neoplastic cells. FDG uptake in malignant tumors depends largely on insulin-independent glucose transporter 1 (GLUT1) and to a lesser extent GLUT3 that are overexpressed in most malignancies (20). GLUT1 is also expressed in inflammatory cells. Cytoplasmic FDG enters the first step of the glycolytic pathway through phosphorylation by hexokinase II, but unlike glucose does not undergo further metabolism and instead gets trapped in the cytosol. The rate of subsequent dephosphorylation and regression from the cell in most tissues is negligible. The degree of FDG accumulation is therefore highly linked to normal glucose metabolism in most tissues although differences in enzymatic reaction rates or affinity of glucose and FDG for passive or active transporters result in some differences in biodistribution in certain organs (most significantly in renal tubular uptake resulting in significant urinary excretion of FDG). A small amount of FDG may also be excreted in biliary system or bowel.

Glucose metabolism and Warburg effect

Otto Warburg observed that malignant cells preferentially metabolize glucose by glycolysis even when sufficient oxygen is present (21). Glycolysis is the primary mean for ATP production in a hypoxic environment due to cancer outgrowing its blood supply or abnormal angiogenesis. Similar changes in glucose metabolism occur in tumor stroma and cancer-associated fibroblasts (22). Glycolysis is an inefficient process compared to oxidation, and together with high energy demand of proliferating cells and inflammatory cells associated with cancer, results in high glucose utilization necessitating over express of glucose transporters and high hexokinase activity.

It is hypothesized that glycolysis enables cancers to synthesize ATP rapidly, promotes flux of metabolites into biosynthetic pathways, alters tissue microenvironment enabling disruption of architecture and immune evasion, and allows for signal transduction (23).

Physiologic biodistribution of FDG

Significant physiologic FDG uptake is seen in normal tissues and can be intense in tissue like brain gray matter or myocardium (24). The biodistribution of FDG is greatly affected by insulin, and a minimum of 4 h of fasting is required to minimize insulin-dependent FDG uptake in skeletal muscles. The one exception is with myocardial viability PET studies with FDG in which insulin is necessary for increasing uptake in viable myocardium. Even small amounts of sugar or simple carbohydrates in "sugar-free" beverages can induce endogenous insulin release (Fig. 14.1). In patients with suboptimally controlled diabetes or patients receiving corticosteroids, high plasma glucose concentration can compete with FDG, resulting in slower intra-cellular uptake and blood pool clearance. The standard PET protocol can be used if plasma glucose level <200 mg/dL prior to injection (25,26). For

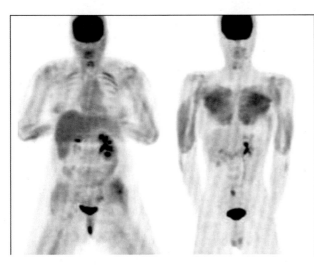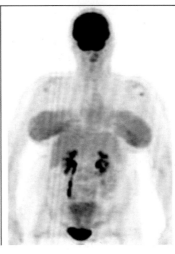

FIG. 14.1 ● Excessive physiologic muscle FDG uptake. Left, the patient had a few chips 2.5 h prior to the study. The plasma glucose level was normal at the time of injection. Middle: patient reported work out at the gym the day prior to the exam. Right: physiologic uptake in breast and uterus in a postpartum patient.

higher glucose levels, the study should be preferably rescheduled until better glycemic control is achieved. If this is not feasible, subcutaneous administration of rapid-acting insulin with injection of FDG after the duration of insulin effect (3–5 h) can be considered. Increasing uptake time can mitigate some of the effects of hyperglycemia. Except for long-acting forms of insulin (duration >18 h) which are equivalent to baseline insulin release, FDG should not be administered within the duration of insulin effect (5–8 h for regular and 12–16 h for intermediate-acting insulin). Although oral hypoglycemic agents may alter the biodistribution of FDG, particularly in the bowels (27), type 2 diabetes mellitus patients controlled by oral medication should generally continue taking their medications. The study can be preferably performed late in the morning after adequate fasting (25). Patients with acute or severe renal disease on metformin who receive intravenous-iodinated contrast may need to temporarily discontinue it (28).

Physical exercise and strenuous activities can temporarily increase insulin-independent uptake in skeletal muscles and should be avoided at least 6 h (preferably 24 h) prior to the study.

High physiologic FDG uptake in the cortical and deep gray matter limits sensitivity of PET for intracranial lesions. Images of the brain should be reviewed carefully for both focal uptake and photopenia, which can indicate vasogenic edema or disruption of cortex. High uptake in spinal gray matter is often not conspicuous (due to partial volume artifact) except in cervical spine and conus.

High physiologic uptake is invariably present in extra-ocular (and occasionally in palpebral) muscles, mylohyoids, and other floor of the mouth muscles, glottis, and cricoarytenoid muscles. Uptake in longus coli and suboccipital muscles and other neck muscles may be seen due to overuse, tension, spasm, or stiffness. Uptake in salivary glands is variable and often mild. Asymmetry may be seen due to atrophy or inflammation. Intense activity is frequently seen in sublingual gland (29) and floor of the mouth muscles (30). A ptotic or transferred submandibular gland may mimic a mass and lymphadenopathy. Masseter or pterygoid uptake may indicate strain or tension. Sucking or chewing immediately before or during uptake time results in intense uptake in buccinator and mastication muscles and should be avoided. Intense uptake in pharyngeal lymphoid tissue can be physiologic in children and young adults. Diffuse thyroid FDG uptake is not normal but frequently represent subclinical thyroiditis.

Physiologic uptake in scalene and intercostal muscles and diaphragm can be seen in patients with difficulty in breathing. Myocardial uptake is highly variable and can be intense even in appropriately fasted patients. To minimize physiologic myocardial activity (necessary in evaluation of cardiac inflammation or masses), a carbohydrate-restricted diet (for 8 and up to 48 h) prior to fasting is helpful. Physiologic uptake can be seen in normal thymus. Thymus is often atrophic after the age of 40 but thymic hyperplasia (rebound) with high physiologic uptake can be seen after chemotherapy.

Normal liver parenchyma is sometimes used as a reference region in FDG PET scan. Hepatic uptake is usually homogeneous and mildly greater than blood pool activity. Liver uptake can be affected by metabolic regulation and conditions such as steatosis. Although hepatocytes are highly metabolically active, low affinity of GLUT2 (the primary glucose transporter in hepatocytes and renal tubules) to FDG and increased dephosphorylation limit physiologic FDG uptake in hepatocytes and cell differentiated hepatocellular carcinomas.

Adrenal and pancreas have uptake less than liver parenchyma. Increased uptake can be seen in adrenal hyperplasia and adenomas (particularly functioning adenomas). Physiologic bowel wall uptake is variable. High uptake primarily in the colon in patients on metformin, after recent enema or use of laxative stimulants can mask lesions. Sphincters may have high physiologic uptake.

Unlike glucose, FDG is poorly reabsorbed from the glomerular filtrate. To minimize the interference of intense activity in the urine with assessment of pelvic organs, patients should empty their bladder prior to PET imaging. If possible, pelvis should be images early to minimize refilling of bladder during acquisition (e.g., by scanning from thighs toward skull-base). Administration of a diuretic 30 min prior to imaging can improve assessment of pelvic or urothelial malignancies.

High physiologic uptake can be seen in degenerating fibroids, postpartum uterus, endometrium during menstruation, and corpus luteum. Uniform mild to moderate physiologic uptake is often present in testes. High physiologic uptake can be seen in breasts during lactation (although FDG is not significantly excreted in milk). Asymmetric uptake can be seen if one of the breasts is preferentially used for lactation.

Mild uptake is typically present in hematopoietic bone marrow in the axial and proximal appendicular skeleton. Focal uptake in red marrow islands in appendicular skeleton mirroring the rest of the red marrow could mimic metastatic lesions. Increased activity and uptake can be seen in response to anemia, recovery from chemotherapy, systemic inflammation, and can be intense within 2 to 3 weeks after administration of colony-stimulating factors, possibly obscuring metastatic involvement. Physiologic uptake in spleen can also increase and exceed that of hepatic uptake due to increased red blood cell turnover. Clinically unexplained increased bone marrow uptake may warrant further evaluation. Fatty marrow replacement with low uptake is seen after external beam radiation.

With proper preparation, physiologic skeletal muscle uptake is minimized. Higher uptake may be seen in muscles used for posture and breathing. Strain, tension, or inflammation can result in high uptake confirming to the anatomy of individual muscle or muscle groups involved. Subcutaneous and visceral adipose tissues typically have minimal uptake although mild uptake can be seen in obesity and metabolic syndrome (31). A distinct distribution of high uptake can be seen due to metabolically active adipose tissue. This is more common in children and young adults, particularly after exposure to cold, and can interfere with detection and quantification of lesional uptake. Avoiding cold exposure, and possibly administration benzodiazepines, or beta-blockers may be necessary to minimize this effect. Focal uptake can be seen due to insults (trauma, injection sites), and fat necrosis. Lipomas often lack uptake, and presence of uptake could indicate an atypical lipomatous tumors or a low-grade liposarcoma. Higher uptake can be seen in brown fat tumors (hibernomas) which are not reliably differentiated from other lesions.

Limitations of FDG

FDG PET has limited sensitivity and diagnostic accuracy in indolent neoplasms with low cellularity (in-situ or minimally invasive pulmonary adenocarcinomas, some ovarian cystadenocarcinomas, mucinous adenocarcinomas) and/or glucose metabolism (e.g., low grade well-differentiated neuroendocrine tumors [NETs]) or malignancies that preferentially utilize other nutrients for ATP production and proliferation (liposarscoma, prostate adenocarcinoma). Hepatocytes and well-differentiated hepatocellular neoplasms can dephosphorylate FDG, which can exit the cell through bidirectional GLUT2, reducing intracellular accumulation. Background uptake (e.g., in the case of brain primary or metastatic lesions) can greatly affect conspicuity of small lesions. However, the most significant limitation of FDG PET is due to the fact that FDG is not specific for cancer and a variety of physiologic conditions and in particular inflammation can result in high uptake. Inflammatory uptake generally reduces the accuracy of FDG PET in most oncological applications although in certain scenarios could be advantageous (e.g., in Hodgkin's lymphoma due to overabundance of reactive cells compared to Hodgkin's or Reed–Sternberg cells).

Technical considerations

Patient preparation (fasting, avoiding strenuous exercise, providing specific recommendations regarding diet or medications) reduces physiologic uptake and increases conspicuity of lesions (25). Blood glucose level must be measured prior to administering FDG. The patient's weight needs to be recorded. For brain metabolism studies, patients should be in a quiet, dimly lit room several minutes before FDG administration and during the uptake phase. The scan is typically done 45 to 75 min after administration of radiotracer. When repeating a study of the same patient for assessment of disease progression or response

to treatment, the delay between injection and scan should ideally vary by less than 10 min. The effective dose from the PET portion of the exam is approximately 7 mSv in adults (for 370 MBq administered activity).

68Ga-DOTATATE

Several ^{68}Ga-labeled somatostatin analogues are in clinical use. SSTRs are present on the cell surface of essentially all cells, but are highly expressed (particularly type 2 receptor, SSRT2) on neuroendocrine cells. DOTA-Tyr3-Octreotate (DOTATATE) which was approved by US Food and Drug Administration (FDA) in 2016 for localization of SSTR-positive NETs in adult and pediatric patients primarily binds to SSTR2. Other SSTR-imaging PET traces also bind avidly to SSRT2 but can additionally bind to SSTR5 (DOTA-octreotide) or SSTR3 and SSTR5 (DOTA-NaI-octreotide). The physiologic biodistribution of these are similar and sensitivity and specificity for well-differentiated neuroendocrine tumors are overall comparable (32–34).

Physiological distribution

High expression of SSTR2 is seen in anterior pituitary (all cell types, but particularly GH-expressing cells), striated ducts of the parotid gland, neuroendocrine/enterochromaffin cells of gastrointestinal (GI) mucosa, enteric ganglia, insulin- and glucagon-secreting cells of the pancreas, reticular zone of the adrenal cortex, glomeruli and tubules of the kidney, luteinized granulosa cells of the ovary, basal parts of testicular tubules, granulocyto-poietic cells of the bone marrow, alveolar macrophages of the lung, and germinal centers of lymph follicles. The degree of uptake on PET depends on both cellularity and expression of SSTR in a tissue, as well as non specific absorption. Similar to ^{111}In-pentetreotide, the highest uptakes are present in the spleen and kidneys (Fig. 14.2). Intense uptake in accessory spleens and splenosis may mimic metastasis from neuroendocrine tumor. Intense physiologic uptake is also seen in pituitary and adrenals. Urinary excreted activity is present in the collecting system and bladder.

Mild to moderate diffuse thyroid uptake is commonly seen. SSTR is overexpressed in both parafollicular cells (C cells) and inflammatory cells that can be present with thyroiditis. Uptake in the GI tract is variable (mild to moderate) and generally highest in the stomach. Moderate physiologic uptake is seen in the pancreas body and tail. Intense focal uptake can be seen in the uncinate process due to high concentration of islet cells. Uptake in breast tissue is variable and can increase in pregnancy or with lactation. Mild to moderate uterine uptake is sometimes seen.

Some benign lesions such as osseous hemangiomas or reactive lymph nodes can have moderate to intense uptake. Other entities that can display high uptake include areas of active infection/inflammation (most white cells express high levels of SSTRs), including inflammatory arthritis, fractures, healing surgical wounds, inflammatory response to radiation, and pneumonia or abscess, prostatitis, and granulomatous reactions (especially if "active"). Osteoblastic activity can also be seen including normal uptake (active epiphyseal plates) and in bone disease (Paget disease, fibrous dysplasia, some bone islands).

Multiple neoplasms are associated with SSTR2 overexpression (Table 14.2) and may have uptake on DOTATATE-PET.

Technical considerations

PET can be performed 40 to 90 min after the intravenous administration of ^{68}Ga-DOTATATE. Longer delays can result

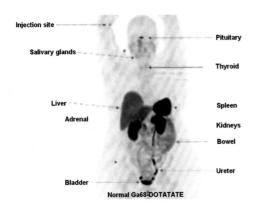

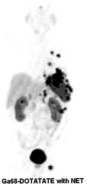

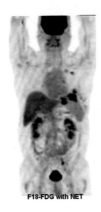

FIG. 14.2 ● Physiological distribution of ⁶⁸Ga-DOTATATE (left). Comparision of ^{68}Ga-DOTATATE (middle) and FDG PET in a patient with metastatic NET.

in deteriorating image quality due to Ga-68 decay. No fasting or restriction of physical activity is necessary prior to administration of radiotracer. The typical administered activity in adults is 4 to 5 mCi (or 2 MBq/kg up to 200 MBq). If the patient is on SST analogs therapy, the nonradioactive SST analogue can competitively bind to SSTR. Some centers hold short-acting SST analogs for 1 day prior to the scan (although this may not be feasible in severely symptomatic patients) or schedule the study 3 to 4 weeks after administration of long-acting SST analogs (typically just before the next scheduled monthly dose of long-acting octreotide analog) (34,35). Hydration before and 1 h after administration of radiotracer is recommended to reduce radiation to the urinary tract. Free gallium is excreted in breast milk, therefore lactating patients are advised to hold breastfeeding for 12 h (~10 half-life of ^{68}Ga). Spleen receives the largest radiation dose (0.109 mGy/MBq). The effective dose from the PET portion of the exam is approximately 4 mSv (0.021 mSv/MBq), which compares favorably to about 12 mSv for ^{111}In-pentetreotide.

Images are interpreted visually in conjunction with clinical history, pathologic grade, and findings on other imaging modalities. Unlike FDG, the degree of uptake and SUV$_{max}$ is not necessarily an indicator of aggressiveness of tumor. High

Table 14.2 NEOPLASMS ASSOCIATED WITH SSTR EXPRESSION

CNS/PNS

Pituitary adenomas	Usually high
• Gonadotroph, corticotroph, and nonfunctioning	Low or absent
• Others	High
Meningiomas	High
Medulloblastomas, neuroblastomas, supratentorial PNETs of childhood, and oligodendrogliomas	High
Astrocytoma	Low, infrequent
Peripheral nerve sheath tumors (especially Schwannomas)	High
Pheochromocytomas and paragangliomas	High (>70%)
Lung and GI	
Gastroenteropancreatic (GEP)-NETs	High
• Gastrinoma	100%
• Carcinoid tumors	86%
• Insulinoma	58%
GIST	High (88%–100%, associated with favorable outcomes)
Colorectal carcinomas, HCCs	Infrequent
Pancreas adenocarcinomas	Low (less than normal pancreatic tissue)
Bronchopulmonary NETs	Variable (32%–56%, lower than GEP NETs)
Other	
Thyroid	
• Medullary thyroid carcinoma	High
• Papillary or follicular thyroid carcinoma	Variable, frequent
NETs of other organs	Variable
• Merkel cell carcinoma	59%
• Thymus, breast, cervix, or prostate	Up to 50%
Prostate cancers	Low (13%, 50% if endocrine differentiation)
Breast, cervical, endometrial, ovarian cancer, melanoma	Infrequent
Lymphoma	Low

GIST, gastrointestinal stromal tumor.

^{68}Ga-DOTATATE uptake generally indicates a well differentiated tumor that is less aggressive. Lack of uptake in a lesion or incidental finding is not necessarily an indicator of benignity or indolence, as poorly differentiated tumors with low uptake are typically associated with a poor prognosis. Krenning score (Table 14.3), which is a visual/qualitative measure originally developed for ^{111}In-Pentetrotide scintigraphy, can be used to describe the activity of lesions. The score based on PET can be higher than the score on scintigraphy particularly for small lesions (35). Tumors with low uptake (Krenning score below 2) are generally better imaged with FDG PET. Heterogeneity of uptake should be evaluated for presence of hemorrhage or necrosis within the lesion versus the possibility of mixed population with different histologic grades. Depending on the degree of uptake in the tumor cells, small lesions within the liver or within or adjacent to organs with similar or higher physiologic uptake (e.g., adrenal glands or spleen) could be better identify on MRI or contrast-enhanced CT.

F-18 FACBC (fluciclovine)

Malignancies are associated with elevated amino-acid metabolism. Glutamate is the second most abundant nutrient in plasma after glucose and can undergo oxidation through the Kreb's cycle to provide energy for cell survival and proliferation. Certain malignancies such as prostate cancer increase amino-acid transporters at the cell membrane. Fluciclovine is a synthetic amino acid (amino-fluorocyclobutane-carboxylic acid) that is preferentially transported through sodium-dependent system ASCT-2, and to a lesser degree via sodium-independent system LAT-1, which are both overexpressed in prostate cancer. ASCT-2 is the most upregulated transporter for glutamine and other amino acids in several different malignancies (36), and the degree of overexpression is associated with aggressive behavior in prostate cancer (37). Androgen receptor signaling and MYC and mTOR oncogenes stimulate ASCT-2 expression is prostate cancer cells (38).

Unlike FDG, fluciclovine is not metabolized in the cytosol, and over time washes out through the same transporters. The biodistribution of fluciclovine therefore changes significantly over time with peak tumors to normal-tissue activity (reflecting mostly first pass uptake due to over expression of amino-acid transporters) within 4 to 10 min. A bolus dose of 370 MBq (10 mCi) is injected intravenously usually with the patient in the scanner and PET is initiated after 3 to 5 min. Increasing physiologic muscle uptake can be noted as the scan proceeds from mid-thigh to the base of skull. Metastatic nodal involvement in prostate cancer is more common in pelvic and retroperitoneal nodes than above the diaphragm. Even with proper flushing,

intense residual activity is sometimes seen in upper extremity veins. Pancreas has the highest physiologic uptake, followed by liver and bone marrow. Urinary excretion is limited, although in patients who voided less than 30 to 60 min prior to the injection, intense activity can be seen in ureters or bladder, and can mimic or mask uptake in retroperitoneal lymph nodes and prostate bed. Mild or moderate physiologic uptake may be present in pituitary, salivary glands, pharyngeal lymphoid tissue, thyroid, breast glandular tissue, gastrointestinal tract, and renal parenchyma (39). Incidental abnormal uptake can be seen in other malignancies (including papillary renal cell carcinoma [RCC]) and benign lesions such as meningioma or schwannoma. Physiologic nodal uptake can be seen with follicular hyperplasia. Symmetric uptake in bilateral axillary, hilar, external iliac, and inguinal lymph nodes in the absence of known prior involvement can be assumed to be physiologic. Nodal uptake in a distribution that is not typical for prostate cancer may represent a different etiology (malignancy or inflammation).

Uptake in recurrent or metastatic prostate cancer is generally significantly greater than bone marrow. Normal L3 vertebral body marrow is typically used a reference for physiologic activity (unless replaced by sclerosis or fatty marrow). Focal uptake in prostate bed or nodes less than bone marrow but greater than blood pool is indeterminate and follow-up is recommended. However, small nodes (long dimension <1 cm) with uptake approaching bone marrow or asymmetric uptake in the seminal vesicles are suspicious for malignancy. Primarily lytic osseous lesions typically demonstrate intense uptake. Mixed lesions may have moderate uptake. Due to high physiologic background uptake in normal bone marrow, primarily sclerotic lesions may not be discretely visible on PET (40). Variable uptake has been reported in various benign and malignant primary bone lesions such as osteoid osteoma and multiple myeloma. Mild uptake associated with degenerative disk disease and facet arthropathy is less than usually seen with FDG.

Technical considerations

Similar to FDG, strenuous exercise should be avoided for at least 1 day prior to the exam, and patients are advised to fast for 4 h. Imaging starts in the pelvic region at 3 to 5 min after intravenous administration. The effective whole-body radiation dose is approximately 8 mSv in an adult, which is slightly higher than the same amount of FDG, noting low renal excretion of fluciclovine (5% in 24 h).

Other positron emission tomography radiopharmaceuticals in oncologic applications

NaF

Fluoride ions get directly incorporated into newly formed hydroxyapatite crystals in the bone matrix as fluoroapatite. First pass uptake is higher than phosphonates due to rapid reaction with hydroxyapatite and minimal binding to plasma proteins. Consequently, skeletal uptake and plasma clearance is faster than in bone scintigraphy using ^{99m}Tc tracers with relatively high uptake in the axial skeleton compared to acro skeleton reflecting a flow-dependent process. Imaging can start as soon as 30 to 45 min after injection although a delay of 90 to 120 min should be considered for imaging of the upper and lower extremities (41). Imaging with simultaneous FDG and NaF injection is possible and may allow for assessment of osseous and extra-osseous

Score	Intensity
0	No uptake
1	Very low
2	Less than or equal to that of liver
3	Greater than that of liver
4	Greater than that of spleen

Table 14.3 **KRENNING SCORE. THE DEGREE OF UPTAKE ON SSTR IMAGING CAN PREDICT RESPONSE TO PRRT (35,143)**

involvement as a single session (42). NaF PET and particularly PET/CT or PET/MRI have higher sensitivity and specificity compared to bone scintigraphy, and allow quantitative/semi-quantitative measurement of bone formation and turnover that can be used for assessment of disease activity and response to treatment in metastatic lesions, Paget's disease and other metabolic bone disorders, infection or inflammatory bone processes, traumatic injuries and acute bone loading, and bone pain. Although the primary clinical indications of NaF are for evaluation of skeleton, it can be used as an investigational molecular marker for evaluation of extra-osseous calcification such as in atherosclerosis.

Prostate specific membrane antigen

Although not approved by the FDA, prostate specific membrane antigen (PSMA) radioligands are in increasing research use in the United States for imaging prostate cancer. PSMA (folate hydrolase or glutamate carboxypeptidase II) is a transmembrane glycoprotein enzyme highly expressed on the surface of prostate cancer cells compared to normal prostate cells. PSMA overexpression is present in the cell surfaces of majority of prostate cancers and correlates with advanced, high-grade, metastatic, androgen-independent disease (43), although it may not be present in some subtypes or lesions and may not parallel Gleason score or prostate-specific antigen (PSA) levels.

Low-molecular-weight substrates that bind with high affinity with the catalytic domain of PSMA have replaced monoclonal antibodies as the preferred targeting agents, due to faster pharmacokinetics and higher tissue penetration, and low non-specific binding to inflammatory cells. Addition of a lipophilic linkage has been shown to further increase binding affinity to PSMA. ^{11}C-DCMC and subsequently ^{18}F-DCFBC have been used for PSMA imaging since 2005 (44,45). ^{18}F-DCPyL is a second-generation radioligand with improved plasma clearance, lower hepatic and skeletal muscle uptake, and higher tumor-to-background uptake ratio compared to DCFBC (46). ^{18}F-PSMA-1007 has similar kinetics to ^{18}F-DCPyL with reduced urinary clearance (47), with high tumor-to-background uptake 2 to 3 h after radiotracer injection (48). Ga-68-labeled lysine-urea-glutamate PSMA inhibitor–chelator conjugates are currently wildly used for prostate cancer imaging throughout the world despite inferior image quality and less suitable half-life of Ga-68 compared to F-18, although interpretation of studies using F-18-labeled PSMA may be more challenging due to higher detection of benign or nonspecific uptake (49). Both F-18- and Ga-68-labeled PSMA agents have higher positivity and tumor-to-background contrast in biochemically recurrent prostate cancer than radiolabeled choline, especially at low-serum PSA levels (<1 ng/mL) (50,51).

Physiologic biodistribution of different PSMA radioligands can be variable but intense uptake is generally present in the renal parenchyma and salivary and lachrymal glands. Intense excreted activity in the urinary tract may obscure adjacent lesions or cause scatter correction artifacts around the bladder. High hepatic uptake in first-generation PSMA radioligands and PSMA-11 reduces sensitivity for hepatic involvement. Uptake can be seen in sympathetic ganglia and variably in the bowel. Benign focal uptake has been reported in mediastinal and hilar lymph nodes with biopsy-proven sarcoidosis, subacute brain infarct, follicular thyroid adenoma, seminal vesicle amyloidosis, and Paget's disease (52). PSMA is overexpressed in neovasculature in malignancies other than prostate cancer. Abnormal uptake has been demonstrated in multiple myeloma, papillary carcinoma of thyroid, gastrointestinal stromal tumor (GIST), squamous cell carcinoma (SCC), and RCC.

Myocardial perfusion positron emission tomography tracers

Cardiac PET images are superior to myocardial perfusion SPECT and enable quantification of myocardial blood flow (in mL/min/g of tissue), and coronary flow reserve. Attenuation artifacts on PET are significantly less but are typically present on SPECT images (even after attenuation correction of SPECT). PET can be particularly useful for minimizing errors due to chest wall attenuation in obese patients or women. Rb-82 chloride and N-13-ammonia are the most commonly used radiopharmaceuticals for myocardial perfusion PET. The primary characteristic of all radiopharmaceuticals used for myocardial perfusion imaging is high first pass myocardial extraction although there are significant technical differences between them (Table 14.4). For example, it is not feasible to do exercise stress using either Rb-82 or O-15 water due to extremely short half-lives. However, due to rapid decay a complete study with rest and post-stress perfusion images can be performed in less than 30 min. Due to longer half-life of N-13, exercise stress can be done prior to placing the patient in the scanner (although exercise stress is not compatible with quantification of myocardial blood flow which requires dynamic imaging starting with radiotracer injection). The rest and stress portion of the study need to be separated by 4 to 5 half-lives (~40 min) to minimize interference between activity from first and second injection, although some centers shorten the delays and increase administered activity for the second injection. Due to long half-life of F-18, the investigational agent, flurpiridaz (binds to mitochondrial complex 1) scan protocols often require different doses for rest and stress (similar to protocols for Tc-99m perfusion agents). A 2-day protocol could allow lower administered activities and decreased effective radiation.

Table 14.4 **PET MYOCARDIAL PERFUSION RADIOTRACERS (53)**

	First pass extraction (rest)	Image resolution (FWHM)	Retention (peak stress)	Image delay	Radiation
Rb-82 chloride	65%	Low (8 mm)	Low (35%)	70–90 s (90–130 s for LVEF<50%)	3 to 6 mSv
N-13 NH$_3$	90%–95%	High (5 mm)	High (50%)	3–5 min (longer in COPD)	2 mSv
O-15 Water	~100%	Intermediate (6 mm)	None	Requires dynamic imaging	1.5 mSv
F-18 Flurpiridaz	95%	High (4 mm)	High (55%)		6 mSv

Rb-82 chloride is an analog of potassium and is extracted efficiently from plasma by myocardial cells via the Na/K exchange pumps, although the first pass extraction is not as high as Tl-201 which has a similar mechanism of uptake. An ^{82}Sr/^{82}Rb generator is eluted every 6 to 10 min, which makes it suitable for centers with high volume of referrals for myocardial perfusion imaging or centers not in proximity of a cyclotron. The generator needs to be replaced every 4 to 8 weeks. Due to high fixed cost of the generator, the cost per dose can be prohibitive for centers with low volume.

Ammonia diffuses passively as NH_3 across cell membranes. In plasma, NH_3 and NH_4 are at equilibrium depending on the pH, whereas within the cytoplasm NH_4 gets trapped through glutamine synthesis. After intravenous injection, NH_3 can dissociate from the plasma in the alveoli and enter the gas phase. A delay of 3 to 5 min between injection and imaging (longer in patients with obstructive airway physiology) helps with the clearance of lung activity. Over time, ^{13}N-labeled metabolites (urea, glutamine, glutamate) accumulate in the blood and account for 40% to 80% of the total activity as early as 5 min after injection of ^{13}N-ammonia. Elimination is primarily through the kidneys (as ^{13}N-urea).

Myocardial perfusion imaging often needs to be performed in conjunction with FDG PET for evaluation of myocardial viability or inflammation (sarcoidosis). Perfusion and FDG uptake provide complementary information and absence of both perfusion and FDG uptake is necessary to confirm infarction or scarring. Although it is possible to compare perfusion SPECT and FDG PET, using PET for perfusion (particularly using NH_3) enables more accurate and more detailed characterization and delineation of regional myocardial abnormalities.

Amyloid and tau tracers in brain imaging

β-amyloid is a key biomarker in Alzheimer's dementia. The deposition of β-amyloid precedes the onset of detectable cognitive symptoms by several years (54). With the introduction of ^{11}C-Pittsburgh Compound B (PiB), in vivo visualization of amyloid deposition in the brain with PET was realized (55). ^{11}C-PiB is an analogue of thioflavin-T, which has been used as a histologic dye for amyloid plaques in vitro. ^{18}F-labeled radiotracers that have been since developed are currently in clinical use and include flutemetamol (Vizamyl^{TM}), which is structurally similar to ^{11}C-PiB and florbetaben (Neuraceq^{TM}) and florbetapir (Amyvid^{TM}), which are stilbene derivatives. These radiotracers are lipophilic and readily cross the blood-brain barrier and bind to the amyloid aggregates in neuritic plaques. Unbound radiotracer washes out from normal gray matter which creates a clear visual contrast with nonspecific retention in white matter due to lipophilic interactions with myelin. Absent or reduced gray–white matter distinction is consistent with moderate to frequent amyloid neuritic plaques. Although there are some differences in administered dosage, recommended delay between injection and imaging, and exact interpretation criteria, ^{18}F-labeled radiotracers are highly concordant with ^{11}C-PiB PET (56). Effective radiation for recommended dose is between 5.8 and 7 mSv.

It has been hypothesized that in the pathogenesis of Alzheimer's disease (AD), amyloid pathology is followed by tau pathology, subsequent neurodegeneration, and eventually cognitive decline (54,57). Tau neurofibrillary tangles are present in several other neurodegenerative disorders such as progressive supranuclear palsy, corticobasal degeneration syndrome, Parkinson's disease dementia, and dementia with Lewy bodies (DLB) (58). Unlike β-amyloid deposits, tau aggregates are primarily intracellular and structurally heterogenous, making it challenging to target using PET tracers (59). β-sheet-binding properties shared between different Tau neurofibrillary tangles have been used for targeting (60). FDDNP was one of the first PET tracer used for in vivo imaging in Alzheimer's dementia and binds to both β-amyloid deposits and tau neurofibrillary tangles (61). Subsequently developed first- and second-generation investigational tau tracers are small molecules, which bind with high affinity to tau β-sheet, but have relatively low affinity to amyloid aggregates and other fibrils (62) although there are some evidence of nonspecific in vivo binding to α-synuclein and TDP-43 deposits. The FDA granted the approval of ^{18}F-flortaucipir (Tauvid^{TM}) in May 2020.

Clinical applications in oncology

FDG PET and other radiotracers are clinically used for diagnosing and staging malignancies, as well as to guide subsequent management after the initial treatment. In diagnosis, the primary indications include differentiation of benign from malignant lesions (e.g., evaluation of a solid noncalcified nodules or solid component in a subsolid nodule larger than 8 mm in diameter [63]), detection of an unknown primary malignancy (in a patient presented with biochemical markers or paraneoplastic syndrome or if metastatic disease is discovered as the first manifestation of cancer), screening patients with multiple endocrine neoplasia (MEN) or other syndromes associated with malignancy, detection of malignant transformation, or planning biopsy target by finding a lesion or a region of the tumor that has optimal compromise between risk associated with biopsy and diagnostic yield. In specific circumstances, PET may be necessary to confirm the diagnosis, for example, ^{68}Ga-DOTATATE PET in patients with anatomic lesions that are suspicious for NET on conventional imaging, particularly when biopsy is not feasible.

The standard of care recognizes the role of PET in staging known malignancies depending on sensitivity and specificity of PET compared to conventional imaging and the a priori probability of metastatic involvement based on histologic and clinical findings. Indications of PET in guiding subsequent treatment strategy include (but are not limited to) early assessment if a treatment is effective (e.g., interim PET after two cycles of chemotherapy in Hodgkin's lymphoma), monitoring the effect of therapy, documenting the degree of response after completion of treatment, characterization of residual abnormalities on physical examination or on other imaging studies following treatment, documenting disease burden prior to initiation of a new treatment, planning adjuvant radiation therapy, or surveillance and detection of cancer recurrence, especially in the presence of elevated tumor markers. For diagnostic-therapeutic (theragnostic) pairs of radiopharmaceuticals such as ^{68}Ga-DOTATATE and ^{177}Lu-DOTATATE, PET can be used to select patients or lesions that could benefit from therapy and may be useful for dosimetry.

In many oncologic applications, the relevant portions of the body are within the torso and imaging is performed from base of the skull to mid-thigh unless there are known or suspicious lesions in other body parts that need to be included. National Comprehensive Cancer Network (NCCN) guidelines recommend skull-base to knees coverage for lung cancer, although the utility of inclusion of lower thighs is unclear and is not consistent with our experience. For brain lesions, coverage is typically limited to the head to allow optimizing resolution and signal to noise. In head and neck malignancies, additional imaging of the head and neck is performed (with arms down to the sides of the patient). Whole-body imaging covering from the top of the head through the feet is necessary in certain applications including melanoma, Merkel cell carcinoma, cutaneous T-cell lymphoma, multiple myeloma, soft-tissue and extremity sarcomas, and malignant peripheral nerve sheet tumors.

It is worth emphasizing that hereafter, the term PET refers to hybrid PET imaging. Anatomic information is crucial for fully utilizing the diagnostic potential of PET, and PET alone systems (which are unable to provide detailed anatomic information) are exceedingly rare in oncologic imaging. PET/CT is the workhorse in oncological imaging. PET/MRI systems are less widely available and there is overall less experience with them than PET/CT. However, the evidence so far suggests that in certain applications PET/MRI is diagnostically superior to PET/CT whereas in most other applications both are diagnostically similar.

Lymphoma

Lymphomas are a heterogeneous group of diseases that develop from lymphocytes, with more than a hundred types and subtypes classified based on histopathologic, immunohistochemical, cytogenetic, and molecular analyses (64), and widely varying clinical behaviors and response profiles. Together, they comprise the most common hematologic malignancy (approximately 5% of all cancers excluding non-melanomatous cutaneous malignancies). A US individual has a 2% lifetime risk of developing lymphoma. The 2016 WHO classification divides mature lymphoid, histiocytic, and dendritic neoplasms into five groups (mature B-cell neoplasms, mature T and NK neoplasms, Hodgkin's lymphoma [HL], posttransplant lymphoproliferative disorders, and histiocytic and dendritic cell neoplasms). HL (approximately 10% of lymphomas) has distinct pathologic features (Hodgkin's or Reed–Steinberg cells), epidemiology (bimodal age distribution with peaks at 15–35 and 60–70 years of age), clinical behavior (contiguous spread), prognosis (86% 5-year overall survival, and as high as 97% in patients younger than 20 years), and treatment is based on stage in contrast to non-Hodgkin's lymphomas (primarily seen after age 60, noncontiguous spread, 71% 5-year overall survival, and treatment primarily based on subtype rather than stage). Nodular lymphocyte predominant Hodgkin's lymphoma is a variant of HL associated with 10% chance of transformation into diffuser large B-cell lymphoma (DLBCL). Most (90%) non-Hodgkin's lymphomas arise from mature B-cells. DLBCL is an aggressive lymphoma that is the most common lymphoid malignancy in the United States (65). Both HL and DLBCL are associated with intense FDG uptake, and disease activity can be characterized based on the degree of uptake on PET by visual assessment (blood pool and liver parenchyma as reference in Deauville or Lugano 5-point scale; Table 14.5). Most lymphomas are FDG avid (uptake greater than blood pool), although the degree of uptake can be variable and in indolent lymphomas such as follicular lymphoma uptake is generally less intense compared to DLBCL. PET/CT is the standard of care for imaging FDG-avid lymphomas. CT can provide complementary staging information and is indicated for non-avid histologies or if PET/CT is not available. For histologies with low or variable FDG avidity, contrast-enhanced CT may be preferable to PET/CT. In the absence of concern for aggressive transformation, PET/CT may have limited value in certain histologies such as chronic lymphocytic leukemia/small lymphocytic lymphoma, lymphoplasmacytic lymphoma/Waldenstrom's macroglobulinemia, mycosis fungoides, or marginal zone lymphomas.

Table 14.5 THE SCORES FOR THE MOST INTENSE UPTAKE IN A SITE OF INITIAL DISEASE (74)

Score	Uptake
1	No uptake (lesion is similar to background on PET)*
2	Uptake ≤ mediastinum
3	Uptake >mediastinum but ≤ liver
4	Uptake moderately higher than liver
5	Uptake markedly higher than liver and/or new lesions
X	New areas of uptake unlikely to be related to lymphoma

*In Waldeyer's ring or extranodal sites with high physiologic uptake or with activation within spleen or marrow (e.g., GCSF), complete metabolic response may be inferred if uptake is less than surrounding normal tissue.

Staging of primary nodal lymphoma is based on extent of nodal and extra-nodal disease, involvement of bone marrow, liver, spleen, and central nervous system, and clinical parameters such as B-symptoms. In limited disease (stage I/II), nodal disease is limited to one side of the diaphragm. Extranodal involvement if present should be limited and contiguous with the involved nodes (a single extranodal lesion without nodal involvement is also stage I). Bulk is an important prognostic factor in some lymphomas. Advanced disease includes nodal or splenic involvement above and below the diaphragm (stage III) or presence of noncontiguous extranodal disease (stage IV). FDG PET/CT has been shown to be more accurate than CT (up-staging in most cases) and can potentially change treatment in 25% to 45% of the patients (66). PET/CT is more sensitive and accurate than bone marrow biopsy in HL (67) and DLBCL although may miss diffuse low cellularity involvement in ~3% of patients with DLBCL (68).

FDG PET/CT has been an integral part of response criteria in FDG-avid lymphomas since 2007 (69). Interim PET (between the second and third cycle of chemotherapy) is highly prognostic in HL (70), and patients with a positive interim PET may benefit from chemotherapy escalation (71). The utility of midtreatment PET in DLBCL is less clear, although patients with a negative PET appear to have better outcomes (72,73). A PET/CT after completion of treatment is however the standard of care to assess for remission in all FDG-avid lymphomas. Because FDG uptake is not specific for malignancy, a biopsy of PET-positive lesions can be performed to confirm presence of disease prior to salvage therapy. PET/CT after salvage chemotherapy is prognostic in refractory and relapsed HL and DLBCL and could be used to select patients for high-dose chemotherapy and stem cell transplant.

Published studies do not support routine surveillance scans after remission. For curable histologies such as HL and DLBCL, the likelihood of relapse decreases over time. However, in follicular, mantle-cell, and other incurable lymphomas, the likelihood of recurrence continues or increases over time, necessitating patients to be observed every few months. Follow-up PET/CT should be prompted by clinical indications. Imaging may be necessary for follow-up in residual intra-abdominal or retroperitoneal disease that cannot be evaluated by clinical exam. Unfortunately, the probability of a false-positive PET can be higher than 20%, limiting the utility of routine surveillance scans.

Head and neck malignancies

Head and neck cancers comprise cancers arising from the mucosa of the upper aerodigestive track (nasal cavity and paranasal sinuses, lips and oral cavity, salivary glands, pharynx, larynx), head- and neck-specific cutaneous cancers, and a variety of other neoplasms (thyroid, lymphoma, paragangliomas, sarcomas, melanoma, and Merkel cell carcinoma). Mucosal head and neck cancers are the sixth most common cancer worldwide (eighth most common in US men). More than half of patients present with locally advanced M0 disease (stages III or IV), which is associated with high morbidity and are often treated with chemoradiation. There is 50% to 60% probability of local recurrence and 20% to 30% probability of discovering distant metastasis within 2 years from treatment.

SCCs are the most common histology in head and neck cancers: 90% to 95% of the lesions in the oral cavity and larynx are SCCs. Risk factors include tobacco smoking (associated with TP53 mutation), EtOH (particularly for cancers of the hypopharynx), and HPV (particularly type 16, up to 70% of oropharyngeal cancers). Other histologies include verrucous carcinoma (a variant of SCC), adenocarcinoma, adenoid cystic carcinoma, mucoepidermoid carcinoma, sinonasal undifferentiated carcinoma, and nonkeratinizing nasopharyngeal carcinoma. The latter is strongly associated with Epstein-Barr virus (EBV) (75% of nasopharyngeal carcinomas in the United States).

The tumor, node, metastasis (TNM) staging system is the basis for assessment of disease status, prognosis, and management of head and neck malignancies. Clinical staging is based on available history, physical examination, and available imaging. Imaging is often performed but is not mandatory for clinical staging. Pathological TNM (pTNM) applies only if the patient undergoes surgery.

FDG PET/CT is an important tool for staging and subsequent management of head and neck malignancies. Glycolysis is highly upregulated in head and neck SCCs. Pathogenesis of SCCs and mutation of P53 gene is associated with increased hypoxia-inducible factor-1 (HIF-1α complex), which binds to the hypoxia response elements in the promoter region and consequently results in GLUT-1 and hexokinase-II overexpression that facilitate accumulation of FDG in malignant cells. High uptake in primary tumor is associated with aggressive behavior. Tumor (T) staging is site specific and in cutaneous and oral cavity cancers requires to measure depth of invasion (DOI), which is difficult to assess on FDG PET. T staging for nasopharyngeal cancers is best assessed with MRI. CT and MRI are both useful for anatomic delineation of primary lesion and assessment of involvement in adjacent structures in other sites. PET/CT and PET/MRI have similar or higher sensitivity compared to CT or MRI for T-staging. False negative can be seen due to small tumors (T1) or high background physiologic activity. Dental artifact is less problematic compared to CT or MRI, and PET has been shown to be superior to MRI for assessment of extent of disease in areas of susceptibility artifact due to dental hardware (75). T4 (Tumor >4 cm with DOI >10 mm or tumor invades adjacent structures) indicates moderate to very advanced local disease and upgrades the stage to IV (except in HPV-mediated oropharyngeal cancers).

Nodal involvement is an important prognostic factor in head and neck malignancies. Nodal staging is based on number, size,

extra-nodal extension (based on clinical exam and pathology but not imaging) and contralateral involvement. Occult nodal involvement has been reported in more than 20% of clinically N0 cancers and its incidence increases with increasing T stage (76). PET/CT and PET/MRI are more sensitive than CT and/ or MRI for nodal staging and can identify metastatic involvement in lymph nodes that are not enlarged by size criteria. The recently published results of ACRIN 6685 trials demonstrate a high negative predictive value (87%) and significant impact in surgical plans in 22% of the patients (77). PET/CT has high sensitivity (84%–88%) and specificity (75%–84%) for nodal staging in occult primary SCCs of the head and neck and can detect the site of primary in 25% to 37% of the cases (78). When the site of primary cancer cannot be identified, P16+ is staged as HPV-mediated oropharyngeal cancer, and EBER+ (Epstein–Barr encoding region) is staged as nasopharyngeal cancer.

FDG PET is increasingly used after chemoradiation and has replaced planned neck dissection in advanced head and neck cancers to document response and assess for residual disease. Patients who underwent PET-CT-guided surveillance has similar survival but required fewer surgeries compared to patients who underwent planned neck dissection (79). Patients who demonstrate complete metabolic response (no visually detectable uptake at prior tumor locations above background) on PET done 3 months after treatment have a very low risk (~5%) of local recurrence (80). PET has very high sensitivity (97% compared to 69% for MRI) and moderate specificity (46% vs. 77%) for recurrent head and neck SCC after radiotherapy or chemoradiotherapy (81). A prospective multicenter study of newly diagnosed patients with locoregionally advanced head and neck cancers (stage IVa/b) show that FDG-PET/CT 12 weeks after completion of chemoradiation has high accuracy for residual disease (defined as focal uptake greater than blood pool and liver parenchyma) and high-negative predictive value (92%) for recurrence within 9 months (82).

The role of FDG PET in evaluation of differentiated thyroid carcinoma is limited but may be considered in staging and evaluation of response to therapy in radioiodine negative high-risk patients with elevated serum Tg (generally >10 ng/ mL) and aggressive histological subtype such as poorly differentiated thyroid cancers, and invasive Hürthle cell carcinomas (83). In anaplastic thyroid carcinomas, FDG PET/CT is recommended for both initial staging and assessment of treatment response 3 to 6 months after initial therapy. Focal FDG uptake within the thyroid is incidentally seen in ~1% to 2% of oncological PETs. FNA is recommended for sonographic ally confirmed nodules >1 cm (35% chance of thyroid carcinoma), or if the possibility of metastatic involvement is considered and can alter management (e.g., in head and neck cancers, lymphoma, or melanoma). For nodules <1 cm or patients with advanced non-thyroid malignancies, active surveillance is alternatively considered (84).

Salivary gland carcinomas are a rare heterogenous group of histologies with different metastatic potential that arise from both major and minor salivary glands. The incidence of occult lymph node metastasis is somewhat lower than SCCs, and the role neck dissection is less well established (85). PET/CT has higher sensitivity (88% vs. 53%) and similar specificity (>90%) compared to contrast-enhanced CT for nodal involvement in salivary gland cancers. The primary lesion typically have intense uptake, although MTV appears to better correlate with survival than the degree of uptake (86). SUV does not reliably differentiate benign versus malignant lesions. Intense uptake can be seen in Warthin's tumor (papillary lymphomatous cystadenoma), which is strongly associated with smoking, male gender, can be bilateral, and is rarely malignant. Pleomorphic adenomas can also have moderate to intense uptake. Incidental focal uptake in parotid gland is often benign (87) except in patients with lymphoma and head and neck malignancies (88).

Head and neck paragangliomas arise from parasympathetic nervous system and chemoreceptors such as carotid body. Unlike pheochromocytoma and sympathetic paragangliomas, head and neck paragangliomas are almost always nonsecretory and most of them are not MIBG avid. They are often discovering incidentally or due to symptoms related to mass effect or involvement of adjacent structures. ^{18}F-FDOPA, and ^{68}Ga-DOTATATE or ^{68}Ga-DOTATOC PET, have higher sensitivity than MIBG scintigraphy for head and neck paragangliomas (89,90). Hereditary head and neck paragangliomas are most commonly associated with germline mutations in one of the SDH subunit genes. FDG PET has a superior sensitivity compared to CT/MRI or MIBG in the localization of primary and metastatic paragangliomas associated with SDH mutation (91).

The PET protocol for head and neck malignancies (if not primarily performed for evaluation of distant metastatic involvement) should include a dedicated head and neck portion with small field of view (FOV) large matrix, and increased time per bed to improved resolution and sensitivity to detect small nodal metastases (92). Arms down, skull vertex (or base) to clavicle is performed to evaluate for distant metastatic involvement. PET/CT for head and neck malignancies are best performed with contrast-enhanced CT. Without iodinated contrast, it is difficult to evaluate for specific sites of disease involvement that might upstage a tumor. (e.g., determining the presence of medial or lateral pterygoid muscle involvement (both T4) by a tonsillar carcinoma is difficult when relying on non-contrast large FOV CT for correlation with FDG uptake.

Lung cancer and other thoracic malignancies

Lung cancer is the leading cause of cancer-related mortality in the United States for both men and women. Pulmonary nodules are frequently identified in asymptomatic high-risk patients undergoing screening chest CTs and can be incidentally identified on ~1% of chest CTs performed for reasons unrelated to cancer (93). The utility of FDG PET in evaluation of incidentally found solid or part solid solitary pulmonary nodules has been extensively studied (94,95). The combination of visual assessment of FDG uptake and pretest factors yields good accuracy (96) and incorporating FDG avidity improves clinical prediction models for assessment of the likelihood of malignancy in pulmonary nodules (97) except for populations within endemic areas for benign inflammatory nodules, such as tuberculosis (98). Per NCCN guidelines, an FDG PET/CT can be performed for evaluation of incidentally found solid pulmonary nodule greater than 8 mm or persistent part-solid nodules with solid component measuring 6 mm or more. Uptake greater than mediastinal blood pool is considered positive. The current data suggest low sensitivity of FDG PET for pulmonary nodules less than 8 mm in diameter (T1a). A false-negative result can also be seen in tumors with low cellularity (e.g., mucinous adenocarcinomas or primarily ground glass lesions), or low uptake typically seen in lesions with indolent behavior and low-grade histology (e.g., carcinoid tumors, carcinoma in situ, and minimally invasive adenocarcinoma).

Non-small cell lung cancer (NSCLC) accounts for 75% to 80% of all lung cancer cases. FDG PET/CT is recommended in pretreatment staging of lung cancer to avoid futile thoracotomies, and is superior to CT in detection of nodal and distant metastases (99,100). PET-negative mediastinal lymph nodes are associated with a low probability of malignant involvement in solid tumors <1 cm and purely nonsolid lesions <3 cm, and pre-resection sampling is optional in these settings. The N stage is based on location of metastatic nodes according to the IASLC lymph node map (N1: ipsilateral peribronchial or hilar nodes, N2: ipsilateral mediastinal or subcarinal nodes, N3: contralateral mediastinal or hilar nodes or any supraclavicular or scalene nodes) (101). N1 disease is considered at least stage IIB, whereas N2 disease is at least stage IIIA category (53% and 36% 5-year survival rates, respectively). N3 disease corresponds to stage IIIB (for primary tumor <5 cm, 26% survival) or IIIC (tumor >5 cm or invasion to adjacent structures or nodule in the same lung; 13% survival) (102).

Extra-thoracic metastasis has major implications for management and prognosis of lung cancer. FDG PET/CT has higher sensitivity and specificity for hepatic and adrenal involvement compared to CT and similar sensitivity and higher specificity compared to bone scintigraphy for osseous involvement. Adrenal nodules are a common incidental finding on CT (103), whereas FDG PET has greater than 90% sensitivity and high specificity for adrenal metastasis (104). Lack of FDG uptake in an adrenal nodule is consistent with a benign adrenal adenoma. FDG PET has limited sensitivity for brain metastasis and MRI brain is recommended in patient with clinical stage II or higher NSCLC.

FDG PET is not currently routinely recommended for surveillance and follow-up of patients with NSCLC. If used as a problem-solving tool after radiation, histopathologic conformation is needed due to possible persistence of postradiation inflammatory uptake for up to 2 years.

Small-cell lung cancers account for 14% of all lung cancers, and are characterized by rapid doubling time, fast growth, and early development of widespread metastasis. Patients typically present with a large hilar mass and mediastinal lymph nodes causing cough and dyspnea. Clinically limited stage disease can be treated with radiation therapy.

FDG PET/CT is recommended by the NCCN for accurate RT planning for both NSCLC and small-cell lung cancer. FDG PET can improve target delineation accuracy from atelectasis and post obstructive consolidation, particularly if IV contrast cannot be administered. A PET/CT (preferably within 4 weeks and no more than 8 weeks prior to therapy, ideally in the same position as treatment) is indicated for staging and target definition.

PET/CT may be considered for staging in clinical stages I to III malignant pleural mesothelioma and epithelial or mixed histology to evaluate for distant metastasis prior to surgery; PET/CT should be performed before pleurodesis. PET/CT may be considered for radiation treatment planning. Intense inflammatory uptake associated with pleurocerids can persist indefinitely (105). With talc pleurodesis, intense uptake typically corresponds to high-attenuation pleural lesions on CT.

FDG PET is a useful tool for evaluation and staging of other intrathoracic malignancies such as thymic neoplasms (106) and can be considered for evaluation of incidentally discovered asymptomatic non-cystic anterior mediastinal masses or unexplained mediastinal lymph nodes larger than 15 mm in short axis without benign texture features on CT and can help guide biopsy planning (107).

Gastrointestinal tract

Malignancies of GI tract (including liver, gallbladder, and pancreas) comprise more than a quarter of new cases of cancers and one third of cancer mortality worldwide (108). The incidence of esophageal cancer is rising in the United States and it is currently the seventh leading cause of cancer death in US men. The prognosis is poor, and the 5-year survival rate varies between 45% (for local disease at the time of diagnosis) and 5% (metastatic disease) (109). Tobacco smoking and alcohol consumption (and particularly combination of both) are major risk factors. SCC is the most common histology worldwide. Adenocarcinoma which commonly occurs in distal esophagus (75%) is the leading cause of esophageal cancer in the United states and is linked to obesity, gastroesophageal reflux disease (GERD), and particularly Barrett's metaplasia. Unlike the rest of the bowel, esophageal lacks serosal barrier to rapid spread of primary tumor into adjacent structures. FDG PET/CT is recommended for initial staging and for assessment of treatment response following both neoadjuvant and definitive chemoradiation >5 to 6 weeks after completion of therapy and could be considered for surveillance of T1b or higher disease, with interval depending on stage (NCCN guideline). FDG PET can aid in better determination of RT volumes and fields borders. Neither PET nor CT can reliably differentiate T1 to T3 tumors. Obliteration of the fat planes between the primary esophageal tumor and adjacent structures on CT can establish a T4 stage tumor but this is less reliable in patients with prior RT or cachectic patients. Assessment of local and regional lymph nodes on PET may be difficult due to intense uptake in the primary esophageal lesion. However, PET has excellent sensitivity for detecting distant nodal and extra-nodal metastasis and can help prevent futile curative-intent surgeries (110,111).

Gastric cancer is a leading cause of cancer death worldwide. The role of FDG PET is staging gastroesophageal junction cancers (particularly for N staging) has been well established. New data confirm that routine FDG PET is also useful for staging of non-junctional gastric cancers (112). PET is more accurate than CT for nodal involvement and is more specific for peritoneal disease, despite low sensitivity. NCCN guidelines recommend the use of FDG PET for initial staging (except if the patient has known distant metastases) and restaging of unresectable or medically unfit patients following primary treatment. A complete metabolic response after therapy correlates with better prognosis (113). The diagnostic performance of FDG PET for early gastric cancers, histologies such as signet ring cell and mucinous types that are associated with low FDG uptake, and peritoneal recurrence is low.

Colorectal malignancies are the second leading cause of cancer-related death in the United States. Diagnosis and staging are primarily done with colonoscopy and contrast-enhanced CT or MRI. MRI is superior to CT for T staging of rectal cancers and assessment of hepatic metastasis. There is insufficient evidence about the use of PET/CT for colorectal cancer staging (114) and PET/CT not routinely indicated for staging colorectal cancers, even though it has higher sensitivity and specificity than conventional imaging (115). FDG PET allows staging patients with contraindication to contrast or MRI. Other indications include evaluation of an equivocal finding on contrast-enhanced CT in patient who are otherwise candidates for curative-intent surgery. The liver is the most common site of metastases in colorectal cancer with up to 25% of patients presenting with hepatic involvement at initial diagnosis. PET/CT scan has high sensitivity for distant metastatic involvement in liver (although sensitivity may be affected by recent chemotherapy) and other organs and in patients with potentially curable M1 disease can help identify other potential sites of involvement that would alter surgical approach or might render patient unresectable for cure. PET scan is not routinely recommended for surveillance or for monitoring progress of therapy. However, it can help identify structural recurrence in patients with negative conventional imaging and colonoscopy who have elevated carcinoembryonic antigen (CEA) (116).

Anal cancer is an uncommon malignancy of the digestive system (109). Most patients present with locoregional involvement that can often be cured with chemoradiation. PET/CT has high diagnostic accuracy (117) and is recommended for initial staging and radiation treatment planning of anal or anal marginal SCC (118,119). Uptake on post-treatment PET is a predictor of recurrence after chemoradiation (120).

Hepatocellular carcinoma is the most common primary liver malignancy in adults and is commonly associated with viral hepatitis or cirrhosis. Dysplastic nodules in cirrhosis have the potential to evolve into carcinoma. Hepatocellular carcinomas demonstrate considerable heterogeneity in clinical and histopathologic features and metabolism. Well-differentiated hepatocellular carcinomas generally have low-FDG uptake but high uptake on ^{11}C-acetate or ^{18}F-choline investigational PETs. High-FDG uptake correlate with high tumor grade and intratumoral fibrosis (121,122), and correlates with recurrence rate after liver transplant (123). PET is not adequate for diagnosis of hepatocellular carcinoma but could be considered for evaluation of metastatic disease (124). A recent meta-analysis of the literature showed moderate sensitivity and high specificity of FDG PET in detecting extrahepatic metastases or local residual/recurrent hepatocellular carcinoma.

PET/CT is not routinely recommended for staging in cholangiocarcinoma or gallbladder adenocarcinoma, although emerging evidence suggests that it may be useful for detection of regional nodal metastases and distant metastatic disease in patients with otherwise potentially resectable disease.

Most pancreatic malignancies including ductal adenocarcinoma are of exocrine origin and are associated with poor prognosis. Contrast-enhanced CT and MRI are the primary modalities for evaluation of pancreatic lesions and staging pancreatic malignancies. The role of FDG PET in pancreatic carcinomas is not fully established. FDG PET is useful in patients presenting with jaundice or pancreatic mass on imaging and equivocal findings on pancreatic protocol CT. PET appears to be more accurate in differentiating benign versus malignant intraductal papillary mucinous neoplasms (IPMN) of the pancreas than CT or MRI (125). High uptake can be seen with some benign conditions such as acute or autoimmune pancreatitis, as well as in solid pseudopapillary tumor of the pancreas, which is a rare neoplasm with low-malignant potential (126). In contrast, mucinous adenocarcinoma or well-differentiated NETs can cause false-negative results on FDG PET. PET/CT or PET/MRI using radiolabeled somatostatin analogs has high diagnostic accuracy for detection and staging in most pancreatic NETs as detailed later in the chapter.

FDG PET is superior to conventional imaging for N and M staging in pancreatic ductal carcinoma (127–129). Patients with localized disease on CT who peruse treatment benefit from staged using FDG PET (130). FDG PET may be considered after dedicated pancreatic CT in high-risk patients to detect extra-pancreatic metastases (NCCN). Patients with resectable locally advanced pancreatic cancer, concurrent or sequential chemoradiation, are the current standard of care. FDG PET can demonstrate response to therapy earlier than CT and is more sensitive for assessment of residual disease (131,132).

GISTs are mesenchymal neoplasms that constitute approximately 1% of all primary gastrointestinal malignancies, typically arising from the stomach and proximal small intestine. FDG PET has high sensitivity for GISTs (133) and can be useful in detecting an unknown primary site, resolving ambiguities on conventional imaging, or as an adjunct staging in patients with marginally resectable disease or potentially resectable disease with risk of considerable morbidity. FDG uptake can markedly decrease as early as 24 h after starting treatment with tyrosine kinase inhibitors such as imatinib (134). Metabolic response precedes structural response and better correlates with progression-free survival and outcome (134,135).

Neuroendocrine neoplasms and paragangliomas

Neuroendocrine neoplasms are a heterogeneous group of neoplasms that arise from endocrine cells within the glands (e.g., adrenomedullary, pituitary, parathyroid) or from endocrine islets in the pancreas, thyroid, respiratory system, and gastrointestinal system (136). The incidence of neuroendocrine neoplasms (NENs) in the past 40 years has continually risen compared to all malignant neoplasms (137). All NENs have malignant potential. However, the likelihood to metastasize or invade the adjacent tissues depends on tumor site and type, and grade. Grade 1 (Ki67 index <3% and mitotic rate <2/10 HPF) has better prognosis than grade 2 (Ki67 of 3%–20% and mitotic rate 2–20/10 HPF) tumors (138). Grade 3 poorly differentiated NENs (Ki67 >20% or mitotic rate>20/10 HPF) are associated with poor prognosis. Classification of NENs was traditionally based on the primary site, although a uniform classification framework has been proposed (139).

Neuroendocrine tumors may be functional (i.e., produce hormones) or nonfunctional. Carcinoid tumors are the most common NENs and are derived from embryonal foregut (including lower respiratory tract and thymus), midgut, or hindgut. Foregut and midgut carcinoids produce 5-HIAA responsible for the "carcinoid" symptoms, such as wheezing, flushing, palpitation, cramps, and diarrhea. Pheochromocytoma is associated with hypertension. Symptoms associated with excess production of gastrin, insulin, glucagon, VIP, somatostatin, or ACT can be present in other gastroenteropancreatic NENs. Somatostatin inhibits and suppresses release of gastrointestinal hormones. Octreotide and other SST analogues such as lanreotide that binds with high affinity to the SSTRs (especially subtypes 2 and 5) can control symptoms with few if any side effects and have and antiproliferative effects on the NET.

Well-differentiated NETs are not typically FDG avid, although FDG PET remains useful in staging primary bronchial and poorly differentiated NENs. SST PET with ^{68}Ga-DOTATATE is a sensitive method of detecting, staging, characterizing the disease, and monitoring the effects of therapy (140). A meta-analysis of 10 studies and 416 patients with NET demonstrated similar high diagnostic accuracy for ^{68}Ga-DOTATOC (biding to both SSTR2 and SSTR5) and ^{68}Ga-DOTATATE 96% (binding with high affinity to SSTR2) PET (34). SSTR imaging using PET has high impact on the management of NET patients compared to conventional imaging or ^{111}In-pentetreotide and ^{123}I-MIBG and can result in changes in management in most patients (141,142). SSTR imaging and FDG PET have complementary roles in evaluation of low-grade well-differentiated NET versus high-grade

poorly differentiated NETs. Poorly differentiated and dedifferentiated NETs and neuroendocrine carcinomas loose SSTR expression on the cell membrane but demonstrate high uptake on FDG PET/CT.

Genitourinary malignancies

Kidneys and bladder

Most PET tracers in clinical use have significant urinary excretion than can interfere with assessment of renal parenchyma, urinary tract, and retroperitoneal and pelvic organs. Sodium/glucose cotransporter 1 and 2 in proximal tubules have low affinity to FDG compared to glucose and FDG remains in glomerular filtrate. With subsequent absorption of water FDG gets concentrated in the urine. Hydration and loop diuretics such as furosemide can reduce urinary activity and increase conspicuity of FDG-avid lesions that would be otherwise obscured or masked by partial volume or scattered activity.

RCC is the most common solid tumor of the kidneys and accounts for 3% to 4% of all malignancies. FDG uptake in primary RCC lesions is variable and can overlap with normal parenchyma and benign lesions such as oncocytoma. The degree of uptake depends on histologic subtype and grade (144,145) and high uptake is associated with aggressive tumors and reduced survival (146). Chromophobe or low-grade clear cell carcinomas are particularly associated with low uptake. Certain uncommon histologies such as succinate dehydrogenase–deficient RCC, mucinous tubular and spindle cell carcinoma, or RCCs with sarcomatoid dedifferentiation typically show intense uptake.

Overall, FDG has limited sensitivity for detection of primary renal lesion and is not considered standard of care in routine staging, although it can be useful to characterize equivocal findings on other modalities and inform decision-making (147). Metastasis to skeleton is seen in one third of patients with advanced RCC and is associated with significant morbidity due to pain, pathologic fracture, spinal cord compression (148). Osseous lesions are typically osteolytic and may be photopenic on bone scintigraphy. FDG PET is superior to bone scan for evaluation of osseous involvement (149) and could be considered in high-risk patients with clinical symptoms or laboratory indicators of bone metastasis, particularly in patient with known or suspected sites of extraosseous metastasis. FDG PET/CT has 85% to 90% sensitivity and specificity for detecting extra-renal metastasis or recurrence after nephrectomy (150,151).

FDG PET can be used in staging muscle-invasive bladder cancer (152) and is more accurate than conventional imaging for nodal or distant metastases (153) although early nodal involvement is frequently missed (154). Patients with stage II or III disease are treated with neoadjuvant chemotherapy followed by radical cystectomy. Persistent FDG uptake in primary tumor following neoadjuvant chemotherapy predicts pathologic residual disease and can inform decision on radical cystectomy (155). PET/CT can be considered after cystectomy (if not previously done or if metastatic disease is suspected [152]), and is accurate for restaging (156) and biopsy planning.

Gynecologic malignancies

FDG PET/CT (and PET/MRI) is increasingly used in initial evaluation, treatment planning, and follow-up in locally advanced or metastatic gynecologic malignancies. SCC, cervical adenocarcinoma, endometrial carcinomas, and high-grade serous or endometrioid ovarian cancers are FDG avid. However, mucinous or papillary carcinomas may have low uptake. The extent of primary tumor and invasion into adjacent structures are best evaluated with gynecologic examination and anatomical imaging such as MRI. The probability of nodal and distant metastasis significantly increases with increasing stage of the primary tumor. Lymph node size or morphology on anatomic imaging cannot reliably detect or exclude metastatic involvement and contrast enhancement or restricted diffusion/apparent diffusion coefficient may provide limited additional information. FDG PET can depict and quantify metabolic activity in tumor and lymph nodes useful for prognostication, assessment of disease burden and activity, and mapping nodal involvement for staging and treatment planning (157), or may identify distant lesions that can lead to a change in patient management necessitating biopsy and/or systemic therapy.

Staging in gynecologic malignancies is primarily based on clinical and pathologic findings. Imaging is not required and was not traditionally used in formal staging of cervical cancer (158) but has been recently allowed in the revised International Federation of Gynecology and Obstetrics (FIGO)-staging system (159). PET has high specificity for evaluation of nodal and extra-pelvic involvement in locally advanced (FIGO stages IB2–IVA) or metastatic cervical cancer (160). The sensitivity for nodal involvement is higher than conventional imaging, although it is considerably lower than sentinel node biopsy or nodal dissection (161,162). The likelihood of nodal metastasis in early stage (FIGO stages IA–IB1) cervical cancer is low and FDG PET may has limited value in pretreatment evaluation (163). In contrast, FDG PET has been reported to affect management in 40% of patients with stage IIIB disease (164). PET-guided intensity-modulated RT can improve survival while decreasing treatment-related toxicity (165).

SCC is the most common histology in vulvar and vaginal cancers. FDG PET/CT is useful in initial staging (except in early stage vulvar carcinomas less than 2 cm in size), RT planning, and evaluation of response to treatment or possible recurrence based on symptoms or examination findings. PET informs prognosis and affect management in a significant number of patients with vulvar and vaginal cancers, even though as with cervical cancer the sensitivity for nodal involvement is limited and does not replace surgical staging in the early disease (166,167). False-positive pelvic lymph node or distant findings may occasionally occur on PET (168).

Endometrial cancer is the most common gynecologic malignancy in developed countries. Staging is surgical (169). FDG PET remains useful in initial staging as clinically indicated if extrauterine disease is suspected and inform prognosis (170), predict which patients benefit from extensive lymph node dissection (171,172), and detect distant metastases particularly in high-grade and non-endometriod tumors (173). PET/CT (and presumably PET/MRI) is the best imaging method to evaluate lymph node and distant metastases (174) and has high specificity but low to moderate sensitivity for nodal or peritoneal involvement in patients with newly diagnosed high-risk endometrial cancer (175). The value of PET in predicting lymph node metastasis in node-negative endometrial cancer on preoperative MRI is not clear (176). Preoperative PET/MRI is more accurate than PET/CT in assessment of myometrial invasion and has slightly better sensitivity for regional lymph node metastasis (177). Posttreatment FDG PET in symptomatic patients or patients with increased tumor biomarkers has high sensitivity and specificity for evaluation of suspected recurrence (172).

Uterine sarcomas account for a small minority of all uterine cancers. Leiomyosarcoma is the most common subtype (excluding carcinosarcomas that are now reclassified as a dedifferentiated or metaplastic form of endometrial carcinoma) (178). Tumor stage is the most important prognostic factor. FDG PET can help characterize uterine lesions (179) but is not able to reliably differentiate high-grade uterine sarcomas from low-grade endometrial stromal sarcomas benign leiomyomas (180). High uptake is nonetheless associated with aggressiveness and is an unfavorable prognostic marker (181). Leiomyosarcoma has poor prognosis even when confined to the uterus. Lung is a frequent site of distant metastasis or recurrence after hysterectomy. PET/CT is recommended for initial staging and surveillance of uterine sarcomas as clinically indicated.

Ovarian cancer is the leading cause of cancer-related death from gynecologic malignancies in the United States. Physiological focal uptake in ovaries is frequently seen in women of child-bearing age, whereas uptake after menopause is worrisome for malignancy. Initial workup for ovarian, fallopian tube, and primary peritoneal cancer is done based on conventional imaging, although FDG PET can be considered for indeterminate lesions that can change management, or extra-abdominopelvic metastasis is suspected (182). Pretreatment FDG PET/CT can inform surgical approaches or alternative treatment options (183). Subsequently, PET can evaluate residual disease after debulking (184), informs decision to perform secondary cytoreductive surgery (185), and can detect recurrence particularly in symptomatic patients with normal cancer antigen (CA)-125 (186) or patients with elevated serum CA-125 levels but inconclusive conventional imaging. As with other gynecologic malignancies, most studies report high specificity and positive predictive value for nodal, peritoneal, and distant metastatic disease, with moderate sensitivity and overall superior accuracy compared to conventional imaging (187).

Prostate

Prostate cancer is the most common malignancy in men and a major cause of cancer death in the United States and worldwide (188). The most common histology is adenocarcinoma, thought to originate from the basal cells of prostate acini. Diagnosis is based on biopsy, although imaging can be performed to guide biopsy or to inform the decision to biopsy or re-biopsy in select cases. Most patients have localized disease at time of diagnosis, although nodal and distant metastases (usually skeleton) are reported to be present in 12% and 6% of patients. The anatomic extent of tumor stage, histologic grading (Gleason score, grade group [189]), and serum PSA are used together for stratification of patients into risk categories (190). Patients in low-risk category are unlikely to have nodal or distant metastatic involvement and may not benefit from systemic staging (191). Gleason score is based on the architectural features and loss of differentiation of the two most prevalent histologic patterns in the prostate tissue specimen (1 = well differentiated; 5 = anaplastic) and correlates closely with clinical behavior and tendency of prostate cancer to metastasize (192). The choice of initial management (active surveillance, definitive therapy, and androgen deprivation therapy) is based on risk category and staging.

Serum PSA is a relatively sensitive and specific biomarker of prostate cancer. A detectable rising PSA after definitive locoregional therapy may represent local and/or distant failure. Biochemical recurrence without visible disease on conventional imaging occurs within 10 years in up to 40% of the patients after prostatectomy (193). With advances in molecular imaging of prostate carcinoma, PET is emerging as a sensitive and accurate diagnostic tool superior to conventional imaging to inform salvage therapies, and as an adjunct to PSA for monitoring disease burden and evaluation of response to systemic therapies such as androgen deprivation therapy, and for selection of patients for radionuclide therapy. Hybrid PET/MRI protocols promise to combine the strengths of multiparametric and whole-body MRI with PET addressing possible limitations of each modality by itself in evaluation of prostate bed, lymph nodes, bone marrow, and other organs. However, large differences in technique and MRI sequences may limit generalization of results in investigational setting to applications in general clinical workflow. The role of PET in theragnostics for metastatic castration-resistant prostate carcinoma is discussed in a separate chapter.

FDG PET has limited utility in prostate carcinomas. High uptake in prostate gland incidentally seen in 1% to 2% of PET studies maybe due to an occult prostate cancer, warranting PSA measurement and possible further investigation, although similar uptake can be seen with more common benign conditions such as prostatitis (194). High uptake is more common in aggressive primary tumors with Gleason score of 8 to 10 (195). Although FDG PET is not indicated in routine staging and management of prostate cancer, it can be helpful in metastatic prostate cancer patients who have known FDG avid lesions (196).

Fluciclovine PET has high sensitivity (>90%) for intermediate or high-risk prostate carcinomas and cancer recurrence in prostate with uptake correlating strongly with Gleason score (197,198). Urinary excretion is low and generally does not interfere with evaluation of prostate and pelvic nodes (Fig. 14.3) (excreted activity in bladder may be seen in patients who void immediately prior to the study). Fluciclovine (Axumin^{TM}) was approved by FDA in 2016 for PET imaging in men with suspected prostate cancer recurrence based on serum PSA following prior treatment. It is not currently recommended for characterization of prostate lesions or initial staging of prostate cancer due to uptake in benign prostatic hyperplasia and limited sensitivity compared to pelvic dissection for pelvic nodal involvement (199). However, in the setting of biochemical recurrence fluciclovine outperforms conventional imaging and In-^{111}Indium-capromab-pendetide (ProstaScint^{TM}) in localization of recurrence with greater than 80% positivity (200) and can impact management in most patients (201). The positivity rate is relatively low for PSA<1 ng/mL (37% vs. 78%–92% for PSA>1 ng/mL) (202). Fluciclovine PET/CT has been reported to be more sensitive than multiparametric MRI for recurrence in prostate in non-prostatectomy patients (100% vs. 15.4%–38.5%) with comparable positive predictive value (62% vs. 50.0%–55.6%) despite uptake in benign lesions (203).

Skeleton is a frequent site of metastatic involvement in high-risk prostate cancer. Currently, bone scintigraphy is the standard test used for detection of bone metastases (191). Due to high physiologic bone marrow uptake and low cellularity and uptake in primarily sclerotic prostate metastases, Fluciclovine is not highly sensitive for evaluation of osseous involvement (40). Fewer lesions are detected on fluciclovine PET compared to bone scan, MRI, or PET/MRI (204). Fluciclovine PET/CT may be sensitive and more accurate than bone scan for osseous lesions (205) due to visibility of sclerotic lesions on CT and higher specificity and lack of uptake in degenerative changes, although CT has limited ability to characterize disease activity and treatment response in sclerotic osseous lesions.

NaF PET outperforms bone scintigraphy and has higher sensitivity and similar diagnostic accuracy to whole-body MRI for evaluation of bone metastases in staging and restaging high-risk prostate cancer (206). In contrast to bone scan, NaF PET can be used for quantitative assessment of response to treatment based on SUV (207,208). Due to the interplay between cancer and bone environment, biochemical markers and PET tracers such as fluciclovine, PSMA ligands, or other tracers that target cancer cells provide complementary information to NaF PET in evaluation of osseous lesions and can be used in conjunction to provide a better picture of osseous disease burden in an individual patient.

PSMA imaging using ^{68}Ga and ^{18}F radiolabeled tracers are increasingly available and are used for clinical or investigational imaging in patients with prostate cancer and have superior diagnostic performance compared to other investigational PET tracers such as ^{11}C-choline or ^{18}F-fluorocholine (209). In biochemically recurrent prostate cancer, PSMA PET enables detection of metastases at lower PSA levels with a positivity rate of 45% for PSA levels between 0.2 and 0.5 ng/mL and 95% for PSA above 2 ng/mL (210), which may outperform fluciclovine (211) and is considerably higher than conventional imaging. In our experience with ^{18}F-DCFPyL (a PSMA PET ligand) PET impacted management in most patients with biochemically recurrent prostate cancer and could frequently identify lesions that could not be identified on CT, MRI, fluciclovine PET, bone scan, or NaF PET (212). Fluciclovine can be superior to PSMA in evaluation of prostatectomy bed and urinary balder (213) (Fig. 14.3). The use of PSMA in theragnostics is discussed in a separate chapter.

Breast cancer

Breast cancer is the most common female malignancy in the Western world. Positron emission mammography or dedicated breast PET is not routinely indicated in screening or diagnosing breast cancer but is a useful diagnostic tool in high-risk women or women with dense breast when contrast-enhanced breast MRI is not feasible (214) or as adjunct to conventional breast imaging for problem solving in indeterminate cases. Focal FDG uptake found incidentally in the breast is associated with malignancy (38%–83%) and referral for dedicated breast imaging is warranted (215). Malignant lesions have generally higher uptake than benign lesions such as fibrocystic change, intraductal papilloma, or fibroadenoma.

FDG PET/CT is recommended by NCCN for initial staging of breast cancer when advanced disease (stage IIIA or higher) is clinically suspected. There is evidence that even in clinical stage II disease, PET can change staging and management in a significant number of patients (216). The most important predictor for survival is axillary lymph node metastases. PET/CT has high specificity for axillary nodal involvement, although cannot replace sentinel node biopsy. Focal FDG uptake in internal mammary lymph nodes is an uncommon finding and likely represents metastatic disease (217). FDG PET has similar sensitivity for osseous metastatic involvement to bone scintigraphy although it is superior in detecting lytic bone metastases. NaF is superior to bone scintigraphy for evaluation of metastatic osseous involvement and provides complementary information to FDG PET. However, when FDG PET/CT clearly indicates bone metastases, bone scan or NaF PET/CT can be superfluous.

Neoadjuvant therapy is frequently administered to patients with locally advanced breast cancer or patients with early-stage cancer if upfront breast-conserving surgery is not possible or could result in poor cosmetic outcome. Patients with aggressive

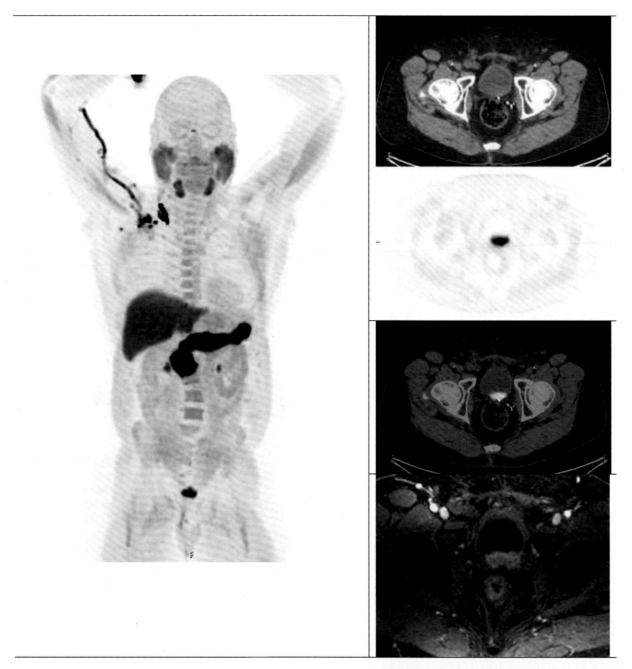

FIG. 14.3 ● Fluciclovine PET/CT. Note residual injected activity in the right upper extremity veins and collateral veins in the right shoulder. Physiologic uptake is seen in the pancreas, liver, and to a lesser extent skeletal and cardiac muscles. A small amount of excreted activity is frequently seen in the kidneys after bolus injection, although subsequent excretion is minimal. Intense activity in the bladder corresponds to a mass, also well seen on axial images and subsequent Gd-enhanced MRI. Lesional uptake was difficult to characterize on a subsequent 8F-DCFPyL PET/CT (not shown) due to intense excreted activity in the bladder.

subtypes such triple-negative or human epidermal growth factor receptor 2 (HER2)-positive cancers with primary tumors greater than 10 mm may also benefit from neoadjuvant therapy. In the absence of clinical suspicion for progression, imaging is often not indicated during neoadjuvant therapy, although multiple studies support a possible future role of FDG PET for early prognostication and identification of non-responders. Most patients with complete metabolic response to neoadjuvant therapy in HER2-positive breast cancer achieve pathologic complete response at the time of surgery. Pathologic complete response

was twice as likely if uptake was reduced by 25% after targeted therapy for 6 weeks (42%–44% vs. 19%–21%) (218). A reduction of SUV_{max} by 42% to 65% (depending on the type of neoadjuvant chemotherapy) after two cycles for triple-negative breast cancer predicts pathologic response and survival (219). The optimal timing and response criteria for response assessment after or during neoadjuvant therapy with PET versus other modalities and implications in management remain topics for research (220,221), noting that FDG PET cannot reliably exclude residual viable tumor (222).

FDG PET is superior to conventional image for detection of breast cancer recurrence or metastasis (223). In one study in patients that underwent PET/CT after completion of therapy, malignancy was detected or excluded with an accuracy of 98%, but resulted in a change in management in less than 7% of patients when it was done without clinical suspicion for recurrence compared to 28% of patients when it was done due to clinical suspicion (224). Other studies have made similar conclusions (e.g., [225]).

Systemic therapies can improve symptoms and quality of life and prolong survival of patients with metastatic breast cancer. Prognosis and choice of therapy is influenced by molecular markers and particularly hormone receptor and HER2 overexpression. PET/CT has been shown to reliably assess metastatic disease burden and response to therapy (226), including bone-only metastasis (227) and is superior to contrast enhanced CT in predicting progression or survival (228,229). A change in SUV has been shown to be an early predictor or response to endocrine therapy (230), targeted HER2 therapy (231), and chemotherapy (232).

Sarcomas and peripheral nerve sheath tumors

Malignant peripheral nerve sheath tumors account for 5% to 10% of all soft-tissue sarcomas and are particularly a significant cause of mortality in neurofibromatosis type 1 (NF-1) patients. Plexiform neurofibromas have potential for sarcomatous transformation. If detected early, surgery can be curative, but prognosis is poor if diagnosis is delayed due to tendency to metastasize early (233). Atypical and malignant lesions in NF-1 have higher cellularity than benign tumors and typically high uptake on FDG PET (more than 2.5–3 times liver parenchyma), in a small subset of benign and malignant lesions uptake may overlap. Morphologic features on MRI and diffusion-weighted imaging can provide complementary information to FDG PET for evaluation of peripheral nerve sheath tumors (234). Both modalities can be used for screening high risk NF-1 patients and FDG-PET/CT is recommended for symptomatic patients for the detection of suspected malignant tumors (235). Neither PET or whole-body MRI is currently recommended for routine imaging of asymptomatic NF-1 patients, although FDG PET/CT can be useful for assessment of whole-body internal tumor burden particularly in patients who have contraindications to MRI or are not able to tolerate a prolonged exam required for whole-body MRI. DOTATATE-PET may be helpful in patients who develop clinical or laboratory evidence of pheochromocytoma or extra-adrenal paragangliomas.

Neurofibromatosis type 2 (NF-2) and Shwanomatosis are clinically and genetically distinct from NF-1. NF-2 is not associated with predisposition to malignancy. Benign peripheral nerve sheath tumors in Shwanomatosis may have high FDG uptake, limiting the utility of FDG PET in these patients (235).

Sarcomas comprise heterogenous malignancies of mesenchymal origin and can arise in different organs. GIST and uterine sarcoma are previously discussed. Other soft-tissue sarcomas can arise throughout the body but are most common in the extremities (particularly lower extremity) in adults (236). Osteosarcoma and other malignant bone tumors are less common than soft-tissue sarcomas except in adolescents and young adults. Although certain histologies such as low-grade liposarcoma or synovial sarcoma are associated with low glucose metabolism (237), FDG PET/CT is generally useful and often superior to conventional imaging for staging, prognostication, and therapy planning (238). High FDG uptake in sarcoma is a predictor of shorter survival and rapid disease progression (239,240). In a retrospective study on 117 patients, FDG PET/CT improved accuracy of staging when combined with conventional imaging with MRI of the tumor location and whole-body CT (241). PET/MR can be used for assessment of tumor, nodal, and distant metastasis in a single session with excellent agreement with conventional staging (242), although PET/MRI may fail to identify sub-centimeter pulmonary metastases. PET is more specific but less sensitive than CT for pulmonary involvement. For bone involvement, FDG PET is complementary to and overall more accurate than bone scintigraphy (243). Combined FDG and NaF PET is feasible and may further increase sensitivity for osseous involvement (42). PET can determine response to neoadjuvant chemotherapy for deep lesions that are larger than 3 cm, and are useful for assessment of response to chemotherapy in metastatic soft-tissue and bone sarcomas (244,245) and metabolic parameters can be used as a biomarker for monitoring new treatments such as kinase inhibitors (246).

Melanoma, Merkel cell carcinoma, and cutaneous T-cell lymphomas

Malignant melanoma arises from melanocytes in the skin, uvea, and mucosal membranes. Cutaneous melanomas are the most aggressive and deadliest skin cancer. For T1b (0.8–1.0 mm in thickness OR ulcerated melanomas <0.8 mm in thickness) or more locally advanced disease with clinically negative regional lymph nodes, sentinel lymph node (SLN) biopsy is used as a staging procedure. Presence of nodal or non-nodal locoregional metastases is associated with worst prognosis (stage III). Stage IV is defined as distant metastasis to skin, subcutaneous tissue and skeletal muscles, non-regional nodes (M1a), lung (M1b), viscera (M1c), and central nervous system (CNS) (M1d). Elevated serum lactate dehydrogenase is associated with reduced treatment response and short survival in metastatic disease (247).

In patients with positive nodal biopsy or clinically advanced disease, FDG PET/CT is superior to anatomic imaging modalities such as CT and MRI for staging although brain MRI should be performed if there concern for CNS involvement. Intense FDG uptake is typically present in melanoma and FDG PET is highly sensitive for nodal and distant metastases except for lesions <5 mm (sensitivity of 23% for nodes <5 mm compared to 83% for 5 to 10 mm lymph nodes [248]). Sensitivity and conspicuity of lesions is lower in organs with high background activity may reduce conspicuity of lesions in certain organs such as heart or bowel (particularly in the setting of metformin use). PET/MRI can improve evaluation of brain, liver, and bone involvement compared to PET/CT (249) although acquisition time is significantly longer. Anatomic information on PET/CT and PET/MR improves sensitivity and specificity compared to PET alone.

Overall, FDG PET/CT has a significant impact on management and can prevent futile surgeries in half of patients with advanced melanoma compared to conventional imaging (250). In patients initially present with stage III melanoma, FDG PET/CT can detect recurrence after surgery earlier than conventional imaging. Many of relapsed patients detected on FDG PET subsequently undergo curative intent resection (251). A negative PET/CT has high negative predictive value and can rule out recurrence (252). NCCN recommends PET/CT or other imaging modalities every 3 to 12 months for surveillance of high-risk patients (initial stage IIB or higher) with no clinical evidence of disease for 5 years.

Besides localization of metastatic disease, FDG PET/CT has utility in assessment of response to therapy. Immune checkpoint inhibitors (ICIs) against cytotoxic T lymphocyte antigen 4 (CTLA-4) and/or programmed death 1 (PD-1) are commonly used for treatment of patients with metastatic melanoma. Immune therapy may initially cause increased uptake in lesions due to mounting inflammatory response or new inflammatory lesions that are detectable on FDG PET (253). A sarcoid-like granulomatous reaction can occur a few weeks to several months after the start of immune therapy (254). Hilar and mediastinal lymph nodes are the most common sites of involvement and typically appear symmetric in distribution, and generally spontaneously resolve a few months after discontinuation of therapy. Although psuedoprogression is not uncommon, it can be distinguished from true progression based on clinical findings and follow up imaging that demonstrate decrease or resolution of uptake in metastatic lesions. Overall, FDG PET remains a powerful tool for assessment of response to immune therapy (253). Complete metabolic response on PET at 1 year is associated with prolonged progression-free survival suggesting ongoing response to therapy (255).

Merkel cell carcinoma is a rare but aggressive neuroendocrine skin tumor with high mortality rate seen typically in white/light-skinned elderly in the seventh and eighth decades of life. It is associated with Merkel cell polyomavirus, ultraviolet (UV) radiation, and immunosuppression. As with melanoma, lesions metastasize locally to satellite skin nodules and lymph nodes, distant metastases can be present at initial diagnosis, and there is a high incidence of local recurrence and distant metastasis after initial therapy. For local and regional disease, surgery and radiotherapy play a major role in management. FDG PET is an integral part of staging Merkle cell carcinoma for tumors >2 cm (stage II) or regional nodal involvement clinically or based on sentinel nodal biopsy (stage III) with high sensitivity for distant metastatic involvement (stage IV). Metastatic disease requires systemic therapy. Checkpoint inhibitor immunotherapy is the first line treatment except in patients with active autoimmune disease or ongoing immune suppression. FDG PET is additionally used for monitoring response to treatment, evaluation of suspected recurrence, and surveillance. A negative PET has a high negative-predictive value for residual disease (256). ^{68}Ga-SSTR PET scintigraphy appears to have similar sensitivity to FDG PET (257) and may be used to determine candidates for ^{177}Lu-DOTATATE peptide receptor RT (258).

Primary cutaneous lymphomas are a heterogeneous group of T-cell (75%) and B-cell (25%) lymphomas that present without evidence of extracutaneous involvement at the time of diagnosis. Mycosis fungoides (and its leukemic variant, Sézary syndrome) are the most common type of cutaneous T-cell lymphomas. Staging and prognosis depends on skin (T), nodal (N), and visceral (M) involvement and presence of Sézary cells in the peripheral blood (B) (259). Most patients present with early stage disease that can be managed with skin-directed therapies and is associated with normal life expectancy. The prognosis of advanced disease is poor although a subset of patients achieves prolonged survival after allogeneic stem cell transplantation (260). T-cell lymphomas are generally FDG avid (261) and FDG PET/CT has high sensitivity for both cutaneous and extracutaneous (nodal and visceral) lesions and can be used for assessment of response to therapy or recurrence, although the ability to characterize cutaneous lesions may be limited (262).

Multiple myeloma and myeloproliferative disorders

Whole-body FDG PET/CT has high sensitivity and specificity for detection of both medullary and extramedullary involvement in multiple myeloma (263). PET/CT is superior to radiographic bone survey for small osseous lesions. Lytic lesions can be seen on the low-mA CT and fulfill the criteria for skeletal damage requiring need to start anti-multiple myeloma therapy. Focal bone FDG uptake greater than physiologic uptake in normal red marrow or liver parenchyma or diffuse bone marrow uptake in the axial and appendicular skeleton greater than liver parenchyma is considered positive on PET. Number of focal lesions, presence of paramedullary (bone lesion with cortical interruption and involvement of surrounding soft tissues) or extramedullary (nodes, liver, spleen, skin) disease, or fractures on CT should be reported. Intense physiologic cortical gray matter FDG uptake can reduce sensitivity of PET for small calvarial lesions. PET may be false negative in a small subgroup of patients with low hexokinase-2 expression (264) and patients with diffuse bone marrow involvement, but it is concordant with MRI in the majority of other cases. Whole-body diffusion-weighted MRI has emerged as the most sensitive modality for imaging multiple myeloma, although the specificity is somewhat lower than FDG PET (265). FDG PET is useful for evaluation of disease burden and metabolic activity of the lesions. More than three focal lesions on baseline PET, high FDG uptake, and extramedullary involvement are associated with reduced progression-free and overall survival.

FDG PET is an excellent tool for assessment of response to treatment and can distinguish between metabolically active and inactive lesions. Presence of multiple FDG-avid lesions after the first cycle of induction chemotherapy is associated with shorter complete response (defined by absence of M-protein) and lower survival, especially in patients with a high-risk gene expression profile (266). A negative PET after treatment precedes and predicts clinical response by several months and is associated with longer progression-free survival. In contrast, signal abnormality on MRI may persist despite complete clinical response and differentiating between vital and necrotic lesions after therapy may not be always possible (267). Patients with a negative FDG PET before starting maintenance therapy have longer progression-free survival and overall survival compared to PET-positive patients, while normalization of MRI does not seem to affect survival (268). FDG PET is useful for detection of minimal residual disease and particularly extramedullary involvement and can provide complementary information to sensitive bone marrow-based assays for assessment of eradication of myeloma cells after treatment.

Smoldering multiple myeloma is an asymptomatic plasma cell disorder that can be a precursor to active multiple myeloma. Patients with smoldering myeloma have a significantly higher risk of progression to malignancy compared to monocolonal gammapathy of undetermined significance (MGUS) (10% vs. 1% per year, respectively). FDG PET/CT is recommended to differentiate smoldering versus active myeloma at the time of diagnosis and can be subsequently used to evaluate for progression. Focal FDG uptake in the absence of lytic lesions is associated with high probability of imminent progression (within 2 years).

A solitary plasmacytoma is a single discrete osteolytic or soft-tissue mass of clonal plasma cells, with absent or minimal (<10% plasma cells) bone marrow plasma-cell infiltration and no end-organ damage. Solitary bone plasmocytomas most frequently occurs in the axial skeleton and are associated with higher probability of progression to multiple myeloma compared to extramedullary plasmacytomas that are usually found in the naso- and oropharynx. FDG PET is recommended for work up of patients with suspect diagnosis of solitary plasmacytomas and can help to confirm the diagnosis by ruling out additional occult sites of proliferating clonal plasma cells (263). Solitary plasmacytomas are often treated with radiation, with chemotherapy considered in cases of bulky disease or in high-risk patients.

Cardiology applications

Myocardial perfusion imaging and flow reserve

The principles, procedures, interpretation, and clinical utility of myocardial perfusion imaging using SPECT are well established as discussed in the chapter on cardiac imaging. Technical differences between different PET perfusion tracers and SPECT are discussed earlier in this chapter. Myocardial-perfusion PET is diagnostically similar or superior to SPECT and provide detailed assessment of distribution of myocardial perfusion at rest and alterations in perfusion with coronary vasodilation (stress) suggestive of ischemia (269,270), particularly in obese patients (271), with less effective radiation dose for the radiotracer administration. Like SPECT, gated imaging provides information about ventricular function, regional contractile dysfunction, and intraventricular synchronism. Quantification of myocardial blood flow and myocardial flow reserve using PET increases specificity for coronary artery disease and adds value in assessment of microvascular disease (272). Flow reserve is generally measured using maximal coronary vasodilation induced by adenosine analogues (53). Normal myocardial perfusion at rest is 0.7 to 1 mL/min/g and increases to 2.5 to 3.5 mL/min/g with maximal pharmacologic vasodilation, consistent with a flow reserve of 3.5 to 4, depending on the technique and radiotracer. Decreased myocardial flow reserve is associated with flow limiting stenosis (>70% angiographic stenosis) and reduced fractional flow reserve (FFR < 0.8) (273) although it can also be seen in non-ischemic cardiomyopathies such as diabetic or hypertrophic cardiomyopathy or cardiac amyloidosis (274), coronary allograft vasculopathy in heart transplant, abnormal microvascular reactivity, or in patients with unusually high resting myocardial flow (53). A global myocardial flow reserve of 2 or higher excludes high-risk coronary artery disease (275) and is associated with low probability of major adverse cardiovascular events.

Myocardial viability

Presence of viable myocardium in ischemic left ventricular dysfunction is associated with improvement in function after treatment (276). FDG PET can be used to identify severely ischemic myocardium that can potentially regain function if ischemia can be corrected and it is superior to SPECT or dobutamine echocardiography for evaluation of extent of viable myocardium. In areas of ischemia, glucose remains readily available for energetic metabolism due to high solubility and diffusibility in extra-cellular water and low-extraction fraction in the tissue. Ischemic myocardium preferentially utilizes glycolysis to sustain basic cellular functions such as Na^+/K^+ pump and retains the ability to uptake and accumulate FDG. In contrast, scar tissue formed in area of infarction has little metabolic activity and FDG uptake. A proportional regional reduction in FDG uptake and myocardial perfusion (i.e., perfusion-metabolism match) signifies nonviable tissue (277). Scar tissue can be directly imagined using pyrophosphate scintigraphy or based on retention of contrast on

late images on cardiac MRI. A scar thickness less than 50% of ventricular wall is considered viable and may benefit from revascularization. FDG PET and delayed contrast-enhancement on cardiac MRI both accurately identify the degree of viability versus scarring (278) although the information they provide is fundamentally complementary (279).

Due to high variability in glucose metabolism and FDG uptake in normal myocardium, assessment of viability using FDG PET is done in conjunction with myocardial perfusion imaging. FDG PET is not necessary to establish viability if rest perfusion is normal. Similarly, assessment of viability is not relevant in myocardium with normal contractile function. Insulin stimulation is necessary to facilitate myocardial FDG uptake and can be done with glucose loading and subsequent insulin administration. Glucose loading is done after a period of fasting but is reduced or omitted if fasting plasma glucose is elevated. Prolonged fasting prior to the study can reduce GLUT1 expression (280) and markedly suppress uptake even in normal myocardium (281). Typically, 1 to 5 units of insulin is administered intravenously depending on plasma glucose level. Plasma glucose level is subsequently monitored if is less than 150 mg/dL FDG is injected. Patients at risk for hypokalemia or hypoglycemia require careful monitoring and may need pretreatment with potassium supplement or treatment with dextrose. Imaging is initiated 45 to 60 min after FDG injection. Patients with insulin resistance and delayed clearance of blood pool activity require administration of additional insulin and repeat acquisition after 20 to 30 min (277). To evaluate for regional perfusion-metabolism mismatch, uptake can be normalized using the segment with the highest count rates on resting perfusion images as the reference region. Quantitative analysis with polar map displays is useful as aid to the visual interpretation. A disproportionately increased FDG uptake (when normalized based on perfusion) signifies viable myocardium with or at-risk for ischemia (corresponding to perfusion defects on rest and post-stress images, respectively). A proportionately decreased FDG uptake signifies scarring. A disproportionately decreased FDG uptake is associated with insulin resistance or suboptimal insulin-simulation (282,283) although it could be seen with ischemic myocardium as well (284). Spuriously decreased FDG uptake in the septum has been described in patients with left bundle branch block (285,286).

Cardiac sarcoidosis

Sarcoidosis is a multisystem disease characterized by presence of noncaseating granuloma of unknown etiology in various organs. Lungs and mediastinal lymph nodes are affected in the majority of patients. Other organs such as heart, liver, spleen, skin, central nervous system, eyes, and skeleton are variably involved. Cardiac involvement is seen in more than 20% of patients. Symptomatic cardiac involvement is seen in only 5% of patients with sarcoidosis (287), manifesting as conduction abnormalities, ventricular arrhythmias, and heart failure. Complete heart block is the most common finding. Lesions are most commonly subepicardial or mid-myocardial (288,289). Although most patients have no or minimal extra-cardiac disease, mortality can be high due to the risk of sudden cardiac death or development of progressive heart failure.

Diagnosis of cardiac sarcoidosis is difficult. Symptoms, electrocardiogram (EKG) and echocardiography findings, and pattern of edema and delayed enhancement on cardiac MRI can be nonspecific. Endomyocardial biopsy has a poor diagnostic yield due to the focal nature of the involvement. However, in patients with histopathologically confirmed extracardiac sarcoidosis, cardiac involvement can be inferred based on clinical evidence (e.g., cardiomyopathy or heart block responding to steroids) or imaging evidence of cardiac involvement. FDG PET is a powerful diagnostic tool for detection and localization of infection or inflammation (290,291). Patchy uptake on cardiac FDG-PET is consistent with cardiac sarcoidosis. Uptake can be seen in early involvement before perfusion abnormalities or scarring develops (292). Furthermore, the degree uptake can distinguish between active and treated disease and can be used for monitoring therapy (293). Patients with focal uptake are at increased risk for ventricular tachycardia and sudden cardiac death (294).

PET and contrast-enhanced MRI provide complementary information in diagnosis and prognostication of cardiac sarcoidosis. PET is particularly useful in patients who cannot tolerate MR or if gadolinium contrast administration is contra-indicated. Diagnostic accuracies of FDG PET and cardiac MR are comparable (295) and accuracy increases if PET and MRI are combined (295). FDG PET is particularly more sensitive in predominantly lymphocytic lesions, which may be visible on MRI as focal T2-abnormality but are not associated with delayed enhancement. Focal FDG uptake in the interventricular septum and septal T2 signal abnormality but not delayed enhancement on MRI correlate with complete heart block and response to treatment (296). Predominantly fibrotic lesions are associated with focal perfusion abnormality and delayed enhancement, but FDG uptake is typically suppressed as is with normal myocardium (297). For this reason, FDG PET should be interpreted in conjunction with resting myocardial perfusion PET or SPECT (Table 14.6). Torso or whole-body PET acquired in the same session as cardiac PET can assess evidence of extra-cardiac sarcoidosis, particularly if biopsy is contemplated.

Physiologic myocardial uptake limits accuracy of FDG PET for evaluation of cardiac lesions including sarcoidosis. Typical fasting (6 h or less) is not sufficient to alter myocardial metabolism and high cardiac activity is frequently evident in oncologic PETs. Prolonged fasting (48 h) can significantly reduce glucose uptake in normal myocardium, but it is not generally feasible. In most patients, a strict lipid-rich carbohydrate-restricted diet for 12 to 24 h prior to the study can minimize physiologic uptake in normal myocardium. Unfortunately, diffuse uptake can persist in

10% to 20% of patients (299). Pattern of uptake can be suggestive of suboptimal suppression of physiologic activity: isolated diffuse uptake in the left ventricular lateral wall without a corresponding perfusion defect is frequently due to physiologic uptake, noting that lateral wall involvement in sarcoidosis is less common than other regions (14% vs. 32% for septum) (288). If PET is non-diagnostic, it can be repeated after 48 to 72 h carbohydrate-restricted diet (281). Preliminary results with other radiotracers such as fluoro-deoxythymidine (a marker of cell proliferations) or SSTR PET tracers such as ^{68}Ga-DOTATATE that have high uptake in inflammatory cells but no or low physiologic cardiac uptake is promising and need to be further validated.

NeuroPET
Dementia
Dementia comprises a heterogenous group of neurological diseases presenting with severe decline in one or more cognitive domain such as memory, language, or executive function (300). Most dementia is caused by a neurodegenerative disease such as AD or DLB. Vascular dementia and other etiologies (alcohol-related, chronic traumatic encephalopathy, normal pressure hydrocephalus, Prion disease, HIV) benefit from specific treatments to slow or halt progression and possibly reverse cognitive decline, although in the presence of coexisting neurodegenerative disease the prognosis remains poor. PET is a valuable investigational and diagnostic tool in evaluation neurodegenerative disorders and can assist in characterization and differential diagnosis of complex or unclear cases.

AD is the most common neurodegenerative disease and the most common cause of dementia (60%–80% of dementia cases in older adults). It has insidious onset and progressive course with eventual severe debilitation and death; 95% of the cases are clinically apparent after age 65, although pathologic changes could precede by a decade or longer (301). The diagnosis of AD is primarily based on clinical assessment and neuropsychologic testing. Brain MRI findings are nonspecific, but it is indicated to exclude alternative or additional diagnoses such as cerebrovascular or structural diseases. Clinical assessment has limited accuracy and 10% to 30% of individuals diagnosed clinically by experts do not have neuropathologic findings of AD at autopsy

Table 14.6 PATTERNS OF FDG UPTAKE AND RESTING PERFUSION DEFECT IN CARDIAC SARCOIDOSIS (ADOPTED BASED ON [297] AND [298])

FDG	Corresponding perfusion	Disease category	Probability of sarcoidosis
No uptake	Normal	Normal myocardium	Very low
No uptake	Mild defect	Nonspecific	Possible
Nonspecific, non-focal	Normal	Likely normal (inadequate preparation)	Indeterminate
Multiple foci (patchy)	Normal or mild defects	Early disease (predominantly lymphocytes)	Probable
Focal on diffuse	Mild to moderate defect	Progressive disease (predominantly granulomas)	Probable
No or minimal uptake	Severe defect	Fibrous disease (predominantly scar)	Possible
Multiple foci	Multiple defects	Progressive disease	Highly probable
Multiple foci + extra cardiac disease	Normal or defects	Progressive disease	Highly probable

(302). FDG and Amyloid PET can support the clinical diagnosis and are particularly useful in patients with young age of onset or atypical presentations (303,304). Although Amyloid PET is not currently recommended for patients who meet the core clinical criteria for probable AD (305), subsequently published evidence suggest that Amyloid PET is of similar diagnostic value in these patients to those who do not meet the criteria (56). Preliminary results from the large multisite Imaging Dementia-Evidence for Amyloid Scanning (IDEAS) study on patients refereed to dementia specialists show that in 25% of patients, diagnosis was changed from AD to non-AD, and in 10% of the patients, it changed from non-AD to AD (306).

In patients who develop Alzheimer's dementia, FDG uptake is characteristically reduced in the medial temporal lobe, followed by parieto-temporal areas, and posterior cingulate cortex. In advanced AD, frontal association cortices also become involved. Glucose metabolism in cerebellum, basal ganglia, and primary sensory and motor cortices is preserved (307). Hypometabolism precedes cognitive decline by several years (308,309) and the degree of metabolic abnormality and cognitive impairment are highly correlated (310). The characteristic topography of metabolic abnormalities has good accuracy in distinguishing AD from other neurodegenerative dementias, vascular dementia, depression, or normal aging without cognitive impairment (311). Age-related hypometabolism primarily involves the anterior cingulate and anterior temporal lobe (312). Pattern of hypometabolism in patients with mild cognitive impairment predict progression to AD versus stable impairment or progression to other neurogenerative dementias (313,314). A meta-analysis compared FDG versus Amyloid PET (using PiB) found that FDG PET is less sensitive (79% vs. 93.5%) bur more specific (74% vs. 56%) in patients with mild cognitive impairment for predicting progression to AD dementia over 1 to 3 years (315). Combination or FDG and Amyloid PET can improve prediction accuracy (316).

DLB is characterized by presence of eosinophilic cytoplasmic inclusions formed from alpha-synuclein aggregates in brainstem nuclei, limbic structures, and subsequently throughout neocortex. Most patients have concomitant AD neuropathologic change (317). Dopaminergic neurons are particularly susceptible to Lewy body formation. Parkinsonian symptoms are present in most

patients and can be as severe as in idiopathic Parkinson's disease. Occipital and in particular pericalcarine (visual cortex) hypometabolism on FDG PET has high sensitivity (90%) and specificity (80%) for diagnosis of DLB (including Lewy body variant of AD) versus AD (318). The degree of occipital hypometabolism correlates with frequency and severity of visual hallucinations which are present in two thirds of patients with DLB (319). It has been suggested that sparing of the posterior cingulate (320) or relative sparing of amygdala can distinguish early DLB from AD (321). Amyloid PET can be positive in a subset of patients but the degree of tracer binding in cortex is less than AD (322).

Frontotemporal lobar degeneration (FTLD) is a common cause of dementia before age 65 and comprises various pathologies primarily involving frontal and/or temporal lobes causing changes in social behavior and personality or aphasia. Abnormal neuronal or glial deposition of Tau, TDP-43, or other proteins are involved in pathogenesis of neurodegeneration although cognitive impairments generally correlate with areas involved rather than histopathologic features. Amyloid and FDG-PET (Fig. 14.4) are helpful in differential diagnosis of AD versus FTLD (304). Pattern of hypometabolism on FDG PET can help differentiate differentiating between AD, DLB, FTLD, or vascular dementia (323) and differentiate between clinical syndromes and subtypes of FTLD (Table 14.7).

In addition to utility for evaluation of patients with clinical features of Alzheimer dementia, amyloid PET has been used to support the diagnosis of cerebral amyloid angiopathy and distinguish it from ischemic microvascular and hypertensive changes (324,325).

Interictal seizure localization

Epilepsy is the most common serious neurologic condition, and the second most significant neurologic cause of morbidity. An epileptic seizure a transient symptomatic episode caused by "abnormal excessive or synchronous neuronal activity in the brain" (331). Epilepsy is defined as a pathologic and enduring tendency to have recurrent seizures and can be diagnosed after two unprovoked seizures. Seizures are classified based on onset to focal (partial), generalized, unknown onset or unclassified (332), and can be subcategorized to motor and non-motor.

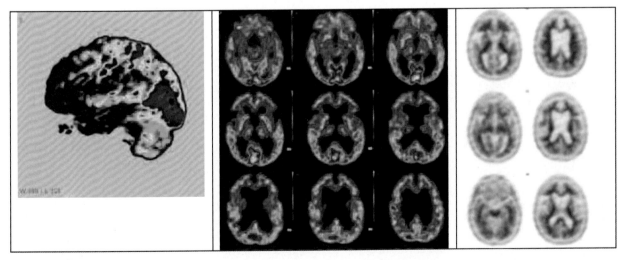

FIG. 14.4 ● FDG PET (left: 3D volume rendering, middle: axial pseudo-colored images at the level of lateral ventricle and basal ganglia) in a patient with frontotemporal dementia showing frontal and temporal hypometabolism compared to cerebellar gray matter. Right: normal florbetapir PET in the same patient.

Table 14.7 CLINICAL AND IMAGING FEATURES IN DEMENTIAS DUE TO NEURODEGENERATIVE DISORDERS (43)

	Clinical features	Imaging findings	Associated pathology
AD	Memory, Executive function, olfactory dysfunction	Temporal and parietal hypometabolism, sparing occipital cortex Amyloid +	Neuritic plaques, Amyloid deposits, Neurofibrillary tangles
PCA	Progressive visuospatial and visuoperceptual impairment, Initially sparing memory, language, executive function	occipitoparietal or occipitotemporal atrophy and hypometabolism. Overlaps with DLB but may be more asymmetric (326,327). Amyloid +	Most have AD Can overlap with CBD or DLB
DLB	Visual hallucinations, REM sleep disorder, parkinsonism	Occipital and limbic hypometabolism. Relative preservation of the mid or posterior cingulate gyrus (cingulate island sign) (320). Amyloid + in a subset of patients	Alpha-synuclein Most have concomitant AD
CBD	Progressive asymmetric movement disorder (limb rigidity, akinesia, dystonia, or myoclonus), cognitive decline	Asymmetric hypometabolism in posterior frontal, sensory moto, inferior parietal, and superior temporal regions, thalamus, and striatum. Amyloid + suggests AD	Tau
PSP	Axial or symmetric limb rigidity/akinesia, urinary incontinence, behavioral changes, vertical gaze abnormality. Preserved olfaction and poor response to levodopa vs. PD	Hummingbird sign on MRI Hypometabolism in the midbrain (earliest sign [328,329]) followed by decreased metabolic activity in the caudate, putamen, and prefrontal cortex	Tau (neurons, oligodendrocytes, and astrocytes)
bvFTD			
fvFTD	Disinhibition, apathy, Hyperorality, compulsion Initially no motor neuron disease	Frontal and temporal hypometabolism	Tau or TDP-43 Less common: FUS (associated with ALS)
rtvFTD	Emotional distance, behavioral changes, later semantic dementia	Right temporal hypometabolism	Commonly TDP-43
PPA			
svPPA	Semantic (anomia, word-finding difficulties, repetitive speech). Preserved language structure and articulation	Left temporal hypometabolism	Commonly TDP-43
nfvPPA	Difficulty with grammar and speech production	Left inferior frontal gyrus (Broca's area) and insula hypometabolism and atrophy	Tau
lvPPA	Verbal working memory impairment, Disproportionate difficulty repeating phrases and sentences versus single words. Decreased spontaneous speech	Left temporo-parietal junction hypometabolism and atrophy Amyloid frequently + (85%) (330)	Amyloid (AD in 76%)

AD, Alzheimer's disease; bvFTD, behavioral variant FTD; CBD, cortical basal degeneration; DLB, dementia with Lewy bodies; FTD, frontotemporal dementia; fvFTD, frontal variant FTD; lvPPA, logopenic variant PPA; nfvPPA, non-fluent variant PCA, posterior cortical atrophy; PD, Parkinson's disease; PPA; PPA, primary progressive aphasia; PSP, progressive supranuclear palsy; svPPA, semantic variant PPA; TDP-43, transactive response DNA-binding 43.

Some patients with focal epilepsy experience impaired awareness, which can occur during any part of the seizure, and can be highly detrimental to quality of life.

The prevalence of active epilepsy is 6 to 7 per 1000 persons (333). The etiology and presentation are different in infants and children versus adults. Genetic epilepsies generally begin in childhood. Neurodevelopmental lesions (including cortical dysplasias, cortical dysgenesis, malformations, heterotopias) represent abnormalities in neuroglial proliferation, migration, or cortical organization, and are associated with seizure in childhood and delayed neurological development. Seizures in children are frequently extratemporal (334). Hippocampal sclerosis can occur in teenagers or even younger children, but it is primarily a cause of seizures in adults (335). New seizure can occur after brain insults such as stroke, trauma, or tumors. The incidence of seizures is particularly high in patients with dementia (336). In

United States, the prevalence of active epilepsy is 1.4% in adults aged 55 to 64 (337). Brain MRI is standard of care for initial workup of new seizure in older individuals to exclude stroke and other structural etiologies.

Seizures in most patients and particularly in children can be well controlled with antiseizure drugs. Discontinuation of treatment can be tried if patient remains seizure free and the estimated risk of seizure recurrence is low. However, a quarter to a third of patients do not achieve satisfactory seizure control with medications (338). Risk factors include poor response to the first antiseizure drug trial (339), and a high number of seizures prior to diagnosis and treatment (340). The primary treatment options for drug-resistant epilepsy include surgery and vagus nerve stimulation. Cortical stimulation is an option in patients with a well-delineated seizure focus. Some patients may benefit from deep brain stimulation and Trigeminal nerve stimulation.

Accurate localization and delineation and complete resection of epileptogenic zone are important for a good outcome after surgery (341). The goal of surgery is to isolate the epileptogenic zone which may variably correspond to a structural lesion (342). In most patients with drug-resistant epilepsy who are referred for PET, video electroencephalogram (EEG) monitoring and MRI has been already performed. Temporal lobe epilepsy is a frequent cause of drug-resistant epilepsy that has favorable outcome in most patients after surgery, particularly if operated on early (343–345). In most patients with temporal lobe epilepsy, MRI can detect and localize hippocampal atrophy due to sclerosis. However, many patients with temporal lobe epilepsy have normal MRI or have only nonspecific findings on MRI, and still benefit from surgery (346,347). Ictal perfusion SPECT has greater than 95% sensitivity for localization of epileptogenic focus in temporal lobe epilepsy (348). However, due to low first pass uptake of FDG and gradual accumulation in gray matter over 15 to 30 min after radiotracer injection, FDG PET does not reliably assess initial ictal metabolism. Perfusion PET (^{15}O-H_2O) is technically and logistically difficult and is not generally available. However, inter-ictal hypometabolism with FDG PET (ideally at least 24 h after last seizure [349]) strongly correlates with the laterality and in most cases the location of epileptogenic focus, even when MRI is equivocal or normal (350). In more than half of patients with temporal lobe epilepsy, interictal PET contributes to surgical decision-making (351). Outcomes for surgery based on inter-ictal PET for MR negative patients is very favorable and is equal to outcomes for patients with hippocampal sclerosis on MRI (352). In patients with unilateral hippocampal sclerosis, bilateral hypometabolism is associated with a higher probability of long-term poor outcome (353).

Extratemporal lobe epilepsy is more frequent in children than adults (335). Frontal lobe epilepsy is more common than parietal or occipital lobe epilepsy (354) and can manifest as psychological disturbances or complex motor movements. FDG PET localizes interictal metabolic abnormalities in most children with frontal lobe epileptic foci (355). In MRI-negative extratemporal epilepsy patients with focal cortical dysplasia, FDG PET can localize the abnormality in most patients (356) and improves surgical outcomes (357). Temporal hypometabolism can be observed in one in five patients with extratemporal epilepsy and vice versa (358). These cases generally have less favorable outcomes after surgery compared to patients with hypometabolism confined to the epileptogenic zone.

Although most published studies focus on interictal cortical hypometabolism, focally increased FDG uptake is reportedly present in approximately 2% of the children, and may help identify the epileptogenic zone (359). Heterotopic gray matter can be similar or hypermetabolic compared to normal cortex (360). It has been suggested that ictal FDG PET may be helpful to evaluate the relationship between heterotopy and epilepsy (361). It needs to be emphasized that the interplay between neuronal activity, connectivity, and neurovascular and neurometabolic couplings in epilepsy is complex, and metabolic manifestations may occur in regions outside of and occasionally distant from the epileptogenic focus. Several PET tracers for evaluation of GABA, opioid, serotonin, and other neurotransmitter receptors are in investigational use for more accurate localization of seizure focus and may provide complementary or superior information to FDG PET (362,363).

Characterization of brain lesions

Contrast-enhanced MRI is the standard of care for imaging and characterization of central nervous system lesions. Compared to MRI, PET and in particular FDG PET have limited sensitivity due to limitations in resolution and tumor to background contrast (although resolution and signal quality is similar or superior to some advanced MR techniques such as arterial spin labeling perfusion or multivoxel MR spectroscopy). Addition of PET in workup of brain lesions provide complementary information that can better characterize lesions and distinguish post-treatment changes from residual or recurrent tumor and can have a significant impact on patient management.

Primary CNS lymphomas are characterized by intense FDG uptake that is significantly higher than physiologic gray matter or other malignant brain tumors (364,365) particularly in the absence or prior treatment with corticosteroids. Uptake is generally higher and more homogeneous than high-grade gliomas and the degree of uptake correlate with survival and is an early predictor of response to treatment (366). Low uptake or nonspecific abnormalities on FDG PET are rare, generally only in patients who present with atypical radiological findings such as disseminated disease or nonenhancing lesions (367,368). PET may identify systemic lymphoma in a subset of patients referred for evaluation of lymphomatous brain lesions (369). The degree of uptake can help distinguish lymphoma from demyelination. In patients with acquired immunodeficiency syndrome, reduced uptake in the lesion helps to distinguish toxoplasmosis from lymphoma. High uptake can be seen in brain abscess and inflammatory conditions such as neurosarcoidosis and can be used to determine biopsy site. The pattern of involvement on whole-body PET may suggest the diagnosis. High uptake can be transiently seen after intracranial hemorrhage (for the first 4 days) and infarction (approximately for 2 weeks) due to inflammatory activity.

Glioma is the second most common primary intracranial neoplasm (after meningioma) and the most common malignant neoplasm in adults, with a median age of 55 to 60 years at diagnosis. High-grade glioma (particularly glioblastoma) is associated with poor survival (370). PET is helpful for differentiation of grades III and IV tumors from non-neoplastic lesions or grades I and II gliomas, and can inform prognosis, biopsy planning, and delineation of tumor prior to surgery or radiotherapy. FDG uptake in low-grade (grade I/II) gliomas is typically less than white matter activity, although high uptake can be seen with pilocytic astrocytoma. High-grade gliomas have uptake greater than white matter and often greater than gray matter. Although there is an overlap between uptake in low- and high-grade gliomas, uptake above that of normal gray matter is highly suggestive of a high-grade tumor. However, unlike lymphoma a tumor to gray matter ratio is rarely above two (371). Uptake and MTV correlate inversely with survival (372,373).

Amino-acid PET tracers are superior to FDG for detection and delineation of brain tumors but have similar performances for glioma grading (374). Abnormal FDG uptake usually does not identifies tumor involvement beyond enhancing lesion on MR (375) whereas amino-acid radiotracers such as fluciclovine can detect tumor in non-enhancing either normal or T2 abnormal brain with high specificity (376). ^{11}C-methionin uptake can be detected up to 40 mm beyond area of T2 abnormality (377). ^{11}C-methionin, ^{18}F-fluoroethyltyrosine, ^{18}F-fluro-DOPA, and fluciclovine all cross the blood–brain barrier and into cells via sodium-independent L (large)-type neutral amino-acid transport system which is overexpressed in tumor vascular endothelium. Flouro-DOPA additionally accumulates in the striatum which could reduce its utility for evaluation of lesions involving basal ganglia. Use of amino-acid PET for radiation treatment planning increases consistency and accuracy in delineation of tumor and may improve outcome compared with planning based on MRI alone (378,379).

High-grade gliomas are treated with maximal safe resection, followed by adjuvant radiation and systemic therapy based on histopathologic and molecular diagnosis. The extent of surgery is balanced with preservation of neurologic function. While maximal resection and adjuvant therapy improves survival, most patients with high-grade gliomas will eventually recur and tumor may transform to a higher grade. Distinguishing treatment-induced imaging changes (pseudoprogression) from progressive disease can be difficult, particularly between 6 weeks and 1 year after completion of radiation therapy. Up to half of patients with new or enlarging enhancement on MRI within the radiation field have pseudoprogression as determined with biopsy or clinical follow up, particularly in asymptomatic patients and patients with MGMT (DNA repair enzyme O[6]-methylguanine-DNA methyltransferase) promoter hypermethylated glioblastoma. FDG and amino-acid PET can be used to inform decision regarding continuing planned adjuvant therapy versus surgical biopsy or debulking, reirradiation, and/or systemic therapy with bevacizumab or other agents.

On FDG PET, lesional uptake similar to or less than normal white matter is compatible with radiation necrosis (380). FDG uptake increases immediately after RT due to inflammation returning to baseline typically by 1 week (381). FDG uptake in the first few weeks after treatment is not predictive of outcome (382). However, persistent intense uptake after 7 weeks is associated with worse survival (383). A new or enlarging enhancing lesion with uptake greater than normal gray matter likely represents tumor recurrence. However, FDG uptake higher than white matter but less than grey matter uptake does not reliably distinguish radiation necrosis from recurrent tumor

(384). Emerging data suggest that amino-acid tracers are more accurate than FDG PET or MRI for differentiating progression from psudoprogression and reliably assess treatment response and prognosis following completion of chemoradiation or after bevacizumab therapy (385) as dexamethasone or antiangiogenic treatment with bevacizumab do not affecting amino acid uptake by brain tumors. Compared to FDG, amino acid uptake is less commonly seen with inflammation, infection, or infarction although prolonged increased uptake maybe seen with hematoma due to glial reaction (386). A tumor to normal brain uptake ratio cut-off of 2.3 for ^{18}F-Fluoroethyl-tyrosine PET has been reported to have 100% sensitivity and 91% specificity for early psuedoprogression (i.e., new or increasing enhancement on MRI within the first 12 weeks after completion of chemoradiation) (387), and a cut-off of 1.9 can differentiate late psuedoprogression (i.e., later than 3 months after completion of radiochemotherapy) from true progression (sensitivity 84%, specificity 86%) (388). Other studies have demonstrated utility of amino-acid PET in detecting pseudoprogression after immunotherapy for gliomas (389) or brain metastases (390).

Meningioma is the most common primary intracranial tumor. Meningiomas can be easily missed on FDG PET due to uptake similar to that of adjacent normal gray matter but are incidentally found in 1% to 2% of amino-acid or SSTR PET examinations (391). SSTR2 is a useful biomarker for meningiomas and ^{68}Ga-DOTATATE can be used to distinguish residual or recurrent meningioma from scar tissue after resection and/or RT (392). SSTR PET has also high sensitivity and diagnostic accuracy for hemangioblastoma in von Hippel–Lindau syndrome and can help differentiate it from other tumors with similar MRI features (393).

Summary

Over the past decade oncologic and other clinical applications of PET expanded significantly and are likely to continue to increase in the future. FDG PET/CT has been the ubiquitous backbone of increased use of PET for diagnostic imaging throughout the years and will remain so despite its limitations. In certain applications such as FDG avid lymphomas, PET/CT is clearly superior to conventional imaging and PET is the modality of choice for staging and/or assessment of response to therapy. In many other applications, PET provides complementary information to other imaging modalities that can affect management and can be highly cost-effective in well selected cases. As more PET radiotracers are translated from investigational to clinical use or become more widely available, imagers and clinicians gain access to more choices and diagnostic tools that can be used as biomarkers for precision medicine. Lack of familiarity with indications and experience in interpretation of novel PET radiotracers, slow adoption in clinical algorithms and guidelines, and difficulties in reimbursement are the main challenges for increased adoption of novel PET radiotracers.

References

1. Velikyan I. Prospective of (6)(8)Ga-radiopharmaceutical development. *Theranostics.* 2013;4(1):47–80.
2. Conti M, Eriksson L. Physics of pure and non-pure positron emitters for PET: a review and a discussion. *EJNMMI Phys.* 2016;3(1):8.
3. Gates VL, et al. Internal pair production of 90Y permits hepatic localization of microspheres using routine PET: proof of concept. *J Nucl Med.* 2011;52(1):72–76.
4. Jodal L, Le Loirec C, Champion C. Positron range in PET imaging: an alternative approach for assessing and correcting the blurring. *Phys Med Biol.* 2012;57(12):3931–3943.
5. Jodal L, Le Loirec C, Champion C. Positron range in PET imaging: non-conventional isotopes. *Phys Med Biol.* 2014;59(23):7419–7434.
6. Badawi RD, et al. First human imaging studies with the EXPLORER total-body PET scanner. *J Nucl Med.* 2019;60(3):299–303.

7. Karp JS, et al. PennPET explorer: design and preliminary performance of a whole-body imager. *J Nucl Med.* 2019.

8. Surti S. Update on time-of-flight PET imaging. *J Nucl Med.* 2015;56(1):98–105.

9. Hsu DFC, et al. Studies of a next-generation silicon-photomultiplier-based time-of-flight PET/CT system. *J Nucl Med.* 2017;58(9):1511–1518.

10. El Fakhri G, et al. Improvement in lesion detection with whole-body oncologic time-of-flight PET. *J Nucl Med.* 2011;52(3):347–353.

11. Lantos J, et al. Standard OSEM vs. regularized PET image reconstruction: qualitative and quantitative comparison using phantom data and various clinical radiopharmaceuticals. *Am J Nucl Med Mol Imaging.* 2018;8(2):110–118.

12. Hofmann M, et al. MRI-based attenuation correction for whole-body PET/MRI: quantitative evaluation of segmentation- and atlas-based methods. *J Nucl Med.* 2011;52(9):1392–1399.

13. Ahn S, et al. Joint estimation of activity and attenuation for PET using pragmatic MR-based prior: application to clinical TOF PET/MR whole-body data for FDG and non-FDG tracers. *Phys Med Biol.* 2018;63(4):045006.

14. de Galiza Barbosa F, et al. Pulmonary nodule detection in oncological patients–value of respiratory-triggered, periodically rotated overlapping parallel T2-weighted imaging evaluated with PET/CT-MR. *Eur J Radiol.* 2018;98:165–170.

15. Burris NS, et al. Detection of small pulmonary nodules with ultrashort echo time sequences in oncology patients by using a PET/MR system. *Radiology.* 2016;278(1):239–246.

16. Lodge MA. Repeatability of SUV in oncologic (18)F-FDG PET. *J Nucl Med.* 2017;58(4):523–532.

17. Im HJ, et al. Current methods to define metabolic tumor volume in positron emission tomography: which one is better? *Nucl Med Mol Imaging.* 2018;52(1):5–15.

18. Morris ED, et al. *Kinetic Modeling in Positron Emission Tomography. Emission Tomography: The Fundamentals of PET and SPECT.* San Diego, CA: *Academic*; 2004.

19. Patlak CS, Blasberg RG. Graphical evaluation of blood-to-brain transfer constants from multiple-time uptake data. *J Cereb Blood Flow Metab.* 1985;5(4):584–590.

20. Meyer H-J, Wienke A, Surov A. Associations between GLUT expression and SUV values derived from FDG-PET in different tumors—a systematic review and meta analysis. *PloS One.* 2019;14(6):e0217781.

21. Warburg O. On the origin of cancer cells. *Science.* 1956;123(3191):309–314.

22. Pavlides S, et al. The reverse Warburg effect: aerobic glycolysis in cancer associated fibroblasts and the tumor stroma. *Cell Cycle.* 2009;8(23):3984–4001.

23. Liberti MV, Locasale JW. The Warburg effect: how does it benefit cancer cells? *Trends Biochem Sci.* 2016;41(3):211–218.

24. Wang Y, et al. Standardized uptake value atlas: characterization of physiological 2-deoxy-2-[18F]fluoro-D-glucose uptake in normal tissues. *Mol Imaging Biol.* 2007;9(2):83–90.

25. Boellaard R, et al. FDG PET/CT: EANM procedure guidelines for tumour imaging: version 2.0. *Eur J Nucl Med Mol Imaging.* 2015;42(2):328–354.

26. American College of Radiology. ACR–SPR practice parameter for performing FDG-PET/CT in oncology. ACR website, 2017.

27. Ozguven MA, et al. Altered biodistribution of FDG in patients with type-2 diabetes mellitus. *Ann Nucl Med.* 2014;28(6):505–511.

28. ACR Committee on Drugs and Contrast Media. ACR manual on contrast media, version 10.3. 2018.

29. Shammas A, Lim R, Charron M. Pediatric FDG PET/CT: physiologic uptake, normal variants, and benign conditions. *Radiographics.* 2009;29(5):1467–1486.

30. Haerle SK, et al. Physiologic [18F]fluorodeoxyglucose uptake of floor of mouth muscles in PET/CT imaging: a problem of body position during FDG uptake? *Cancer Imaging.* 2013;13:1–7.

31. Tahara N, et al. Clinical and biochemical factors associated with area and metabolic activity in the visceral and subcutaneous adipose tissues by FDG-PET/CT. *J Clin Endocrinol Metab.* 2015;100(5):E739–E747.

32. Poeppel TD, et al. 68Ga-DOTATOC versus 68Ga-DOTATATE PET/CT in functional imaging of neuroendocrine tumors. *J Nucl Med.* 2011;52(12):1864–1870.

33. Kabasakal L, et al. Comparison of (6)(8)Ga-DOTATATE and (6)(8)Ga-DOTANOC PET/CT imaging in the same patient group with neuroendocrine tumours. *Eur J Nucl Med Mol Imaging.* 2012;39(8):1271–1277.

34. Yang J, et al. Diagnostic role of Gallium-68 DOTATOC and Gallium-68 DOTATATE PET in patients with neuroendocrine tumors: a meta-analysis. *Acta Radiol.* 2014;55(4):389–398.

35. Hope TA, et al. (111)In-pentetreotide scintigraphy versus (68)Ga-DOTATATE PET: impact on Krenning scores and effect of tumor burden. *J Nucl Med.* 2019;60(9):1266–1269.

36. Scalise M, et al. The human SLC1A5 (ASCT2) amino acid transporter: from function to structure and role in cell biology. *Front Cell Dev Biol.* 2018;6:96.

37. Li R, et al. Expression of neutral amino acid transporter ASCT2 in human prostate. *Anticancer Res.* 2003;23(4):3413–3418.

38. White MA, et al. Glutamine transporters are targets of multiple oncogenic signaling pathways in prostate cancer. *Mol Cancer Res.* 2017;15(8):1017–1028.

39. Parent EE, Schuster DM. Update on 18F-Fluciclovine PET for prostate cancer imaging. *J Nucl Med.* 2018;59(5):733–739.

40. Savir-Baruch B, Zanoni L, Schuster DM. Imaging of prostate cancer using fluciclovine. *PET Clin.* 2017;12(2):145–157.

41. Beheshti M, et al. (18)F-NaF PET/CT: EANM procedure guidelines for bone imaging. *Eur J Nucl Med Mol Imaging.* 2015;42(11):1767–1777.

42. Moradi F, Iagaru A. Dual-tracer imaging of malignant bone involvement using PET. *Clin Transl Imaging.* 2015;3(2):123–131.

43. Ross JS, et al. Correlation of primary tumor prostate-specific membrane antigen expression with disease recurrence in prostate cancer. *Clin Cancer Res.* 2003;9(17):6357–6362.

44. Foss CA, et al. Radiolabeled small-molecule ligands for prostate-specific membrane antigen: in vivo imaging in experimental models of prostate cancer. *Clin Cancer Res.* 2005;11(11):4022–4028.

45. Mease RC, et al. N-[N-[(S)-1,3-Dicarboxypropyl]carbamoyl]-4-[18F]fluorobenzyl-L-cysteine, [18F]DCFBC: a new imaging probe for prostate cancer. *Clin Cancer Res.* 2008;14(10):3036–3043.

46. Szabo Z, et al. Initial evaluation of [(18)F]DCFPyL for prostate-specific membrane antigen (PSMA)-targeted PET imaging of prostate cancer. *Mol Imaging Biol.* 2015;17(4):565–574.

47. Giesel FL, et al. Intraindividual comparison of (18)F-PSMA-1007 and (18)F-DCFPyL PET/CT in the prospective evaluation of patients with newly diagnosed prostate carcinoma: a pilot study. *J Nucl Med.* 2018;59(7):1076–1080.

48. Giesel FL, et al. F-18 labelled PSMA-1007: biodistribution, radiation dosimetry and histopathological validation of tumor lesions in prostate cancer patients. *Eur J Nucl Med Mol Imaging.* 2017;44(4):678–688.

49. Rauscher I, et al. Matched-pair comparison of (68)Ga-PSMA-11 and (18)F-PSMA-1007 PET/CT: frequency of pitfalls and detection efficacy in biochemical recurrence after radical prostatectomy. *J Nucl Med.* 2019.

50. Treglia G, et al. Radiolabelled choline versus PSMA PET/CT in prostate cancer restaging: a meta-analysis. *Am J Nucl Med Mol Imaging.* 2019;9(2):127–139.

51. Schwenck J, et al. Comparison of (68)Ga-labelled PSMA-11 and (11)C-choline in the detection of prostate cancer metastases by PET/CT. *Eur J Nucl Med Mol Imaging.* 2017;44(1):92–101.

52. Sahoo MK. (68)Ga-prostate-specific membrane antigen positron emission tomography/computed tomography: how much specific it is? *World J Nucl Med.* 2017;16(4):338–339.

53. Murthy VL, et al. Clinical quantification of myocardial blood flow using PET: joint position paper of the SNMMI cardiovascular council and the ASNC. *J Nucl Med.* 2018;59(2):273–293.

54. Jack CR Jr, et al. Hypothetical model of dynamic biomarkers of the Alzheimer's pathological cascade. *Lancet Neurol.* 2010;9(1):119–128.

55. Klunk WE, et al. Imaging brain amyloid in Alzheimer's disease with Pittsburgh Compound-B. *Ann Neurol.* 2004;55(3):306–319.

56. Johnson KA, et al. Appropriate use criteria for amyloid PET: a report of the Amyloid Imaging Task Force, the Society of Nuclear Medicine and Molecular Imaging, and the Alzheimer's Association. *J Nucl Med.* 2013;54(3):476–490.

57. Jack CR Jr, et al. Tracking pathophysiological processes in Alzheimer's disease: an updated hypothetical model of dynamic biomarkers. *Lancet Neurol.* 2013;12(2):207–216.

58. Leuzy A, et al. Tau PET imaging in neurodegenerative tauopathies-still a challenge. *Mol Psychiatry.* 2019;24(8):1112–1134.

59. Robertson JS, Rowe CC, Villemagne VL. Tau imaging with PET: an overview of challenges, current progress, and future applications. *Q J Nucl Med Mol Imaging.* 2017;61(4):405–413.

60. Harada R, et al. Characteristics of tau and its ligands in PET imaging. *Biomolecules.* 2016;6(1):7.

61. Small GW, et al. PET of brain amyloid and tau in mild cognitive impairment. *N Engl J Med.* 2006;355(25):2652–2663.

62. Marquie M, et al. Validating novel tau positron emission tomography tracer [F-18]-AV-1451 (T807) on postmortem brain tissue. *Ann Neurol.* 2015;78(5):787–800.

63. MacMahon H, et al. Guidelines for management of incidental pulmonary nodules detected on CT images: from the Fleischner Society 2017. *Radiology.* 2017;284(1):228–243.

64. Swerdlow SH, et al. The 2016 revision of the World Health Organization classification of lymphoid neoplasms. *Blood.* 2016;127(20):2375–2390.

65. Teras LR, et al. 2016 US lymphoid malignancy statistics by World Health Organization subtypes. CA Cancer J Clin. 2016;66(6):443–459.

66. Raanani P, et al. Is CT scan still necessary for staging in Hodgkin and non-Hodgkin lymphoma patients in the PET/CT era? *Ann Oncol.* 2005;17(1):117–122.

67. El-Galaly TC, et al. Routine bone marrow biopsy has little or no therapeutic consequence for positron emission tomography/computed tomography-staged treatment-naive patients with Hodgkin lymphoma. *J Clin Oncol.* 2012;30(36):4508–4514.

68. Adams HJ, et al. FDG PET/CT for the detection of bone marrow involvement in diffuse large B-cell lymphoma: systematic review and meta-analysis. *Eur J Nucl Mol Imaging.* 2014;41(3):565–574.

69. Cheson BD, et al. Revised response criteria for malignant lymphoma. *J Clin Oncol.* 2007;25(5):579–586.

70. Hutchings M, et al. In vivo treatment sensitivity testing with positron emission tomography/computed tomography after one cycle of chemotherapy for Hodgkin lymphoma. *J Clin Oncol.* 2014;32(25):2705–2711.

71. Gallamini A, et al. Early chemotherapy intensification with escalated BEACOPP in patients with advanced-stage Hodgkin lymphoma with a positive interim positron emission tomography/computed tomography scan after two ABVD cycles: long-term results of the GITIL/FIL HD 0607 trial. *J Clin Oncol.* 2018;36(5):454–462.

72. Kitajima K, et al. Predictive value of interim FDG-PET/CT findings in patients with diffuse large B-cell lymphoma treated with R-CHOP. *Oncotarget.* 2019;10(52):5403–5411.

73. Burggraaff CN, et al. Predictive value of interim positron emission tomography in diffuse large B-cell lymphoma: a systematic review and meta-analysis. *Eur J Nucl Med Mol Imaging.* 2019;46(1):65–79.

74. Barrington SF, et al. Role of imaging in the staging and response assessment of lymphoma: consensus of the International Conference on Malignant Lymphomas Imaging Working Group. *J Clin Oncol.* 2014;32(27):3048–3058.

75. Hong HR, et al. Clinical values of (18) F-FDG PET/CT in oral cavity cancer with dental artifacts on CT or MRI. *J Surg Oncol.* 2014;110(6):696–701.

76. Pillsbury HC III, Clark M. A rationale for therapy of the N0 neck. *Laryngoscope.* 1997;107(10):1294–1315.

77. Lowe VJ, et al. Multicenter trial of [(18)F]fluorodeoxyglucose positron emission tomography/computed tomography staging of head and neck cancer and negative predictive value and surgical impact in the N0 neck: results from ACRIN 6685. *J Clin Oncol.* 2019;37(20):1704–1712.

78. Golusinski P, et al. Evidence for the approach to the diagnostic evaluation of squamous cell carcinoma occult primary tumors of the head and neck. *Oral Oncol.* 2019;88:145–152.

79. Mehanna H, et al. PET-CT surveillance versus neck dissection in advanced head and neck cancer. *N Engl J Med.* 2016;374(15):1444–1454.

80. de Ridder M, et al. FDG-PET/CT improves detection of residual disease and reduces the need for examination under anaesthesia in oropharyngeal cancer patients treated with (chemo-) radiation. *Eur Arch Oto-Rhino-Laryngol.* 2019;276(5):1447–1455.

81. Driessen JP, et al. Prospective comparative study of MRI including diffusion-weighted images versus FDG PET-CT for the detection of recurrent head and neck squamous cell carcinomas after (chemo) radiotherapy. *Eur J Radiol.* 2019;111:62–67.

82. Van den Wyngaert T, et al. Fluorodeoxyglucose-positron emission tomography/computed tomography after concurrent chemoradiotherapy in locally advanced head-and-neck squamous cell cancer: the ECLYPS study. *J Clin Oncol.* 2017;35(30):3458–3464.

83. Haugen BR, et al. 2015 American Thyroid Association management guidelines for adult patients with thyroid nodules and differentiated thyroid cancer: the American Thyroid Association guidelines task force on thyroid nodules and differentiated thyroid cancer. *Thyroid.* 2016;26(1):1–133.

84. Pattison DA, et al. (18)F-FDG-avid thyroid incidentalomas: the importance of contextual interpretation. *J Nucl Med.* 2018;59(5):749–755.

85. Thielker J, et al. Contemporary management of benign and malignant parotid tumors. *Front Surg.* 2018;5:39.

86. Park MJ, et al. 18F-FDG PET/CT versus contrast-enhanced CT for staging and prognostic prediction in patients with salivary gland carcinomas. *Clin Nucl Med.* 2017;42(3):e149–e156.

87. Makis W, Ciarallo A, Gotra A. Clinical significance of parotid gland incidentalomas on (18)F-FDG PET/CT. *Clin Imaging.* 2015;39(4):667–671.

88. Casselden E, Sheerin F, Winter SC. Incidental findings on 18-FDG PET-CT in head and neck cancer. A retrospective case-control study of incidental findings on 18-FDG PET-CT in patients with head and neck cancer. *Eur Arch Otorhinolaryngol.* 2019;276(1):243–247.

89. Naji M, et al. 68Ga-DOTA-TATE PET vs. 123I-MIBG in identifying malignant neural crest tumours. *Mol Imaging Biol.* 2011;13(4):769–775.

90. Kroiss AS, et al. (68)Ga-DOTATOC PET/CT in the localization of head and neck paraganglioma compared with (18)F-DOPA PET/CT and (123)I-MIBG SPECT/CT. *Nucl Med Biol.* 2019;71:47–53.

91. Blanchet EM, et al. 18F-FDG PET/CT as a predictor of hereditary head and neck paragangliomas. *Eur J Clin Invest.* 2014;44(3):325–332.

92. Rodrigues RS, et al. Comparison of whole-body PET/CT, dedicated high-resolution head and neck PET/CT, and contrast-enhanced CT in preoperative staging of clinically M0 squamous cell carcinoma of the head and neck. *J Nucl Med.* 2009;50(8):1205–1213.

93. Alzahouri K, et al. Management of SPN in France. Pathways for definitive diagnosis of solitary pulmonary nodule: a multicentre study in 18 French districts. *BMC Cancer.* 2008;8:93.

94. Gould MK, et al. Accuracy of positron emission tomography for diagnosis of pulmonary nodules and mass lesions: a meta-analysis. *JAMA.* 2001;285(7):914–924.

95. Divisi D, et al. Diagnostic performance of fluorine-18 fluorodeoxyglucose positron emission tomography in the management of solitary pulmonary nodule: a meta-analysis. *J Thorac Dis.* 2018;10 (Suppl 7):S779–S789.

96. Herder GJ, et al. Clinical prediction model to characterize pulmonary nodules: validation and added value of 18F-fluorodeoxyglucose positron emission tomography. *Chest.* 2005;128(4):2490–2496.

97. Al-Ameri A, et al. Risk of malignancy in pulmonary nodules: a validation study of four prediction models. *Lung Cancer.* 2015;89(1):27–30.

98. Yang B, et al. Comparison of four models predicting the malignancy of pulmonary nodules: a single-center study of Korean adults. *PLoS One.* 2018;13(7):e0201242.

99. van Tinteren H, et al. Effectiveness of positron emission tomography in the preoperative assessment of patients with suspected non-small-cell lung cancer: the PLUS multicentre randomised trial. *Lancet.* 2002;359(9315):1388–1393.

100. Silvestri GA, et al. Methods for staging non-small cell lung cancer: diagnosis and management of lung cancer, 3rd ed: American College of Chest Physicians evidence-based clinical practice guidelines. *Chest.* 2013;143(5 Suppl):e211S–e250S.

101. Rusch VW, et al. The IASLC lung cancer staging project: a proposal for a new international lymph node map in the forthcoming seventh edition of the TNM classification for lung cancer. *J Thorac Oncol.* 2009;4(5):568–577.

102. Carter BW, et al. Revisions to the TNM staging of lung cancer: rationale, significance, and clinical application. *Radiographics.* 2018;38(2):374–391.

103. Mayo-Smith WW, et al. Management of incidental adrenal masses: a white paper of the ACR Incidental Findings Committee. *J Am Coll Radiol.* 2017;14(8):1038–1044.

104. Kumar R, et al. 18F-FDG PET in evaluation of adrenal lesions in patients with lung cancer. *J Nucl Med.* 2004;45(12):2058–2062.

105. Fanggiday JC, et al. Persistent inflammation in pulmonary granuloma 48 years after talcage pleurodesis, detected by FDG-PET/CT. *Case Rep Med.* 2012;2012:686153.

106. Sung YM, et al. 18F-FDG PET/CT of thymic epithelial tumors: usefulness for distinguishing and staging tumor subgroups. *J Nucl Med.* 2006;47(10):1628–1634.

107. Munden RF, et al. Managing incidental findings on thoracic CT: mediastinal and cardiovascular findings. a white paper of the ACR Incidental Findings Committee. *J Am College Radiol.* 2018;15(8):1087–1096.

108. Bray F, et al. Global cancer statistics 2018: GLOBOCAN estimates of incidence and mortality worldwide for 36 cancers in 185 countries. *CA Cancer J Clin.* 2018;68(6):394–424.

109. Siegel RL, Miller KD, Jemal A. Cancer statistics, 2019. *CA Cancer J Clin.* 2019;69(1):7–34.

110. Barber TW, et al. 18F-FDG PET/CT has a high impact on patient management and provides powerful prognostic stratification in the primary staging of esophageal cancer: a prospective study with mature survival data. *J Nucl Med.* 2012;53(6):864–871.

111. You JJ, et al. Clinical utility of 18F-fluorodeoxyglucose positron emission tomography/computed tomography in the staging of patients with potentially resectable esophageal cancer. *J Thorac Oncol.* 2013;8(12):1563–1569.

112. Findlay JM, et al. Routinely staging gastric cancer with (18)F-FDG PET-CT detects additional metastases and predicts early recurrence and death after surgery. *Eur Radiol.* 2019;29(5):2490–2498.

113. Yun M. Imaging of gastric cancer metabolism using 18 F-FDG PET/CT. *J Gastric Cancer.* 2014;14(1):1–6.

114. Bruening W, et al. *AHRQ Comparative Effectiveness Reviews, in Imaging Tests for the Staging of Colorectal Cancer.* Rockville, MD: Agency for Healthcare Research and Quality (US); 2014.

115. Whiteford MH, et al. Usefulness of FDG-PET scan in the assessment of suspected metastatic or recurrent adenocarcinoma of the colon and rectum. *Dis Colon Rectum.* 2000;43(6):759–767; discussion 767–770.

116. Flamen P, et al. Unexplained rising carcinoembryonic antigen (CEA) in the postoperative surveillance of colorectal cancer: the utility of positron emission tomography (PET). *Eur J Cancer.* 2001;37(7):862–869.

117. Mahmud A, Poon R, Jonker D. PET imaging in anal canal cancer: a systematic review and meta-analysis. *Br J Radiol.* 2017;90(1080):20170370.

118. Engstrom PF, et al. NCCN clinical practice guidelines in oncology. Anal carcinoma. *J Natl Compr Canc Netw.* 2010;8(1):106–120.

119. Glynne-Jones R, et al. Anal cancer: ESMO-ESSO-ESTRO clinical practice guidelines for diagnosis, treatment and follow-up. *Eur J Surg Oncol.* 2014;40(10):1165–1176.

120. Jones MP, et al. FDG-PET parameters predict for recurrence in anal cancer—results from a prospective, multicentre clinical trial. *Radiat Oncol.* 2019;14(1):140.

121. Torizuka T, et al. In vivo assessment of glucose metabolism in hepatocellular carcinoma with FDG-PET. *J Nucl Med.* 1995;36(10):1811–1817.

122. Wudel LJ Jr, et al. The role of [18F]fluorodeoxyglucose positron emission tomography imaging in the evaluation of hepatocellular carcinoma. *Am Surg.* 2003;69(2):117–124; discussion 124–126.

123. Kornberg A, et al. Patients with non-[18 F]fludeoxyglucose-avid advanced hepatocellular carcinoma on clinical staging may achieve long-term recurrence-free survival after liver transplantation. *Liver Transpl.* 2012;18(1):53–61.

124. Lin CY, et al. 18F-FDG PET or PET/CT for detecting extrahepatic metastases or recurrent hepatocellular carcinoma: a systematic review and meta-analysis. *Eur J Radiol.* 2012;81(9):2417–2422.

125. Sultana A, et al. What is the best way to identify malignant transformation within pancreatic IPMN: a systematic review and meta-analyses. *Clin Transl Gastroenterol.* 2015;6:e130.

126. Kim YI, et al. Comparison of F-18-FDG PET/CT findings between pancreatic solid pseudopapillary tumor and pancreatic ductal adenocarcinoma. *Eur J Radiol.* 2014;83(1):231–235.

127. Kauhanen SP, et al. A prospective diagnostic accuracy study of 18F-fluorodeoxyglucose positron emission tomography/computed tomography, multidetector row computed tomography, and magnetic resonance imaging in primary diagnosis and staging of pancreatic cancer. *Ann Surg.* 2009;250(6):957–963.

128. Asagi A, et al. Utility of contrast-enhanced FDG-PET/CT in the clinical management of pancreatic cancer: impact on diagnosis, staging, evaluation of treatment response, and detection of recurrence. *Pancreas.* 2013;42(1):11–19.

129. Joo I, et al. Preoperative assessment of pancreatic cancer with FDG PET/MR imaging versus FDG PET/CT plus contrast-enhanced multidetector CT: a prospective preliminary study. *Radiology.* 2017;282(1):149–159.

130. O'Reilly D, et al. Diagnosis and management of pancreatic cancer in adults: a summary of guidelines from the UK National Institute for Health and Care Excellence. *Pancreatology.* 2018;18(8):962–970.

131. Yoshioka M, et al. Role of positron emission tomography with 2-deoxy-2-[18F]fluoro-D-glucose in evaluating the effects of arterial infusion chemotherapy and radiotherapy on pancreatic cancer. *J Gastroenterol.* 2004;39(1):50–55.

132. Dalah E, et al. PET-based treatment response assessment for neoadjuvant chemoradiation in pancreatic adenocarcinoma: an exploratory study. *Transl Oncol.* 2018;11(5):1104–1109.

133. Cho MH, et al. Clinicopathologic features and molecular characteristics of glucose metabolism contributing to (1)(8) F-fluorodeoxyglucose uptake in gastrointestinal stromal tumors. *PLoS One.* 2015;10(10):e0141413.

134. Prior JO, et al. Early prediction of response to sunitinib after imatinib failure by 18F-fluorodeoxyglucose positron emission tomography in patients with gastrointestinal stromal tumor. *J Clin Oncol.* 2009;27(3):439–445.

135. Van den Abbeele AD, et al. ACRIN 6665/RTOG 0132 phase II trial of neoadjuvant imatinib mesylate for operable malignant gastrointestinal stromal tumor: monitoring with 18F-FDG PET and correlation with genotype and GLUT4 expression. *J Nucl Med.* 2012;53(4):567–574.

136. Kulke MH, et al. Neuroendocrine tumors, version 1.2015. *J Natl Compr Canc Netw.* 2015;13(1):78–108.

137. Dasari A, et al. Trends in the incidence, prevalence, and survival outcomes in patients with neuroendocrine tumors in the United States. *JAMA Oncol.* 2017;3(10):1335–1342.

138. Lloyd RV, et al. WHO classification of tumours of endocrine organs. *International Agency for Research on Cancer;* 2017.

139. Rindi G, et al. A common classification framework for neuroendocrine neoplasms: an International Agency for Research on Cancer (IARC) and World Health Organization (WHO) expert consensus proposal. *Mod Pathol.* 2018;31(12):1770–1786.

140. Hofman MS, Lau WF, Hicks RJ. Somatostatin receptor imaging with 68Ga DOTATATE PET/CT: clinical utility, normal patterns, pearls, and pitfalls in interpretation. *Radiographics*. 2015;35(2):500–516.

141. Herrmann K, et al. Impact of 68Ga-DOTATATE PET/CT on the management of neuroendocrine tumors: the referring physician's perspective. *J Nucl Med*. 2015;56(1):70–75.

142. Hofman MS, et al. High management impact of Ga-68 DOTATATE (GaTate) PET/CT for imaging neuroendocrine and other somatostatin expressing tumours. *J Med Imaging Radiat Oncol*. 2012;56(1):40–47.

143. Krenning EP, et al. Scintigraphy and radionuclide therapy with [indium-111-labelled-diethyl triamine penta-acetic acid-D-Phe1]-octreotide. Ital J Gastroenterol Hepatol. 1999;31 Suppl 2:S219–S223.

144. Nakajima R, et al. Evaluation of renal cell carcinoma histological subtype and fuhrman grade using (18)F-fluorodeoxyglucose-positron emission tomography/computed tomography. *Eur Radiol*. 2017;27(11):4866–4873.

145. Takahashi M, et al. Preoperative evaluation of renal cell carcinoma by using 18F-FDG PET/CT. *Clin Nucl Med*. 2015;40(12):936–940.

146. Pankowska V, et al. FDG PET/CT as a survival prognostic factor in patients with advanced renal cell carcinoma. *Clin Exp Med*. 2019;19(1):143–148.

147. Lakhani A, et al. FDG PET/CT pitfalls in gynecologic and genitourinary oncologic imaging. *Radiographics*. 2017;37(2):577–594.

148. Chen SC, Kuo PL. Bone metastasis from renal cell carcinoma. Int J Mol Sci. 2016;17(6):987.

149. Wu HC, et al. Comparing whole body 18F-2-deoxyglucose positron emission tomography and technetium-99m methylene diphosphate bone scan to detect bone metastases in patients with renal cell carcinomas—a preliminary report. J Cancer Res Clin Oncol. 2002;128(9):503–506.

150. Wang HY, et al. Meta-analysis of the diagnostic performance of [18F]FDG-PET and PET/CT in renal cell carcinoma. *Cancer Imaging*. 2012;12:464–474.

151. Ma H, et al. Diagnostic performance of 18F-FDG PET or PET/CT in restaging renal cell carcinoma: a systematic review and meta-analysis. *Nucl Med Commun*. 2017;38(2):156–163.

152. Flaig TW, et al. NCCN guidelines insights: bladder cancer, version 5.2018. *J Natl Compr Canc Netw*. 2018;16(9):1041–1053.

153. Soubra A, et al. The diagnostic accuracy of 18F-fluorodeoxyglucose positron emission tomography and computed tomography in staging bladder cancer: a single-institution study and a systematic review with meta-analysis. *World J Urol*. 2016;34(9):1229–1237.

154. Ha HK, Koo PJ, Kim SJ. Diagnostic accuracy of F-18 FDG PET/CT for preoperative lymph node staging in newly diagnosed bladder cancer patients: a systematic review and meta-analysis. *Oncology*. 2018;95(1):31–38.

155. Soubra A, et al. FDG-PET/CT for assessing the response to neoadjuvant chemotherapy in bladder cancer patients. *Clin Genitourin Cancer*. 2018;16(5):360–364.

156. Ozturk H, Karapolat I. Efficacy of (18)F-fluorodeoxyglucose-positron emission tomography/computed tomography in restaging muscle-invasive bladder cancer following radical cystectomy. *Exp Ther Med*. 2015;9(3):717–724.

157. Pano B, et al. Pathways of lymphatic spread in gynecologic malignancies. Radiographics. 2015;35(3):916–945.

158. Koh WJ, et al. Cervical cancer, version 3.2019, NCCN clinical practice guidelines in oncology. *J Natl Compr Canc Netw*. 2019;17(1):64–84.

159. Bhatla N, et al. Revised FIGO staging for carcinoma of the cervix uteri. *Int J Gynaecol Obstet*. 2019;145(1):129–135.

160. Gee MS, et al. Identification of distant metastatic disease in uterine cervical and endometrial cancers with FDG PET/CT: analysis from the ACRIN 6671/GOG 0233 multicenter trial. *Radiology*. 2018;287(1):176–184.

161. Tanaka T, et al. Which is better for predicting pelvic lymph node metastases in patients with cervical cancer: fluorodeoxyglucose-positron emission tomography/computed tomography or a sentinel node biopsy? A retrospective observational study. *Medicine (Baltimore)*. 2018;97(16):e0410.

162. Gouy S, et al. Prospective multicenter study evaluating the survival of patients with locally advanced cervical cancer undergoing laparoscopic para-aortic lymphadenectomy before chemoradiotherapy in the era of positron emission tomography imaging. *J Clin Oncol*. 2013;31(24):3026–3033.

163. Driscoll DO, et al. 18F-FDG-PET/CT is of limited value in primary staging of early stage cervical cancer. *Abdom Imaging*. 2015;40(1):127–133.

164. Morkel M, et al. Evaluating the role of F-18 fluorodeoxyglucose positron emission tomography/computed tomography scanning in the staging of patients with stage IIIB cervical carcinoma and the impact on treatment decisions. *Int J Gynecol Cancer*. 2018;28(2):379–384.

165. Kidd EA, et al. Clinical outcomes of definitive intensity-modulated radiation therapy with fluorodeoxyglucose-positron emission tomography simulation in patients with locally advanced cervical cancer. *Int J Radiat Oncol Biol Phys*. 2010;77(4):1085–1091.

166. Cohn DE, et al. Prospective evaluation of positron emission tomography for the detection of groin node metastases from vulvar cancer. *Gynecol Oncol*. 2002;85(1):179–184.

167. Crivellaro C, et al. 18F-FDG PET/CT in preoperative staging of vulvar cancer patients: is it really effective? *Medicine (Baltimore)*. 2017;96(38):e7943.

168. Lin G, et al. Computed tomography, magnetic resonance imaging and FDG positron emission tomography in the management of vulvar malignancies. *Eur Radiol*. 2015;25(5):1267–1278.

169. Hagemann IS, et al. Controversies in gynecologic cancer staging: an AJCC cancer staging manual, perspective. *AJSP Rev Rep*. 2018;23(3):118–128.

170. Erdogan M, et al. Prognostic value of metabolic tumor volume and total lesion glycolysis assessed by 18F-FDG PET/CT in endometrial cancer. *Nucl Med Commun*. 2019;40(11):1099–1104.

171. Asicioglu O, et al. A novel preoperative scoring system based on 18-FDG PET-CT for predicting lymph node metastases in patients with high-risk endometrial cancer. *J Obstet Gynaecol*. 2019;39(1):105–109.

172. Kadkhodayan S, et al. Accuracy of 18-F-FDG PET imaging in the follow up of endometrial cancer patients: systematic review and meta-analysis of the literature. *Gynecol Oncol*. 2013;128(2):397–404.

173. Kulkarni R, et al. Role of positron emission tomography/computed tomography in preoperative assessment of carcinoma endometrium-a retrospective analysis. *Indian J Surg Oncol*. 2019;10(1):225–231.

174. Lin MY, et al. Role of imaging in the routine management of endometrial cancer. *Int J Gynaecol Obstet*. 2018;143 Suppl 2:109–117.

175. Stewart KI, et al. Preoperative PET/CT does not accurately detect extrauterine disease in patients with newly diagnosed high-risk endometrial cancer: a prospective study. *Cancer*. 2019;125(19):3347–3353.

176. Park JY, et al. The value of preoperative positron emission tomography/computed tomography in node-negative endometrial cancer on magnetic resonance imaging. *Ann Surg Oncol*. 2017;24(8):2303–2310.

177. Bian LH, et al. Comparison of integrated PET/MRI with PET/CT in evaluation of endometrial cancer: a retrospective analysis of 81 cases. *PeerJ*. 2019;7:e7081.

178. Mbatani N, Olawaiye AB, Prat J. Uterine sarcomas. *Int J Gynaecol Obstet*. 2018;143 Suppl 2:51–58.

179. Kusunoki S, et al. Efficacy of PET/CT to exclude leiomyoma in patients with lesions suspicious for uterine sarcoma on MRI. *Taiwan J Obstet Gynecol*. 2017;56(4):508–513.

180. Nakagawa M, et al. A multiparametric MRI-based machine learning to distinguish between uterine sarcoma and benign leiomyoma: comparison with (18)F-FDG PET/CT. *Clin Radiol*. 2019;74(2):167.e1–167.e7.

181. Park JY, et al. Prognostic significance of preoperative (1)(8)F-FDG PET/CT in uterine leiomyosarcoma. *J Gynecol Oncol*. 2017;28(3):e28.

182. Khiewvan B, et al. An update on the role of PET/CT and PET/MRI in ovarian cancer. *Eur J Nucl Med Mol Imaging*. 2017;44(6):1079–1091.

183. Han S, et al. Performance of pre-treatment (1)(8) F-fluorodeoxyglucose positron emission tomography/computed tomography for detecting metastasis in ovarian cancer: a systematic review and meta-analysis. *J Gynecol Oncol*. 2018;29(6):e98.

184. Roze JF, et al. Positron emission tomography (PET) and magnetic resonance imaging (MRI) for assessing tumour resectability in advanced epithelial ovarian/fallopian tube/primary peritoneal cancer. *Cochrane Database Syst Rev*. 2018;10:Cd012567.

185. Amit A, et al. The role of F18-FDG PET/CT in predicting secondary optimal de-bulking in patients with recurrent ovarian cancer. *Surg Oncol*. 2017;26(4):347–351.

186. Bhosale P, et al. Clinical utility of positron emission tomography/computed tomography in the evaluation of suspected recurrent ovarian cancer in the setting of normal CA-125 levels. *Int J Gynecol Cancer*. 2010;20(6):936–944.

187. Lee YJ, et al. Diagnostic value of integrated (1)(8)F-fluoro-2-deoxyglucose positron emission tomography/computed tomography in recurrent epithelial ovarian cancer: accuracy of patient selection for secondary cytoreduction in 134 patients. *J Gynecol Oncol*. 2018;29(3):e36.

188. Howlader N eds., et al. *SEER Cancer Statistics Review, 1975–2016*. Bethesda, MD: National Cancer Institute. https://seer.cancer.gov/csr/1975_2016/, based on November 2018 SEER data submission, posted to the SEER web site, April 2019.

189. Epstein JI, et al. A contemporary prostate cancer grading system: a validated alternative to the gleason score. *Eur Urol*. 2016;69(3):428–435.

190. Buyyounouski MK, et al. Prostate cancer–major changes in the American Joint Committee on Cancer eighth edition cancer staging manual. *CA Cancer J Clin*. 2017;67(3):245–253.

191. Coakley FV, et al. ACR appropriateness criteria® prostate cancer—pretreatment detection, surveillance, and staging. *J Am College Radiol*. 2017;14(5):S245–S257.

192. Antonarakis ES, et al. The natural history of metastatic progression in men with prostate-specific antigen recurrence after radical prostatectomy: long-term follow-up. BJU Int. 2012;109(1):32–39.

193. Isbarn H, et al. Long-term data on the survival of patients with prostate cancer treated with radical prostatectomy in the prostate-specific antigen era. BJU Int. 2010;106(1):37–43.

194. Makis W, Ciarallo A. Clinical significance of (18) F-fluorodeoxyglucose avid prostate gland incidentalomas on positron emission tomography/computed tomography. *Mol Imaging Radionucl Ther*. 2017;26(2):76–82.

195. Beauregard JM, et al. FDG-PET/CT for pre-operative staging and prognostic stratification of patients with high-grade prostate cancer at biopsy. *Cancer Imaging*. 2015;15:2.

196. Fox JJ, et al. Positron emission tomography/computed tomography-based assessments of androgen receptor expression and glycolytic activity as a prognostic biomarker for metastatic castration-resistant prostate cancer. *JAMA Oncol*. 2018;4(2):217–224.

197. Suzuki H, et al. Diagnostic performance and safety of NMK36 (trans-1-amino-3-[18F]fluorocyclobutanecarboxylic acid)-PET/CT in primary prostate cancer: multicenter Phase IIb clinical trial. *Jpn J Clin Oncol*. 2016;46(2):152–162.

198. Jambor I, et al. Prospective evaluation of (18)F-FACBC PET/CT and PET/MRI versus multiparametric MRI in intermediate- to high-risk prostate cancer patients (FLUCIPRO trial). *Eur J Nucl Med Mol Imaging*. 2018;45(3):355–364.

199. Selnaes KM, et al. (18)F-Fluciclovine PET/MRI for preoperative lymph node staging in high-risk prostate cancer patients. *Eur Radiol*. 2018;28(8):3151–3159.

200. Schuster DM, et al. Anti-3-[(18)F]FACBC positron emission tomography-computerized tomography and (111)In-capromab pendetide single photon emission computerized tomography-computerized tomography for recurrent prostate carcinoma: results of a prospective clinical trial. *J Urol*. 2014;191(5):1446–1453.

201. Andriole GL, et al. The impact of positron emission tomography with 18F-Fluciclovine on the treatment of biochemical recurrence of prostate cancer: results from the LOCATE trial. *J Urol*. 2019;201(2):322–331.

202. Odewole OA, et al. Recurrent prostate cancer detection with anti-3-[(18)F]FACBC PET/CT: comparison with CT. *Eur J Nucl Med Mol Imaging*. 2016;43(10):1773–1783.

203. Akin-Akintayo O, et al. Prospective evaluation of fluciclovine ((18) F) PET-CT and MRI in detection of recurrent prostate cancer in non-prostatectomy patients. *Eur J Radiol*. 2018;102:1–8.

204. Amorim BJ, et al. Performance of (18)F-Fluciclovine PET/MR in the evaluation of osseous metastases from castration-resistant prostate cancer. *Eur J Nucl Med Mol Imaging*. 2019.

205. Chen B, et al. Comparison of 18F-Fluciclovine PET/CT and 99mTc-MDP bone scan in detection of bone metastasis in prostate cancer. *Nucl Med Commun*. 2019;40(9):940–946.

206. Sheikhbahaei S, et al. (18)F-NaF-PET/CT for the detection of bone metastasis in prostate cancer: a meta-analysis of diagnostic accuracy studies. *Ann Nucl Med*. 2019;33(5):351–361.

207. Harmon SA, et al. Quantitative assessment of early [(18)F]sodium fluoride positron emission tomography/computed tomography response to treatment in men with metastatic prostate cancer to bone. *J Clin Oncol*. 2017;35(24):2829–2837.

208. Velez EM, Desai B, Jadvar H. Treatment response assessment of skeletal metastases in prostate cancer with (18)F-NaF PET/CT. *Nucl Med Mol Imaging*. 2019;53(4):247–252.

209. Morigi JJ, et al. Prospective comparison of 18F-Fluoromethylcholine versus 68Ga-PSMA PET/CT in prostate cancer patients who have rising PSA after curative treatment and are being considered for targeted therapy. *J Nucl Med*. 2015;56(8):1185–1190.

210. Perera M, et al. Gallium-68 prostate-specific membrane antigen positron emission tomography in advanced prostate cancer-updated diagnostic utility, sensitivity, specificity, and distribution of prostate-specific membrane antigen-avid lesions: a systematic review and meta-analysis. *Eur Urol*. 2019.

211. England JR, et al. 18F-Fluciclovine PET/CT detection of recurrent prostate carcinoma in patients with serum PSA </= 1 ng/mL after definitive primary treatment. *Clin Nucl Med*. 2019;44(3):e128–e132.

212. Song H, et al. Prospective evaluation in an academic center of (18) F-DCFPyL PET/CT in biochemically recurrent prostate cancer: a focus on localizing disease and changes in management. *J Nucl Med*. 2019.

213. Pernthaler B, et al. A prospective head-to-head comparison of 18F-Fluciclovine with 68Ga-PSMA-11 in biochemical recurrence of prostate cancer in PET/CT. *Clin Nucl Med*. 2019;44(10):e566–e573.

214. Narayanan D, Berg WA. Dedicated breast gamma camera imaging and breast PET: current status and future directions. *PET Clin*. 2018;13(3):363–381.

215. Kang BJ, et al. Clinical significance of incidental finding of focal activity in the breast at 18F-FDG PET/CT. *Am J Roentgenol*. 2011;197(2):341–347.

216. Nursal GN, et al. Is PET/CT necessary in the management of early breast cancer? *Clin Nucl Med*. 2016;41(5):362–365.

217. Wang CL, et al. (18)F-FDG PET/CT-positive internal mammary lymph nodes: pathologic correlation by ultrasound-guided fine-needle aspiration and assessment of associated risk factors. *Am J Roentgenol*. 2013;200(5):1138–1144.

218. Gebhart G, et al. 18F-FDG PET/CT for early prediction of response to neoadjuvant lapatinib, trastuzumab, and their combination in HER2-positive breast cancer: results from Neo-ALTTO. *J Nucl Med*. 2013;54(11):1862–1868.

219. Groheux D, et al. (1)(8)F-FDG PET/CT for the early evaluation of response to neoadjuvant treatment in triple-negative breast cancer: influence of the chemotherapy regimen. *J Nucl Med*. 2016;57(4):536–543.

220. Connolly RM, et al. TBCRC026: phase II trial correlating standardized uptake value with pathologic complete response to pertuzumab and trastuzumab in breast cancer. *J Clin Oncol*. 2019;37(9):714–722.

221. Paydary K, et al. The evolving role of FDG-PET/CT in the diagnosis, staging, and treatment of breast cancer. *Mol Imaging Biol.* 2019;21(1):1–10.

222. Dose-Schwarz J, et al. Assessment of residual tumour by FDG-PET: conventional imaging and clinical examination following primary chemotherapy of large and locally advanced breast cancer. *Br J Cancer.* 2010;102(1):35–41.

223. Isasi CR, Moadel RM, Blaufox MD. A meta-analysis of FDG-PET for the evaluation of breast cancer recurrence and metastases. *Breast Cancer Res Treat.* 2005;90(2):105–112.

224. Taghipour M, et al. Value of fourth and subsequent post-therapy follow-up 18F-FDG PET/CT scans in patients with breast cancer. *Nucl Med Commun.* 2016;37(6):602–608.

225. Chang HT, et al. Role of 2-[18F] fluoro-2-deoxy-D-glucose-positron emission tomography/computed tomography in the post-therapy surveillance of breast cancer. *PLoS One.* 2014;9(12):e115127.

226. Constantinidou A, et al. Positron emission tomography/computed tomography in the management of recurrent/metastatic breast cancer: a large retrospective study from the Royal Marsden Hospital. *Ann Oncol.* 2011;22(2):307–314.

227. Park S, et al. Prognostic utility of FDG PET/CT and bone scintigraphy in breast cancer patients with bone-only metastasis. *Medicine (Baltimore).* 2017;96(50):e8985.

228. Riedl CC, et al. Comparison of FDG-PET/CT and contrast-enhanced CT for monitoring therapy response in patients with metastatic breast cancer. *Eur J Nucl Med Mol Imaging.* 2017;44(9):1428–1437.

229. Helland F, et al. FDG-PET/CT versus contrast-enhanced CT for response evaluation in metastatic breast cancer: a systematic review. *Diagnostics (Basel).* 2019;9(3).

230. Mortazavi-Jehanno N, et al. Assessment of response to endocrine therapy using FDG PET/CT in metastatic breast cancer: a pilot study. *Eur J Nucl Med Mol Imaging.* 2012;39(3):450–460.

231. Lin NU, et al. Phase II study of lapatinib in combination with trastuzumab in patients with human epidermal growth factor receptor 2-positive metastatic breast cancer: clinical outcomes and predictive value of early [18F]Fluorodeoxyglucose positron emission tomography imaging (TBCRC 003). *J Clin Oncol.* 2015;33(24):2623–2631.

232. Zhang FC, et al. (18)F-FDG PET/CT for the early prediction of the response rate and survival of patients with recurrent or metastatic breast cancer. *Oncol Lett.* 2018;16(4):4151–4158.

233. Tovmassian D, Abdul Razak M, London K. The role of [(18)F] FDG-PET/CT in predicting malignant transformation of plexiform neurofibromas in neurofibromatosis-1. *Int J Surg Oncol.* 2016;2016:6162182.

234. Broski SM, et al. Evaluation of (18)F-FDG PET and MRI in differentiating benign and malignant peripheral nerve sheath tumors. *Skeletal Radiol.* 2016;45(8):1097–1105.

235. Ahlawat S, et al. Current status and recommendations for imaging in neurofibromatosis type 1, neurofibromatosis type 2, and schwannomatosis. *Skeletal Radiol.* 2019.

236. Lawrence W Jr, et al. Adult soft tissue sarcomas. A pattern of care survey of the American College of Surgeons. *Ann Surg.* 1987;205(4):349–359.

237. Sambri A, et al. The role of 18F-FDG PET/CT in soft tissue sarcoma. *Nucl Med Commun.* 2019;40(6):626–631.

238. von Mehren M, et al. Soft tissue sarcoma, version 2.2018, NCCN clinical practice guidelines in oncology. *J Natl Compr Canc Netw.* 2018;16(5):536–563.

239. Eary JF, et al. Sarcoma tumor FDG uptake measured by PET and patient outcome: a retrospective analysis. *Eur J Nucl Med Mol Imaging.* 2002;29(9):1149–1154.

240. Kubo T, et al. Prognostic significance of (18)F-FDG PET at diagnosis in patients with soft tissue sarcoma and bone sarcoma; systematic review and meta-analysis. *Eur J Cancer.* 2016;58:104–111.

241. Tateishi U, et al. Bone and soft-tissue sarcoma: preoperative staging with fluorine 18 fluorodeoxyglucose PET/CT and conventional imaging. *Radiology.* 2007;245(3):839–847.

242. Platzek I, et al. FDG PET/MR in initial staging of sarcoma: initial experience and comparison with conventional imaging. *Clin Imaging.* 2017;42:126–132.

243. Harrison DJ, Parisi MT, Shulkin BL. The role of (18)F-FDG-PET/CT in pediatric sarcoma. *Semin Nucl Med.* 2017;47(3):229–241.

244. Schuetze SM, et al. Use of positron emission tomography in localized extremity soft tissue sarcoma treated with neoadjuvant chemotherapy. *Cancer.* 2005;103(2):339–348.

245. Eary JF, et al. Sarcoma mid-therapy [F-18]fluorodeoxyglucose positron emission tomography (FDG PET) and patient outcome. *J Bone Joint Surg Am.* 2014;96(2):152–158.

246. Sachpekidis C, et al. Neoadjuvant pazopanib treatment in high-risk soft tissue sarcoma: a quantitative dynamic (18)F-FDG PET/CT study of the German Interdisciplinary Sarcoma Group. *Cancers (Basel).* 2019;11(6):790.

247. Gershenwald JE, et al. Melanoma staging: evidence-based changes in the American Joint Committee on Cancer eighth edition cancer staging manual. *CA Cancer J Clin.* 2017;67(6):472–492.

248. Crippa F, et al. Which kinds of lymph node metastases can FDG PET detect? A clinical study in melanoma. *J Nucl Med.* 2000;41(9):1491–1494.

249. Buchbender C, et al. Oncologic PET/MRI, part 2: bone tumors, soft-tissue tumors, melanoma, and lymphoma. *J Nucl Med.* 2012;53(8):1244–1252.

250. Forschner A, et al. Impact of (18)F-FDG-PET/CT on surgical management in patients with advanced melanoma: an outcome based analysis. *Eur J Nucl Med Mol Imaging.* 2017;44(8):1312–1318.

251. Lewin J, et al. Surveillance imaging with FDG-PET/CT in the post-operative follow-up of stage 3 melanoma. *Ann Oncol.* 2018;29(7):1569–1574.

252. Vensby PH, et al. The value of FDG PET/CT for follow-up of patients with melanoma: a retrospective analysis. *Am J Nucl Med Mol Imaging.* 2017;7(6):255–262.

253. Ito K, et al. (18)F-FDG PET/CT for monitoring of ipilimumab therapy in patients with metastatic melanoma. *J Nucl Med.* 2019;60(3):335–341.

254. Gkiozos I, et al. Sarcoidosis-like reactions induced by checkpoint inhibitors. *J Thorac Oncol.* 2018;13(8):1076–1082.

255. Tan AC, et al. FDG-PET response and outcome from anti-PD-1 therapy in metastatic melanoma. *Ann Oncol.* 2018;29(10):2115–2120.

256. Ben-Haim S, et al. Metabolic assessment of Merkel cell carcinoma: the role of 18F-FDG PET/CT. *Nucl Med Commun.* 2016;37(8):865–873.

257. Taralli S, et al. 18 F-FDG and 68 Ga-somatostatin analogs PET/CT in patients with Merkel cell carcinoma: a comparison study. *EJNMMI Res.* 2018;8(1):64.

258. Basu S, Ranade R. Favorable response of metastatic Merkel cell carcinoma to targeted 177Lu-DOTATATE therapy: will PRRT evolve to become an important approach in receptor-positive cases? *J Nucl Med Technol.* 2016;44(2):85–87.

259. Olsen EA, et al. Clinical end points and response criteria in mycosis fungoides and Sezary syndrome: a consensus statement of the International Society for Cutaneous Lymphomas, the United States Cutaneous Lymphoma Consortium, and the Cutaneous Lymphoma Task Force of the European Organisation for Research and Treatment of Cancer. *J Clin Oncol.* 2011;29(18):2598–2607.

260. Trautinger F, et al. European Organisation for Research and Treatment of Cancer consensus recommendations for the treatment of mycosis fungoides/Sezary syndrome—update 2017. *Eur J Cancer.* 2017;77:57–74.

261. Feeney J, et al. Characterization of T-cell lymphomas by FDG PET/CT. *Am J Roentgenol.* 2010;195(2):333–340.

262. Qiu L, et al. The role of 18F-FDG PET and PET/CT in the evaluation of primary cutaneous lymphoma. *Nucl Med Commun.* 2017;38(2):106–116.

263. Cavo M, et al. Role of (18)F-FDG PET/CT in the diagnosis and management of multiple myeloma and other plasma cell disorders: a consensus statement by the International Myeloma Working Group. *Lancet Oncol.* 2017;18(4):e206–e217.

264. Rasche L, et al. Low expression of hexokinase-2 is associated with false-negative FDG-positron emission tomography in multiple myeloma. *Blood.* 2017;130(1):30–34.

265. Gariani J, et al. Comparison of whole body magnetic resonance imaging (WBMRI) to whole body computed tomography (WBCT) or (18)F-fluorodeoxyglucose positron emission tomography/CT ((18)F-FDG PET/CT) in patients with myeloma: systematic review of diagnostic performance. *Crit Rev Oncol Hematol.* 2018;124:66–72.

266. Usmani SZ, et al. Prognostic implications of serial 18-fluorodeoxyglucose emission tomography in multiple myeloma treated with total therapy 3. *Blood.* 2013;121(10):1819–1823.

267. Hillengass J, Merz M, Delorme S. Minimal residual disease in multiple myeloma: use of magnetic resonance imaging. *Semin Hematol.* 2018;55(1):19–21.

268. Moreau P, et al. Prospective evaluation of magnetic resonance imaging and [(18)F]Fluorodeoxyglucose positron emission tomography-computed tomography at diagnosis and before maintenance therapy in symptomatic patients with multiple myeloma included in the IFM/DFCI 2009 trial: results of the IMAJEM study. *J Clin Oncol.* 2017;35(25):2911–2918.

269. Danad I, et al. Comparison of coronary CT angiography, SPECT, PET, and hybrid imaging for diagnosis of ischemic heart disease determined by fractional flow reserve. *JAMA Cardiol.* 2017;2(10):1100–1107.

270. Mc Ardle BA, et al. Does rubidium-82 PET have superior accuracy to SPECT perfusion imaging for the diagnosis of obstructive coronary disease? A systematic review and meta-analysis. *J Am Coll Cardiol.* 2012;60(18):1828–1837.

271. Chow BJ, et al. Prognostic value of PET myocardial perfusion imaging in obese patients. *JACC Cardiovasc Imaging.* 2014;7(3):278–287.

272. Chen K, Miller EJ, Sadeghi MM, PET-based imaging of ischemic heart disease. *PET Clin.* 2019;14(2):211–221.

273. Danad I, et al. Quantitative assessment of myocardial perfusion in the detection of significant coronary artery disease: cutoff values and diagnostic accuracy of quantitative [(15)O]H2O PET imaging. *J Am Coll Cardiol.* 2014;64(14):1464–1475.

274. Majmudar MD, et al. Quantification of coronary flow reserve in patients with ischaemic and non-ischaemic cardiomyopathy and its association with clinical outcomes. *Eur Heart J Cardiovasc Imaging.* 2015;16(8):900–909.

275. Naya M, et al. Preserved coronary flow reserve effectively excludes high-risk coronary artery disease on angiography. *J Nucl Med.* 2014;55(2):248–255.

276. Panza JA, et al. Myocardial viability and long-term outcomes in ischemic cardiomyopathy. *N Engl J Med.* 2019;381(8):739–748.

277. Dilsizian V, et al. ASNC imaging guidelines/SNMMI procedure standard for positron emission tomography (PET) nuclear cardiology procedures. *J Nucl Cardiol.* 2016;23(5):1187–1226.

278. Wu YW, et al. Comparison of contrast-enhanced MRI with (18)F-FDG PET/201Tl SPECT in dysfunctional myocardium: relation to early functional outcome after surgical revascularization in chronic ischemic heart disease. *J Nucl Med.* 2007;48(7):1096–1103.

279. Hunold P, et al. Accuracy of myocardial viability imaging by cardiac MRI and PET depending on left ventricular function. *World J Cardiol.* 2018;10(9):110–118.

280. Laybutt DR, et al. Selective chronic regulation of GLUT1 and GLUT4 content by insulin, glucose, and lipid in rat cardiac muscle in vivo. *Am J Physiol.* 1997;273(3 Pt 2):H1309–H1316.

281. Kraegen EW, et al. Glucose transporters and in vivo glucose uptake in skeletal and cardiac muscle: fasting, insulin stimulation and immunoisolation studies of GLUT1 and GLUT4. *Biochem J.* 1993;295 (Pt 1):287–293.

282. Hansen AK, et al. Reverse mismatch pattern in cardiac 18F-FDG viability PET/CT is not associated with poor outcome of revascularization: a retrospective outcome study of 91 patients with heart failure. *Clin Nucl Med.* 2016;41(10):e428–e435.

283. Sarikaya I, et al. Status of F-18 fluorodeoxyglucose uptake in normal and hibernating myocardium after glucose and insulin loading. *J Saudi Heart Assoc.* 2018;30(2):75–85.

284. Kitsiou AN, et al. 13N-ammonia myocardial blood flow and uptake: relation to functional outcome of asynergic regions after revascularization. *J Am Coll Cardiol.* 1999;33(3):678–686.

285. Thompson K, et al. Is septal glucose metabolism altered in patients with left bundle branch block and ischemic cardiomyopathy? *J Nucl Med.* 2006;47(11):1763–1768.

286. Wang JG, et al. Septal and anterior reverse mismatch of myocardial perfusion and metabolism in patients with coronary artery disease and left bundle branch block. *Medicine (Baltimore).* 2015;94(20):e772.

287. Birnie DH, et al. Cardiac Sarcoidosis. *J Am Coll Cardiol.* 2016;68(4):411–421.

288. Tavora F, et al. Comparison of necropsy findings in patients with sarcoidosis dying suddenly from cardiac sarcoidosis versus dying suddenly from other causes. *Am J Cardiol.* 2009;104(4):571–577.

289. Roberts WC, McAllister HA Jr, Ferrans VJ. Sarcoidosis of the heart. A clinicopathologic study of 35 necropsy patients (group 1) and review of 78 previously described necropsy patients (group 11). *Am J Med.* 1977;63(1):86–108.

290. Jamar F, et al. EANM/SNMMI guideline for 18F-FDG use in inflammation and infection. *J Nucl Med.* 2013;54(4):647–658.

291. Vaidyanathan S, et al. FDG PET/CT in infection and inflammation—current and emerging clinical applications. *Clin Radiol.* 2015;70(7):787–800.

292. Okumura W, et al. Usefulness of fasting 18F-FDG PET in identification of cardiac sarcoidosis. *J Nucl Med.* 2004;45(12):1989–1998.

293. Genovesi D, et al. The role of positron emission tomography in the assessment of cardiac sarcoidosis. *Br J Radiol.* 2019;92(1100):20190247.

294. Blankstein R, et al. Cardiac positron emission tomography enhances prognostic assessments of patients with suspected cardiac sarcoidosis. *J Am Coll Cardiol.* 2014;63(4):329–336.

295. Ohira H, et al. Myocardial imaging with 18F-fluoro-2-deoxyglucose positron emission tomography and magnetic resonance imaging in sarcoidosis. *Eur J Nucl Med Mol Imaging.* 2008;35(5):933–941.

296. Orii M, et al. Comparison of cardiac MRI and 18F-FDG positron emission tomography manifestations and regional response to corticosteroid therapy in newly diagnosed cardiac sarcoidosis with complet heart block. *Heart Rhythm.* 2015;12(12):2477–2485.

297. Bravo PE, et al. Advanced cardiovascular imaging for the evaluation of cardiac sarcoidosis. *J Nucl Cardiol.* 2019;26(1):188–199.

298. Skali H, Schulman AR, Dorbala S. 18F-FDG PET/CT for the assessment of myocardial sarcoidosis. *Curr Cardiol Rep.* 2013;15(4):352.

299. Osborne MT, et al. Patient preparation for cardiac fluorine-18 fluorodeoxyglucose positron emission tomography imaging of inflammation. *J Nucl Cardiol.* 2017;24(1):86–99.

300. American Psychiatric Association. *Diagnostic and Statistical Manual of Mental Disorders: DSM-5™.* Arlington, VA: American Psychiatric Publishing, Inc; 2013.

301. Vermunt L, et al. Duration of preclinical, prodromal, and dementia stages of Alzheimer's disease in relation to age, sex, and APOE genotype. *Alzheimers Dement.* 2019;15(7):888–898.

302. Nelson PT, et al. Alzheimer's disease is not "brain aging": neuropathological, genetic, and epidemiological human studies. *Acta Neuropathol.* 2011;121(5):571–587.

303. Foster NL, et al. FDG-PET improves accuracy in distinguishing frontotemporal dementia and Alzheimer's disease. *Brain.* 2007;130(Pt 10):2616–2635.

304. Rabinovici GD, et al. Amyloid vs. FDG-PET in the differential diagnosis of AD and FTLD. *Neurology.* 2011;77(23):2034–2042.

305. Johnson KA, et al. Appropriate use criteria for amyloid PET: a report of the Amyloid Imaging Task Force, the Society of Nuclear Medicine and Molecular Imaging, and the Alzheimer's Association. *J Nucl Med.* 2013;54(3):476–490.

306. Rabinovici GD, et al. Association of amyloid positron emission tomography with subsequent change in clinical management among medicare beneficiaries with mild cognitive impairment or dementia. *JAMA.* 2019;321(13):1286–1294.

307. Mosconi L, et al. Pre-clinical detection of Alzheimer's disease using FDG-PET, with or without amyloid imaging. *J Alzheimers Dis.* 2010;20(3):843–854.

308. Mosconi L, et al. Hippocampal hypometabolism predicts cognitive decline from normal aging. *Neurobiol Aging.* 2008;29(5):676–692.

309. Mosconi L, et al. FDG-PET changes in brain glucose metabolism from normal cognition to pathologically verified Alzheimer's disease. *Eur J Nucl Med Mol Imaging.* 2009;36(5):811–822.

310. Blass JP. Alzheimer's disease and Alzheimer's dementia: distinct but overlapping entities. *Neurobiol Aging.* 2002;23(6):1077–1084.

311. Mosconi L, et al. Multicenter standardized 18F-FDG PET diagnosis of mild cognitive impairment, Alzheimer's disease, and other dementias. *J Nucl Med.* 2008;49(3):390–398.

312. Curiati PK, et al. Age-related metabolic profiles in cognitively healthy elders: results from a voxel-based [18F]fluorodeoxyglucose-positron-emission tomography study with partial volume effects correction. *Am J Neuroradiol.* 2011;32(3):560–565.

313. Caminiti SP, et al. FDG-PET and CSF biomarker accuracy in prediction of conversion to different dementias in a large multicentre MCI cohort. *Neuroimage Clin.* 2018;18:167–177.

314. Smailagic N, et al. 18F-FDG PET for prediction of conversion to Alzheimer's disease dementia in people with mild cognitive impairment: an updated systematic review of test accuracy. *J Alzheimers Dis.* 2018;64(4):1175–1194.

315. Zhang S, et al. Diagnostic accuracy of 18 F-FDG and 11 C-PIB-PET for prediction of short-term conversion to Alzheimer's disease in subjects with mild cognitive impairment. *Int J Clin Pract.* 2012;66(2):185–198.

316. Iaccarino L, et al. A cross-validation of FDG- and amyloid-PET biomarkers in mild cognitive impairment for the risk prediction to dementia due to Alzheimer's disease in a clinical setting. *J Alzheimers Dis.* 2017;59(2):603–614.

317. Jellinger KA, Attems J. Prevalence and impact of vascular and Alzheimer pathologies in Lewy body disease. *Acta Neuropathol.* 2008;115(4):427–436.

318. Minoshima S, et al. Alzheimer's disease versus dementia with Lewy bodies: cerebral metabolic distinction with autopsy confirmation. *Ann Neurol.* 2001;50(3):358–365.

319. Firbank MJ, Lloyd J, O'Brien JT. The relationship between hallucinations and FDG-PET in dementia with Lewy bodies. *Brain Imaging Behav.* 2016;10(3):636–639.

320. Lim SM, et al. The 18F-FDG PET cingulate island sign and comparison to 123I-beta-CIT SPECT for diagnosis of dementia with Lewy bodies. *J Nucl Med.* 2009;50(10):1638–1645.

321. Pillai JA, et al. Amygdala sign, a FDG-PET signature of dementia with Lewy Bodies. *Parkinsonism Relat Disord.* 2019;64:300–303.

322. Donaghy P, Thomas AJ, O'Brien JT. Amyloid PET imaging in Lewy body disorders. *Am J Geriatr Psychiatry.* 2015;23(1):23–37.

323. Nobili F, et al. European Association of Nuclear Medicine and European Academy of Neurology recommendations for the use of brain (18) F-fluorodeoxyglucose positron emission tomography in neurodegenerative cognitive impairment and dementia: Delphi consensus. *Eur J Neurol.* 2018;25(10):1201–1217.

324. Johnson KA, et al. Imaging of amyloid burden and distribution in cerebral amyloid angiopathy. *Ann Neurol.* 2007;62(3):229–234.

325. Gurol ME, et al. Florbetapir-PET to diagnose cerebral amyloid angiopathy: a prospective study. *Neurology.* 2016;87(19):2043–2049.

326. Spehl TS, et al. Syndrome-specific patterns of regional cerebral glucose metabolism in posterior cortical atrophy in comparison to dementia with Lewy bodies and Alzheimer's disease—a [F-18]-FDG pet study. *J Neuroimaging.* 2015;25(2):281–288.

327. Whitwell JL, et al. (18)F-FDG PET in posterior cortical atrophy and dementia with Lewy bodies. *J Nucl Med.* 2017;58(4):632–638.

328. Mishina M, et al. Midbrain hypometabolism as early diagnostic sign for progressive supranuclear palsy. *Acta Neurol Scand.* 2004;110(2):128–135.

329. Blin J, et al. Positron emission tomography study in progressive supranuclear palsy. Brain hypometabolic pattern and clinicometabolic correlations. *Arch Neurol.* 1990;47(7):747–752.

330. Bergeron D, et al. Prevalence of amyloid-beta pathology in distinct variants of primary progressive aphasia. *Ann Neurol.* 2018;84(5):729–740.

331. Fisher RS, et al. ILAE official report: a practical clinical definition of epilepsy. *Epilepsia.* 2014;55(4):475–482.

332. Fisher RS, et al. Operational classification of seizure types by the International League Against Epilepsy: position paper of the ILAE commission for classification and terminology. *Epilepsia.* 2017;58(4):522–530.

333. Fiest KM, et al. Prevalence and incidence of epilepsy: a systematic review and meta-analysis of international studies. *Neurology.* 2017;88(3):296–303.

334. Englot DJ, et al. Seizure outcomes after resective surgery for extratemporal lobe epilepsy in pediatric patients. *J Neurosurg Pediatr.* 2013;12(2):126–133.

335. Wyllie E, et al. Seizure outcome after epilepsy surgery in children and adolescents. *Ann Neurol.* 1998;44(5):740–748.

336. Vossel KA, et al. Epileptic activity in Alzheimer's disease: causes and clinical relevance. *Lancet Neurol.* 2017;16(4):311–322.

337. Sapkota S, et al. Close to 1 million US adults aged 55years or older have active epilepsy-National Health Interview Survey, 2010, 2013, and 2015. *Epilepsy Behav.* 2018;87:233–234.

338. Kalilani L, et al. The epidemiology of drug-resistant epilepsy: a systematic review and meta-analysis. *Epilepsia.* 2018;59(12):2179–2193.

339. Perucca P, Hesdorffer DC, Gilliam FG. Response to first antiepileptic drug trial predicts health outcome in epilepsy. *Epilepsia.* 2011;52(12):2209–2215.

340. Del Felice A, et al. Early versus late remission in a cohort of patients with newly diagnosed epilepsy. *Epilepsia.* 2010;51(1):37–42.

341. Rosenow F, Luders H. Presurgical evaluation of epilepsy. *Brain.* 2001;124(Pt 9):1683–1700.

342. Dallas J, Englot DJ, Naftel RP. Neurosurgical approaches to pediatric epilepsy: indications, techniques, and outcomes of common surgical procedures. *Seizure.* 2018.

343. Wiebe S, et al. A randomized, controlled trial of surgery for temporal-lobe epilepsy. *N Engl J Med.* 2001;345(5):311–318.

344. McIntosh AM, Wilson SJ, Berkovic SF. Seizure outcome after temporal lobectomy: current research practice and findings. *Epilepsia.* 2001;42(10):1288–1307.

345. Janszky J, et al. Temporal lobe epilepsy with hippocampal sclerosis: predictors for long-term surgical outcome. *Brain.* 2005;128(Pt 2):395–404.

346. Arya R, et al. Long-term seizure outcomes after pediatric temporal lobectomy: does brain MRI lesion matter? *J Neurosurg Pediatr.* 2019;24(2):200–208.

347. Mariani V, et al. Prognostic factors of postoperative seizure outcome in patients with temporal lobe epilepsy and normal magnetic resonance imaging. *J Neurol.* 2019;266(9):2144–2156.

348. Devous MD Sr, et al. SPECT brain imaging in epilepsy: a meta-analysis. *J Nucl Med.* 1998;39(2):285–293.

349. Leiderman DB, et al. The dynamics of metabolic change following seizures as measured by positron emission tomography with fludeoxyglucose F 18. *Arch Neurol.* 1994;51(9):932–936.

350. Gok B, et al. The evaluation of FDG-PET imaging for epileptogenic focus localization in patients with MRI positive and MRI negative temporal lobe epilepsy. *Neuroradiology.* 2013;55(5):541–550.

351. Menon RN, et al. Does F-18 FDG-PET substantially alter the surgical decision-making in drug-resistant partial epilepsy? *Epilepsy Behav.* 2015;51:133–139.

352. Capraz IY, et al. Surgical outcome in patients with MRI-negative, PET-positive temporal lobe epilepsy. *Seizure.* 2015;29:63–68.

353. Shin JH, et al. Prognostic factors determining poor postsurgical outcomes of mesial temporal lobe epilepsy. *PLoS One.* 2018;13(10):e0206095.

354. D'Argenzio L, et al. Seizure outcome after extratemporal epilepsy surgery in childhood. *Dev Med Child Neurol.* 2012;54(11):995–1000.

355. da Silva EA, et al. Identification of frontal lobe epileptic foci in children using positron emission tomography. *Epilepsia.* 1997;38(11):1198–1208.

356. Chassoux F, et al. Type II focal cortical dysplasia: electroclinical phenotype and surgical outcome related to imaging. *Epilepsia.* 2012;53(2):349–358.

357. Chassoux F, et al. FDG-PET improves surgical outcome in negative MRI Taylor-type focal cortical dysplasias. *Neurology.* 2010;75(24):2168–2175.

358. Tomas J, et al. The predictive value of hypometabolism in focal epilepsy: a prospective study in surgical candidates. *Eur J Nucl Med Mol Imaging.* 2019;46(9):1806–1816.

359. Schur S, et al. Significance of FDG-PET hypermetabolism in children with intractable focal epilepsy. *Pediatr Neurosurg.* 2018;53(3):153–162.

360. Morioka T, et al. Functional imaging in periventricular nodular heterotopia with the use of FDG-PET and HMPAO-SPECT. *Neurosurg Rev.* 1999;22(1):41–44.

361. Calabria FF, et al. Ictal 18F-FDG PET/MRI in a patient with cortical heterotopia and focal epilepsy. *Clin Nucl Med.* 2017;42(10):768–769.

362. Vivash L, et al. 18F-flumazenil: a gamma-aminobutyric acid A-specific PET radiotracer for the localization of drug-resistant temporal lobe epilepsy. *J Nucl Med.* 2013;54(8):1270–1277.

363. Sarikaya I. PET studies in epilepsy. *Am J Nucl Med Mol Imaging.* 2015;5(5):416–430.

364. Yamaguchi S, et al. The diagnostic role of (18)F-FDG PET for primary central nervous system lymphoma. *Ann Nucl Med.* 2014;28(7):603–609.

365. Zhou W, et al. (18)F-FDG PET/CT in immunocompetent patients with primary central nervous system lymphoma: differentiation from glioblastoma and correlation with DWI. *Eur J Radiol.* 2018;104:26–32.

366. Kawai N, et al. Prognostic value of pretreatment 18F-FDG PET in patients with primary central nervous system lymphoma: SUV-based assessment. *J Neurooncol.* 2010;100(2):225–232.

367. Li L, Rong JH, Feng J. Neuroradiological features of lymphomatosis cerebri: a systematic review of the English literature with a new case report. *Oncol Lett.* 2018;16(2):1463–1474.

368. Kawai N, et al. Use of PET in the diagnosis of primary CNS lymphoma in patients with atypical MR findings. *Ann Nucl Med.* 2010;24(5):335–343.

369. Malani R, et al. Staging identifies non-CNS malignancies in a large cohort with newly diagnosed lymphomatous brain lesions. *Leuk Lymphoma.* 2019;60(9):2278–2282.

370. Ostrom QT, et al. Adult glioma incidence and survival by race or ethnicity in the United States from 2000 to 2014. *JAMA Oncol.* 2018;4(9):1254–1262.

371. Kosaka N, et al. 18F-FDG PET of common enhancing malignant brain tumors. *Am J Roentgenol.* 2008;190(6):W365–W369.

372. Tralins KS, et al. Volumetric analysis of 18F-FDG PET in glioblastoma multiforme: prognostic information and possible role in definition of target volumes in radiation dose escalation. *J Nucl Med.* 2002;43(12):1667–1673.

373. Zhang Q, et al. Prognostic value of MTV, SUVmax and the T/N ratio of PET/CT in patients with glioma: a systematic review and meta-analysis. *J Cancer.* 2019;10(7):1707–1716.

374. Dunet V, et al. Performance of 18F-FET versus 18F-FDG-PET for the diagnosis and grading of brain tumors: systematic review and meta-analysis. *Neuro Oncol.* 2016;18(3):426–434.

375. Gross MW, et al. The value of F-18-fluorodeoxyglucose PET for the 3-D radiation treatment planning of malignant gliomas. *Int J Radiat Oncol Biol Phys.* 1998;41(5):989–995.

376. Wakabayashi T, et al. Diagnostic performance and safety of positron emission tomography using (18)F-Fluciclovine in patients with clinically suspected high- or low-grade gliomas: a multicenter phase IIb trial. *Asia Ocean J Nucl Med Biol.* 2017;5(1):10–21.

377. Grosu AL, et al. L-(methyl-11C) methionine positron emission tomography for target delineation in resected high-grade gliomas before radiotherapy. *Int J Radiat Oncol Biol Phys.* 2005;63(1):64–74.

378. Miwa K, et al. Re-irradiation of recurrent glioblastoma multiforme using 11C-methionine PET/CT/MRI image fusion for hypofractionated stereotactic radiotherapy by intensity modulated radiation therapy. *Radiat Oncol.* 2014;9:181.

379. Zhao F, et al. (18)F-Fluorothymidine PET-CT for resected malignant gliomas before radiotherapy: tumor extent according to proliferative activity compared with MRI. *PLoS One.* 2015;10(3):e0118769.

380. Law I, et al. Joint EANM/EANO/RANO practice guidelines/SNMMI procedure standards for imaging of gliomas using PET with radiolabelled amino acids and [(18)F]FDG: version 1.0. *Eur J Nucl Med Mol Imaging.* 2019;46(3):540–557.

381. Rozental JM, et al. Early changes in tumor metabolism after treatment: the effects of stereotactic radiotherapy. *Int J Radiat Oncol Biol Phys.* 1991;20(5):1053–1060.

382. Spence AM, et al. 2-[(18)F]Fluoro-2-deoxyglucose and glucose uptake in malignant gliomas before and after radiotherapy: correlation with outcome. *Clin Cancer Res.* 2002;8(4):971–979.

383. Charnley N, et al. Early change in glucose metabolic rate measured using FDG-PET in patients with high-grade glioma predicts response to temozolomide but not temozolomide plus radiotherapy. *Int J Radiat Oncol Biol Phys.* 2006;66(2):331–338.

384. Nihashi T, Dahabreh IJ, Terasawa T. Diagnostic accuracy of PET for recurrent glioma diagnosis: a meta-analysis. *Am J Neuroradiol.* 2013;34(5):944–950.

385. Albert NL, et al. Response Assessment in Neuro-Oncology Working Group and European Association for Neuro-Oncology recommendations for the clinical use of PET imaging in gliomas. *Neuro Oncol.* 2016;18(9):1199–1208.

386. Ogawa T, et al. Carbon-11-methionine PET evaluation of intracerebral hematoma: distinguishing neoplastic from non-neoplastic hematoma. *J Nucl Med.* 1995;36(12):2175–2179.

387. Galldiks N, et al. Diagnosis of pseudoprogression in patients with glioblastoma using O-(2-[18F]fluoroethyl)-L-tyrosine PET. *Eur J Nucl Med Mol Imaging.* 2015;42(5):685–695.

388. Kebir S, et al. Late pseudoprogression in glioblastoma: diagnostic value of dynamic O-(2-[18F]fluoroethyl)-L-tyrosine PET. *Clin Cancer Res.* 2016;22(9):2190–2196.

389. Chiba Y, et al. Use of (11)C-methionine PET parametric response map for monitoring WT1 immunotherapy response in recurrent malignant glioma. *J Neurosurg.* 2012;116(4):835–842.

390. Kebir S, et al. Dynamic O-(2-[18F]fluoroethyl)-L-tyrosine PET imaging for the detection of checkpoint inhibitor-related pseudoprogression in melanoma brain metastases. *Neuro Oncol.* 2016;18(10):1462–1464.

391. Parghane RV, Talole S, Basu S. Prevalence of hitherto unknown brain meningioma detected on (68)Ga-DOTATATE positron-emission tomography/computed tomography in patients with metastatic neuroendocrine tumor and exploring potential of (177)Lu-DOTATATE peptide receptor radionuclide therapy as single-shot treatment approach targeting both tumors. *World J Nucl Med.* 2019;18(2):160–170.

392. Ivanidze J, et al. Gallium-68 DOTATATE PET in the evaluation of intracranial meningiomas. *J Neuroimaging.* 2019;29(5):650–656.

393. Papadakis GZ, et al. 18F-FDG and 68Ga-DOTATATE PET/CT in von Hippel-Lindau disease-associated retinal hemangioblastoma. *Clin Nucl Med.* 2017;42(3):189–190.

CHAPTER SELF-ASSESSMENT QUESTIONS

1. Which statement is false in relation to PET/CT and PET/MRI?

   A. PET/MRI is associated with higher radiation exposure.

   B. PET/MRI may be preferred over PET/CT where the unique features of MRI provide more robust imaging evaluation in certain clinical settings.

   C. Radiotracers that can be used with PET/CT can also generally be used with PET/MRI.

2. PET/CT with a relevant radiotracer is useful in the imaging evaluation of:

   A. Alzheimer's disease

   B. Myocardial viability

   C. Prostate cancer

   D. All of the above

3. Which pairing is incorrect:

   A. Florbetapir & Alzheimer

   B. FDG and myocardial viability

   C. Flurpiridaz & prostate cancer

   D. NaF & bone

Answers to Chapter Self-Assessment Questions

1. A. PET/MRI is in fact associated with less radiation exposure in view of lack of CT radiation. Answers B and C are true statements.

2. D. PET/CT may be used in the imaging evaluation of AD with a number of radiotracers including FDG, amyloid agents (e.g., florbetapir) and tau agents (e.g., flortaucipir). Myocardial viability is assessed with FDG PET. There are also a number of PET tracers relevant to imaging evaluation of prostate cancer (e.g., radiocholine-, fluciclovine-, PSMA-based agents)

3. C. Flurpiridaz is an investigation PET agent for myocardial perfusion imaging. All the other pairing of PET radiotracer and clinical condition is correct.

Lymphoscintigraphy

15

Patrick M. Colletti

LEARNING OBJECTIVES

1. Describe the principles of lymphoscintigraphy.
2. Explain cancer lymphatic drainage and the principle of sentinel node biopsy.
3. Interpret lymphoscintigraphy in patients with lymphedema.
4. Explain the principles for reverse lymphatic mapping.

LYMPHOSCINTIGRAPHY PRINCIPLES

Lymphoscintigraphy radiopharmaceuticals are radioactive particles that enter and move along lymphatic channels upon intradermal, subcutaneous, or intratissue injection.

Classical cancer surgery most often involved removal of the primary tumor and excision of the lymph nodes in the tumor's most likely nodal drainage basins. While more complete nodal excisions statistically resulted in improved outcomes, the majority of the excised nodes did not harbor cancer cells. Moreover, a substantial number of patients developed lymphedema in the extremities that shared nodal drainage basins with the tumor. Thus, surgeons began to perform nodal labeling with injected methylene blue at the time of surgery. The idea was to tag, locate, and sample only the primary or sentinel nodes draining the tumor (1). If these sentinel nodes were positive, nodal resection was performed; if not, no further nodal dissection was performed. While lymph node labeling with methylene blue is practical, it may be difficult to locate deeper nodes with this visual technique. Thus, lymphoscintigraphy was developed with the use of radioactive particle scintigraphy and intraoperative localization with the use of surgical gamma probes. Figure 15.1 demonstrates how an abdominal melanoma may spread along lymphatics to either axilla or groin nodes. Generally, if the first or sentinel node is cancer free, secondary nodes will also be cancer free and therefore do not require surgical sampling (2).

Table 15.1 compares the ^{99m}Tc-based radiopharmaceutical agents that have been used for lymphoscintigraphy (3). Filtered ^{99m}Tc-sulfur colloid is most commonly used in the United States, while other colloids such as antimony trisulfide (Lymph-Flo®) and nanocolloidal albumin (Nanocoll®) are more commonly used in Europe. These agents are radioactive nanoparticles and when injected into tissue, they are mobilized along lymphatic channels. Smaller particles move more rapidly than larger particles with typical lymphatic flow rates of 30 mm/min.

^{99m}Tc-tilmanocept (Lymphoseek®) is an alternative small molecule (7 nm) agent which binds to CD206 receptor specific

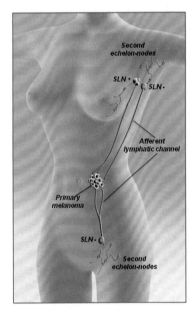

FIG. 15.1 ● Schematic representation of the sentinel lymph node (SLN) concept, defined as the lymphatic station first encountered by tumor cells entering the lymphatic circulation. Photograph shows a primary cutaneous melanoma of the left abdominal wall and some afferent lymphatic channels draining to a left inguinal SLN (negative for the presence of metastases [SLNj]) and to two left axillary SLNs (one of which is positive for the presence of melanoma cells [SLN+]). SLN+, SLN positive for the presence of melanoma cells; SLNj, SLN negative for the presence of melanoma cells. Reprinted with permission from Manca et al. (2).

to reticuloendothelial cells including lymph nodes. As a small molecule, tilmanocept moves more rapidly than nanoparticles. As a CD206 receptor binding agent, tilmanocept may tag less

Table 15.1 **CHARACTERISTICS OF [99M]TC-BASED RADIOPHARMACEUTICALS**

Agent	Maximum Particle Size (nm)	Particle Size Range (nm)
Tilmanocept (Lymphoseek®)	About 7 (equivalence)	About 7 (equivalence)
Antimony trisulfide (Lymph-Flo®)	80	5–30
Sulfide nanocolloid (Lymphoscint®)	100	10–50
Nanocolloidal albumin (Nanocoll®)	100	5–80
Rhenium sulfide (Nanocis®)	500	50–200
Tin colloid	800	30–250
Labeled dextran	800	10–400
Hydroxyethyl starch	1,000	100–1,000
Stannous phytate	1,200	200–400
Sulfur colloid (Sulfur colloid®)	5,000 (unfiltered)	100–200 (filtered)
Comparison of Nuclear Medicine-Labeled Particles		
Technigas™	3,000 (with clumping)	30–60
DTPA radioaerosol	1,000	200–1,000
Red blood cell	7,000	7,000
MAA	90,000	20,000–50,000
SIR-Spheres® Y-90 resin microspheres	60,000	20,000–60,000
TheraSphere® Glass Microspheres	25,000	20,000–30,000

This table shows the comparison of the ^{99m}Tc-based radiopharmaceutical agents that have been used for lymphoscintigraphy. Other particle-like nuclear medicine agents are also included for comparison. Reprinted by permission of Springer: Bluemel et al. (3). Copyright © 2015 Springer Nature.

DTPA, diethylene triamine pentaacetic acid; MAA, macro-aggregated albumin.

secondary nodes, thus potentially sparing less fruitful nodal excisions (4).

In addition, many patients find the small volume intradermal and subcutaneous injections of tilmanocept to be less painful as compared to filtered ^{99m}Tc-sulfur colloid.

Cancer lymphatic drainage

Classically, lymphoscintigraphy was initially applied to breast cancer and melanoma sentinel nodal identification. The tracer injection may be administered in the operating room without imaging or in the nuclear medicine department immediately before or the day before surgery with or without imaging. The dose is typically 1 mCi if surgery is to be performed immediately, while 2 to 4 mCi may be given if surgery is to be delayed for one or more ^{99m}Tc half-life.

Breast lymphoscintigraphy as shown in Figure 15.2 is generally performed with subareolar tracer administration followed by scintigraphy and intraoperative gamma probe in-situ detection and confirmation (5).

Melanoma lymphoscintigraphy is performed with intradermal tracer administration followed by gamma camera views of all possible draining lymph node basins (6,7).

Figure 15.3 demonstrates lymphoscintigraphy images of a patient with a melanoma in the center of her back. Posterior views demonstrate multiple radioactive lymph channels draining to multiple nodes in both axillae. Anterior views of the pelvis and groin show no sentinel nodes in either inguinal area. Thus, the surgeon sampled the multiple nodes in both axillae without sampling any inguinal nodes.

While intradermal radiocolloid administration is typically performed for melanoma lymph node mapping, breast cancer may also be mapped via intradermal tracer administration,

though with more patient discomfort and less opportunity to demonstrate internal mamillary nodal drainage.

Other tumors including head and neck cancers, thyroid cancer, and pelvic cancers may be lymph nodal mapped with intra- or per-tumoral injections.

LYMPHEDEMA

Lymphedema is caused by the accumulation of lymph fluid within tissues at a rate greater than the capacity for drainage (Fig. 15.4).

Lymphoscintigraphy for lymphedema is typically performed with the administration of tracer into the web spaces of the hand or foot of the extremities of interest. Sequential gamma camera views of the extremities of interest demonstrate lymphatic drainage.

The lymphoscintigraphic demonstration of lymphedema is based on the identification of (Figs. 15.5 and 15.6) (8):

1. delayed or asymmetric lymph transport;
2. "dermal backflow" to dermal lymphatics;
3. collateral lymphatic channels;
4. non-visualized or reduced lymph channels or nodes; and
5. crossover nodal filling.

REVERSE LYMPHATIC MAPPING

Reverse lymphatic mapping is performed by injecting radiotracer into the hands or feet of interest. The lymph nodes draining the extremity of interest are identified in the operating room with the use of a gamma probe. These radioactive nodes are not sampled or harvested for vascularized lymph node transplant, thus

FIG. 15.2 ● Routine breast lymphoscintigraphy. **(A)** The initial right breast injection with identification of the main draining lymph channel. **(B)** The injection site and lymphatic channel with transmission scan body localization. **(C)** The injection site, main lymphatic, and the single right axillary node. **(D)** The injection site out of view with clear identification of the right axillary sentinel node.

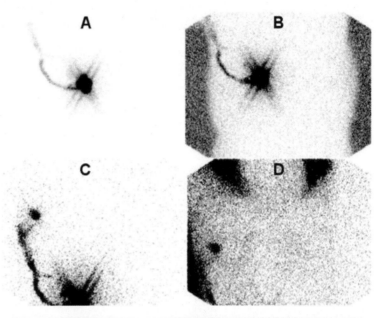

FIG. 15.3 ● Lymphoscintigraphy images of a patient with a melanoma in the center of her back. Posterior view (right) demonstrates multiple radioactive lymph channels draining to multiple nodes in both axillae. Anterior views (left) of the head, neck, and chest show axillary nodes bilaterally (arrows), whereas abdomen, pelvis, and groin views show no sentinel nodes. Thus, the surgeon sampled multiple nodes in both axillae without sampling any inguinal nodes.

RT.

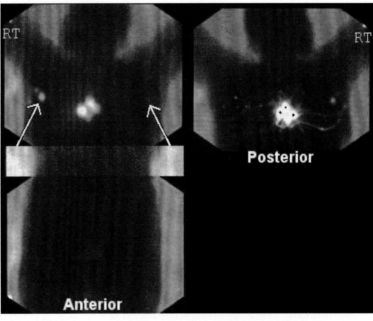

FIG. 15.4 ● Mass balance for lymphatic flow.

SV.

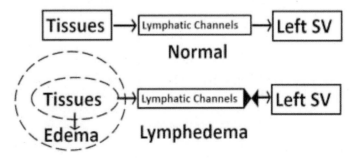

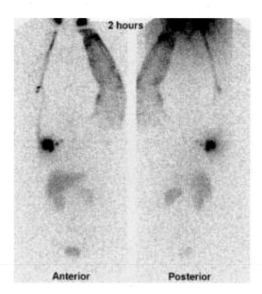

FIG. 15.5 ● Anterior and posterior views show left upper extremity lymphedema after axillary dissection for breast cancer. The right upper extremity shows normal lymph channels and axillary lymph nodes.

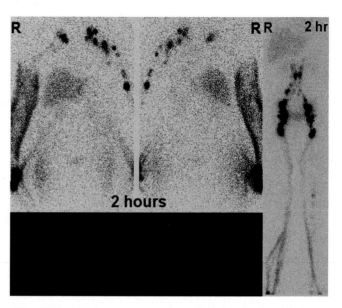

FIG. 15.7 ● Demonstrates upper extremity lymphedema (left) and lower extremity reverse mapping (right). The reverse mapping labels the radioactive nodes which drain the lower extremities. The surgeon harvested a nonradioactive node for vascular nodal transplant into the patient's right axilla. R, right side.

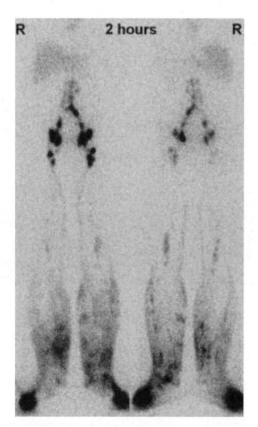

FIG. 15.6 ● Bilateral swollen lower extremities with lymphedema and dermal backflow of unknown cause. R, right side.

reducing the risk of further post-procedural lymphedema (9,10). Figure 15.7 demonstrates upper extremity lymphedema and lower extremity reverse mapping. The reverse mapping demonstrates the radioactive nodes which drain the lower extremities. The surgeon harvested a nonradioactive node for vascular nodal transplant into the patient's right axilla.

References

1. Nieweg OE, Tanis PJ, Kroon BB. The definition of a sentinel node. *Ann Surg Oncol.* 2001;8:538–541.
2. Manca G, Rubello D, Romanini A, Boni G, Chiacchio S, Tredici M, Mazzarri S, Duce V, Colletti PM, Volterrani D, Mariani G. Sentinel lymph node mapping in melanoma: the issue of false-negative findings. *Clin Nucl Med.* 2014;39:e346–e354.
3. Bluemel C, Herrmann K, Giammarile F, et al. EANM practice guidelines for lymphoscintigraphy and sentinel lymph node biopsy in melanoma. *Eur J Nucl Med Mol Imaging.* 2015;42(11):1750–1766.
4. Wallace AM, Hoh CK, Limmer KK, Darrah DD, Schulteis G, Vera DR. Sentinel lymph node accumulation of Lymphoseek and Tc-99m-sulfur colloid using a "2-day" protocol. *Nucl Med Biol.* 2009;36(6):687–692.
5. Kim T, Giuliano AE, Lyman GH. Lymphatic mapping and sentinel lymph node biopsy in early-stage breast carcinoma: a metaanalysis. *Cancer.* 2006 Jan 1;106(1):4–16.
6. Morton DL, Thompson JF, Cochran AJ, et al. Sentinel-node biopsy or nodal observation in melanoma. *N Engl J Med.* 2006;355:1307–1317.
7. Morton DL, Wen DR, Wong JH, et al. Technical details of intraoperative lymphatic mapping for early stage melanoma. *Arch Surg.* 1992;127:392–399.
8. Kleinhans E, Baumeister RGH, Hahn D, et al. Evaluation of transport kinetics in lymphoscintigraphy: follow-up study in patients with transplanted lymphatic vessels. *Eur J Nucl Med.* 1985;10:349–352.
9. Weiss M, Baumeister RG, Hahn K. Dynamic lymph flow imaging in patients with oedema of the lower limb for evaluation of the functional outcome after autologous lymph vessel transplantation: an 8-year follow-up study. *Eur J Nucl Med.* 2003;30:202–206.
10. Gandhi SJ, Satish C, Sundaram PS, et al. Axillary reverse mapping using ^{99m}Tc-SC: a case illustration. *Clin Nucl Med.* 2014 Oct;39(10):e428–e430.
11. Uçmak Vural G, Şahiner I, Demirtaş S, Efetürk H, Demirel BB. Sentinel lymph node detection in contralateral axilla at initial presentation of a breast cancer patient: case report. *Mol Imaging Radionucl Ther.* 2015;24(2):90–93.
12. Manca G, Volterrani D, Mazzarri S, et al. Sentinel lymph node mapping in breast cancer: a critical reappraisal of the internal mammary chain issue. *Q J Nucl Med Mol Imaging.* 2014;58(2):114–126.

CHAPTER SELF-ASSESSMENT QUESTIONS

1. In the image earlier, which letter represents aberrant lymphatic drainage?

2. In the image earlier, which letter represents internal mammillary drainage?

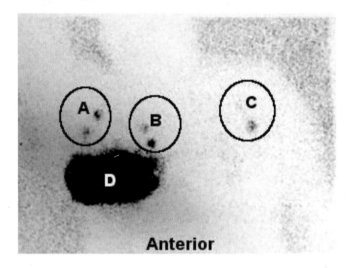

Anterior

Answers to Chapter Self-Assessment Questions

1. A   represents right axillary sentinel lymph nodes.

2. B   represents the ipsilateral internal mammary sentinel lymph nodes.

3. C   represents aberrant contralateral sentinel lymph nodes.

4. D   is the injection sites in right breast. The diffuse configuration is due to tracer spreading after massage.

Thus, the best answer to question 1 is "C", contralateral breast sentinel lymph nodes.

The best answer to question 2 is "B", ipsilateral internal mammary sentinel lymph nodes.

Radio-Theranostics 16

Carina Mari Aparici and Farshad Moradi

LEARNING OBJECTIVES

1. Define radio-theranostics and how it can contribute to precision medicine.
2. Provide several examples of radio-theranostics in various clinical settings.
3. Describe advantages and limitations of radio-theranostics.

INTRODUCTION

The term theranostics or theragnostics is a portmanteau word derived from the Greek meaning therapy (therapo) and diagnosis/knowledge (gnosis) (1).

Emerging as a specific, safe, and efficient molecular-targeted discipline, theranostics focuses on patient-centered care. It provides a transition from conventional medicine to personalized medicine at the molecular diagnostic and therapeutic level. In the theranostics approach, the first phase is diagnostic, whereas a molecular probe is introduced in the body to obtain high-quality images of a disease (usually malignancies) based on the targeting of a specific biomarker. This phase is followed by the delivery of personalized therapy to the patient, based on the introduction in the body of the same molecular probe (therefore identical biodistribution) although this time with therapeutic properties. The ability to image the molecular and biological pathways of specific diseases/malignancies in the body with these paired probes allows the development of a more selective diagnostic and therapeutic plan tailored to every individual's disease.

The term theranostics started to appear sporadically in the medical literature at the end of the last century and has steadily increased in frequency of usage (2). Although there are theoretically several theranostic platforms, such as radio-theranostics (the use of radioactive material in the theranostic domain), nanotheranostics, optotheranostics, and magnetotheranostics; radio-theranostics (also known as theranostics by itself), is the only one that is used in the everyday clinical arena. Its unique approach of using targeted-probes already known to the body, in less than microgram levels, labeled with diagnostic or therapeutic natural radiation-emitters of high or low penetration, allows to diagnose or produce a very efficient treatment by trying to target each cell individually, with as low toxicity as possible to healthy (non-targeted) tissues. Thus, theranostics is a holistic evolution from trial and error medicine to informative, predictive, and personalized medicine. In that sense, it achieves the goal of precision medicine, by tailoring and optimizing therapies based on specific characteristics and biology of an individual patient's disease at the molecular level.

Radio-theranostic pairs

The "concept" of theranostics is not novel to Nuclear Medicine and Molecular Imaging, since radio-theranostics has been an integral part of it since its inception. The backbone of radio-theranostics is the use of a "*pair*" of chemically and structurally identical or nearly identical radiopharmaceuticals labeled with different isotopes, one for molecular diagnostic imaging and other for molecular targeted radionuclide therapy (TRT) of the same disease. A general approach is to use different radioisotopes of the same periodic element (e.g., I^{124} for diagnosis and I^{131} for therapeutics), or the same molecular probe, and label it with different radionuclides based on their diagnostic versus therapeutic properties.

From a puristic point of view, radiolabeling can somehow affect reaction rates and uptake properties of biochemicals compounds; however, as long as the relevant reaction rates (e.g., binding affinity to the receptor) remain fairly similar (e.g., ^{68}Ga-DOTATATE and ^{177}Lu-DOTATATE), it follows the theranostic principle. Theoretically, as the degree of similarity between diagnostic and therapeutic chemicals decreases (even with change in domains that do not directly participate in the reactions), their potential to be used in theranostic applications can be affected. Therefore, the "ideal" theranostic pair would use different isotopes of the same element that are optimal for imaging and therapy (e.g., ^{86}Y and ^{90}Y), respectively. In this case, there is virtually no difference in chemical properties for different isotopes of the same element (excluding hydrogen/deuterium). These "ideal" theranostic pairs have identical reaction rates in the body. The only difference in physical and physiological effects will be due to differences in physical half-life and decay limiting the time course of pharmacokinetics of the radiopharmaceutical and its metabolites.

The quality of the emitting radiation of the radionuclides involved in the theranostic pair is key in their selection for diagnosis or therapy. Each element of the pair should have the radio-emission properties that make it more ideal for a diagnostic or therapeutic purpose of the same molecular target. Gamma rays are useful for imaging (diagnosis) since they have very low tissue

Table 16.1 **RADIONUCLIDES OF POSSIBLE USE IN THERAPEUTIC THERANOSTICS**

Radionuclide	Half-life	Energy (MeV)	Max range	Other
^{131}I	8 d	0.606 (β^-)	2 mm	γ (81%, 364 keV)
^{177}Lu	6.65 d	0.498 (β^-)	1.7 mm	γ (17%, 130/208 keV)
^{90}Y	2.7 d	2.28 (β^-)	11 mm	Bremsstrahlung radiation
^{223}Ra	11.4 d	5–7.5 (α)	<100 µm	β^- (3.6%), γ (1.1%)
^{225}Ac	10 d	5.9 (α)	<100 µm	β^-, γ (218 keV, 440 keV)
^{213}Bi	46 min	6 (α)	<100 µm	γ (440 keV)

absorption and energy transfer, and very long path lengths, resulting in lower radiation to the target and increased but low-level energy radiation to surrounding tissue (emitted for example by ^{123}I). Beta particles on the other hand (emitted for example by ^{131}I, ^{177}Lu, and ^{90}Y) have higher energy transfer to the target (0.2–2 keV/µm) at path lengths that can be up to 11 mm (Table 16.1). Alpha particles (emitted for example by ^{223}Ra) have very high energy transfer (80 keV/µm) and very short path lengths (<100 µm), which are usually the diameter of a few cells. Beta emitters have been proposed for large-/mid-size metastases for the reasons discussed earlier, whereas alpha emitters are considered more advantageous in non-solid tumors and micrometastases. Auger electron emitters (emitted for example by ^{111}In) can be used for therapy as well, although Auger electrons are generally less effective due to very short path length (2–500 nm) and low energy deposition (4–26 keV/mm), and the radionuclide usually needs to be intra-cellular to be effective. Having said all that, rarely a radionuclide has a single type of emission. Most of them have a combination of two or more types of emissions with different abundancies. This property actually makes some of these radionuclides amenable, although not ideal, for both diagnostic and therapeutic purposes. For instance, some beta emitters used for therapy also emit gamma photons and can be used to confirm the molecular targeting after therapy or even dosimetry (e.g., ^{131}I and ^{177}Lu).

Targeted radionuclide therapy—the "thera" component of the pair

Targeted radionuclide therapy (TRT) is currently a growing treatment option for malignancies. High-affinity molecular probes that carry the radionuclide with therapeutic properties to specific tumor cells based on targeted biomarkers can minimize accumulation of radionuclide in non-target tissues, and therefore significantly reduce side effects. The ideal carrier should have high affinity and specificity for the biomarker expressed by these targeted cells. Commonly used carriers in TRT may include analogs, agonists, or antagonists to selective transporters (e.g., ^{131}I-MIBG acting as a norepinephrine analogue), to selective peptide receptors (e.g., somatostatin receptors type 2 [SSTR2] in PRRT [peptide receptor radiation therapy] with ^{177}Lu-DOTATATE), ligands of membrane proteins/enzymes (e.g., ^{177}Lu-PSMA) or monoclonal antibodies (e.g., radioimmunotherapy with ^{90}Y-ibritumomab tiuxetan).

Internalization and trapping of the radionuclide inside the cell can potentiate the effect of the therapy although is not a requirement. Radiolabeled ligands and small peptides have significant pharmacokinetics advantages to larger molecules such as antibodies or antibody fragments due to faster uptake, more rapid clearance from blood pool activity (particularly resulting in lower radiation to bone marrow), and better penetration in tumors with reduced vascularity, therefore increasing effectiveness and reducing radiation to benign tissues and possible side effect.

The therapeutic effect of ionizing radiation is due to irreversible DNA strand breaks and free radicals. A double-strand break often results in failure to repair DNA and non-viable cells die through induced programmed cell death (apoptosis) (3). Alpha-particles cause irreversible DNA damage if two to three tracks transit the cross-section of the DNA structure, compared to 100 to 1000 tracks for beta-particles (4). Beta-emitting radionuclides are considered to have lower efficacy for tumor micro-deposits than alpha-emitting radionuclides due to its lower linear energy transfer. However, for larger lesions, the "cross-fire" effect between neighboring cells significantly increases the probability of ionization and DNA damage. The "cross-fire" effect is very effective in tumors that have mixed cellularity, some of which no longer expresses the desired molecular target. However, as long as these cells can be within the range of the emitting radiation of the targeted cells, they will also be treated. In addition, radiation and disruption of tumor stroma further contribute to the therapeutic effect. In certain circumstances, long-range penetration is crucial as penetrating radiation can reach cells within the tumor that are difficult to access by the radionuclide, for example, in cases of poorly vascularized tumoral cells. The "cross-fire" effect however is also responsible for causing collateral damage to adjacent benign cells within the range of ionizing radiation from targeted cells, which therefore may cause clinical toxicity and has to be accounted for. The "cross-fire" effect obviously increases with the range of the emitting therapeutic radiation (^{90}Y >> ^{131}I > ^{177}Lu >> ^{223}Ra).

Pseudo–radio-theranostic pairs

Generally, as the degree of similarity between diagnostic and therapeutic chemicals decreases (even with change in domains that do not directly participate in the reactions), their potential to be used in theranostic applications can be affected. In contrast, different biomarkers that target closely linked molecular mechanisms are sometimes very useful as diagnostic–therapeutic pairs. An example is ^{99m}Tc-methylene diphosphonate (a bisphosphonate) and ^{223}Ra-dichloride (a calcium analogue). Both have high uptake in areas of bone remodeling and bind to new bone formation, and therefore can be used for diagnosis and treatment of osteoblastic osseous metastatic lesions, respectively. Although the "strict" definition of radio-theranostics does not encompass these compounds, they definitely seem to work "functionally" as a theranostic tandem or what could be called a "pseudo-theranostic" pair.

Tc^{99m}-biphosphonate-radium^{223} — bone-seeking pseudo-theranostic pairs

There is a long history of radionuclides being used for imaging and treatment of osteoblastic bone lesions and their pain. The skeleton is a common site of metastasis for certain cancers such as breast and prostate carcinoma, and in most malignancies, they result in increased osseous turnover at the site of the lesion (osteoblastic metastases). This property enables radiopharmaceuticals such as Tc^{99m}-biphosphonates, ^{18}F-NaF, or calcium analogues that get incorporated into the newly formed bone matrix to achieve high uptake in skeletal metastases. Tc^{99m}-biphosphonates, such as Tc^{99m}-MDP, are still the most commonly used radiopharmaceuticals for bone scintigraphy despite the diagnostic superiority of ^{18}F-NaF. They have high sensitivity and specificity compared to conventional imaging for detection and characterization of malignant osteoblastic involvement.

^{223}Ra-dichloride (Xofigo®) is currently the most commonly used radionuclide for bone-targeted therapies. Xofigo® is the first alpha-emitter approved in 2013 by the food and drug administration (FDA) for clinical use. Although ^{223}Ra-dichloride has been approved for treatment of symptomatic bone metastases in castration-resistant prostate cancer whereas, it can also potentially provide a therapeutic alternative in osteoblastic bone metastases of any other malignancy. As a calcium analogue, radium binds to newly formed hydroxyapatite crystals in areas of increased osseous turnover without directly targeting cancer cells but placing itself intimately adjacent to them. Due to the very short path length of the alpha particle emission, its therapeutic effect is primarily due to the disruption of tumor–stroma interaction rather than radiation to malignant cells (5). Consequently, tumor markers such as prostate specific antigen (PSA) are not reliable for response assessment and may lag treatment effects such as reduced bone pain (typically seen after 2 weeks) or decreased alkaline phosphatase. Although flare phenomenon (increased uptake in skeletal lesions on metabolic bone scanning) can initially be seen on imaging, true progression of bone involvement during ^{223}Ra-dichloride treatment is relatively rare.

^{99m}Tc-biphosphonates or ^{18}F-NaF can also be paired with therapeutic bone-seeking agents that emit beta radiation. Although internal targeted radiation therapies for osseous lesions using beta-emitting radionuclides strontium-89 (^{89}Sr) and samarium-153 (^{153}Sm-EDTMP) can improve pain in most patients (6–8), the effect on survival is limited. Palliation occurs within 4 to 28 days after administration of ^{89}Sr and typically lasts for 3 to 6 months. ^{223}Ra-dichloride administration has a dose-dependent effect in reducing pain, with more than 50% of patients experiencing relief or decreased need for pain medication after intravenous injection of 55 kBq/kg (9).

In a randomized double-blinded multinational phase III clinical trial (ALSYMPCA), patients treated with six injections of ^{223}Ra-dichloride at 4-week intervals had improved survival (14.9 months median overall survival vs. 11.3 months in placebo group), and increased time to symptomatic skeletal events (10). ^{223}Ra-dichloride was safe and effective when used before or after chemotherapy with docetaxel. Concurrent ^{223}Ra-dichloride therapy and chemotherapy are however currently not recommended. Although ^{223}Ra can generally be given safely with abiraterone or enzalutamide (11), adding ^{223}Ra therapy to combination of abiraterone and prednisone does not improve skeletal symptoms and has been associated with increased incidence of pathologic fractures and mortality [ERA-223 trial: 806 patients, increased incidence of fracture 28.6% vs. 11.4%]. ^{223}Ra-dichloride, however, can be considered and appears to be safe in patients who have adequate marrow function after chemotherapy. Recently published results from a small clinical trial suggested that patients who had been previously treated with ^{223}Ra-dichloride and progressed afterwards can be retreated (12). In a 2-year follow–up after retreatment, no serious drug-related adverse events were observed.

The short path length of the emitted alpha particles minimizes hematopoietic marrow toxicity compared to beta-emitting radionuclides (13,14). Although hematopoietic toxicity, gastrointestinal adverse reactions, and peripheral edema were the most common side effects compared to placebo group in the ^{223}Ra-dichloride phase III clinical trial, ^{223}Ra-dichloride therapy is safe and very well tolerated. Severe (grades 3–4) hematologic abnormalities can nonetheless occur in some cases (lymphocytopenia: 20%, anemia: 6%, thrombocytopenia: 3%), and blood count tests are therefore mandatory in the follow-up care of these patients.

Selective internal radiation therapy and pairing

Molecular targeted internal radiation can use biochemical and biological mechanisms to target specific molecules in the lesions to be treated following oral or parenteral administration of a radiolabeled target-specific molecular probe. However, radiolabeled molecular probes can also be delivered via vehicles that can be mechanically placed in the lesion and have an effect in the malignant cells due to proximity (such as brachytherapy, intra-arterial radioembolization, or intra-cavity radionuclide therapy).

Intra-arterial radioembolization of liver lesions has become a common practice nowadays. This practice is based on the unique dual blood supply of the liver and the radiosensitivity principle of malignant tissues (liver metastases and hepatocellular carcinomas are more radiosensitive than normal hepatic parenchyma). Since malignant tissues in the liver preferentially utilize the hepatic artery as their blood supply, intra-arterial internal radiotherapies can achieve significantly higher concentration of radionuclide in the tumors compared to the benign liver parenchyma (which receives 75%–90% of its blood supply from the portal vein). Although these therapies are not molecular targeted, they are lesion selective by virtue of differences in blood supply. Both resin and glass microspheres impregnated with ^{90}Y have been used for selective internal radiation therapy. Even though the radionuclide remains trapped within the microspheres intravascularly, the high energy and "relatively" long path length of the emitted beta particles provide good penetration into the immediately adjacent malignant tumor tissue. Resin and glass microspheres are fairly similar in diameter (30–35 um vs. 20–30 um, respectively). However, the activity per particle is significantly higher with glass microspheres (2500 Bq vs. 50 Bq), requiring fewer particles and lower embolic potential to provide similar radiation levels. Another technical difference is that high specific gravity of glass particles requires high pressure during administration compared to resin microspheres.

Extrahepatic adverse effects with this therapy are usually due to arterial collaterals or arteriovenous shunts associated with the tumors or cirrhosis (15). In fact, these tumors tend to recruit vessels from the diaphragm and adjacent organs such as stomach, duodenum, or pancreas. As a fraction of microspheres enters systemic circulation through these arteriovenous shunts and blood supply of adjacent organs, they may cause pneumonitis, cholecystitis, gastritis, duodenitis, and pancreatitis. A radiation dose of 30 Gy (or a cumulative dose of 50 Gy) to the lung is associated with pneumonitis, and long-term significant morbidity due to eventual development of pulmonary fibrosis. Therefore, prior to intra-arterial radioembolization of liver lesions, the hepatic arterial anatomy has to be mapped with catheter angiography and collaterals to other organs visualized, so that they can be coiled. The degree of hepatopulmonary shunting from the macro and microcirculation also has to be mapped and quantitated prior to hepatic arterial embolization via intra-arterial administration of ^{99m}Tc-macro aggregated albumin (MAA) and subsequent imaging. The administered radioactivity by means of microspheres may need to be limited if there is significant shunting to the lungs or if there is any activity in other abdominopelvic viscera that cannot be corrected by coil embolization. In that sense, this practice works in tandem with a diagnostic image that guides the therapeutic component. Although not molecularly targeted or using the same molecular probe for diagnostic and therapeutic purposes, the utility of this combination of diagnostic/therapeutic pair is necessary, used in this case more to avoid undesirable and preventable side effects than to assess the effectiveness of the therapy. In that sense, intra-arterial MAA is a surrogate for microspheres.

Radiation-induced liver disease (RILD) is an uncommon complication that can occur 60 to 90 days posttreatment presenting with jaundice, ascites, and elevated bilirubin levels. Small livers (<1.5 kg) or reduced hepatic reserve in the setting of prior liver-directed therapy, steatosis, steatohepatitis, hepatitis or cirrhosis, and low tumor burden (<5%) are the risk factors associate with RILD. Pretreatment with steroids may reduce the risk.

Radio-theranostics in the clinic

In this section, we focus on the radio-theranostic pairs which are either used currently in the clinic or are anticipated to be approved for use soon. Significant research is currently undergoing to develop new theranostic pairs and expand the clinical radio-theranostic applications. Promising results from multiple clinical trials studying diagnostic/therapeutic radio-probes for various cancers including for example prostate carcinoma (targets such as PSMA and gastrin-releasing peptide receptor), lymphoproliferative malignancies (various targets including chemokine receptor type 4, CD20, and CD37), ovarian and breast cancers (targeting human epidermal growth factor receptor 2) are becoming more and more available.

Radioiodine

Radioactive iodine has been used for diagnosis and treatment of benign and malignant thyroid disorders since 1940s, and it is by definition the first radio-theranostic agent used (16). The molecular mechanism is based on the fact that thyroid follicular cells take up iodine (radioactive or non-radioactive) from the blood via the sodium-iodide symporters (NIS) localized in the basolateral membrane, which cotransports two sodium ions along with one iodide ion inside the cell via NIS (17). Thyroid hormone biosynthesis requires iodide efflux through the apical membrane via pendrins into the follicular lumen, with subsequent oxidation, organification, and incorporation in tyrosyl residues of thyroglobulin at the cell-colloid interface. Iodinated thyroglobulin enters the cell via pinocytosis and undergoes hydrolysis, and T3 and T4 are subsequently secreted into the bloodstream at the basolateral membrane (18). NIS is used by the radioiodine family to get inside the cancer cell and follow the subsequent iodine metabolism. This molecular mechanism can be used for diagnostic and therapeutic radioiodine purposes. Of all 37 known iodine isotopes, all except one (^{127}I) are radioactive, and several of which (^{123}I, ^{124}I, ^{125}I, and ^{131}I) are commercially available for diagnostic and therapeutic purposes depending on their emissions (Table 16.2). All of them follow NIS for their diagnostic or therapeutic interactions with benign or malignant thyroid cells.

Thyroid-stimulating hormone (TSH) and iodide modulate NIS activity via transcriptional and posttranscriptional mechanisms. High concentrations of iodide lead to reduction in both NIS mRNA and protein levels and inhibit organification of iodine (Wolff-Chaikoff effect). It is however unclear if a low-iodine diet (defined by an intake of <50 μg/day for 1–2 weeks) can increase NIS expression independent of TSH. The TSH receptor is the major controller of thyroid cell proliferation, differentiation, and function via activation of the cAMP cascade (19). Stimulation of TSH receptors by autoantibodies in Graves' disease or weak binding by human chorionic gonadotropin (hCG) in gestational hyperthyroidism results in increased iodine uptake.

Several combinations of radioiodine theranostic pairs can be used for the treatment of benign as well as malignant thyroid. ^{123}I is used for diagnosing and radioiodine therapy planning in Graves' disease, toxic adenoma, and toxic multinodular goiter. These conditions are associated with elevated radioiodine uptake (particularly Graves' disease) in contrast to other etiologies of hyperthyroidism. Quantification of uptake and retention at 24 h allows for delivery of a precise dose of ^{131}I to the target tissue (e.g., 0.15–0.2 mCi/g [20]).

Radioactive iodine is a critical tool for staging, surveillance, and treatment in well-differentiated thyroid carcinomas.

Table 16.2 **COMMONLY USED IODINE ISOTOPES IN THERANOSTICS**

Isotope	Half-life	Decay mode, emissions	Main application
^{123}I	13 h	EC, γ (159 keV)	Diagnostic
^{124}I	4.18 d	EC, β$^+$	Diagnostic-positron emission tomography (PET)
^{125}I	59.40 d	EC, IC and Auger electrons, γ (35 keV)	(Brachy)therapy/Diagnostic pre-clinical
^{127}I	Stable	None	Thyroid blockade
^{131}I	8.02 d	β$^-$, γ (364 keV)	Diagnostic/Therapy

EC, electron capture; IC, internal conversion.

Differentiated thyroid cancer which includes papillary and follicular histology is a common malignancy and has a favorable prognosis and very low mortality compared with most other malignancies. Differentiated thyroid cancer (papillary thyroid carcinoma being the most common comprising 70%–75% of differentiated thyroid carcinomas, followed by follicular thyroid carcinoma in 10%–15% of cases in the United States and 17%–20% in the world) expresses NIS. Hurthle cell carcinoma is an aggressive variant of follicular carcinoma and is associated with low avidity for radioiodine in most patients (21). In general, NIS expression is lower in cancer than in normal thyroid follicular cells and may be even lower in metastatic lesions than in the primary cancer tissue. Therefore, stimulation of TSH release in patients with history of thyroid cancer and total thyroidectomy via withdrawal of thyroid hormone intake, or intramuscular administration of recombinant human TSH (rhTSH, thyrotropin) is used to increase radioiodine uptake in residual/recurrent/metastatic thyroid cancer for diagnostic (^{123}I and ^{124}I) and therapeutic purposes (^{131}I) using theranostic pairs of the iodine family. Poorly differentiated and dedifferentiated thyroid cancer have reduced functional NIS expression at the cellular membrane and loses the ability to trap Iodine. Therefore, the utility of theranostics with radioiodine pairs also decreases. Nevertheless, some medications such as selumetinib are now known to induce re-differentiation of these cancer cells and increase radioiodine uptake again (22). The clinical utility of these medications prior to ^{124}I/^{131}I diagnostic/treatment is being evaluated (23) and already used currently in some Institutions (Fig. 16.1).

Somatostatin receptor

Epithelial neoplasms with predominant neuroendocrine differentiation can arise in a variety of different organs. All neuroendocrine neoplasms have malignant potential, but well-differentiated neuroendocrine tumors (NETs) generally have a more indolent course and much better prognosis compared to poorly differentiated neuroendocrine carcinomas. The histological grading is based on mitotic count and the Ki-67 labeling index. Lower-grade well-differentiated NETs and certain other malignancies that arise from tissues derived embryologically from the neural crest overexpress somatostatin receptors (SSTR), a group of G-coupled membrane proteins that bind to endogenous somatostatin and have been used both as diagnostic imaging biomarker and more recently as a therapeutic target for peptide receptor radionuclide therapy (PRRT), therefore forming a theranostic pair for somatostatin receptor-expressing tumors.

Somatostatin is a very short-lived but important regulator of endocrine system that inhibits the release of numerous secondary hormones such as growth hormone, insulin, and glucagon. Octreotide is a synthetic 8-amino acid peptide that mimics larger natural somatostatins by binding with different affinities to the five types of somatostatin receptors (primarily SSTR type 2) but degrades less quickly in the plasma than the native form. Octreotide was initially used for treatment of functioning NETs to reduce symptoms associated with the release of serotonin (for carcinoid syndrome), or other hormones/hormonally active peptides produced by other functioning gastropancreatic NETs. With

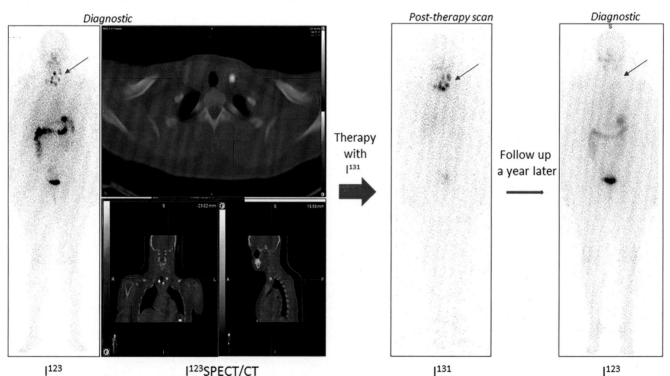

FIG. 16.1 ● Radioiodine theranostics. The left panel shows a patient with papillary thyroid cancer post-thyroidectomy with radioiodine (^{123}I)-avid nodal metastases in the neck seen on both diagnostic planar scintigraphy and single photon computed tomography (SPECT)/computed tomography (CT). The patient was treated with 100 mCi ^{131}I with the post-therapy planar scintigraphy (middle panel) demonstrating the nodal metastases with improved conspicuity. One year later, the ^{123}I diagnostic scan (right panel) shows no residual radioiodine-avid disease.

demonstration of antineoplastic and antiproliferative effects, the treatment was expanded to nonfunctioning tumors (24,25) since more than 80% of gastroenteropancreatic neuroendocrine tumors (including most of the nonfunctioning tumors) overexpress SSTR2, which is associated with a favorable prognosis.

Radiolabeled somatostatin analogues ideal for somatostatin receptor imaging (SRI) were introduced in the clinic for diagnosis of NET in the 1990s (26). In tumors with high SSTR expression, ^{111}In-pentetreotide (Octreoscan®) was found to have higher sensitivity and specificity compared to other imaging modalities (27) and high impact on treatment decisions (28,29). The possible use of radiolabeled somatostatin analogues for systemic molecular targeted radiotherapy of patients with inoperable or metastasized neuroendocrine tumors also started in the late 1990s with ^{111}In-pentetreotide. Although ^{111}In produces Auger electrons that can be used to cause DNA damage, limited electron range and efficiency, and potential toxicity associated with the needed high-doses of ^{111}In-pentetreotide limited its therapeutic potential and success rate (30).

Other theranostics agents have been introduced in the clinic for SRI since then. ^{68}Ga-DOTATATE is a compound of tyrosine3-octreotate and a macrocyclic chelating agent (DOTA, tetraxetan). Tyrosine3-octreotate is a variant of octreotide with very high affinity to SSTR2 (after compounding with ^{68}Ga-DOTA) and decreased binding to SSTR3 and SSTR5. ^{68}Ga-DOTATATE (Netspot®) and ^{177}Lu-DOTATATE (Lutathera®) were approved by FDA in 2016 and in 2018, respectively, for diagnosis and therapy of gastroenteropancreatic neuroendocrine tumors. DOTA compounds of octreotide variants such as DOTATATE, DOTANOC, and DOTATOC allow them to be conjugated with [68]Ga (a positron emission tomography (PET) radionuclide) for imaging and alpha-/beta-emitting radionuclide such as [225]Ac, ^{90}Y, or ^{177}Lu for PRRT. [68]Ga- or ^{18}F-based SSTR imaging agents are superior to ^{111}In-pentetrotide imaging in terms of diagnostic accuracy and evaluation of tumor burden (31,32). The degree of uptake on SSTR imaging by these diagnostic molecular agents is known to predict response to PRRT (33) and change in uptake after treatment can predict time to progression (34).

DOTA compounds of somatostatin analogues labeled with alpha- and beta-emitting radionuclide for PRRT have proven to be more effective at lower doses and provided lower side effects compared to ^{111}In-pentetreotide. PRRT with both ^{90}Y-DOTATOC (35) and ^{177}Lu-DOTATATE (36) or even a combination of them in tandem (37) has shown favorable results and improved survival. [90]Y has a shorter half-life (2.7 days) and higher particle energy and range (11 mm maximum range in soft tissue) compared to [177]Lu (6.6 days half-life, average 0.23 mm, max. 1.7 mm range in soft tissue). [177]Lu (but not ^{90}Y) produces gamma rays useful for posttreatment imaging to confirm molecular targeting of lesions and dosimetry. Although the longer range of beta particles allow ^{90}Y to be more effective for large tumors and tumors with areas of low vascularity, it also provides it with higher renal and marrow radiotoxicity. The shorter path length of the ^{177}Lu may provide less off-target radiation and deposit a larger fraction of radiation within the lesion, which is more suitable for treatment of sub-centimeter metastases.

Over the past three decades, there has been increasing evidence for efficacy and safety of PRRT. In 2017, the preliminary results of the first multicenter randomized controlled phase III clinical trial (NETTER-1 study) were published (36). This study compared PRRT with ^{177}Lu-DOTATATE (7.4 GBq /200 mCi every 8 weeks, for a total of four cycles) plus best supportive care versus administration of long-acting octreotide in patients with advanced midgut (gastroenteropancreatic) neuroendocrine tumors who had disease progression during first-line therapy with somatostatin analogues, and all of the target lesions were SSTR positive on SRI. PRRT increased progression-free survival from 11% at 20 months in the control group to 65% and was associated with a significant improvement in quality of life compared with high-dose octreotide. Many patients experienced only mild adverse effects related to PRRT including nausea and vomiting attributable mainly to concomitant infusion of an amino-acid solution for renal radioprotection, which now has been optimized. Other mild common adverse events included fatigue or asthenia, abdominal pain, and diarrhea. A small subset of patients developed grades 3 to 4 bone marrow toxicity manifesting as neutropenia, thrombocytopenia, and lymphopenia (in 1%, 2%, and 9% of patients, respectively, vs. no patients in the control group). Although kidneys can receive significant radiation, no severe renal toxicity was reported with the use of amino acids. This and other studies confirm that proper renal protection (typically starting 30 min before infusion of ^{177}Lu-DOTATATE) minimizes renal toxicity even in patients with a single kidney (38) or reduced baseline glomerular filtration rate (GFR) (39). Large studies in The Netherlands on patients with SSTR positive gastroenteropancreatic and bronchial neuroendocrine tumors demonstrated that long-term bone marrow toxicity is infrequent (40,41) whereas no therapy-related long-term renal or hepatic failure was observed. In patients who progress after PRRT and have exhausted other treatment alternatives, salvage PRRT appears to be safe and can provide antineoplastic effect, although may be less effective than the original PRRT cycles (42) (Fig. 16.2).

Although most clinical experience with PRRT is in patients with gastroenteropancreatic (GEP) NETs and to a lesser extent bronchopulmonary and other foregut and hindgut NETs, there is evidence of high expression of SSTR2 by SRI in other NETs and there are preliminary results supporting potential utility of PRRT in Merkel cell carcinoma (43), inoperable or metastatic NETs of rare sites such as uterus (44), and in refractory or relapsed high-risk neuroblastoma (45).

Several PRRT strategies under active research include the use of alpha-emitting radiolabeled somatostatin antagonists (46), or pretreatment with chemotherapy to increase SSTR expression in low-expressing neuroendocrine tumors. Short-range and high linear energy transfer of alpha emissions can theoretically increase effectiveness while reducing toxicity. For instance, initial results support tolerability of [225]Ac-DOTATOC for targeted alpha therapy in patients with NETs (47). Other alpha-emitting somatostatin analogues are mainly in preclinical studies (48). Liver is a frequent site of metastasis in gastroenteropancreatic tumors. Intra-arterial PRRT (particularly using an alpha-emitter such as [213]Bi-DOTATOC) (49) can deliver high radiation dose to neuroendocrine tumor hepatic metastases while reducing hepatic radiotoxicity. It has been suggested that an increased number of binding sites in tumor cells for somatostatin antagonists compared to agonists and lower uptake in normal liver parenchyma and hematopoietic cells may improve the safety window of PRRT (50,51).

Meta-iodobenzylguanidine, iobenguane

Neuroblastoma, which is the most common extracranial solid tumor of childhood, arises from the primitive neural crest cells found in the adrenal glands or in sympathetic ganglia. The

Theranostics of somatostatin receptors

Theranostic pair:
Ga^{68}-DOTATATE – Lu^{177}- DOTATATE

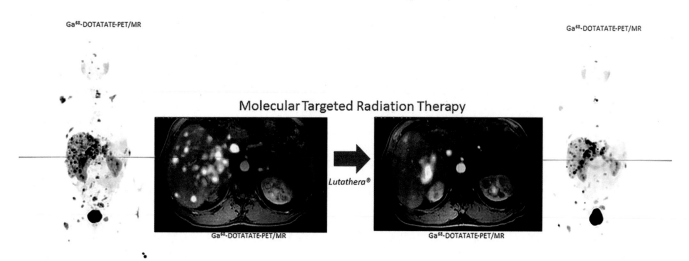

FIG. 16.2 ● Somatostatin receptor theranostics. The left panel images show maximum intensity projection (MIP) and fused ^{68}Ga-DOTATATE PET/MRI of a patient with metastatic neuroendocrine tumor involving the liver, nodes, and bone. The right panel images show decline in number and conspicuity of lesions compatible with partial response after treatment with ^{177}Lu-DOTATATE.

prognosis and outcomes in neuroblastoma are widely divergent ranging from spontaneous regression in some infants to a progressive course in children 18 months or older at diagnosis, to indolent but fatal disease in adolescents and adults despite multimodality therapy (52,53). Pheochromocytomas and paragangliomas are neuroendocrine tumors arising from the adrenal medulla and extra-adrenal paraganglia, respectively. These tumors can be malignant and 15% to 20% of patients can develop metastatic disease, and a subset of tumors causes symptoms due to catecholamine release.

Tumors of neural crest origin express high levels of norepinephrine transporter on cell membrane. Ninety percent of neuroblastoma tumors (54) and 50% to 60% of pheochromocytomas and paragangliomas (55), respectively, overexpress norepinephrine transporters. This expression can be low in head and neck paragangliomas. High expression of norepinephrine transporter has occasionally been observed in other malignancies such as GEP neuroendocrine tumors, medullary thyroid carcinomas, other neuroendocrine lesions (Merkel cell carcinoma, ganglioneuroma), and rarely in adrenocortical adenoma or carcinoma, retroperitoneal angiomyolipoma, and hemangioma (56).

Iobenguane is a norepinephrine analogue and is taken up by the norepinephrine transporter in adrenergic nerve terminals present in ganglia, adrenal medulla and sympathetically innervated organs such as the brown adipose tissue, heart, lungs, salivary glands, liver, and spleen. Physiologic uptake is significantly reduced in patients with high circulating catecholamine levels (57). In contrast to norepinephrine, MIBG (Meta Iodine Benzyl Guanidine) has low affinity for adrenergic receptors reducing physiological side effects (58). ^{131}I-MIBG and ^{123}I-MIBG (the radioiodinated versions of MIBG) have been used for several decades for imaging evaluation of

neuroblastoma, pheochromocytoma, and paragangliomas. High-specific-activity, carrier-free ^{131}I-MIBG has enabled high uptake and retention of radiopharmaceutical while minimizing pharmacologic effects due to saturation of norepinephrine transporters that were common with the use of low-specific activity preparations in the past (59). MIBG is stored in the cytosol in neurosecretory granules via vesicular monoamine transporters 1 and 2 (60). MIBG uptake and its anticancer effect are primarily driven by retention in chromaffin cells rather than the degree of catecholamine transporters expression (61). Poorly differentiated paragangliomas may have low uptake due to low expression of vesicular monoamine transporters (62).

^{131}I-iobenguane for therapeutic purposes, however, was approved in the United States very recently in 2018 for treatment of patients 12 years and older with MIBG scan positive, unresectable, locally advanced, or metastatic pheochromocytoma or paraganglioma. The approval of ^{131}I-iobenguane (Azedra®) was based on the results of an open-label, single-arm, multicenter clinical trial showing a 50% or greater reduction of all antihypertensive medication for at least 6 months in 25% of the patients and radiologic response (RECIST 1.0) in 22% of the patients (63). Most patients experienced some hematologic adverse reaction including severe (grades 3–4) lymphopenia (78%), neutropenia (59%), and thrombocytopenia (50%). In some patients (12%) treatment was discontinued due to persistent severe myelosuppression or other non-hematologic adverse reactions such as nausea. Myelodysplastic syndrome or acute leukemias were reported in ~7% of the patients. Worsening hypertension occurred in 11% of the patients. The results of this clinical trial are in line with previously published results supporting the utility of ^{131}I-MIBG for therapy despite the possibility of serious toxicity (64). Patients with SDHB (succinate dehydrogenase complex iron sulfur subunit B) mutations may respond particularly very well to therapy (64).

Patient preparation requires discontinuation of medications that affect norepinephrine transport for at least five half-lives prior to MIBG injection (either for imaging or therapy) through at least 7 days after therapy. The medication list includes certain blood pressure medications (combined alpha/beta-blocker labetalol and calcium channel blockers), antidepressants, tramadol, and decongestants (pseudoephedrine). ^{131}I-MIBG therapy requires adequate bone marrow function (platelet count 80,000 × 10^9/L or higher and absolute neutrophil count 1,200 × 10^9/L). The recommended therapeutic dose is 296 MBq/kg (8 mCi/kg) up to 18.5 GBq (500 mCi). The dose can be adjusted based on dosimetry in an individual patient. The dose is repeated once after 90 days. To reduce radioiodine uptake in the thyroid, blockade is started at least 24 h before therapy and should continue for 10 days after MIBG injection. Iobenguane is eliminated mostly unmetabolized through kidneys (approximately half by 24 h and >80% within 4–5 days after administration (65)) (Fig. 16.3).

Multiple clinical trials have used ^{131}I-MIBG for treatment of neuroblastoma in the past three decades. Although most neuroblastomas overexpress norepinephrine transporters and have high uptake on MIBG scintigraphy, therapeutic response is typically seen in only one third of patients (66). Myelosuppression is not an uncommon adverse effect, and hematopoietic stem cell support is often needed to allow for administration of the high activity needed to achieve therapeutic radiation doses in the targeted lesions. To minimize radiation to caregivers and family, hospitalization in a lead-lined room and strict radiation precautions are necessary (67).

Prostate-specific membrane antigen

Prostate-specific membrane antigen (PSMA), also known as folate hydrolase or glutamate carboxypeptidase II, is a transmembrane glycoprotein and a metalloenzyme belonging to the M28 peptidase family. PSMA was initially found in prostate cancer

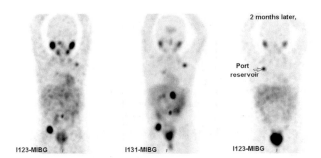

FIG. 16.3 • *MIBG theranostics. Maximum intensity projection (MIP) images of ^{123}I-MIBG SPECT in a 5-year-old female with history of neuroblastoma. A surveillance scan (left) showed multiple new lesions (left scapula, left posterior element of L4, and right iliac bone) and mild focal uptake in midline of the abdomen in a periaortic lymph node and persistent abnormal uptake in the right posterior sixth rib. The patient was subsequently treated with two cycles of ^{131}I-MIBG for refractory disease. The posttreatment scan (middle, ^{131}I window) performed approximately 1 month after the ^{123}I-MIBG scan and 7 days after receiving 427 mCi ^{131}I-MIBG shows intense focal uptake in the same lesions. Note better image quality due to high counts and better washout of background activity. A follow-up ^{123}I-MIBG study (right) 2 months after the second cycle of therapy shows complete resolution of abnormal uptake in all disease sites. The focal activity projected over the right upper chest indicates residual activity in a port reservoir. Physiologic parotid salivary gland uptake is also noted.*

cells. Despite the name, and although it is highly expressed in nearly all prostate cancers, PSMA is also robustly expressed in neo-vasculature of a variety of solid tumors including glioblastomas, suggesting a role in tumor angiogenesis (68,69). In normal prostate cells, a truncated variant of PSMA is primarily in the cytosol and not available for binding to extracellular targeting agents such as antibodies or small molecules that do not cross the cell membrane (70,71). PSMA overexpression on the cell membrane correlates with advanced, high-grade, metastatic, androgen-independent disease (72). PSMA has low expression in some normal tissues such as the duodenal mucosa, proximal renal tubules, and salivary glands (73,74).

The large differential surface expression of PSMA in prostate cancer versus normal prostate cells has caused extensive interest in PSMA as a target for theranostics in prostate carcinoma and particularly in metastatic castration-resistant prostate cancer (mCRPC). Initial clinical results from the PSMA-targeted imaging were disappointing due to radiolabeled monoclonal antibodies (^{111}In-capromab pendetide) binding to the intracellular epitope of PSMA. Subsequent studies using a humanized monoclonal antibody J591 that targeted the extracellular domain of PSMA were superior to ^{111}In-capromab pendetide. Novel PSMA-targeting agents are based on high-affinity low-molecular-weight ligands that bind to either folate hydrolase or glutamate carboxypeptidase II catalytic domains. The ligand–PSMA complex subsequently can internalize through endocytosis resulting in accumulation and retention of radionuclide within the cancer cells (70). Low-molecular-weight ligands have better pharmacokinetics, and faster and higher tumor penetration compared to large targeting molecules such as radiolabeled antibodies (75), and unlike antibodies, has little binding to receptors in inflammatory cells of prostatitis or benign prostatic hyperplasia.

PSMA inhibitors based on the lysine-urea-glutamate motif are currently the most commonly used/studied PSMA-targeting agents for theranostics. Addition of a lipophilic linking region as in PSMA-11 and PSMA-617 further increases binding affinity of the ligand to PSMA. Conjugation of ligand with DOTA chelator enables labeling with positron-, gamma-, beta-, or alpha-emitting radionuclides such as ^{68}Ga, ^{111}In, ^{90}Y, ^{177}Lu, ^{213}Bi, and ^{225}Ac, allowing for optimal theranostic pairing based on the selection of the radiolabeling isotope. PSMA-617 is the best studied radioligand in therapy and has been used in small clinical trials with both beta-emitting ^{177}Lu and alpha-emitting ^{225}Ac. PSMA-617 has high internalization and prolonged tumor retention. Rapid renal clearance of PSMA-617 compared to other PSMA ligands has shown to reduce radiation to the kidneys (76). Slow pharmacokinetics compared to ^{68}Ga half-life makes PSMA-617 less suitable for diagnostic imaging, although high-quality imaging can be obtained using ^{44}Sc (half-life of 4 h) (77).

Multiple compassionate use publications and prospective Phase II clinical trials have examined and demonstrated safety and effectiveness of ^{177}Lu-labeled PSMA ligands in patients with mCRPC with high expression of PSMA in target lesions. Xerostomia is a common but usually transient side effect with >80% of patients experiencing primarily grade 1 dry mouth. Severe (grades 3–4) asymptomatic hematological adverse effects are reported in up to 10% of the patients. The therapeutic effects include PSA response (78), decreased size of soft-tissue lesions (79), improved progression-free and overall survival (79,80), and improved pain control and quality of life (81). PSA response is seen in most patients after the first treatment and is a predictor of longer overall survival (82). PSA decline often continues after each subsequent treatment (83). PSMA radioligand therapy is effective and well tolerated in patients with metastatic disease limited to lymph nodes (84). Presence of visceral metastasis seems to correlate with poor PSA response and shorter survival after treatment (85).

Summary

Theranostics with its combination of targeted molecular imaging and molecular radiotherapy offers knowledge-based precision medicine. The field is moving forward rapidly and it is anticipated to play a significant role in the clinic, particularly in the care of patients with cancer. However, support for research and specific education in radio-theranostics is going to be crucial to position theranostics in the everyday cutting-edge clinical medicine. Expertise in radiobiology, diagnostic imaging, dosimetry, and bedside clinical care, is going to be critical to determine the most optimal diagnostic/therapeutic algorithms for radio-theranostics. In addition, the regulatory and reimbursement agencies should be encouraged to match the rapid pace of theranostics in order to allow a rapid transition of promising pairs to clinical trials and to the clinic.

References

1. Frangos S, Buscombe JR. Why should we be concerned about a "g"? *Eur J Nucl Med Mol Imaging.* 2019;46(2):519.
2. Herrmann K, Larson SM, Weber WA. Theranostic concepts: more than just a fashion trend—introduction and overview. *J Nucl Med.* 2017;58(Supplement 2):1S–2S.
3. Cannan WJ, Pederson DS. Mechanisms and consequences of double-strand DNA break formation in chromatin. *J Cell Physiol.* 2016;231(1):3–14.
4. Gudkov SV, et al. Targeted radionuclide therapy of human tumors. *Int J Mol Sci.* 2015;17(1):33.
5. Cheetham PJ, Petrylak DP. Alpha particles as radiopharmaceuticals in the treatment of bone metastases: mechanism of action of radium-223 chloride (Alpharadin) and radiation protection. *Oncology (Williston Park).* 2012;26(4):330–337, 341.
6. Robinson RG, et al. Strontium 89 therapy for the palliation of pain due to osseous metastases. *JAMA.* 1995;274(5):420–424.
7. Liepe K, Kotzerke J. A comparative study of 188Re-HEDP, 186Re-HEDP, 153Sm-EDTMP and 89Sr in the treatment of painful skeletal metastases. *Nucl Med Commun.* 2007;28(8):623–630.
8. Jong JM, et al. Radiopharmaceuticals for palliation of bone pain in patients with castration-resistant prostate cancer metastatic to bone: a systematic review. *Eur Urol.* 2016;70(3):416–426.
9. Nilsson S, et al. A randomized, dose-response, multicenter phase II study of radium-223 chloride for the palliation of painful bone metastases in patients with castration-resistant prostate cancer. *Eur J Cancer.* 2012;48(5):678–686.
10. Parker C, et al. Alpha emitter radium-223 and survival in metastatic prostate cancer. *N Engl J Med.* 2013;369(3):213–223.
11. Saad F, et al. Radium-223 and concomitant therapies in patients with metastatic castration-resistant prostate cancer: an international, early access, open-label, single-arm phase 3b trial. *Lancet Oncol.* 2016;17(9):1306–1316.
12. Sartor O, et al. Re-treatment with radium-223: 2-year follow-up from an international, open-label, phase 1/2 study in patients with castration-resistant prostate cancer and bone metastases. *Prostate.* 2019;79(14):1683–1691.
13. Parker CC, et al. Three-year safety of radium-223 dichloride in patients with castration-resistant prostate cancer and symptomatic bone metastases from phase 3 randomized alpharadin in symptomatic prostate cancer trial. *Eur Urol.* 2017;73(3):427–435.
14. Uemura H, et al. Three-year follow-up of a phase II study of radium-223 dichloride in Japanese patients with symptomatic castration-resistant prostate cancer and bone metastases. *Int J Clin Oncol.* 2019;24(5):557–566.
15. Khan AN, et al. Pulmonary vascular complications of chronic liver disease: pathophysiology, imaging, and treatment. *Ann Thorac Med.* 2011;6(2):57–65.
16. Silberstein EB. Radioiodine: the classic theranostic agent. *Semin Nucl Med.* 2012;42(3):164–170.
17. Dohan O, et al. The sodium/iodide Symporter (NIS): characterization, regulation, and medical significance. *Endocr Rev.* 2003;24(1):48–77.
18. Braverman L, Kopp P, Utiger R. *Thyroid Hormone Synthesis: Thyroid Iodine Metabolism, in Werner and Ingbar's the Thyroid: A Fundamental and Clinical Text.* Philadelphia, PA: Lippincott, Williams & Wilkins; 2005:52–76.
19. Tuncel M. Thyroid stimulating hormone receptor. *Mol Imaging Radionucl Ther.* 2017;26(Suppl 1):87–91.
20. Ross DS, et al. 2016 American Thyroid Association guidelines for diagnosis and management of hyperthyroidism and other causes of thyrotoxicosis. *Thyroid.* 2016;26(10):1343–1421.
21. Ahmadi S, et al. Hurthle cell carcinoma: current perspectives. *Onco Targets Ther.* 2016;9:6873–6884.
22. Hong CM, Ahn BC. Redifferentiation of radioiodine refractory differentiated thyroid cancer for reapplication of I-131 therapy. *Front Endocrinol (Lausanne).* 2017;8:260.
23. Brown SR, et al. Investigating the potential clinical benefit of Selumetinib in resensitising advanced iodine refractory differentiated thyroid cancer to radioiodine therapy (SEL-I-METRY): protocol for a multicentre UK single arm phase II trial. *BMC Cancer.* 2019;19(1):582.
24. Rinke A, et al. Placebo-controlled, double-blind, prospective, randomized study on the effect of octreotide LAR in the control of tumor growth in patients with metastatic neuroendocrine midgut tumors: a report from the PROMID Study Group. *J Clin Oncol.* 2009;27(28):4656–4663.
25. Oberg K, et al. Neuroendocrine gastro-entero-pancreatic tumors: ESMO clinical practice guidelines for diagnosis, treatment and follow-up. *Ann Oncol.* 2012;23 Suppl 7:vii124–30.
26. Krenning EP, et al. Somatostatin receptor scintigraphy with [111In-DTPA-d-Phe1]- and [123I-Tyr3]-octreotide: the Rotterdam experience with more than 1000 patients. *Eur J Nucl Med.* 1993;20(8):716–731.
27. Gibril F, et al. Somatostatin receptor scintigraphy: its sensitivity compared with that of other imaging methods in detecting primary and metastatic gastrinomas. A prospective study. *Ann Intern Med.* 1996;125(1):26–34.
28. Lebtahi R, et al. Clinical impact of somatostatin receptor scintigraphy in the management of patients with neuroendocrine gastroentero-pancreatic tumors. *J Nucl Med.* 1997;38(6):853–858.
29. Jamar F, et al. Somatostatin receptor imaging with indium-111-pentetreotide in gastroenteropancreatic neuroendocrine tumors: safety, efficacy and impact on patient management. *J Nucl Med.* 1995;36(4):542–549.
30. Anthony LB, et al. Indium-111-pentetreotide prolongs survival in gastroenteropancreatic malignancies. *Semin Nucl Med.* 2002;32(2):123–132.
31. Buchmann I, et al. Comparison of 68Ga-DOTATOC PET and 111In-DTPAOC (Octreoscan) SPECT in patients with neuroendocrine tumours. *Eur J Nucl Med Mol Imaging.* 2007;34(10):1617–1626.
32. Hope TA, et al. (111)In-pentetreotide scintigraphy versus (68)Ga-DOTATATE PET: impact on Krenning scores and effect of tumor burden. *J Nucl Med.* 2019;60(9):1266–1269.

33. Kratochwil C, et al. SUV of [68Ga]DOTATOC-PET/CT predicts response probability of PRRT in neuroendocrine tumors. *Mol Imaging Biol*. 2015;17(3):313–318.

34. Haug AR, et al. 68Ga-DOTATATE PET/CT for the early prediction of response to somatostatin receptor-mediated radionuclide therapy in patients with well-differentiated neuroendocrine tumors. *J Nucl Med*. 2010;51(9):1349–1356.

35. Valkema R, et al. Survival and response after peptide receptor radionuclide therapy with [90Y-DOTA0,Tyr3]octreotide in patients with advanced gastroenteropancreatic neuroendocrine tumors. *Semin Nucl Med*. 2006;36(2):147–156.

36. Strosberg J, et al. Phase 3 trial of (177)Lu-Dotatate for midgut neuroendocrine tumors. *N Engl J Med*. 2017;376(2):125–135.

37. Kunikowska J, et al. Long-term results and tolerability of tandem peptide receptor radionuclide therapy with (90)Y/(177)Lu-DOTATATE in neuroendocrine tumors with respect to the primary location: a 10-year study. *Ann Nucl Med*. 2017;31(5):347–356.

38. Ranade R, Basu S. 177Lu-DOTATATE PRRT in patients with metastatic neuroendocrine tumor and a single functioning kidney: tolerability and effect on renal function. *J Nucl Med Technol*. 2016;44(2):65–69.

39. Naik C, Basu S. (177)Lu-DOTATATE peptide receptor radionuclide therapy in patients with borderline low and discordant renal parameters: treatment feasibility assessment by sequential estimation of triple parameters and filtration fraction. *World J Nucl Med*. 2018;17(1):12–20.

40. Brabander T, et al. Long-term efficacy, survival, and safety of [(177) Lu-DOTA(0),Tyr(3)]octreotate in patients with gastroenteropancreatic and bronchial neuroendocrine tumors. *Clin Cancer Res*. 2017;23(16):4617–4624.

41. Bergsma H, et al. Persistent hematologic dysfunction after peptide receptor radionuclide therapy with (177)Lu-DOTATATE: incidence, course, and predicting factors in patients with gastroenteropancreatic neuroendocrine tumors. *J Nucl Med*. 2018;59(3):452–458.

42. van Essen M, et al. Salvage therapy with (177)Lu-octreotate in patients with bronchial and gastroenteropancreatic neuroendocrine tumors. *J Nucl Med*. 2010;51(3):383–390.

43. Kasi PM, Sharma A, Jain MK. Expanding the indication for novel theranostic 177Lu-dotatate peptide receptor radionuclide therapy: proof-of-concept of PRRT in Merkel cell cancer. *Case Rep Oncol*. 2019;12(1):98–103.

44. Thapa P, Parghane R, Basu S. (177)Lu-DOTATATE peptide receptor radionuclide therapy in metastatic or advanced and inoperable primary neuroendocrine tumors of rare sites. *World J Nucl Med*. 2017;16(3):223–228.

45. Kong G, et al. Initial experience with gallium-68 DOTA-octreotate PET/CT and peptide receptor radionuclide therapy for pediatric patients with refractory metastatic neuroblastoma. *J Pediatr Hematol Oncol*. 2016;38(2):87–96.

46. Fani M, Nicolas GP, Wild D. Somatostatin receptor antagonists for imaging and therapy. *J Nucl Med*. 2017;58(Suppl 2):61s–66s.

47. Kratochwil C, et al. Ac-225-DOTATOC-an empiric dose finding for alpha particle emitter based radionuclide therapy of neuroendocrine tumors. *J Nucl Med*. 2015;56(supplement 3):1232–1232.

48. Stallons TAR, et al. Preclinical investigation of (212)Pb-DOTAMTATE for peptide receptor radionuclide therapy in a neuroendocrine tumor model. *Mol Cancer Ther*. 2019;18(5):1012–1021.

49. Kratochwil C, et al. (2)(1)(3)Bi-DOTATOC receptor-targeted alpha-radionuclide therapy induces remission in neuroendocrine tumours refractory to beta radiation: a first-in-human experience. *Eur J Nucl Med Mol Imaging*. 2014;41(11):2106–2119.

50. Nicolas GP, et al. Biodistribution, pharmacokinetics, and dosimetry of (177)Lu-, (90)Y-, and (111)In-labeled somatostatin receptor antagonist OPS201 in comparison to the agonist (177)Lu-DOTATATE: the mass effect. *J Nucl Med*. 2017;58(9):1435–1441.

51. Wild D, et al. Comparison of somatostatin receptor agonist and antagonist for peptide receptor radionuclide therapy: a pilot study. *J Nucl Med*. 2014;55(8):1248–1252.

52. Whittle SB, et al. Overview and recent advances in the treatment of neuroblastoma. *Expert Rev Anticancer Ther*. 2017;17(4):369–386.

53. Franks LM, et al. Neuroblastoma in adults and adolescents: an indolent course with poor survival. *Cancer*. 1997;79(10):2028–2035.

54. Carlin S, et al. Development of a real-time polymerase chain reaction assay for prediction of the uptake of meta-[(131)I]iodobenzyl-guanidine by neuroblastoma tumors. *Clin Cancer Res*. 2003;9(9):3338–3344.

55. Tan TH, et al. Diagnostic performance of (68)Ga-DOTATATE PET/CT, (18)F-FDG PET/CT and (131)I-MIBG scintigraphy in mapping metastatic pheochromocytoma and paraganglioma. *Nucl Med Mol Imaging*. 2015;49(2):143–151.

56. Taieb D, et al. EANM 2012 guidelines for radionuclide imaging of phaeochromocytoma and paraganglioma. *Eur J Nucl Med Mol Imaging*. 2012;39(12):1977–1995.

57. Sinclair AJ, et al. Pre- and post-treatment distribution pattern of 123I-MIBG in patients with phaeochromocytomas and paragangliomas. *Nucl Med Commun*. 1989;10(8):567–576.

58. Wieland DM, et al. Radiolabeled adrenergi neuron-blocking agents: adrenomedullary imaging with [131I]iodobenzylguanidine. *J Nucl Med*. 1980;21(4):349–353.

59. Jimenez C, Erwin W, Chasen B. Targeted radionuclide therapy for patients with metastatic pheochromocytoma and paraganglioma: from low-specific-activity to high-specific-activity iodine-131 metaiodobenzylguanidine. *Cancers (Basel)*. 2019;11(7):1018.

60. Bomanji J, et al. Uptake of iodine-123 MIBG by pheochromocytomas, paragangliomas, and neuroblastomas: a histopathological comparison. *J Nucl Med*. 1987;28(6):973–978.

61. van Berkel A, et al. Semiquantitative 123I-metaiodobenzylguanidine scintigraphy to distinguish pheochromocytoma and paraganglioma from physiologic adrenal uptake and its correlation with genotype-dependent expression of catecholamine transporters. *J Nucl Med*. 2015;56(6):839–846.

62. Fottner C, et al. 6-18F-fluoro-L-dihydroxyphenylalanine positron emission tomography is superior to 123I-metaiodobenzyl-guanidine scintigraphy in the detection of extraadrenal and hereditary pheochromocytomas and paragangliomas: correlation with vesicular monoamine transporter expression. *J Clin Endocrinol Metab*. 2010;95(6):2800–2810.

63. Pryma DA, et al. Efficacy and safety of high-specific-activity (131) I-MIBG therapy in patients with advanced pheochromocytoma or paraganglioma. *J Nucl Med*. 2019;60(5):623–630.

64. Gonias S, et al. Phase II study of high-dose [131I]metaiodobenzyl-guanidine therapy for patients with metastatic pheochromocytoma and paraganglioma. *J Clin Oncol*. 2009;27(25):4162–4168.

65. Sisson JC, Wieland DM. Radiolabeled meta-iodobenzylguanidine: pharmacology and clinical studies. *Am J Physiol Imaging*. 1986;1(2):96–103.

66. Wilson JS, et al. A systematic review of 131I-meta iodobenzylguanidine molecular radiotherapy for neuroblastoma. *Eur J Cancer*. 2014;50(4):801–815.

67. Cougnenc O, et al. High-dose 131I-MIBG therapies in children: feasibility, patient dosimetry and radiation exposure to workers and family caregivers. *Radiat Prot Dosimetry*. 2017;173(4):395–404.

68. Spatz S, et al. Comprehensive evaluation of prostate specific membrane antigen expression in the vasculature of renal tumors: implications for imaging studies and prognostic role. *J Urol*. 2018;199(2):370–377.

69. Wernicke AG, et al. Prostate-specific membrane antigen as a potential novel vascular target for treatment of glioblastoma multiforme. *Arch Pathol Lab Med*. 2011;135(11):1486–1489.

70. Ghosh A, Heston WD. Tumor target prostate specific membrane antigen (PSMA) and its regulation in prostate cancer. *J Cell Biochem*. 2004;91(3):528–539.

71. Mannweiler S, et al. Heterogeneity of prostate-specific membrane antigen (PSMA) expression in prostate carcinoma with distant metastasis. *Pathol Oncol Res*. 2009;15(2):167–172.

72. Ross JS, et al. Correlation of primary tumor prostate-specific membrane antigen expression with disease recurrence in prostate cancer. *Clin Cancer Res*. 2003;9(17):6357–6362.

73. Silver DA, et al. Prostate-specific membrane antigen expression in normal and malignant human tissues. *Clin Cancer Res*. 1997;3(1):81–85.

74. Sheikhbahaei S, et al. Pearls and pitfalls in clinical interpretation of prostate-specific membrane antigen (PSMA)-targeted PET imaging. *Eur J Nucl Med Mol Imaging.* 2017;44(12):2117–2136.
75. Haberkorn U, et al. New strategies in prostate cancer: prostate-specific membrane antigen (PSMA) ligands for diagnosis and therapy. *Clin Cancer Res.* 2016;22(1):9–15.
76. Benesova M, et al. Preclinical evaluation of a tailor-made DOTA-conjugated PSMA inhibitor with optimized linker moiety for imaging and endoradiotherapy of prostate cancer. *J Nucl Med.* 2015;56(6):914–920.
77. Eppard E, et al. Clinical translation and first in-human use of [(44)Sc]Sc-PSMA-617 for PET imaging of metastasized castrate-resistant prostate cancer. *Theranostics.* 2017;7(18):4359–4369.
78. Ahmadzadehfar H, et al. Early side effects and first results of radioligand therapy with 177Lu-DKFZ-617 PSMA of castrate-resistant metastatic prostate cancer: a two-centre study. *EJNMMI Res.* 2015;5(1):36.
79. Kulkarni HR, et al. PSMA-based radioligand therapy for metastatic castration-resistant prostate cancer: the Bad Berka experience since 2013. *J Nucl Med.* 2016;57(Suppl 3):97S–104S.
80. Rahbar K, et al. PSMA targeted radioligandtherapy in metastatic castration resistant prostate cancer after chemotherapy, abiraterone and/or enzalutamide. A retrospective analysis of overall survival. *Eur J Nucl Med Mol Imaging.* 2018;45(1):12–19.
81. Hofman MS, et al. [(177)Lu]-PSMA-617 radionuclide treatment in patients with metastatic castration-resistant prostate cancer (LuPSMA trial): a single-centre, single-arm, phase 2 study. *Lancet Oncol.* 2018;19(6):825–833.
82. Kim YJ, Kim YI. Therapeutic responses and survival effects of 177Lu-PSMA-617 radioligand therapy in metastatic castrate-resistant prostate cancer: a meta-analysis. *Clin Nucl Med.* 2018;43(10):728–734.
83. Rahbar K, et al. Delayed response after repeated (177)Lu-PSMA-617 radioligand therapy in patients with metastatic castration resistant prostate cancer. *Eur J Nucl Med Mol Imaging.* 2018;45(2):243–246.
84. Edler von Eyben F, et al. (177)Lu-PSMA radioligand therapy of predominant lymph node metastatic prostate cancer. *Oncotarget.* 2019;10(25):2451–2461.
85. Heck MM, et al. Treatment outcome, toxicity, and predictive factors for radioligand therapy with (177)Lu-PSMA-I&T in metastatic castration-resistant prostate cancer. *Eur Urol.* 2019;75(6):920–926.

 CHAPTER SELF-ASSESSMENT QUESTIONS

1. Which statement below best describes theranostics?
   A. Diagnostics and therapeutics using the same or similar biological target
   B. Is only limited to care of patients with cancer
   C. Is only limited to use of radioactive agents
   D. Has been established in the past few years

2. Which of the following pairs constitute a theranostics pair?
   A. FDG and 131I-MIBG
   B. ^{177}Lu-PSMA-617 and ^{68}Ga-PSMA-11
   C. ^{68}Ga-DOTATATE and ^{131}I
   D. ^{131}I-iobenguane and ^{177}Lu-DOTATATE

3. Which of the following biological targets for theranostics and disease processes relate?
   A. SSTR2 and melanoma
   B. PSMA and neuroendocrine tumor
   C. Norepinephrine and pheochromocytoma
   D. Sodium iodide symporter and prostate cancer

Answers to Chapter Self-Assessment Questions

1. A Theranostics is generally defined as diagnostics and therapeutics using the same or similar biological target. Answer B, C, and D are incorrect. While currently theranostics focuses on cancer, but there is no theoretical limitation for theranostic to be used in a broad range of other disease processes. Theranostics domain may include nanotheranostics, optotheranostics, and magnetotheranostics and radio-theranostics. The latter term uses radioactive agents. Radio-theranostics was established in early 1940s after the first radioiodine administration for thyroid disorder.

2. The correct pairing is B (^{177}Lu-PSMA-617 and ^{68}Ga-PSMA-11). All other pairings are incorrect.

3. The correct pairing is C (norepinephrine and pheochromocytoma). All other pairings are incorrect.

Essentials of Pediatric Nuclear Medicine

17

Hedieh Khalatbari, Barry L. Shulkin, Helen R. Nadel, and Marguerite T. Parisi

LEARNING OBJECTIVES

1. Differentiate the scintigraphic patterns in neonates with congenital hypothyroidism.
2. Use renal scintigraphy to identify the subset of patients with congenital dilation of the renal collecting system that will benefit from surgical intervention.
3. Apply the interpretive criteria for distinguishing biliary atresia from other causes of prolonged neonatal cholestatic jaundice on hepatobiliary scans.
4. Discuss the optimal approach to performing a Meckel scan in children.
5. Describe the modified Curie score and its significance when interpreting iodine-labeled metaiodobenzylguanidine scans for patients with neuroblastoma.

INTRODUCTION

Children are not small adults. There are age-related developmental changes as well as physiologic variants in children that can be mistaken for pathology. Further, the disease processes encountered in the pediatric population differ from those in adults. Even when similar pathologies are encountered, the causes and the sites of involvement vary between adults and children. One such example is osteomyelitis. Osteomyelitis is classified as *hematogenous* osteomyelitis, *contiguous focus* osteomyelitis from trauma, surgery, prosthetic material, or soft tissue spread, and *vascular insufficiency* osteomyelitis (1). Hematogenous osteomyelitis predominates in children where the metaphases of the long bones are most commonly involved (2,3). In younger adults, osteomyelitis is often related to trauma or surgery, that is, contiguous focus osteomyelitis. In older adults, contiguous focus osteomyelitis and vascular insufficiency osteomyelitis predominate (3).

Interpretation of pediatric nuclear medicine (NM) studies requires a knowledge of the patient's history, clinical presentation as well as the indication for the requested study. Findings on anatomic imaging modalities should be reviewed and correlated with those identified on NM studies. Additionally, one must be cognizant of the physiologic biodistribution of the administered radiopharmaceutical to ensure that unexpected findings that may alter patient diagnosis or treatment are not overlooked. While the radiopharmaceuticals used are the same as in adults, there are physiologic and developmental changes that occur in the growing child and adolescent that must be recognized and not confused with pathology (Fig. 17.1).

This chapter will focus on the studies performed in a typical pediatric NM practice, the practicalities of performing these studies (Tables 17.1 and 17.2), and illustrative examples (4–38).

RADIOPHARMACEUTICAL DOSAGE AND RADIATION DOSE

There are technical aspects of performing NM studies that must be adjusted for the pediatric patient. Children are more sensitive to radiation than their adult counterparts and they have a longer life expectancy in which to exhibit adverse effects of radiation (39). Consequently, concerted efforts must be made to optimize radiopharmaceutical administered doses and hybrid-imaging techniques in this vulnerable population to allow for decreased patient radiation exposure while maintaining diagnostic efficacy (39,40). There has been an emphasis in the literature on the potential carcinogenic risks of ionizing radiation, particularly in the pediatric population. There are several models to predict relative radiation risks and the linear-no-threshold hypothesis is the most widely used (41). This hypothesis indicates that exposure to ionizing radiation at any level has the potential to increase the likelihood of the development of malignancy later in life (42). Therefore, NM and positron-emission tomography/computed tomography (PET/CT) studies are to be performed only when clearly clinically indicated and using weight-based radiopharmaceutical administered activities in accordance with the North American and European Association of Nuclear Medicine (EANM) guidelines (12,13). In addition, in diagnostic pediatric NM studies, the use iodine-123 (I-123) and I-123 metaiodobenzylguanidine (MIBG) is preferred over iodine-131 (I-131) and I-131 MIBG in thyroid disease and neuroblastoma respectively, due to their shorter half-life, improved image quality due to the energy of the emitted photons, and lower effective patient radiation dose. Finally, there are various techniques that can be used to reduce radiation when performing NM and PET/CT studies; these are summarized in Table 17.3 (12,13,35,43,44).

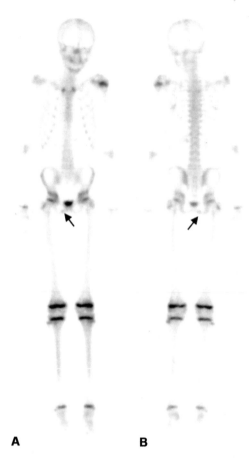

A   **B**

FIG. 17.1 ● Asymmetry of ischiopubic synchondrosis and physiologic uptake in growth plates. 10-year-old male with history of localized osteosarcoma of the right proximal humerus; he is status post chemotherapy and right proximal humeral resection with bone graft reconstruction. Surveillance Tc-99m MDP bone scan was performed. **A and B:** Anterior (A) and posterior (B) whole-body bone scans demonstrate a photopenic defect in the right proximal humerus consistent with history of right proximal humeral resection with bone graft reconstruction. No osseous metastases or local recurrence is present. Intense physiological radiopharmaceutical accumulation is seen in the growth plates. The asymmetry of the ischiopubic synchondrosis is a developmental variant and may be seen in children before puberty during the fusion of ischial and pubic bones. Ischiopubic synchondrosis asymmetry is seen as asymmetric enlargement of the synchondrosis on radiographs and may demonstrate increased radiopharmaceutical uptake on bone scan and 18F-FDG PET/CT that should not be mistaken for trauma, infection, or tumor.

DISTRACTION TECHNIQUES, SEDATION, AND GENERAL ANESTHESIA

Unlike most adults, younger children, children with developmental delay, or children with multiple prior exposures to painful or anxiety-provoking medical procedures may not be able to comprehend instructions, hold still, or otherwise cooperate during the performance of NM examinations. Thus, for the pediatric patient, one must ensure that the requested study is "the right test, for the right patient, using the right dose, at the right time." (36,45). In addition to tailoring the NM study protocol to the specific indication, the use of pharmacologic approaches to reducing pain during venous access (46) as well as distraction and immobilization techniques to minimize the incidence and thus the risks

of sedation and general anesthesia are part of the best practices we will discuss in the ensuing pages (Table 17.4) (47). An example of a pharmacologic approach for reducing pain during venous access is the J-Tip system (J-Tip needleless injection system, National Medical Products, Inc, Irvine, CA). The J-Tip is a small, disposable, needle-free injector device that uses pressurized carbon dioxide to infiltrate a solution of lidocaine into subcutaneous tissue (46). Immobilization devices are used keep a body part or the entire body in a fixed position for an extended period during an imaging procedure. Swaddling devices (papooses) are available in multiple sizes. The older child may be swaddled in a blanket which is then secured with safety straps. While swaddling techniques work for infants, children younger than 6 years of age will typically need to undergo sedation or general anesthesia for studies such as single-photon-emission computed tomography (SPECT), SPECT/computed tomography (SPECT/CT), PET/CT, and PET/magnetic resonance imaging (PET/MRI) which require longer periods of immobilization. However, the use of sedation and general anesthesia needs to be carefully considered as the potential risks include the immediate medical consequences of cardiopulmonary depression and the potentially deleterious long-term neurocognitive effects on the developing brain from repeated sedative/anesthetic drug exposure (42).

THYROID

Congenital hypothyroidism

Congenital hypothyroidism (CH), the most common preventable cause of mental retardation, can be categorized as transient or permanent. Transient hypothyroidism, typically resolving within weeks to years, is due to transplacental maternal thyrotropin receptor-blocking antibodies, iodine deficiency during pregnancy, excess iodine exposure in iodine-sufficient countries, or maternal ingestion of drugs such as propylthiouracil. Permanent hypothyroidism is caused either by abnormal thyroid formation during embryogenesis (thyroid dysgenesis), abnormal thyroid hormone production (dyshormonogenesis), or resistance to thyroid-stimulating hormone (TSH) binding or signaling (48). Thyroid dysgenesis includes thyroid ectopy, agenesis, hypoplasia, and hemiagenesis (17,48). Dyshormonogenesis denotes hereditary disorders of thyroid hormone synthesis and secretion.

As the vast majority of CH patients are asymptomatic at birth, newborn screening programs for detection of CH have been established in many countries. Most commonly, TSH level is screened through heel stick blood sample (49). If there is an elevated TSH in the screening sample, a serum sample is obtained to confirm TSH findings and obtain a thyroxine (T4) level. Treatment with levothyroxine should begin as soon as the diagnosis is confirmed to prevent or ameliorate permanent neurologic damage and the other physical defects that can occur if CH is left untreated.

Imaging for those with CH has not been recommended by the American Academy of Pediatrics. While imaging findings may not change immediate patient management in most cases, they may determine the etiology of the problem and have implications for treatment decisions, prognosis, and counseling for parents regarding the natural history and course of CH (50). Such complementary imaging studies include thyroid ultrasound (US) and scintigraphy using either technetium-99m (Tc-99m) pertechnetate or I-123 (14). While US can identify the presence and size of the thyroid gland when in eutopic position, it is less efficacious in

Table 17.1 **NUCLEAR MEDICINE STUDIES OF THE PEDIATRIC URINARY TRACT**

Nuclear medicine study	Radiopharmaceutical*	Comments
Renal—dynamic renal scintigraphy (4,5)	Tc-99m-labeled tubular agents are preferred to glomerular agents due to more efficient extraction: Tc-99m mercaptoacetyltriglycine (MAG3) Tc-99m ethylenecysteine (EC) Tc-99m diethylenetriaminepentaacetic acid (DTPA)**	**SNMMI and EANM Procedural Guidelines:** **Hydration:** 5% dextrose, 0.33 normal saline, or other solution per institutional policy at 15–20 mL/kg (about two thirds of it should be given before furosemide injection) administered intravenously (IV). However, many children can achieve adequate hydration by age-appropriate oral intake of fluids (milk, water, or juice) **Bladder catheterization:** advised in infants and children with megaureter, posterior urethral valves, known vesicoureteral reflux or neuropathic bladder **Furosemide administration:** **(a) Timing:** F-0 or F+(*20 or 30*) protocols refer to the timing of furosemide administration relative to the radiopharmaceutical; that is, either concomitantly or after *20 or 30* min. However, furosemide may be given earlier or later with fast drainage or inadequate filling of the outflow tracts respectively **(b) Dose:** 1 mg/kg (maximum dose of 40 mg) IV. Consistent timing of administration for each patient on follow-up imaging **Dynamic imaging, phases:** *perfusion, cortical, and pre-furosemide drainage* for a total duration of 20–30 min: *post-furosemide drainage* (typically imaged for 20–30 min) **Planar images, gravity-assisted drainage or post-void images:** **(a) Gravity-assisted drainage images:** planar 1-min posterior images are obtained before and after the patient is kept upright for a standardized period of time (e.g., 10 or 15 min) **(b) post-void images:** planar 1-min image is obtained at a standardized time period (60 min or longer) after the injection of the radiopharmaceutical **Image processing:** **(a)** Calculation of *differential renal function*, typically at 60–120 s, with C-shaped regions of interest (ROIs) for background correction **(b)** *Post-furosemide drainage curve* generated with ROIs drawn to include the maximally dilated outflow tract **(c)** Calculation of several drainage parameters from the post-furosemide drainage curve: *washout half-time* and *percentage drainage* at the end of image acquisition **(d)** *Gravity assisted drainage* = [(ROI counts in pre-upright image)–(ROI counts in post-upright image)] / (ROI counts in pre-upright image)
Renal—cortical renal scintigraphy (6–10)	Tc-99m dimercaptosuccinic acid (DMSA)	Planar images with parallel hole collimation: posterior, right posterior oblique, and left posterior oblique Processing: ROI around each kidney to calculate differential function (with ROIs for background correction) Optional: SPECT, SPECT/CT, or pinhole collimation
Bladder and outflow tracts—direct radionuclide cystography (11)	Tc-99m sulfur colloid Tc-99m DTPA Tc-99m pertechnetate ***	Radiopharmaceutical preparation and instillation via urinary bladder catheter, options: **(a)** Injected into a 500 mL bag of normal saline that is hung 100 cm above the imaging table **(b)** Injected directly into urinary bladder after instilling 10–20 mL of normal saline into the bladder

* According to North American and EANM guidelines (12,13).

** Tc-99m DTPA, a glomerular agent, may be used when Tc-99m MAG3 and Tc-99m EC are not available (4).

***Tc-99m pertechnetate may be absorbed into the bloodstream from the bladder wall, especially if inflamed. The radiopharmaceutical can then accumulate in the renal collecting system and result in a false positive study (11).

Abbreviations: cm, centimeters; DMSA, dimercaptosuccinic acid; DTPA, diethylenetriaminepentaacetic acid; EC, ethylenecysteine; IV, intravenous; MAG3, mercaptoacetyltriglycine; ROI, region of interest; SPECT, single-photon-emission computed tomography; SPECT/CT, single-photon-emission computed tomography/computed tomography; Tc-99m, technetium-99m.

From References 4–13.

Table 17.2 **NUCLEAR MEDICINE DIAGNOSTIC STUDIES OF OTHER SYSTEMS IN PEDIATRICS**

Nuclear medicine study	Radiopharmaceutical*	Comments
Thyroid—congenital hypothyroidism (14,15)	(a) Tc-99m pertechnetate (IV) (b) I-123 (oral)	Patient should not be on thyroid hormone replacement for more than 7 days prior to the study No iodine-containing intravenous contrast administration in the prior 6 weeks
Thyroid—hyperthyroidism (16,17)	Scan and uptake: I-123	Scan and uptake: at 2–6 h (early imaging); percent uptake calculated at 2–6 and 24 h
Hepatobiliary scan—neonatal jaundice (18,19)	Tc-99m bromo-iminodiacetic acid	Premedication: phenobarbital (5 mg/kg/day for 5 days in two divided doses) to achieve a serum phenobarbital level of ≥15 mcg/mL 60-min anterior dynamic imaging followed by static anterior and right lateral images of the abdomen at 2, 4, 6, and 8 h till biliary excretion is demonstrated or up to a maximum of 24 h post-injection
Liver spleen scan—functional splenic tissue (20)	Tc-99m sulfur colloid	SPECT/CT aids in localizing the radiopharmaceutical uptake
Meckel scan (21,22)	Tc-99m pertechnetate	Fasting for 4–6 h Premedication: H2 antagonists or proton pump inhibitors 60-min of anterior dynamic imaging, followed by lateral and post-void images Ectopic gastric mucosa usually appears at the same time as gastric mucosa but delayed appearance (up to 40–50 min) is possible
Gastroesophageal reflux and liquid gastric emptying (23,24)	Tc-99m sulfur colloid Tc-99m DTPA	2–4 h fast depending on age and clinical circumstances Meal composition: cow's milk or formula similar in volume to the patient's usual meals Route of administration: orally, nasogastric tube, or percutaneous gastrostomy tube Calculate gastric emptying: acquire static anterior images of the abdomen at 1 h and 2 or 3 h. Percent gastric emptying = [counts in the bowel/(counts in the bowel + counts in the stomach)] x 100
Gastric emptying, solid (25,26)	Tc-99m sulfur colloid Tc-99m DTPA	4–6 h fast No standardized meal, no universal reference gastric emptying percent values Discontinue drugs that interfere with gastric motility unless the scan is performed to evaluate their efficacy
Radionuclide salivagram (27)	Tc-99m sulfur colloid	No preparation is necessary Volume and route of administration: small volume of radiopharmaceutical is placed on the tongue 60-min of posterior dynamic imaging of the chest is acquired
Bone scintigraphy (28–32)	Tc-99m-labeled radiopharmaceuticals from the bisphosphonate family**	**Types of bone scintigraphy:** (a) Delayed whole-body planar images in anterior and posterior projections: in younger children (especially when under anesthesia) this is acquired as multiple overlapping spot acquisitions to improve image resolution. The whole-body images may be supplemented with spot views in other projection. (b) Multiphase (two- or three-phase) bone scintigraphy: blood flow images (phase 1), immediate blood pool images (phase 2), and delayed images (phase 3). A two-phase bone scintigraphy includes phases 2 and 3 (c) SPECT or SPECT/CT (d) Late-phase images up to 24 h

Nuclear medicine study	Radiopharmaceutical*	Comments
MIBG scan	I-123 MIBG	Whole-body planar images in anterior and posterior projection or multiple overlapping spot acquisitions for improved image resolution. SPECT/CT of the primary tumor (33,34). In infants the neck, chest, abdomen, and pelvis are included in one SPECT acquisition.
18F-FDG PET/CT in neoplasms	18F-FDG	Typically includes whole-body scanning from vertex to toes Different options for the CT portion include, low-dose for attenuation correction only, diagnostic CT, or a combination thereof (32,35,36)
18F-FDG PET/CT in infection and inflammation	18F-FDG	Typically includes whole-body scanning from vertex to toes (37)
18F-FDG PET/CT in epilepsy (38)	18F-FDG	EEG hooked up Review the PET images fused to MR images
NM CSF shunt study	Tc-99m pertechnetate Tc-99m DTPA	Review prior anatomical imaging and NM CSF shunt studies Identify type of valve and expected normal CSF opening pressure

*According to North American and EANM guidelines (12,13).

** Methylene diphosphonate, hydroxy- ethylene diphosphonate, 2,3-dicarboxypropane-1, and 1-diphosphonate.

Abbreviations: 18F, fluorine-18; 18F-FDG, fluorine-18 fluorodeoxyglucose; CSF, cerebrospinal fluid; EEG, electroencephalogram; MAG3, Mercaptoacetyltriglycine; MDP, methylene diphosphonate; MIBG, Metaiodobenzylguanidine; MR, magnetic resonance; PET, positron-emission tomography; PET/CT, positron-emission tomography/computed tomography; SPECT/CT, single photon-emission computed tomography/ computed tomography; Tc-99m, technetium-99m.

From References (12–38).

Table 17.3 DOSE REDUCTION STRATEGIES FOR PEDIATRIC NUCLEAR MEDICINE (PLANAR AND SPECT/CT) AND 18F-FDG PET/CT STUDIES

Strategies	Comments
Eliminate unnecessary studies or choose alternative imaging modality that is associated with no or lower radiation (43)	PET/MR rather than PET/CT when available
Reduce injected dose of radiopharmaceutical (12,13)	Refer to North American or EANM guidelines (12,13) Increase time per bed position to obtain more counts
CT methodology—match methodology to purpose for acquisition (35)	**Purpose of CT acquisition:** – attenuation correction – anatomic colocalization – diagnostic interpretation – a combination of above
CT acquisition— optimize to reduce radiation dose (44)	**Scan parameters:** X-ray tube current, X-ray tube potential, image quality index, gantry rotation speed, and helical pitch **Image production methods**: image filters, reconstruction algorithm, and section thickness **Utilize proper scan technique:** optimize scan length and position patient at center of gantry – PET/CT scan length: whole-body; rarely "eyes to thigh" image acquisition – SPECT/CT length: only include the area of interest in the CT portion of the study

From References (12,13,35,43,44).

Table 17.4 **DISTRACTION TECHNIQUES**	
Techniques	**Description**
Interactive games	Age-appropriate applications displayed on a tablet device can be used to divert the patient's attention during the procedure.
Music	Music is a powerful calming tool. Children can listen to their favorite song(s) on a phone, tablet or other available device.
Reading	Age-appropriate books are one of the most useful pediatric distraction methods. The stories can be read out loud to the child and they can further be engaged by asking them questions about the story.
Movies and cartoons	Children can be distracted with age-appropriate movies and cartoons displayed on a tablet device or television.
Light-up toys and stuffed animals	Infants and toddlers can be distracted with stuffed animals and toys that light up, buzz, or play music.
Rewards	Before starting the procedure let the child know that he/she will receive a reward after the procedure is completed and engage the child by asking what sort of prize, he/she would like. A treasure chest containing games, books, toys and stuffed animals is available in many pediatric imaging facilities. Alternatively, the accompanying adult may already have a reward planned and they can engage the child by talking about the reward.

From Trottier et al. (47).

cases of thyroid ectopia (14). Most importantly, unlike scintigraphy, US cannot assess thyroid function.

Tc-99m pertechnetate is preferred for neonatal thyroid scintigraphy due to availability, lower cost, lower radiation dose to thyroid gland, image acquisition within 30 min of injection, and higher image quality when compared to I-123. However, Tc-99m pertechnetate only reflects thyroid trapping and does not undergo further metabolism, namely organification. Another limitation to the use of I-123 in this population is that neonates cannot swallow a capsule. To administer I-123 in a liquid form, a fume hood is required which may not available in all NM facilities (14,15,17).

Thyroid scintigraphy should be performed within 7 days of initiating thyroid hormone replacement. Otherwise, the resultant suppressed TSH will result in lack of accumulation of radiopharmaceutical in the thyroid gland. The interpretation of NM thyroid scans in neonates with primary CH exemplifies the pattern approach in imaging. The five main patterns on NM thyroid scans include *absent thyroid uptake, decreased eutopic uptake, increased eutopic uptake, ectopic uptake,* and *thyroid hemiagenesis patterns* (Fig. 17.2 and Table 17.5) (14,17,48,51,52). A normal NM thyroid scan, while uncommon, may be seen in patients with transient CH whose thyroid function test results have normalized.

Graves' disease

The most common cause of hyperthyroidism in pediatrics is Graves' disease. Similar to adults, NM thyroid scans may be used to differentiate the etiologies of hyperthyroidism (53–55). The only indication for I-131 thyroid ablation in pediatric hyperthyroidism is Graves' disease. As in adults, the patient should not be breastfeeding or pregnant and the patient and family should be able to adhere to radiation safety precautions. I-131 thyroid ablation is not a therapeutic option for children with autonomous thyroid nodules or toxic multinodular goiters due to concerns for a mutagenic effect of low-activity radioiodine and a higher risk of incidentally discovered differentiated thyroid cancer (DTC) in these entities in the pediatric population (16,56). Surgical

resection is usually recommended for children with an autonomous thyroid nodule (17).

There are specific considerations for I-131 ablation in pediatric Graves' disease. I-131 thyroid ablation is not performed in patients younger than 5 years of age. The maximum I-131 dose in patients between 5 and 10 years of age is 10 mCi. Ablation is not performed in patients with a thyroid gland weight of ≥80 g (16). I-131 ablation may be used as first-line therapy or after a trial of methimazole. The administered dose is either a fixed dose between 10 and 15 mCi or a calculated dose based on gland weight to deliver 200 to 300 μCi/g of thyroid tissue (16,17). Thyroid US is recommended, not only to estimate gland size for radioiodine dose determination but to ensure that the patient does not have an associated thyroid nodule present that would necessitate the performance of a total thyroidectomy to treat both Graves' disease and the potentially neoplastic thyroid nodule.

Differentiated thyroid cancer

While the incidence of thyroid nodules is higher in adults than in children, the risk of malignancy within a thyroid nodule is greater in children (16,56). Similar to adults, DTCs is the most common type of thyroid cancer. Papillary thyroid carcinoma (PTC) and follicular thyroid carcinoma (FTC) account for 95% and 5% of the DTCs. DTCs are often iodine-avid and highly sensitive to TSH (57). Unlike adults, children often present with advanced disease at diagnosis. Despite this, they have a better long-term prognosis than adults. For these and other reasons, pediatric-specific guidelines were created to diagnose and treat children with thyroid nodules and DTC (58). Again, as opposed to adults, total or near-total thyroidectomy, as opposed to lobectomy, is the recommended surgery for DTC in children, with central and lateral neck dissection as indicated (59). After total thyroidectomy, a staging whole-body I-123 scan is performed only in patients classified as intermediate or high-risk as defined by the American Thyroid Association (Fig. 17.3) (59). SPECT/CT is recommended to aid in localization of foci of

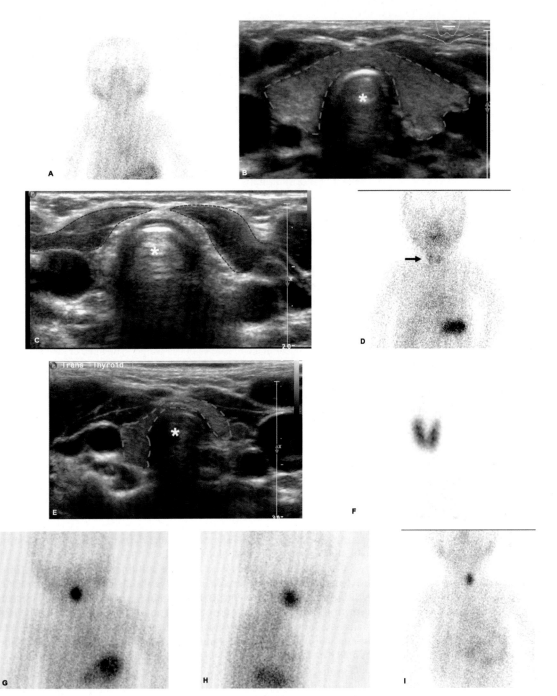

FIG. 17.2 ● **Thyroid uptake patterns on scintigraphy in congenital hypothyroidism.** Technetium-99m pertechnetate thyroid scans (A, D, F, G, and I are anterior images; H is a lateral image) demonstrate the five scintigraphic patterns in different neonates. Transverse thyroid ultrasound images (B, C, and E) demonstrate the corresponding appearance of the thyroid gland; asterisks denote the tracheal airway (in B, C, and E). **A–C: Absent thyroid uptake pattern.** Physiologic distribution of Tc-99m pertechnetate is seen in the salivary glands, mediastinal blood pool, and stomach. There is no accumulation of radiopharmaceutical in the thyroid bed or ectopically in the neck (A). This scintigraphic pattern may be associated with either a eutopic thyroid gland on ultrasound (dashed lines in B) or an absent thyroid gland on ultrasound (dashed line outlines the strap muscles in C). In patients with absent thyroid uptake pattern on scintigraphy, US differentiates between thyroid agenesis and the other etiologies (Table 17.5). **D and E: Decreased eutopic uptake pattern with hypoplastic thyroid gland on US** (hypoplasia in situ). The bilobed butterfly-shaped thyroid gland is eutopic in position but appears small with subjectively decreased uptake on NM thyroid scan (arrow in D). This may be secondary to either small thyroid gland size (hypoplasia) or decreased uptake secondary to other etiologies. Ultrasound confirms a small thyroid gland in expected position (dashed lines in E). In patients with decreased eutopic uptake pattern on scintigraphy, US differentiates between thyroid hypoplasia in situ and the other etiologies (Table 17.5). **F: Increased eutopic uptake pattern with dyshormonogenesis.** Maternal and neonatal history as well as subsequent clinical course differentiates the etiologies of this scintigraphic uptake pattern. Clinical and laboratory follow-up confirmed permanent hypothyroidism with lifelong requirement of thyroid hormone replacement. **G and H: Ectopic uptake pattern.** Thyroid scan in the anterior (G) and lateral (H) projections demonstrate radiopharmaceutical uptake in an ectopic thyroid gland located at the tongue base (lingual thyroid) with absence of radiopharmaceutical uptake in the thyroid bed. Ectopic thyroid gland may be located anywhere between the foramen cecum at the base of the tongue and the thyroid bed; uptake is typically unifocal but may be multifocal. **I: Hemiagenesis pattern.** Thyroid scan in the anterior projection demonstrates radiopharmaceutical uptake in the left thyroid lobe and absence of uptake in the right thyroid lobe. Agenesis of the left thyroid lobe is much more frequent representing 87.5% of cases in one series (From Ruchala et al. [51]). Thyroid hemiagenesis is usually an incidental finding but may be associated with hypothyroidism (From Szczepanek-Parulska et al. [52]).

Table 17.5 THE MAIN DIFFERENTIAL DIAGNOSES OF THREE OF THE UPTAKE PATTERNS IN PRIMARY CONGENITAL HYPOTHYROIDISM ON NM THYROID SCANS[τ]

Pattern	Differential diagnoses

Absent thyroid uptake*	1. Thyroid agenesis
	2. Scintigraphy may show no uptake despite the presence of a eutopic thyroid gland on ultrasound with
	   a. Dyshormonogenesis (i.e., inactivating mutations in the sodium/iodide symporter)
	   b. Maternal TSH receptor-blocking antibodies
	   c. TSH receptor mutations
	   d. Excess iodine intake through exposure (e.g., from antiseptic preparations)
	   e. TSH suppression from levothyroxine treatment

Decreased eutopic uptake**	1. Hypoplasia in situ 2. Dyshormonogenesis (i.e., mutations in the sodium/iodide symporter) 3. Maternal TSH receptor-blocking antibodies 4. TSH receptor mutations
Increased eutopic uptake	1. Dyshormonogenesis 2. Maternal anti-thyroid medication use*** 3. Chronic iodine deficiency***

[τ] Ectopic thyroid and hemiagenesis do not have a differential diagnosis.

* Thyroid ultrasound can differentiate athyreosis from the remainder of the etiologies of this pattern. The three uptake patterns of *no thyroid uptake decreased eutopic uptake, increased eutopic uptake* may be seen with dyshormonogenesis. For example, mutations in the sodium-iodide symporter result in either *no thyroid uptake* or *decreased eutopic uptake* (14).

**Thyroid ultrasound can differentiate hypoplasia in situ from the remainder of the etiologies of this pattern.

***The endocrinologist correlates with maternal history to differentiate these etiologies.

From Leger et al. (14); Giovanella et al. (17); Peters et al. (48).

abnormal uptake (57,60). I-131 therapy is indicated for iodine-avid persistent, unresectable locoregional or nodal disease and iodine-avid distant metastases (57,59,61). As children are more sensitive to the effects of thyroid hormone withdrawal than are adults, recombinant human thyroid-stimulating hormone (rhTSH) may be used, rather than levothyroxine withdrawal, to prepare the patient for both the whole-body I-123 post-thyroidectomy staging study and the subsequent I-131 therapy if indicated (57,59).

URINARY TRACT

Congenital anomalies of the kidneys and urinary tracts

Congenital anomalies of the kidneys and urinary tracts (CAKUT) are common and are the underlying etiology in 30% to 50% of cases of chronic kidney disease in children that ultimately require dialysis and/or renal transplant. Anomalies may be unilateral or bilateral and several anomalies may coexist (62–64). CAKUT may be classified as (i) renal parenchymal malformations (Fig. 17.4), (ii) anomalies of renal embryonic migration (Fig. 17.5), and (iii) outflow abnormalities (Figs. 17.6–17.10, Table 17.6) (65,66). With the increasing use of prenatal US, the most common abnormalities of the urinary tract in the fetus and neonate are dilation of the renal collecting system or concomitant dilation of the renal collecting system and ureter. Postnatally, these patients may be symptomatic, presenting with a urinary tract infection (UTI) or palpable abdominal mass, or asymptomatic. The natural course of dilation of the outflow tracts is variable and it may resolve, improve, stabilize, or worsen with resultant loss of renal function (4). The main

goal of NM renography is to identify that subset of patients that will benefit from surgical intervention. Such patients include those with (i) impaired split renal function (<40%), (ii) a decrease of split renal function of >10% in subsequent studies, or (iii) poor drainage after the administration of furosemide (4,67,68).

NM studies of the kidneys and urinary tracts evaluate renal function, drainage of the outflow tracts, and vesicoureteral reflux (VUR). **Relative renal function** is assessed with technetium-99m mercaptoacetyltriglycine (Tc-99m MAG3) or Tc-99m dimercaptosuccinic acid (Tc-99m DMSA) (Fig. 17.9). The relative function of *renal units* is assessed, that is, right versus left kidney and additionally, in duplicated collecting systems, the upper versus the lower moiety (Fig. 17.6). The renal unit may be nonfunctional or have decreased function secondary to dysplasia or a multicystic dysplastic kidney (MCDK). The **drainage of the dilated outflow tracts,** that is the renal collecting system or the combination of the renal collecting system and ureter in patients with a megaureter (Fig. 17.8), is assessed with Tc-99m MAG3 dynamic renal scintigraphy. Furosemide is administered to augment urine production and urine flow and to assess drainage of the radiopharmaceutical from the outflow tract (4). Serial dynamic images and the time-activity curve (TAC) are evaluated to assess drainage. With normal drainage, the TAC should rapidly decline from peak. With abnormal drainage, the TAC may ascend, plateau, or descend but not to baseline. The addition of planar gravity-assisted drainage images (Fig. 17.7), after the acquisition of dynamic images, may provide additional information about the drainage of the outflow tracts (69).

Magnetic resonance urography may also be used to assess function and drainage of the kidneys and is particularly useful

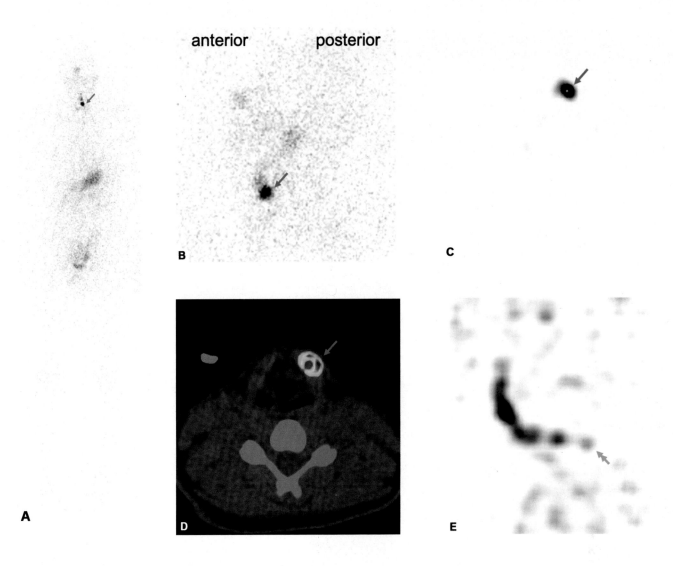

anterior   posterior

A   B   C

D   E

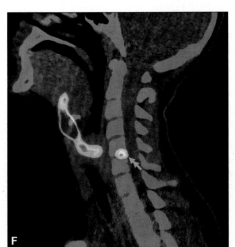

F

FIG. 17.3 ● **Metastatic thyroid cancer.** 16-year-old male presents with diffuse thyroid enlargement and cervical lymphadenopathy. Neck US (not shown) demonstrated a diffusely enlarged thyroid gland with microcalcifications and pathological lymphadenopathy in bilateral levels 2–4 and level 6. Chest CT (not shown) demonstrated level 7 lymphadenopathy but no pulmonary metastases. Patient underwent total thyroidectomy, bilateral lateral modified radical neck dissection at levels 2A, 3, and 4, as well as bilateral level 6 and 7 central neck dissection. The tumor had invaded into bilateral Berry's ligaments (suspensory ligaments that pass from the thyroid gland to the trachea). Pathology demonstrated papillary thyroid carcinoma, diffuse sclerosing variant (multifocal involvement of bilateral thyroid lobes and the isthmus), with positive surgical margins, angioinvasion, and lymphatic invasion; 36/54 positive lymph nodes; pathologic classification pT3b pN1b, American Thyroid Association high-risk group. Anti-thyroglobulin antibody was present (>3000 IU/mL). Staging whole-body I-123 scan with SPECT/CT of the head and neck was performed. **A and B:** Anterior whole-body (A) and left lateral spot images of the head and neck (B) demonstrate several foci of abnormal uptake in the neck that are best localized to the left strap muscles and thyroid cartilage (arrows in A and B) with SPECT/CT (refer to C and D). Additionally, there is abnormal uptake in the C5 vertebral body (refer to E and F), the thyroid bed, and right cricothyroid cartilage (corresponding SPECT and SPECT/CT images not shown). **C and D:** Paired axial SPECT (C) and SPECT/CT (D) of the thyroid cartilage demonstrates uptake in the left strap muscles and thyroid cartilage (arrow). **E and F:** Paired sagittal SPECT (E) and SPECT/CT (F) of the cervical spine demonstrates focal uptake in the inferior C5 vertebral body (double arrow); there was no corresponding abnormality on low-dose CT (not shown). The patient weighed 89 kg and 194 mCi of I-131 was administered. Post-therapy whole-body scans (not shown) demonstrated additional osseous metastases in the sternum and two ribs.

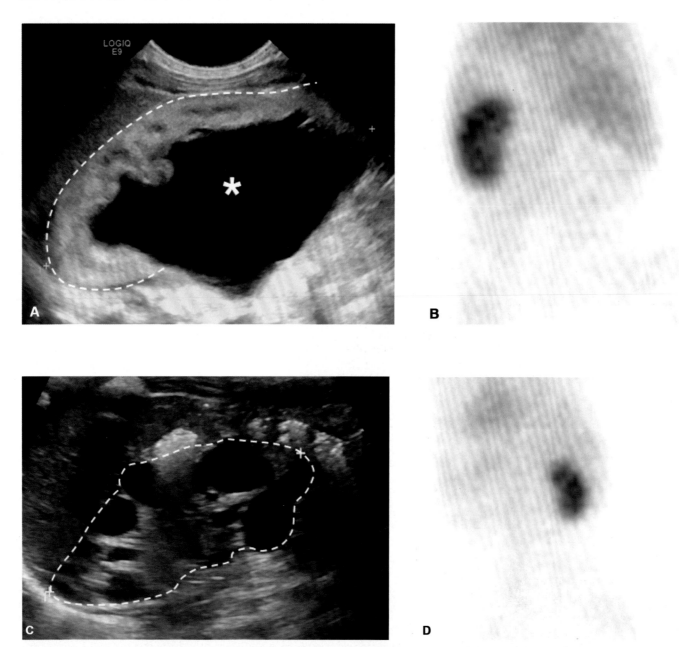

FIG. 17.4 ● Nonfunctional kidneys in two different infants. Obstructive renal dysplasia. **A:** Ultrasound on day one of life (DOL) in an infant male with history of in-utero hydronephrosis demonstrates dilation of the right renal pelvis (*) and calyces associated with increased renal parenchymal echogenicity and loss of corticomedullary differentiation. Voiding cystourethrogram (VCUG) performed on DOL 6 (not shown) was normal without evidence of vesicoureteral reflux (VUR). **B:** Tc-99m MAG3 renogram was performed at 1.5 months of age. Posterior cortical phase image (composite of all frames acquired between 60–120 s) demonstrates lack of radiopharmaceutical accumulation in the right renal fossa consistent with a non-functioning right kidney due to obstructive renal dysplasia. **Multicystic dysplastic kidney. C:** One-day-old infant female with a diagnosis of CAKUT on fetal ultrasound undergoes renal ultrasound which demonstrates multiple, varying-sized, non-connecting cysts without normal intervening renal parenchyma in the left renal fossa, the typical appearance of a multicystic dysplastic kidney (MCDK). VCUG (not shown) performed of 1 month of age was normal, without VUR identified. **D:** Tc-99m MAG3 renogram was performed at 3 months of age. Posterior cortical phase image demonstrates lack of radiopharmaceutical accumulation in the left renal fossa, confirming a non-functioning, multicystic dysplastic left kidney.

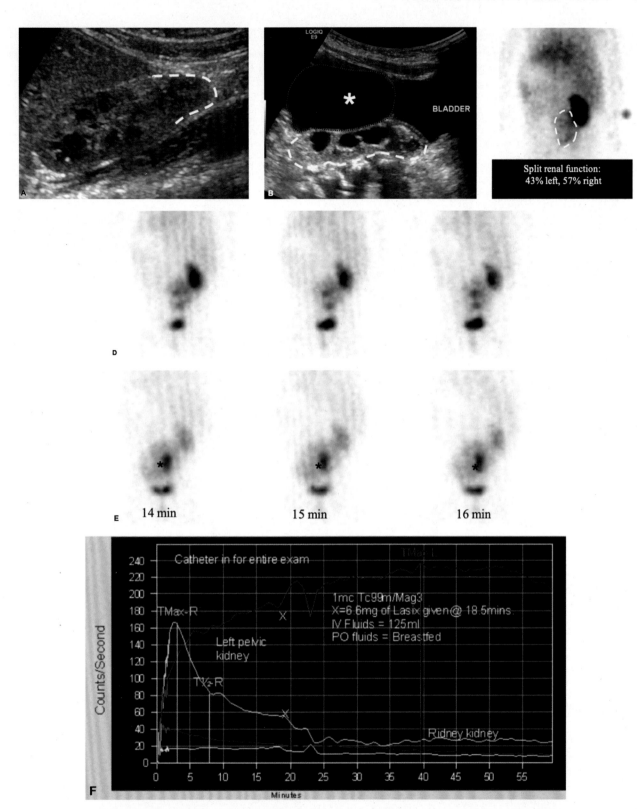

FIG. 17.5 ● **Ectopic left kidney with outflow tract abnormality.** 2-month-old male with left, malrotated pelvic kidney and dilation of the left collecting system on fetal ultrasound presents for renal ultrasound and Tc-99m MAG3 renogram with furosemide. **A and B:** Longitudinal ultrasound images of the kidneys demonstrate a eutopic right kidney (A); the lower pole is well-delineated (dashed line in A) and therefore, the kidneys are not fused. The left pelvic kidney (B) is malrotated with the dilated renal pelvis (asterisk and outlined with dotted line) located anteriorly and immediately superior to the urinary bladder. **C–F:** Posterior cortical phase image (C) from Tc-99m MAG3 renogram study demonstrates the left pelvic kidney (dashed outline in C) with differential renal function (DRF) of 43% on the left and 57% on the right. In patients with anomalies of renal embryonic migration (fusion anomalies or renal ectopia), the initial images should be acquired with a dual-detector camera to calculate geometric means for DRF, if feasible. However, posterior dynamic images are adequate for evaluation of the post-diuresis drainage (4). Dynamic posterior images from 4 to 6 min (D) and 14 to 16 min (E) demonstrate accumulation of radiopharmaceutical in the left dilated collecting system (asterisk in E). Furosemide was administered at 18.5 min and the post-furosemide renogram curve (F) of the left kidney (red line) was ascending and subsequently plateaued. Findings are consistent with a urodynamically significant obstruction of the left outflow tract. There is normal right renal drainage.

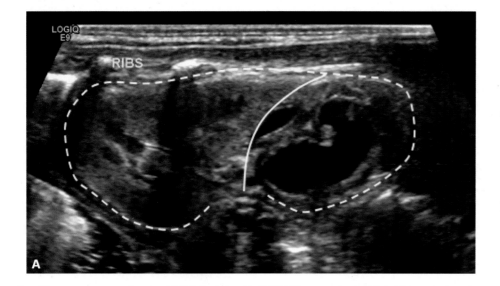

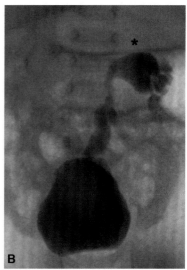

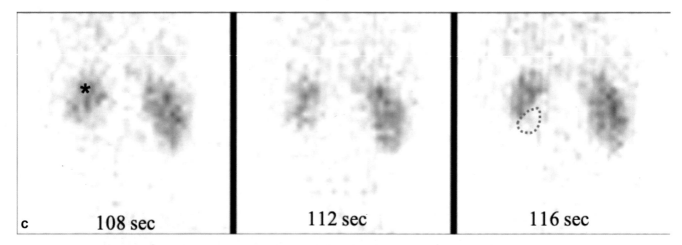

FIG. 17.6 ● **Duplicated left renal collecting system with nonfunctional lower moiety.** One-day-old infant female with CAKUT on fetal ultrasound. **A:** Renal US on DOL 1 demonstrates a duplicated left renal collecting system. The left kidney is outlined with a dashed line and the solid line separates the upper from the lower moiety. The lower moiety has a dilated collecting system with dysplastic parenchyma. **B:** VCUG performed at 1 month of age demonstrates grade IV reflux into the lower moiety of the duplicated left renal collecting system ("drooping lily sign"). There is no reflux of contrast into the upper moiety (expected location demarcated with an asterisk). **C–F:** Tc-99m MAG3 renogram was performed when the patient was 5 months of age. The urinary bladder was catheterized given history of high-grade reflux; furosemide was not administered. Three posterior frames (108–116 s) from the cortical phase (C) and dynamic posterior images from 4 to 6 min (D) and 24 to 26 min (E) demonstrate a truncated appearance of the lower pole of the left kidney. There is absent perfusion to and uptake by the lower pole moiety of the left kidney consistent with a nonfunctional lower pole moiety. There is prompt radiopharmaceutical perfusion, uptake and excretion from the upper-pole moiety (asterisk in C and D). There is delayed visualization of the radiopharmaceutical in the smaller lower moiety (dashed line in E) representing indirect evidence of VUR into the dilated lower moiety collecting system. Regions of interest were drawn around the right kidney and the left upper moiety (F) in the posterior cortical phase image to calculate DRF of 35% on the left and 65% on the right.

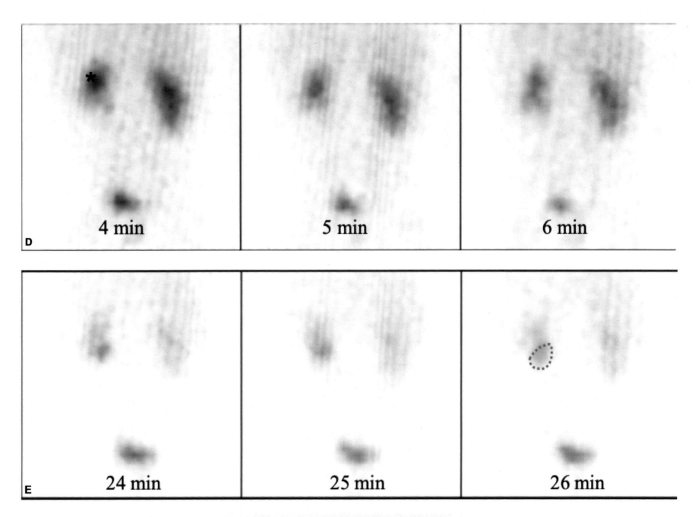

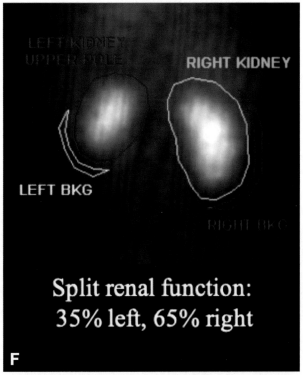

FIG. 17.6 ● (Continued)

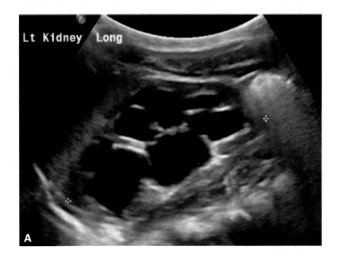

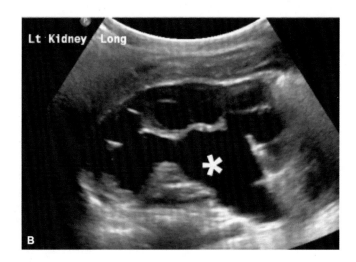

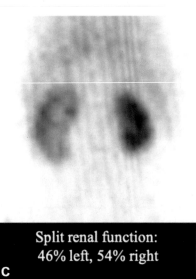

FIG. 17.7 • **Ureteropelvic junction obstruction.** 6-month-old male with prenatal diagnosis of a dilated left renal collecting system. Tc-99m MAG3 renogram (not shown) was initially performed at 1 month of age and demonstrated preserved left renal function (DRF of 55% on the left and 45% on the right) with a post-furosemide drainage of 75% at 30 min after the injection of diuretic. Serial renal ultrasounds demonstrated worsening dilation of the renal collecting system, leading to repeat US and Tc-99m MAG3 renogram with furosemide at 6 months of age. **A and B:** Longitudinal renal US images of the left kidney demonstrates marked dilation of the renal calyces and pelvis (asterisk in B) with diffuse parenchymal thinning. The right kidney (not shown) was normal. **C–G:** Tc-99m MAG3 renogram with furosemide was performed. Furosemide was administered at 21.5 min and the urinary bladder was catheterized to ensure appropriate drainage. Posterior cortical phase image (C) demonstrates a DRF of 46% on the left and 54% on the right. Dynamic posterior images from 18 to 20 min (D), 28 to 20 min (E), and 54 to 56 min (F) demonstrate retention of radiopharmaceutical in the dilated left collecting system. The post-diuretic time-activity curve (G) for the left kidney demonstrates a descending curve (red line) after the administration of furosemide that subsequently plateaus above baseline. There is a post-furosemide drainage of 50% at 30 min after the injection of diuretic. **H:** Posterior gravity-assisted drainage images, obtained before and after holding the infant upright for 15 min to improve drainage of the outflow tract, demonstrate an additional 21% emptying of the left renal collecting system. Gravity-assisted drainage is calculated by using the difference between the counts in the ROIs drawn around the dilated outflow tract on the pre-upright and post-upright images and dividing it by the pre-upright counts; it can be expressed as a ratio or a percentage (as in this case) (From Majd et al. [4]). Based on the constellation of findings of interval decreased relative function of the left kidney and the configuration and drainage of the post-diuretic and gravity-assisted drainage images, the patient has a urodynamically significant (i.e., critical) ureteropelvic junction obstruction. **I:** Retrograde ureterogram obtained during surgery demonstrates a transition point (arrow) between the proximal ureter and a markedly dilated renal pelvis (asterisk).

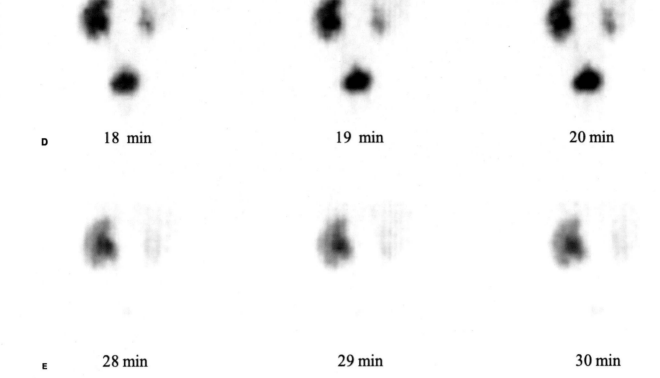

D   18 min   19 min   20 min

E   28 min   29 min   30 min

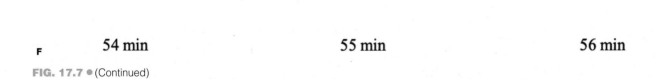

F   54 min   55 min   56 min

FIG. 17.7 ● (Continued)

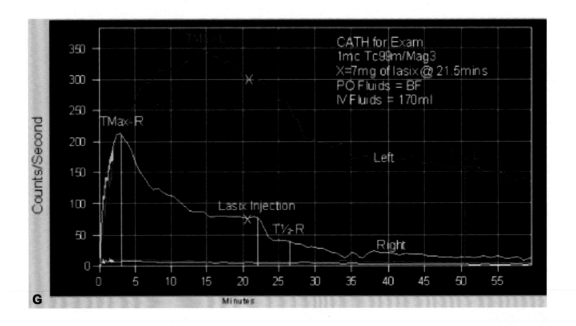

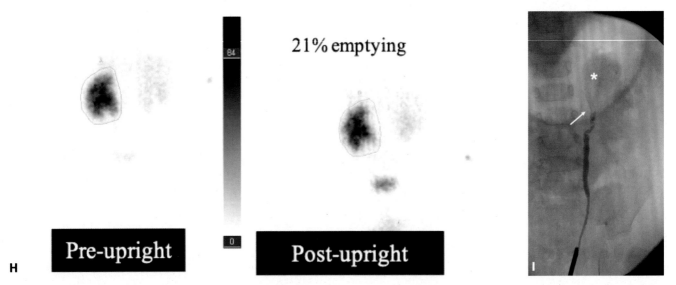

FIG. 17.7 ● (Continued)

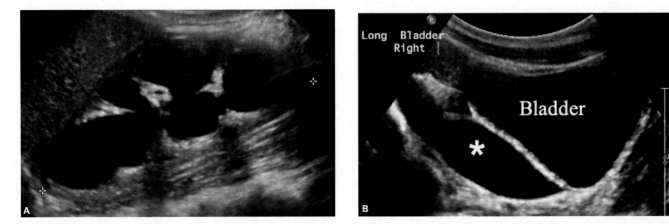

FIG. 17.8 ● **Congenital obstructive megaureter.** 8-year-old male presents with an acute episode of right flank and lower quadrant pain. **A and B:** Abdominal US demonstrates dilation of the right renal collecting system associated with marked parenchymal thinning (A) as well as a right megaureter (asterisk in B). The right and left kidneys measured 12.9 cm and 9 cm in length respectively.

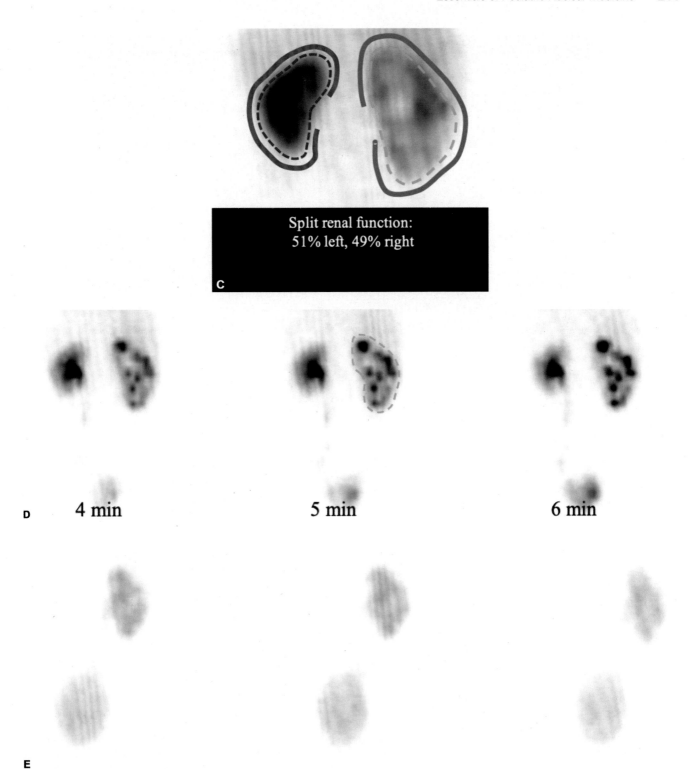

FIG. 17.8 ● (Continued) **Congenital obstructive megaureter. C:** Tc-99m MAG3 renogram with furosemide was performed; furosemide was administered at 17 min. As the patient was able to cooperate with voiding he was not catheterized; the study was paused at 32 min for the patient to void in the restroom and subsequently resumed. Schematic of the posterior cortical phase image demonstrates the appropriately drawn regions of interest (ROIs) for each kidney as well as the preferred C-shaped ROI for background correction. There is an asymmetrically larger right kidney with a DRF of 51% on the left and 49% on the right. The function of the hydronephrotic right kidney may be overestimated secondary to technical issues such as background subtraction (From Capone et al. [64]). The DRF is calculated using the composite image with the maximum accumulation of the radiopharmaceutical in the parenchyma and no radiopharmaceutical transit to the collecting system (e.g., 60–120 s). A C-shaped region of interest is drawn around each kidney for subtraction of background counts from the liver and spleen blood-pool activity (From Majd et al. [4]). **D and E:** Dynamic posterior images from 4 to 6 min (D) and 54 to 56 min (E) demonstrate parenchymal thinning and partial drainage of the dilated right collecting system. Parenchymal thinning of the right kidney is appreciated by the proximity of the calyces to the outer renal contour (dashed line in D).

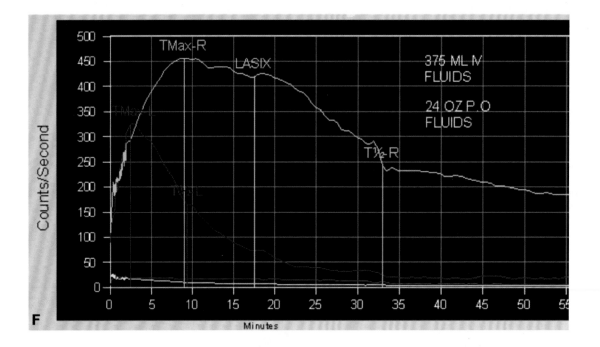

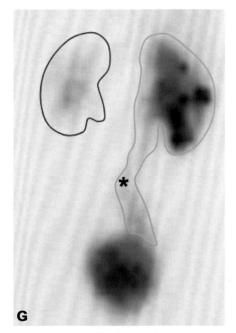

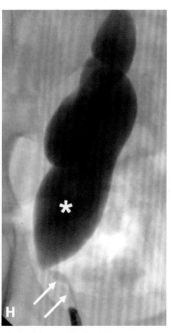

FIG. 17.8 ● (Continued) **Congenital obstructive megaureter. F and G:** The post-diuretic time-activity curve (F) for the right kidney is initially descending (green curve in F) and subsequently plateaus well above baseline. Schematic diagram (G) demonstrates the appropriate ROIs for evaluation of the drainage of the left (red ROI) and right (green ROI) outflow tracts. The ROIs for generation of the drainage time-activity curve must include the entire dilated outflow tract and should be drawn on the images with maximal dilatation of the outflow tract (From Majd et al. [4]). On the posterior composite image (G) the time-activity curve for the right outflow tract is generated by drawing the region of interest (green ROI in G) to surround the right kidney and right ureter (asterisk in G). **H:** Retrograde ureterogram obtained during surgery demonstrates short segment stenosis (arrows) with severe upstream dilation of the ureter (asterisk). The ureter was reimplanted. Ureterovesical junction obstruction denotes "partial obstruction and is due to narrowing of the distal ureter, duplication with ectopic ureterocele, or ectopic insertion of the ureter" (From Majd et al. [4]).

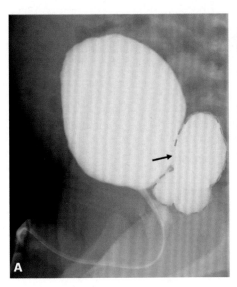
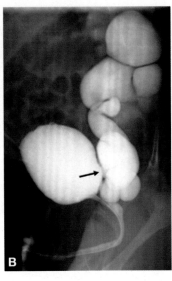
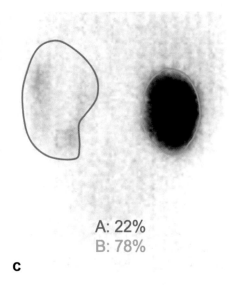

A: 22%
B: 78%

FIG. 17.9 ● **Refluxing megaureter with congenital reflux nephropathy.** 1-month-old male presents for VCUG. He had a prenatal diagnosis of dilation of the left renal collecting system and ureter. This was confirmed on post-natal US performed on DOL 1 (not shown) which demonstrated severe dilation of the left renal collecting system, marked parenchymal thinning, and a left megaureter. **A and B:** Anterior oblique images (A and B) from VCUG demonstrate a large bladder diverticulum (dashed line in A) arising from the posterior bladder (arrows in A and B indicate the neck of the diverticulum). There is grade V reflux of contrast into a dilated and tortuous left ureter that inserts into the bladder diverticulum. There is marked dilation of the collecting system. **C:** Cortical renal scintigraphy with DMSA was performed at 3 months of age to assess left renal function. Posterior image demonstrates decreased function of the left kidney with a differential function of 22% on the left and 78% on the right. The dilated left collecting system is appreciated as a central photopenic defect. There is diffusely decreased radiopharmaceutical accumulation in the left kidney consistent with renal dysplasia secondary to congenital reflux nephropathy.

when there is complex anatomy to be defined, such as occurs in those with genitourinary anomalies (59,70).

DIMERCAPTOSUCCINIC ACID

Cortical renal scintigraphy with Tc-99m dimercaptosuccinic acid (DMSA) is the gold standard for identifying renal scars or foci of acute pyelonephritis. Both renal scarring and acute pyelonephritis result in areas of reduced radiopharmaceutical uptake. In renal scarring, there is a well-defined photopenic defect with volume loss and change in the adjacent renal contour. In acute pyelonephritis, the photopenic defects may be patchy and there is no associated volume loss or change in renal contour (6,71).

DMSA scintigraphy performed *early* on, within 7 days of symptom onset, can diagnose acute pyelonephritis in clinically misleading cases. Scarring is best identified when DMSA scintigraphy is performed *4 to 6 months* after a UTI (71,72). Two main approaches have been proposed for the controversial workup of patients with UTI and suspected VUR. These include the *top–down approach* and the *bottom–up approach*. In the *top–down approach*, the DMSA scan is performed before the voiding cystourethrogram (VCUG) in order to reliably detect children at greatest risk for kidney damage and to decrease the numbers of unnecessary VCUGs. In the *bottom–up approach*, a VCUG is performed first followed eventually by DMSA scintigraphy (71–73). The American College of Radiology appropriateness criteria for imaging of UTIs in children was published in 2017 (74). In children with recurrent or atypical UTI, cortical scintigraphy is rated as 6 (i.e., may be appropriate) and direct radionuclide voiding cystography is rated as 7 (i.e., usually appropriate, especially in girls).

Radiation dose to the kidneys is higher with Tc-99m DMSA cortical scintigraphy compared to Tc-99m MAG3 dynamic renal scintigraphy. In a 1-year-old child the radiation dose to the kidneys is 0.77 and 0.016 mGy/MBq with Tc-99m DMSA and Tc-99m MAG3 respectively (75). Therefore, in infants, when the clinical question is to evaluate the function of a kidney (such as in MCDK or obstructive dysplasia), Tc-99m MAG3 dynamic renal scintigraphy is the preferred exam.

Voiding cystography

Imaging options for the evaluation of VUR include fluoroscopic VCUG, direct or indirect radionuclide voiding cystography (Fig. 17.10), and contrast-enhanced voiding urosonography (ceVUS) (76–78). ceVUS has similar or better accuracy in detecting VUR compared to VCUG without the use of ionizing radiation (77–79). Some authors have reported increased sensitivity in detection of VUR with cyclic direct radionuclide voiding cystography compared to a single cycle of bladder filling (80,81).

The effective radiation dose during fluoroscopic VCUG may be lower than direct radionuclide voiding cystography with the use of modern image acquisition tools and an optimized protocol (82). However, direct radionuclide-voiding cystography is easily performed, allows continuous monitoring of the bladder filling and emptying cycle, and is highly sensitive for the detection of VUR (83,84). Direct radionuclide voiding cystography does not provide anatomical detail about the bladder or the urethra and can only distinguish three grades of VUR, as opposed to five grades on VCUG. On direct radionuclide voiding cystography, the severity of reflux is graded as one to three: (I) reflux restricted to the ureter, (II) reflux reaches the renal pelvis, and (III) reflux reaches the renal pelvis with associated dilation of the renal collecting system (79). Similar to VCUG, the NM report should

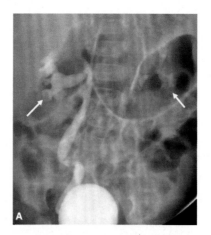

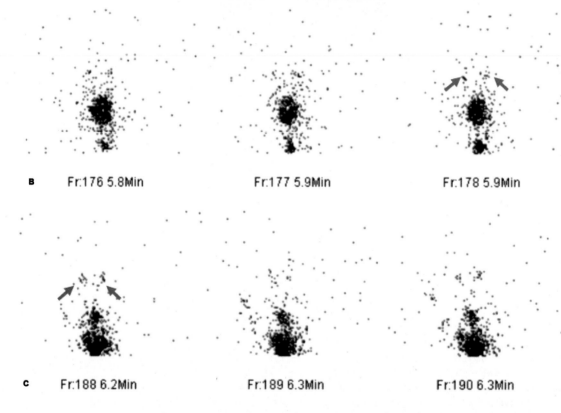

B   Fr:176 5.8Min   Fr:177 5.9Min   Fr:178 5.9Min

C   Fr:188 6.2Min   Fr:189 6.3Min   Fr:190 6.3Min

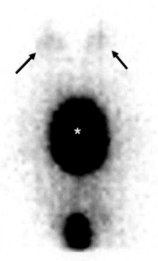

D

FIG. 17.10 ● **Bilateral vesicoureteral reflux on VCUG and direct radionuclide cystography.** 6-week-old male with a history of urinary tract infection treated with a course of acute as well as prophylactic antibiotics presents for a VCUG. Renal ultrasound (not shown) was normal. **A:** AP view from a VCUG demonstrates grade III right and grade II left vesicoureteral reflux that initially occurred during filling phase. **B–D:** Prophylactic antibiotics were continued for another year after which the patient undergoes direct radionuclide cystography at 1 year of age to re-evaluate vesicoureteral reflux. One mCi of Tc-99m sulfur colloid was admixed with 500 mL of normal saline. The catheterized bladder was filled with 100 mL of this admixed solution and posterior dynamic images were acquired at 2 s per frame during filling and voiding for total duration of 6.5 min. The patient started micturition at 5.6 min. Sequential 2 s/frame images at 5.9 min (B, during filling) and 6.2 min (C, during voiding) demonstrate reflux of radiopharmaceutical into the bilateral renal collecting systems (arrows in B and C) during voiding. Asterisks in B and D demarcate the urinary bladder; the ovoid focus of radiopharmaceutical inferior to the urinary bladder (in B–D) is the accumulation of radiopharmaceutical in the diaper after voiding. A composite image of the filling and voiding phases (D) better demonstrates reflux extending into dilated bilateral renal collecting systems (arrows).

Table 17.6 CLASSIFICATION OF CONGENITAL ANOMALIES OF THE KIDNEYS AND URINARY TRACTS

CAKUT Classification	Categories
Renal parenchymal malformations	Renal agenesis Simple renal hypoplasia Renal dysplasia and hypodysplasia Multicystic dysplastic kidney Renal tubular dysgenesis Genetic cystic disease – autosomal dominant polycystic kidney disease – autosomal recessive polycystic kidney disease – nephronophthisis
Anomalies of renal embryonic migration	Renal ectopia Fusion anomalies
Outflow abnormalities	Duplicated collecting system Ureteropelvic junction obstruction Megaureter: (a) obstructive, (b) refluxing, (c) obstructive and refluxing, and d) non-obstructive and non-refluxing Vesicoureteral reflux Posterior urethral valves

From Murugapoopathy and Gupta (65).

indicate whether reflux was present during the filling phase, the voiding phase, or both phases of direct radionuclide voiding cystography.

HEPATOBILIARY SYSTEM AND SPLEEN

Neonatal biliary atresia

Prolonged cholestatic jaundice in the neonate is most commonly due to neonatal hepatitis or biliary atresia. Untreated biliary atresia results in cirrhosis. Kasai portoenterostomy results in successful biliary drainage when performed before 60 days of life in approximately 80% of cases. The success rate of surgery decreases to 20% when performed after 90 days of life (85). Consequently, neonatal hepatobiliary scintigraphy is a critical tool which, when performed correctly, can noninvasively distinguish between these two entities in infants under 3 months of age. Absence of biliary or gut excretion up to 24 h after radiopharmaceutical injection associated with normal hepatic radiopharmaceutical uptake is highly suggestive of biliary atresia (19,86,87). The gold standard for the diagnosis of biliary atresia is an intraoperative cholangiogram. A liver biopsy may be obtained to aid in the diagnosis (87).

Kwatra et al. (19) used two interpretive criteria to define three hepatobiliary scan patterns in infants with prolonged cholestatic jaundice. The interpretive criteria are (i) presence or absence of radiopharmaceutical in the gallbladder, biliary tree or bowel in images obtained up to 24 h (i.e., biliary excretion) and (ii) normal or decreased hepatic uptake. The hepatic uptake is determined by comparing the intensity of radiopharmaceutical in the liver to the cardiac blood pool at 5 min after injection of the radiopharmaceutical. In *decreased hepatic uptake*, the intensity is lower in the liver than in the cardiac blood pool. The three scan patterns are: (a) **presence of biliary excretion** (with normal or decreased hepatic uptake), (b) **absence of biliary excretion with decreased hepatic uptake,** and (c) **absence of biliary excretion with normal hepatic uptake.** The *presence of biliary excretion*

is interpreted as cholestasis from causes other than biliary atresia. *Absence of biliary excretion with decreased hepatic uptake is* interpreted as cholestasis from causes other than biliary atresia in infants up to 3 months of age. In infants older than 3 months, this pattern may be seen in children with biliary atresia with compromised liver function. *Absence of biliary excretion with normal hepatic uptake* is highly suggestive of biliary atresia (Fig. 17.11). Using their strict interpretive criteria, these authors have demonstrated 100% sensitivity and 94% specificity in distinguishing biliary atresia from other causes of neonatal cholestatic jaundice.

Several groups have evaluated the use of SPECT in the neonatal hepatobiliary scan and have suggested that it has a higher accuracy than planar imaging. Further, with the addition of SPECT imaging at 4–6 h, planar imaging at 24 h or the standard pretreatment with phenobarbital prior to performance of hepatobiliary scintigraphy for this indication may not be necessary (88,89).

Other pediatric-specific hepatobiliary and splenic pathologies

Historically, the hepatobiliary scan has been used in the diagnosis of choledochal cyst (90,91). The filling of an intra- or extrahepatic cystic lesion with radiopharmaceutical in a hepatobiliary scan identifies the structure as a choledochal cyst (Fig. 17.12). With the more widespread availability of MRI and the exquisite anatomical detail of the biliary system seen on magnetic resonance cholangiopancreatography (MRCP), the role of hepatobiliary scans in this disease entity has waned (92).

Liver spleen scans with Tc-99m sulfur colloid (reticuloendothelial imaging) may be used to identify functional splenic tissue in suspected anatomic or functional asplenia as well as in hyposplenism. Disease processes that lead to atrophy, infarction, engorgement, or infiltration of the spleen may result in either *hyposplenism* or *functional asplenia*. *Anatomic asplenia* is most often due to surgical removal of the spleen, although it can also be

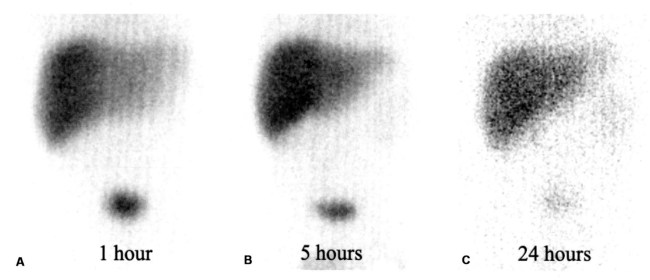

FIG. 17.11 ● **Biliary atresia.** 25-day-old female with persistent jaundice presents for a phenobarbital-enhanced hepatobiliary scan. **A–C:** Dynamic anterior images obtained over 60 min (not shown) demonstrated prompt hepatic uptake and prompt clearance of radiopharmaceutical from the blood pool but lack of visualization of the biliary tree, gallbladder or small bowel. Anterior planar images obtained at 1 (A), 5 (B), and 24 (C) h following radiopharmaceutical administration demonstrate retention of radiopharmaceutical in the liver parenchyma with no bowel excretion. There is renal excretion of the radiopharmaceutical. Findings are highly suggestive of, but not diagnostic for, biliary atresia. The differential diagnosis includes paucity of intrahepatic bile ducts and neonatal hepatitis, although prompt hepatic uptake as well as prompt clearance of radiopharmaceutical from the blood pool makes neonatal hepatitis less likely. Biliary atresia was confirmed with intraoperative cholangiography and liver biopsy and the patient underwent a Kasai portoenterostomy.

congenital in those with heterotaxy and bilateral right-sidedness (93,94). In pediatrics, liver spleen scans can be obtained to identify functional splenic tissue in entities such as sickle cell anemia (95), heterotaxy (20,96) (Fig. 17.13), following splenic trauma, with a wandering spleen (97), suspected accessory spleen(s) or ectopic splenosis in the thorax, abdomen, pelvis or scrotal sac (98–100) (Fig. 17.14).

GASTROINTESTINAL TRACT

Gastroesophageal reflux scintigraphy, gastric emptying scintigraphy, and radionuclide salivagram

Gastroesophageal reflux (GER), the passage of gastric contents into the esophagus, is a normal physiologic process that occurs in healthy infants, children, and adults. Most episodes of GER are brief and do not cause symptoms, esophageal injury, or other complications. When the GER episodes are associated with symptoms or complications, such as esophagitis or poor weight gain, GER disease (GERD) is present (101). Monitoring esophageal pH (pH probe) and/or impedance can quantify esophageal reflux but is invasive (102). A fluoroscopic upper gastrointestinal series may be used in selected cases to rule out anatomic abnormalities such as malrotation; however, it has no role in identifying or quantifying GER (102).

According to the Pediatric Gastroesophageal Reflux Clinical Practice Guidelines: Joint Recommendations of the respective North American and European Societies, the standards for the interpretation of NM studies for GERD are poorly established (102). Although these studies may detect pulmonary aspiration, a negative test does not necessarily exclude pulmonary aspiration. The presence of GER on scintigraphic studies is not sufficient for a diagnosis of GERD. Scintigraphic studies are only recommended

to evaluate gastric emptying in patients with symptoms of gastric retention (102).

GER scintigraphy or "milk scan" is typically performed by admixing a radiopharmaceutical, either Tc-99m sulfur colloid or Tc-99m diethylenetriaminepentaacetic acid (DTPA), with milk or formula similar in volume and composition to the child's customary feeds. Posterior dynamic images of the chest and upper abdomen are obtained for 60 min. The number of episodes of reflux as well as the level of reflux in the esophagus and the duration for each episode of reflux should be reported. GER may be graded as mild, moderate or severe based on a combination of the number, level, and clearance of the episodes of GER during dynamic imaging (24). Regions of interest may be drawn around the esophagus to generate a time-activity curve. Gastric emptying and pulmonary aspiration may also be evaluated (26).

Kwatra et al. (24) performed a retrospective review to determine age-specific liquid gastric emptying values at 1 and 3 h in children ≤5 years of age. In their retrospective patient cohort, they identified 205 patients who were closest to normal healthy children (i.e., fed orally and without GER). In this group, the median percent gastric emptying at 1 h and 3 h was 43% (interquartile range of 34%–52%) and 91% (interquartile range of 81%–98%), respectively. The authors proposed a 3-h gastric emptying cutoff value of ≥80% for a normal study in infants and children ≤5 years of age. Percent gastric emptying at 1 h is variable and may not be a reliable measure of gastric emptying (23,24).

In the older child gastric emptying is evaluated with a radiolabeled solid meal in which Tc-99m sulfur colloid is added to a beaten egg or egg white and cooked. Planar images are obtained, at a minimum, at 0, 1, 2, and 4 h after meal ingestion as described originally (25). In our practice, we obtain anterior planar images at 0, 15, 30, and 45 min in addition to the 1, 2, and 4-h time intervals. However, due to the variability in meal composition and

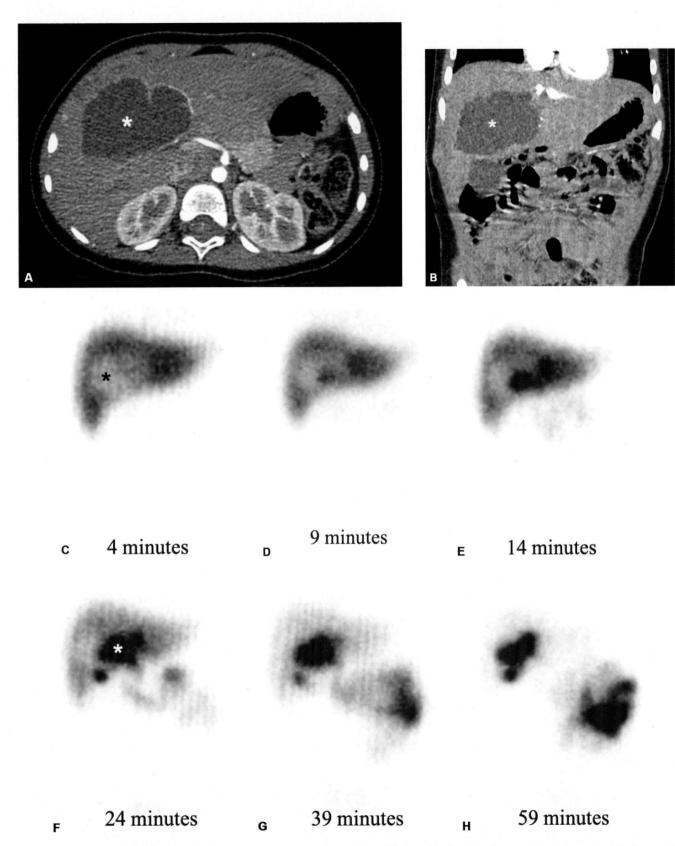

FIG. 17.12 ● Choledochal cyst. 14-month-old female presents for further evaluation of an intrahepatic cyst detected on prenatal ultrasound. **A and B:** Axial (A) and coronal (B) images from a contrast-enhanced CT of the abdomen demonstrate a thin-walled intrahepatic cystic lesion (asterisks in A and B). **C–H:** Hepatobiliary scan was performed with 60 min of dynamic imaging. Anterior frames at 4 (C), 9 (D), 14 (E), 24 (F), 39 (G), and 59 (H) min demonstrate progressive radiopharmaceutical accumulation within the intrahepatic cyst (asterisks in C and F), first appreciated as a photopenic defect at 4 min. Findings are consistent with an intrahepatic choledochal cyst, Todani classification type V. There is appropriate clearance of radiopharmaceutical from the blood pool and liver parenchyma with transit into the bile ducts and bowel.

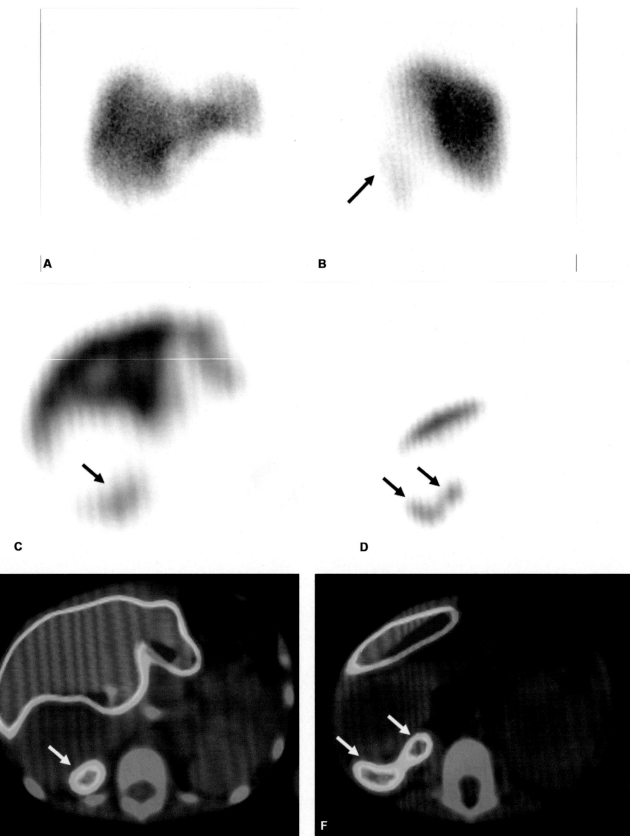

FIG. 17.13 ● **Heterotaxy with midline transverse liver and polysplenia.** 3-year-old male with heterotaxy. Tc-99m sulfur colloid liver–spleen scan was performed to evaluate for functional splenic tissue. **A and B:** Anterior and right lateral planar images demonstrate a transverse configuration of the liver. Additional focus of radiopharmaceutical uptake is seen in the right upper quadrant (arrow in B). **C–F:** Corresponding axial SPECT (C and E) and fused SPECT/CT (D and F) images of the upper abdomen localize radiopharmaceutical uptake in the posterior right upper quadrant to three splenules (arrows in C–E) consistent with functional splenic tissue in polysplenia.

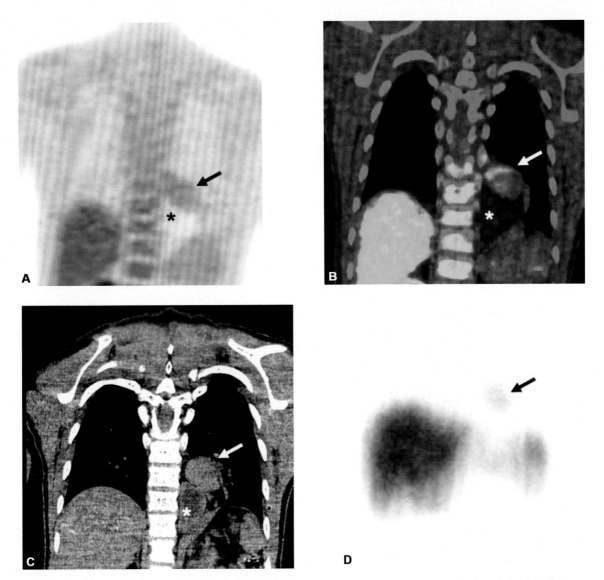

FIG. 17.14 ● Splenosis in a para-esophageal hernia. 14-year-old male with an aggressive osseous lesion of the right fibula presents for 18F-FDG PET/CT. Patient has a past surgical history of a Nissen fundoplication. **A–C:** Corresponding coronal PET (A), fused PET/CT (B), and low-dose CT (C) demonstrate a para-esophageal hernia (asterisks in A–C) associated with a 5 × 3.5 cm adjacent ovoid, mildly FDG-avid mass (arrows in A–C). The18F-FDG uptake of this ovoid mass is similar to that of normal spleen located in the left upper quadrant. **D:** Anterior spot image of the chest and upper abdomen from a Tc-99m sulfur colloid scan demonstrates physiologic distribution of the radiopharmaceutical in the liver and spleen as well as in the ovoid intrathoracic mass (arrow). Constellation of findings are consistent with splenosis in a para-esophageal hernia. Reproduced with permission from Khalatbari H. Society of Pediatric Radiology Unknown Case # 229: Splenule in a hiatal hernia. http://www.pedrad.org/Education/Unknown-Case

preparation, there is no universal reference standard value for solid gastric emptying studies in pediatrics.

A radionuclide salivagram can be performed to evaluate for aspiration of saliva into the tracheobronchial tree or lungs (Fig. 17.15) (27,103–105).

Ectopic gastric mucosa in a Meckel diverticulum

Meckel diverticulum, the incomplete obliteration of the ompha-lomesenteric duct, is the most common congenital anomaly of the gastrointestinal tract. When a Meckel diverticulum contains ectopic gastric mucosa, the patient may present with lower gas-trointestinal bleeding. Tc-99m pertechnetate accumulates in the surface cells of gastric mucosa and can be used to detect the

presence of ectopic gastric mucosa in a Meckel diverticulum (21). When performed using a meticulous technique including premedication with H2 antagonists or proton pump inhibitors, pertechnetate scintigraphy has a high sensitivity and specificity (up to 100%) in diagnosing a Meckel diverticulum containing ectopic gastric mucosa in the pediatric population (Fig. 17.16) (106). This is in contradistinction to adults where a much lower accuracy of 21% was reported in one series of 35 adult patients with a bleeding Meckel diverticulum (107). In patients with a high clinical suspicion for a bleeding Meckel diverticulum but a negative initial study, the Meckel scan may be repeated, especially if the initial scan was performed with no or inade-quate pre-medication (108). After the initial 60 min of anterior dynamic images, additional planar, post-void images should

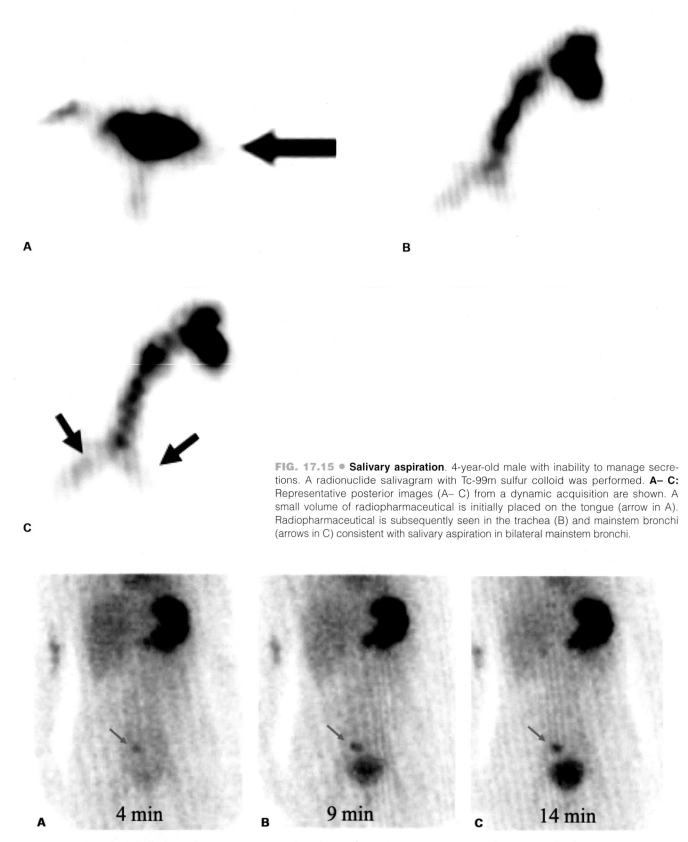

A

B

C

FIG. 17.15 ● **Salivary aspiration**. 4-year-old male with inability to manage secretions. A radionuclide salivagram with Tc-99m sulfur colloid was performed. **A– C:** Representative posterior images (A– C) from a dynamic acquisition are shown. A small volume of radiopharmaceutical is initially placed on the tongue (arrow in A). Radiopharmaceutical is subsequently seen in the trachea (B) and mainstem bronchi (arrows in C) consistent with salivary aspiration in bilateral mainstem bronchi.

A 4 min   **B** 9 min   **C** 14 min

FIG. 17.16 ● **Meckel diverticulum containing ectopic gastric mucosa.** 6-year-old female presents with painless bright red blood per rectum. A Tc-99m pertechnetate Meckel scan was performed. **A–C:** Anterior frames from minutes 4 (A), 9 (B), and 14 (C) of imaging demonstrate a focus (arrows) of radiopharmaceutical accumulation in the right lower quadrant that appeared coincident with uptake in the gastric mucosa and persisted throughout the entirety of the study, increasing in intensity, similar to the gastric mucosa. Lateral views at 1 h (not shown) confirmed anterior location of the abnormal focus of radiopharmaceutical uptake. Scintigraphic findings of a Meckel diverticulum containing ectopic gastric mucosa were confirmed at surgery.

be obtained in the anterior and lateral projections not only to detect a Meckel diverticulum obscured by the bladder but to aid in differentiating focal uptake from false-positive findings, such as physiologic excretion in the renal collecting system (109). In suspicious cases with focal radiopharmaceutical accumulation, the uptake may be localized through the addition of SPECT or SPECT/CT images, increasing accuracy as well as confidence in the diagnosis (110).

MUSCULOSKELTAL SYSTEM

Radiopharmaceuticals for bone imaging include Tc-99m methylene diphosphonate (MDP) and fluorine-18 sodium fluoride (18F-NaF). In pediatrics, typically two- or three-phase whole-body imaging is performed, often with the addition of spot images, SPECT, or SPECT/CT (111). A three-phase bone scan includes an (i) angiographic phase (dynamic imaging for 60 s), (ii) soft tissue or blood pool phase (3-min planar image), and (iii) a delayed phase (whole-body and/or spot planar images at 2–4 h). The information in the angiographic and soft-tissue phases is similar and demonstrates the presence or absence of preferential hyperemia (112). Hence, a two-phase bone scan, comprised of soft-tissue and delayed phases, will yield information similar to a three-phase bone scan. Some authors have advocated routinely obtaining a two-phase whole-body bone scan in all pediatric patients regardless of the clinical indication as the soft-tissue phase depicts *marrow infiltrative processes* such as leukemia which may present with bone pain (Fig. 17.17) (111,113). Kwatra et al. (111) demonstrated that marrow infiltrative processes are best appreciated on the soft-tissue phase images. Further, in children, the increased physiologic uptake of radiopharmaceutical in the growth plates (Fig.17.1) may obscure lesions in the adjacent epiphysis or metaphysis on the delayed phase images. The soft tissue phase increases the accuracy for detecting metaphyseal lesions.

In contradistinction, in adults, bone scintigraphy is typically comprised of delayed phase images only. The main indications for a three-phase bone scan in adults are differentiation of osteomyelitis and cellulitis, assessment of hardware loosening and osteomyelitis after hip or knee arthroplasty, complex regional pain syndrome (CRPS), assessment of bone viability in avascular necrosis, and assessment of viability of flap reconstruction (112).

The primary pathologies evaluated on bone scan in children are different from those in adults. Common indications for bone scintigraphy in children include the evaluation of primary benign or malignant osseous tumors (including osteoid osteoma and Langerhans cell histiocytosis) (Fig. 17.18), osseous metastases, osteomyelitis and chronic recurrent multifocal osteomyelitis (114,115) (Fig. 17.19), stress fractures and spondylolysis (116–119), traumatic (Fig. 17.20) or pathologic fractures, and fibrous dysplasia (monostotic versus polyostotic) (Fig. 17.21). Bone scans may serve as a problem-solving tool, especially in children presenting with bone pain, where it may be the first study to suggest the diagnosis of entities such as leukemia (Fig. 17.17) (31). Since children cannot localize pain well, whole-body imaging is indicated for all children undergoing bone scintigraphy.

With the more widespread utilization of MRI and fluorine-18 fluorodeoxyglucose (18F-FDG) PET/CT some of the aforementioned indications for bone scan are now evaluated with other imaging modalities. Previously bone scans were frequently obtained for the diagnosis, staging, therapeutic response monitoring, and surveillance of both the primary tumor and osseous metastases in osteosarcoma (Fig. 17.22), Ewing sarcoma (Fig. 17.23), soft-tissue sarcomas, and Langerhans cell histiocytosis, among others. More recently, 18F-FDG PET/CT, or 18F-FDG PET/MR when available, has replaced the bone scan for these indications, given its greater sensitivity in detection, its ability to rapidly normalize with response to treatment or surgery, as well as its increasing role in outcomes prognostication in these tumors. Currently, bone scans are most often obtained as surveillance imaging after tumoral surgical excision and reconstruction have been performed, although 18F-FDG PET /CT or PET/MR imaging can also supersede this role (31).

Bone stress injuries: Stress reactions and stress fractures

Bone fractures may be complete or incomplete and are usually readily apparent on radiographs. Specific types of bone injury include stress injury (stress fracture and stress reaction), insufficiency fracture, and pathologic fracture. Bone stress injuries encompass a wide spectrum. On one end of the spectrum is asymptomatic stress reaction visible on MRI as bone marrow edema. On the other end are clinically symptomatic stress fractures with fracture lines seen on imaging which may progress to chronic nonunion (Fig. 17.24) (120). Tibial stress injuries are the most common stress injuries.

Medial tibial stress syndrome (MTSS), commonly known as shin splints, is an overuse injury or repetitive-stress injury of the shin (121,122). MTTS presents as diffuse pain along the medial border of the tibia that is related to activity. It is characterized by diffuse tibial anteromedial or posteromedial periostitis, most often near the junction of the mid and distal thirds of the tibia, usually in conjunction with underlying cortical bone edema and microtrauma (121). There is controversy regarding the relationship between MTSS and *tibial stress injuries*. It is unclear whether they represent a continuum of injury or are two separate entities. On two- or three-phase bone scans, MTTS is described as increased uptake of radiopharmaceutical in the cortical bone, showing a characteristic longitudinal pattern on the delayed phase only (123). Acute stress fractures appear as discrete, localized, sometimes linear areas of increased uptake on all three phases (angiographic, soft tissue, and delayed phases) of a Tc-99m MDP bone scan.

Historically, when radiographs were not diagnostic, two- or three-phase bone scans were key in identifying and differentiating MTSS and tibial stress injuries. However, bone scans have largely been replaced by MRI (124). In patients with suspected tibial stress injuries findings on MRI include periosteal edema, bone marrow edema, and intracortical signal abnormality or fracture lines (Fig. 17.24) (125,126). A system to grade stress fracture severity based on extent of cortical uptake on bone scintigraphy was developed in 1987 (127); this system may be updated to reflect the medullary radiopharmaceutical uptake in the soft-tissue and delayed phases which correspond to the bone marrow edema seen on MRI (Fig. 17.24).

Back pain and spondylolysis

The most common etiologies of back pain in children and adolescents are spondylolysis, spondylolisthesis, Scheuermann's kyphosis, disk herniations, infections, and tumors (128). Spondylolysis accounts for approximately 12% to 16% of back pain in adolescents presenting to specialty clinics with back pain (129,130).

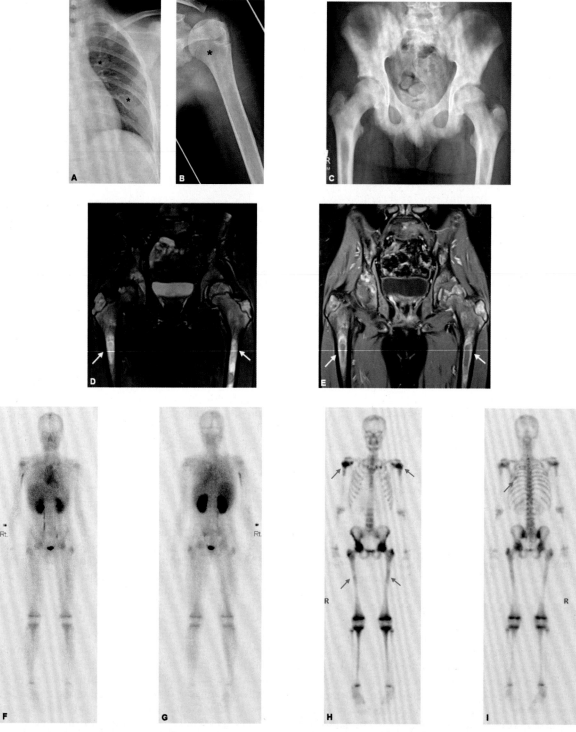

FIG. 17.17 ● Leukemia. 11-old- male present with a 10-month history of multifocal bone pain as well as a 30- to 40-pound weight loss. Routine blood chemistries demonstrated elevated CRP, elevated ESR, and anemia. A radiographic bone survey was performed followed by MRI of the pelvis and a two-phase whole-body Tc-99m MDP bone scan 2 weeks later. **A–C:** Anteroposterior radiographs of the chest (A), proximal left humerus (B), and pelvis (C) demonstrate expansile lesions in the left fifth and seventh ribs (asterisks in A), subtle lucency in the proximal left humeral metaphysis (asterisk in B), and diffuse heterogeneous sclerosis with lucencies in the pelvis and proximal femurs. Findings are suggestive a bone marrow infiltrative process such as leukemia, lymphoma, or metastases. **D and E:** Coronal short tau inversion recovery (STIR, D) and coronal T1-weighted fat-saturated post-contrast (E) images demonstrate multiple foci of high STIR signal with heterogeneous enhancement in the pelvis and bilateral proximal femurs (arrows) including the bilateral greater trochanters. **F–I:** Anterior (F) and posterior (G) whole-body blood pool images and corresponding delayed (H and I) images demonstrate multifocal lesions with increased radiopharmaceutical uptake in the axial and appendicular bones (arrows in H). Soft tissue phase images demonstrate increased radiopharmaceutical uptake in the proximal humeri, multiple vertebrae, pelvis, and lower extremities. There are multifocal rib lesions; the left seventh expansile rib lesion corresponds to the radiographic findings (arrow in I). Bone marrow aspirate and biopsy demonstrated pre-B acute lymphoblastic leukemia. Skin biopsy was sent for germline p53 testing and the results were consistent with Li Fraumeni syndrome (germline p53 mutation).

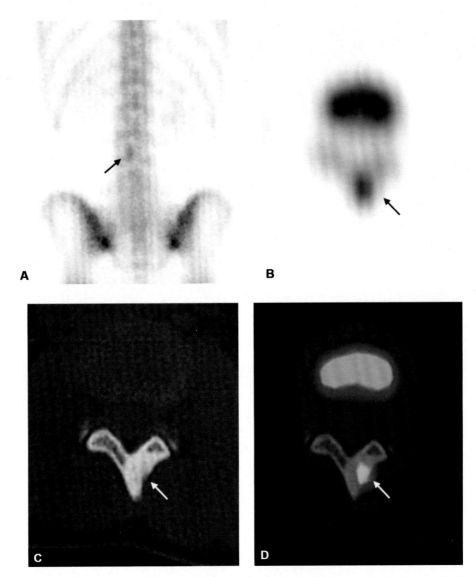

FIG. 17.18 ● Osteoid osteoma. 14-year-old female presents with a 1-year history of lumbar pain. Whole-body Tc-99m MDP bone scan with SPECT/CT of the lumbar spine was performed; the extent of the low-dose CT was limited to L2 to L4 vertebrae. **A:** Posterior spot image of the lumbar spine demonstrate focally increased radiopharmaceutical uptake in the posterior elements of L3 (arrow). **B–D:** Corresponding axial SPECT (B), low-dose CT (C), and fused SPECT/CT (D) images demonstrate sclerosis and expansion of the left L3 lamina and spinous process associated with focally increased radiopharmaceutical uptake consistent with the nidus of an osteoid osteoma (arrows in B–D).

Spondylolysis, a unilateral or bilateral fracture in the vertebral pars interarticularis, usually occurs in the lower lumbar vertebrae, most commonly the isthmus in L5. Spondylolisthesis is the anterior slipping of the upper vertebral body that may occur with bilateral pars defects. Spondylolysis results from recurrent microtrauma with lumbar hyperextension or lumbar flexion and extension, typically in sports such as gymnastics, dancing, weightlifting, etc. (128), or with acute overload injury (131).

The imaging workup for suspected spondylitis starts with lateral and anteroposterior radiographs of the lumbar spine. If these are not confirmatory and the clinical suspicion for spondylolysis remains high after two to three weeks of rest, advanced imaging, either bone scan with SPECT or SPECT/CT or MRI of the lumbar spine, is obtained (119,132). Bone scintigraphy with SPECT/CT is superior to MRI in distinguishing stress reaction from stress fracture and in the diagnosis of complete versus incomplete acute spondylolysis (133). On bone scintigraphy,

acute spondylolysis demonstrates increased radiopharmaceutical uptake while chronic spondylolysis does not; however, the accompanying low-dose CT will demonstrate a pars defect with adjacent sclerosis in chronic spondylolysis (Fig. 17.25). The addition of low-dose CT to the SPECT acquisition allows for more precise localization of the site and etiology of increased radiopharmaceutical uptake in bone as well as the identification of osseous abnormalities on CT without associated increased radiopharmaceutical uptake on SPECT (119,132).

Non-accidental trauma

The Federal Child Abuse Prevention and Treatment Act defines the term *child abuse and neglect* as "at a minimum, any recent act or failure to act on the part of a parent or caretaker, which results in death, serious physical or emotional harm, sexual abuse or exploitation, or an act or failure to act which presents an imminent risk of serious harm" (134). This act provides

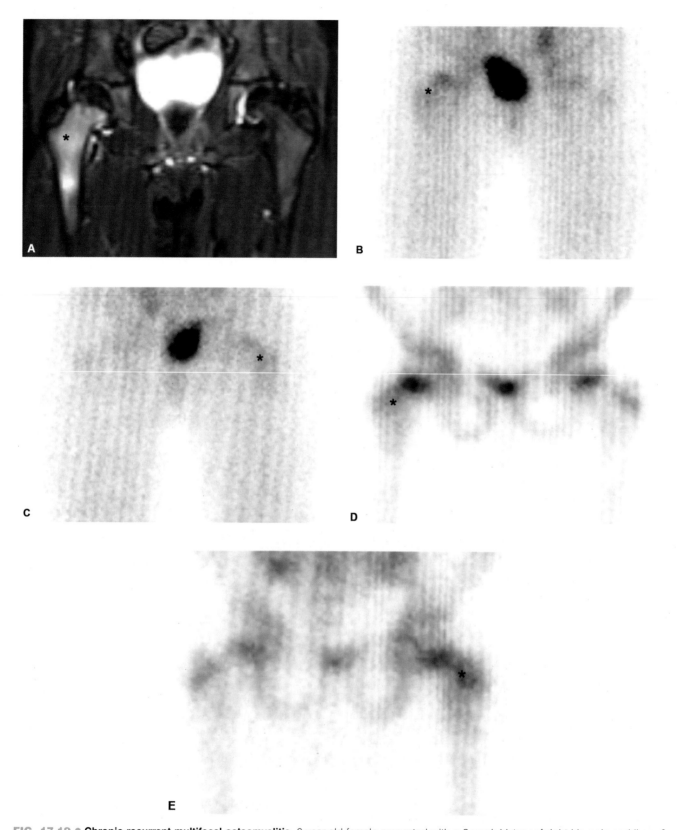

FIG. 17.19 ● **Chronic recurrent multifocal osteomyelitis.** 6-year-old female presented with a 3-week history of right hip pain and limp. **A:** MRI of the lower extremities was performed. Coronal STIR image of the proximal femurs demonstrates high STIR signal (asterisk) in the proximal right femur extending from the epiphysis to the junction of the proximal and mid-third of the shaft. There was mild enhancement on post-contrast images (not shown); no periosteal reaction, cortical breakthrough or associated soft tissue mass was present. **B–E:** Two-phase whole-body Tc-99m MDP bone scan was performed. Anterior and posterior soft tissue phase (B and C) and corresponding delayed phase (D and E) spot images of the pelvis demonstrate hyperemia on the soft tissue phase images (asterisks in B and C) as well as mildly increased radiopharmaceutical uptake on delayed phase images (asterisks in D and E) in the right proximal femur. No additional osseous lesions were seen. After an extensive workup including negative blood cultures and bone biopsy, the patient was diagnosed with chronic recurrent multifocal osteomyelitis.

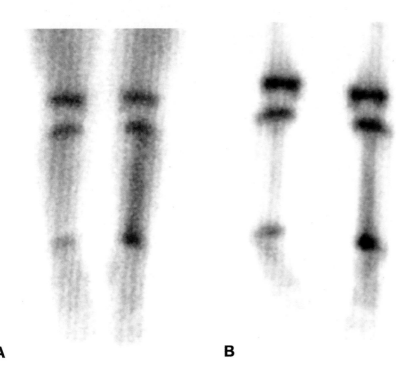

A   **B**

FIG. 17.20 • **Toddler fracture.** 2.5-year-old afebrile female presents with left leg pain. Radiographs were unremarkable. Two-phase whole-body Tc-99m MDP bone scan was performed. **A and B**: Anterior images from soft tissue (A) and delayed (B) phases demonstrate diffusely increased uptake in the left tibial diaphysis. Upon further questioning, parents and child reported that a fall had occurred 2 days prior to presentation. Toddler fractures are nondisplaced spiral fractures of the tibia that are most commonly seen between 9 months and 3 years of age.

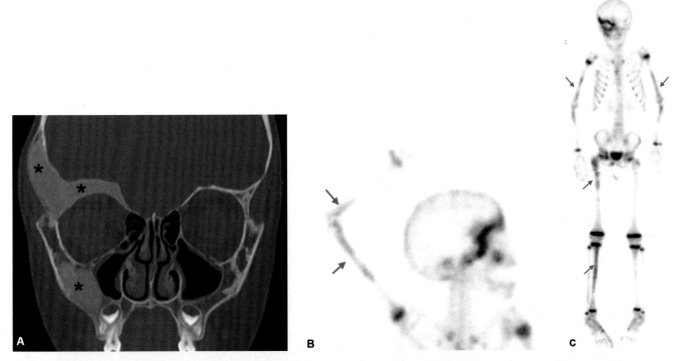

A   **B**   **C**

FIG. 17.21 • **Polyostotic fibrous dysplasia inMcCune–Albright syndrome.** 4-year-old female presents with a 4-week history of a bump over the right eyebrow. **A:** Coronal non-contrast CT image of the face in bone windows demonstrate expansile lesions (asterisks) with ground glass density in the right orbital roof, right frontal bone and right maxilla. Several additional lesions were present in the skull base (not shown). **B and C:** Delayed-phase whole-body Tc-99m MDP bone scan was performed. Lateral spot view of the skull and right upper extremity (C) and stitched anterior spot views of the whole body (C) demonstrate multifocal lesions in the skull and appendicular skeleton (several of which are indicated with arrows in B and C) consistent with polyostotic fibrous dysplasia. On physical exam the patient had multiple café-au-lait spots. She had an abnormal response of growth hormone levels to oral glucose tolerance test which was consistent with growth hormone excess. Constellation of findings of polyostotic fibrous dysplasia, café-au-lait-spots, and acromegaly are consistent with McCune-Albright syndrome.

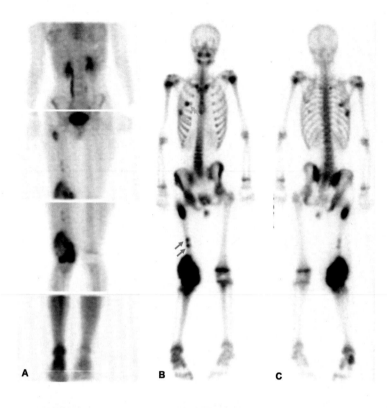

FIG. 17.22 ● Metastatic osteosarcoma. 13-year-old female with right knee pain and shortness of breath. Two-phase whole-body Tc-99m MDP bone scan was performed. **A–C:** Anterior (A) soft-tissue phase spot images and anterior (B) and posterior (C) delayed phase images demonstrate the primary mass in the distal right femur, skip lesions in the right femoral diaphysis (arrows in B), osseous metastases in the pelvis and proximal right femoral diaphysis, and metastatic pulmonary nodules (double arrows in B).

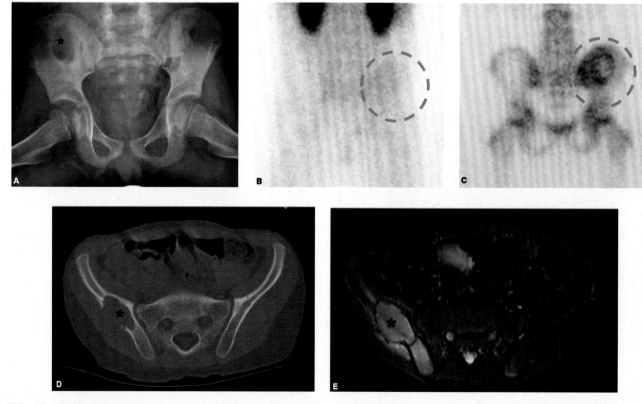

FIG. 17.23 ● Ewing sarcoma. 4-year-old male presents with left hip pain. **A:** Radiographs of the pelvis were obtained at presentation (not shown) and repeated 2-weeks later (A). Anterior radiograph of the pelvis in frog position was interpreted as normal. **B and C:** Two-phase whole-body Tc-99m MDP bone scan was performed. Posterior spot images of the abdomen, pelvis and thighs on the blood pool (B) and delayed phases (C) demonstrate mildly increased radiopharmaceutical accumulation in the blood pool phase (dashed circle in B) associated with a rim of increased radiopharmaceutical accumulation in the delayed phase (dashed circle in C) in the right iliac wing. In retrospect, these abnormalities correspond to a lytic lesion in the right iliac wing (asterisks in a) initially attributed to an overlying loop of bowel on pelvic radiograph. **D and E:** Axial CT (D) and axial STIR (E) MR images demonstrate an expansible lytic lesion (asterisks in D and E) with lateral cortical breakthrough and high STIR signal. The increased high STIR signal in the adjacent right iliac wing represent bone marrow edema and corresponds to the diffusely increased radiopharmaceutical uptake seen in the right iliac wing in C (secondary to hyperemia). Ewing sarcoma was diagnosed at biopsy. Bone scan may be utilized as a problem-solving tool in pediatric patients with bone pain.

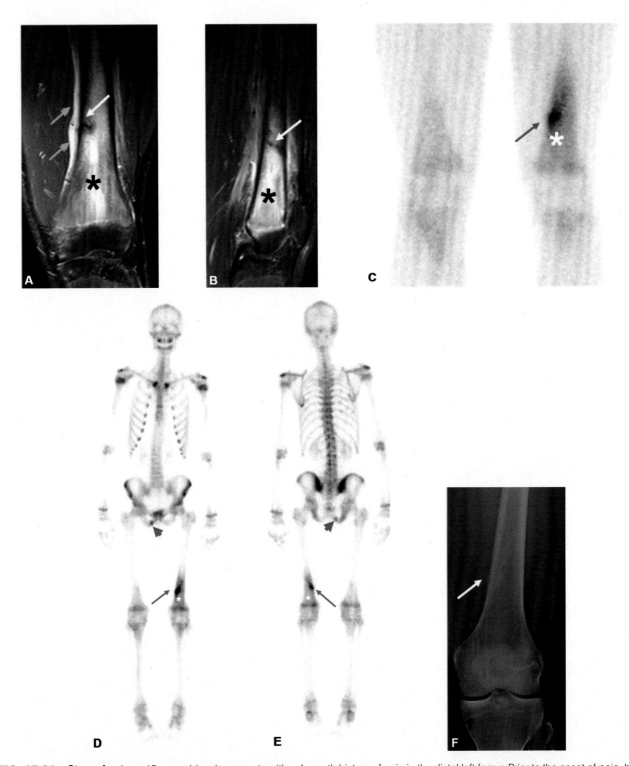

FIG. 17.24 ● **Stress fracture.** 15-year-old male presents with a 1-month history of pain in the distal left femur. Prior to the onset of pain, he had recently returned to high school football after a 1-year hiatus due to an L5 pars fracture (acute spondylolysis). Radiographs of the left knee were normal. MRI of the left knee to evaluate for internal derangement (not shown) demonstrated edema in the distal left femur leading to the immediate performance of an MRI of the left thigh. **A and B:** Coronal (A) and (B) sagittal STIR images of the distal left femur demonstrate high STIR signal in the bone marrow (asterisks in A and B) and the periosteum (double arrows in A) consistent with bone marrow edema and periosteal reaction. There is a dark, oblique line in the medial aspect of the distal femoral diaphysis (arrows in A and B) consistent with a stress fracture. This corresponds to grade IV tibial stress fracture in the Fredericson classification (125,126). However, this outside study was initially interpreted as concerning for tumor or osteomyelitis, prompting referral to our institution for further evaluation. **C–E:** Two-phase whole-body Tc-99m MDP bone scan was performed. Anterior spot blood pool images (C) and anterior (D) and posterior (E) whole-body images demonstrate focal, linear increased radiopharmaceutical accumulation (arrow in C–E) corresponding to the oblique fracture line seen on MRI. There is mild increased radiopharmaceutical accumulation in the distal left femoral diaphysis and metaphysis secondary to hyperemia corresponding to the bone marrow edema seen on MRI (asterisks in C–E). The asymmetry of the ischiopubic synchondrosis (arrowheads in D and E) is a benign developmental variant that should not be mistaken for pathology. **F:** Radiographs of the left femur were repeated and demonstrated subtle sclerosis and periosteal reaction corresponding to the focal uptake on bone scan. Constellation of findings is consistent with a stress fracture.

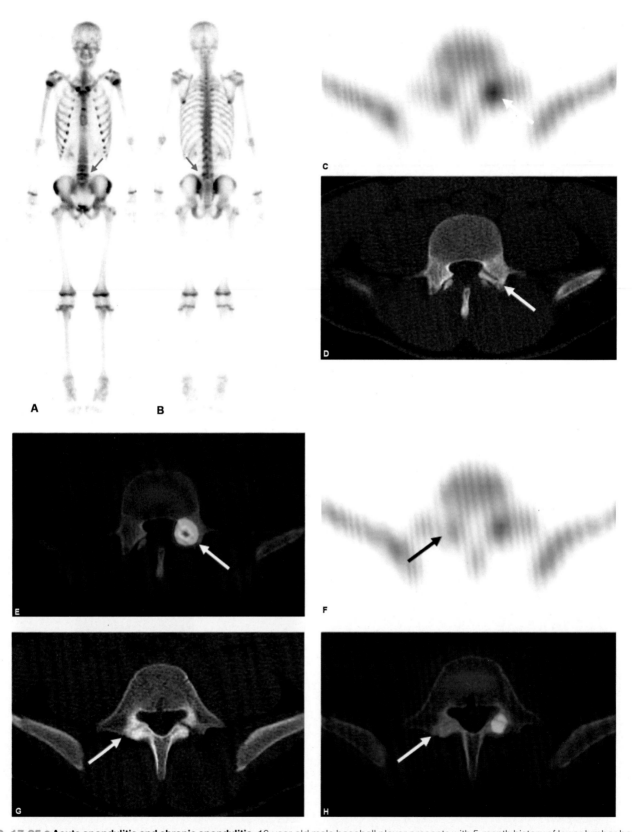

FIG. 17.25 ● **Acute spondylitis and chronic spondylitis.** 16-year-old male baseball player presents with 5-month history of lower lumbar back pain. Delayed whole-body Tc-99m MDP bone scan with SPECT of the lumbar spine was performed. The extend of the low-dose CT performed in conjunction with SPECT was limited to L4 to S1. **A and B:** Anterior (A) and posterior (B) whole-body images demonstrate focal increased uptake at left L5 pars interarticularis. **C–E:** Corresponding axial SPECT (C), low-dose CT (D), and fused SPECT/CT (E) images demonstrate focally increased radiopharmaceutical uptake with a corresponding complete fracture in the left L5 pars interarticularis on CT consistent with acute spondylolysis (arrows in C–E). **F–H:** Corresponding axial SPECT (F), low-dose CT (G), and fused SPECT/CT (H) images demonstrate a complete fracture with surrounding sclerosis but no abnormally increased radiopharmaceutical uptake in the right L5 pars interarticularis consistent with a chronic spondylolysis at the right L5 pars interarticularis (arrows in F–H). The addition of SPECT/CT leads to improved identification and characterization of causes of low back pain. From Trout et al. (119).

minimum standards to the states for defining maltreatment with each state defining child physical abuse within its own civil and criminal statutes (135). The clinical workup in cases of suspected child abuse includes medical history, physical examination, and diagnostic testing and documentation. The diagnostic imaging workup recommended by the American Academy of Pediatrics includes (i) radiographic skeletal survey in all patients, (ii) MRI of the brain and spine (or CT of the head which may be more expeditious in some institutions) in patients with suspected head trauma, and (iii) CT of the abdomen in patients with suspected abdominal trauma (135). Repeat radiographic skeletal surveys are recommended in high-risk cases and bone scintigraphy may be used to complement radiographic skeletal surveys (135). The American College of Radiology appropriateness criteria for suspected physical child abuse published in 2017 also recommends bone scintigraphy as a problem-solving study rather than a first-line imaging study (136). PET/CT with 18F-NaF has a higher resolution than bone scans with Tc-99m MDP (Fig. 17.26) and is used as an alternative in some institutions.

Complex regional pain syndrome

CRPS, pain that is out of proportion to the history and physical findings, is associated with at least one sign and one symptom of autonomic dysfunction. Signs of autonomic dysfunction include temperature asymmetry, skin color change, edema, sweating asymmetry, and dystrophic changes (137). Symptoms of autonomic dysfunction included allodynia, hyperalgesia, and motor dysfunction. The pain typically occurs in a single extremity but may occur at multiple sites (137). CRPS is categorized into two types. In CRPS type 1, no defined nerve lesion is present and in CRPS type 2, a defined nerve lesion is present. CRPS type 1 is the common category in pediatrics. The etiology of CRPS is not well understood.

The main role of imaging in patients with suspected CRPS it to exclude other etiologies such as tumor (including osteoid osteoma), stress fracture, or osteomyelitis. The classical appearance of CRPS on three-phase bone scans in adults is that of asymmetrically increased uptake on angiographic, soft-tissue, and delayed phases, with increased periarticular activity on the delayed phased images (138). In the original study by Mackinnon et al. (138) the angiographic, blood pool, and delayed phases were positive in 45%, 52%, and 96% of the cases respectively. In the "cold variant" of CRPS, the pattern most commonly seen in children, there is asymmetrically decreased uptake on angiographic, soft-tissue, and delayed phases in the affected extremity (Fig. 17.27) (139,140). However, presence of a normal two- or three-phase bone scan does not exclude the diagnosis of CRPS in children (141).

FUNCTIONAL IMAGING IN PEDIATRIC ONCOLOGY

Metaiodobenzylguanidine in neuroblastoma

Neuroblastoma is an embryonal neoplasm derived from neural crest cells (142). The most common solid extra-cranial tumor of childhood, neuroblastoma has an incidence of 10.5 per million

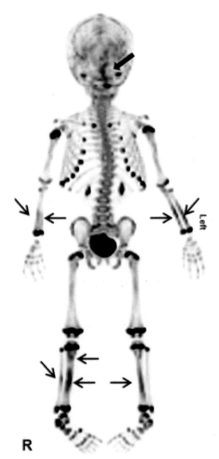

FIG. 17.26 ● **Nonaccidental trauma (NAT).** A 15-month-old girl presents with suspected NAT. Anterior maximum intensity projection image from 18F-NaF PET/CT demonstrates multiple foci of increased uptake in the calvarium and extremities. These include linear uptake in the left occipital bone (thick arrow), bilateral radii and ulnas (thin arrows on upper extremities), bilateral tibias, and right fibula (thin arrows on lower extremities). These are highly concerning for nonaccidental trauma. Many of these fractures had none or subtle correlates on the radiographic skeletal survey (not shown). On the radiographic skeletal survey, classic metaphyseal lesions in multiple extremity bones and left eighth costochondral junction fracture were also seen. These are not appreciated on 18F-NaF PET/CT due to proximity to the physiologic radiopharmaceutical accumulation in the adjacent growth plates. Radiographic skeletal survey and 18F-NaF PET/CT scan are complementary in detecting osseous injuries in patients with suspected NAT. Reprinted from Khalatbari et al. (194). Copyright © 2018 Elsevier.

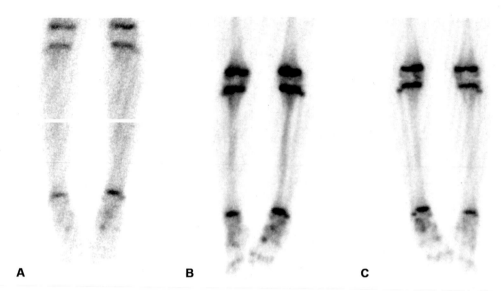

FIG. 17.27 • **Complex regional pain syndrome, cold variant**. 10-year-old female presents with right foot pain, allodynia, and swelling. Two-phase whole-body Tc-99m MDP bone scan was performed. **A–C:** Anterior soft tissue phase spot images (A) and anterior (B) and posterior (C) delayed phase spot images demonstrate decreased radiopharmaceutical accumulation in the right leg and foot in a predominantly peri-articular distribution consistent with the cold variant of complex regional pain syndrome. The cold variant of complex regional pain syndrome is more common than the hot variant in the pediatric age group.

children less than 15 years of age each year. While neuroblastoma represents 8% to 10% of all childhood tumors, it accounts for approximately 15% of all pediatric cancer mortalities. Approximately 40% of patients with neuroblastoma are younger than 1 year of age at diagnosis while less than 5% of those with neuroblastoma present at age 10 years or older (143).

Neuroblastic tumors include neuroblastoma, ganglioneuroblastoma, and ganglioneuroma. Neuroblastic tumors most frequently arise in the adrenal (47%) and abdominal/retroperitoneal (24%,) regions, with the remainder arising along the sympathetic chain in the neck, thorax, and pelvis (144).

Presenting signs and symptoms may relate to the primary tumor or to sites of metastases, which are present in approximately 50% of patients at diagnosis. For example, patients may present with a palpable mass; alternatively, proptosis, periorbital ecchymoses, or bone pain due to osteomedullary metastases may be the initial presentation. Associated paraneoplastic syndromes include opsoclonus-myoclonus-ataxia syndrome and refractory diarrhea among others (145–148). At diagnosis, the most common metastatic sites are bone marrow (56%), bone (47%), lymph nodes (24%), and liver (21%) (149).

The definitive diagnosis of neuroblastoma requires histologic confirmation either from incisional biopsy of the primary tumor or bone marrow biopsy/aspirate in individuals with suspected bone marrow involvement (150). The disease spectrum in neuroblastoma is highly variable with clinical course ranging from spontaneous regression to refractory metastatic tumors associated with poor survival (151,152). The intensity of the therapeutic regimen is determined after staging and risk stratification.

MIBG is a norepinephrine analogue most commonly radiolabeled with either I-131 or preferably, I-123. I-123 MIBG is the cornerstone of functional imaging for diagnosis, staging, therapeutic response monitoring, prognostication, and the detection of recurrence in patients with neuroblastoma (Fig. 17.28) (153).

More than 90% of individuals with neuroblastoma demonstrate uptake of radiolabeled MIBG (154,155). The specificity of radiolabeled MIBG for neuroblastoma and pheochromocytoma approaches 100% (156). The radiopharmaceutical uptake resolves when a tumor is necrotic, involutes, dedifferentiates, or when maturation into a more differentiated tumor type occurs (157).

High-dose I-131 MIBG, typically in conjunction with autologous stem cell transplant, has been used successfully as a systemic therapeutic agent for patients with high-risk neuroblastoma or pheochromocytoma with recurrent or refractory disease (153). High-dose I-131 MIBG is also increasingly used as an up-front therapeutic option in this patient population (153).

The European Association of Nuclear Medicine first published procedure guidelines for tumor imaging with MIBG-labeled with 131I or 123I in 2010. These guidelines were recently updated in 2018 (33,34). Patient preparation and precautions include considerations related to pregnancy, breastfeeding, thyroid blockade, and potential drug interferences.

MIBG images are interpreted both qualitatively and semiquantitatively. There is physiologic an uptake of 123I-MIBG in the salivary glands, nasal mucosa, myocardium, liver, bowel, and urinary bladder. Additional sites of variable normal uptake include lungs, spleen, uterus, and gallbladder (158,159). There may also be uptake in brown fat, particularly in the supraclavicular regions, as well as in normal adrenal glands. There is no accumulation of MIBG in the normal bone or bone marrow. Hence, the ease of detection of osseous metastases with this radiopharmaceutical. Qualitative interpretation is done by observing the distribution of the radiopharmaceutical in the primary mass as well as in osteomedullary and soft-tissue metastases (Fig. 17.28). SPECT, SPECT/CT, and fused SPECT/MR-registered images improve detection, characterization, and localization of MIBG-avid lesions. Semiquantitative scoring systems for evaluating MIBG were developed to assess the

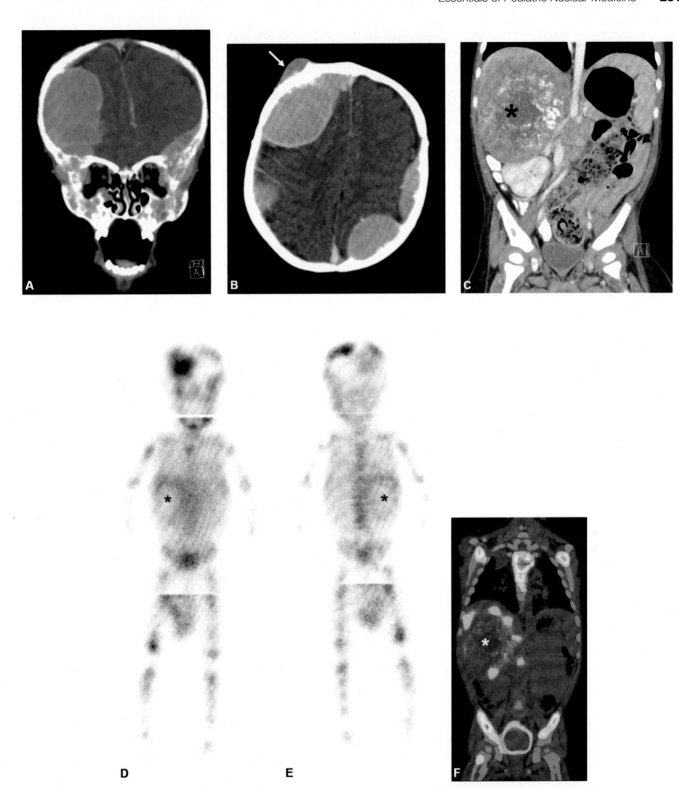

FIG. 17.28 ● Metastatic neuroblastoma. 14-month old male presents with a 2-month history of an enlarging lump in the right forehead, proptosis of the left eye, and a 2-day history of limping. **A–C:** CT of the head, chest, abdomen and pelvis with intravenous and oral contrast. Coronal (A) and axial (B) images of the head and coronal image of the abdomen and pelvis (C) demonstrate multiple calvarial metastases with associated epidural extension. The palpable mass on the right forehead corresponds to a subperiosteal soft tissue mass (arrow in B) associated with a large right frontal osseous metastasis. There are extensive bilateral periorbital metastases. The primary mass in the right suprarenal region (asterisk in C) demonstrates central necrosis and calcification. **D–F:** Anterior (D) and posterior (E) stitched spot images of the whole-body and coronal SPECT/CT image of the chest, abdomen, and pelvis (F) from an I-123 MIBG scan demonstrate the primary soft tissue mass (asterisks in D–F) with central photopenia secondary to necrosis. There are extensive osseous metastases involving the majority of the axial and appendicular skeleton. The urine-soaked diaper is lying between the patient's thighs on the planar images.

extent of disease and response to chemotherapy through the use of reliable, reproducible, and easily learned techniques (153,160–162). One such system, the modified Curie score, divides the skeleton into nine segments, each of which is assigned a score of 0 to 3 to assess the extent of osteomedullary involvement. An additional 10th segment assesses soft tissue involvement (160,163).

In the early 2000s, the International Society of Pediatric Oncology European Neuroblastoma (SIOPEN) Research Network developed the SIOPEN semi-quantitative score which is the other most commonly used semiquantitative scoring system to assess degree of osteomedullary involvement in those with neuroblastoma (162,164). According to the SIOPEN semi-quantitative scoring method, the skeleton is divided into 12 anatomical osteomedullary body segments and each segment is scored 0 to 6 scale to discriminate between focal discrete lesions and patterns of more diffuse infiltration with a maximum score of 72 (162,164).

The modified Curie as well as the SIOPEN scores has been shown to have prognostic significance in individuals with high-risk neuroblastoma. In these patients, MIBG scores at diagnosis (165–168), at mid-cycle during induction therapy (160,161,163,169) and at completion of induction therapy (170,171), have prognostic significance as does the presence of MIBG-avid disease at the end of induction or before myeloablative therapy (166,172,173). At diagnosis, a Curie score ≤2 and a SIOPEN score ≤4 are associated with a significantly better event-free and overall survival compared with higher scores (167). After four cycles of chemotherapy, overall survival was significantly better for MIBG-negative patients compared with those with any residual MIBG-positive metastases (167). A postinduction Curie as well as SIOPEN score of >2 is associated with poor event-free survival (170).

There are two staging systems for neuroblastoma. The International Neuroblastoma Staging System (INSS) was created in 1988 and revised in 1993, is implemented after surgical resection and cannot be used to risk-stratify individuals prior to treatment (150,174). In 2004, the International Neuroblastoma Risk Group (INRG) adopted the SIOPEN image-defined risk factors for neuroblastoma staging (175). This system allows risk-stratification of patients at the time of initial diagnosis and is used alongside INSS to define pre-treatment cohorts in clinical trials (150). This staging system mandates either CT or MR imaging of the primary tumor and first-line functional imaging with radioiodine-labeled MIBG. 18F-FDG PET/CT is reserved for those with non-MIBG-avid tumors (149). Somatostatin receptors are expressed in the majority of neuroblastoma cells. Somatostatin receptor imaging with Gallium-68 DOTA-DPhel-Tyr^3-octreotate (68Ga DOTATE), a positron emitter that is used for PET/CT imaging, is a promising alternative functional imaging option in non or poorly-MIBG-avid neuroblastomas patients (176).

The INRG classification system stratifies individuals into several pre-treatment risk groups (very low, low, intermediate and high) (174,177–179). Individuals with very low-risk, low-risk and intermediate-risk diseases have excellent outcomes and high survival rates, whereas individuals with aggressive high-risk disease are at significant risk for disease progression or death (153). Treatment options are tailored to risk group stratification and include expectant observation, surgical resection, chemotherapy, autologous stem cell transplantation, radiation therapy, immunotherapy, and I-131 MIBG systemic therapy (152).

18F-FDG PET/CT in pediatric neoplasms

Pediatric cancers are rare compared to the incidence of cancers in adults. Most pediatric tumors are mesenchymal (leukemia, lymphoma, and sarcoma) or neuroectodermal (brain tumors and neuroblastoma) in origin, whereas in adults the majority are of epithelial origin. NM functional imaging studies are routinely used to evaluate neuroblastomas, osseous and soft-tissue sarcomas, lymphomas, and Langerhans cell histiocytosis in pediatrics (180–182).

There are unique differences between children and adults including age-related developmental and physiologic variants that may mimic pathology. These include increased 18-F FDG uptake in the growth plates, Waldeyer ring, thymus, and activated brown adipose tissue (Fig. 17.29) (183–188). Moreover, the primary neoplasms and their patterns of metastases are different in pediatrics and mandate whole-body PET/CT or PET/MR imaging. An altered biodistribution of 18F-FDG in white adipose tissue may be seen on post-induction PET/CT images which has been attributed to the effects of corticosteroids administered as part of the induction treatment (189).

18F-FDG PET/CT is routinely used for initial staging, therapeutic response monitoring response, surveillance, and as a prognostic indicator in many pediatric tumors including Hodgkin and non-Hodgkin lymphoma (Fig. 17.30 and 17.31), osteosarcoma (Fig. 17.32), Ewing sarcoma, soft-tissue sarcomas (Fig. 17.33), Langerhans cell histiocytosis (Fig. 17.34), and non or poorly MIBG-avid neuroblastomas (31,149,190–194). An additional imaging modality for evaluation of pediatric neoplasms is 18F-FDG PET/MR. However, PET/MR scanners need to become more widely distributed in order to become accessible to the majority of pediatric cancer patients (195–197).

INFECTION AND INFLAMMATION

Although radionuclide imaging can provide useful information in children with known or suspected infectious or inflammatory conditions, it has largely been superseded by MRI. Historically, Tc-99m MDP bone scintigraphy had been used for detection and localization of osteomyelitis. In patients with sickle cell disease, a combination of bone and bone marrow scanning is be needed to distinguish osteomyelitis from bone infarct and performs better than MRI in distinguishing between these two entities (37).

Since, activated inflammatory cells use glucose as an energy source, there is increased 18F-FDG accumulation at sites of infection and inflammation. On the molecular level, this is due to the over-expression of glucose transporter 1 receptors in stimulated macrophages, neutrophils and lymphocytes. Not only has 18F-FDG PET/CT been shown to localize sites of suspected infectious and inflammatory conditions in children (Fig. 17.35) and adults, it has proven particularly helpful in establishing the diagnosis in children presenting with fever of unknown origin. Its role in detection and therapeutic response monitoring in those with infectious processes continues to evolve (37,198).

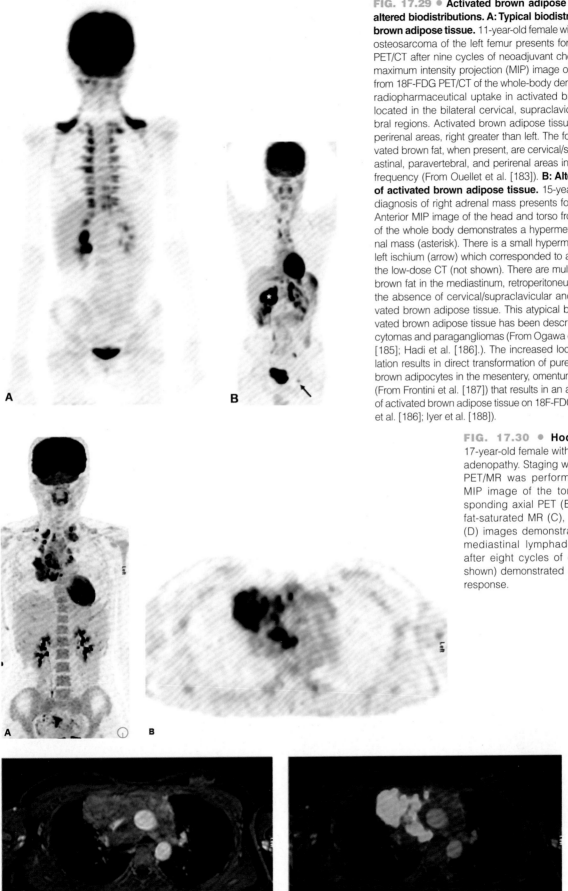

FIG. 17.29 ● **Activated brown adipose tissue, typical and altered biodistributions. A: Typical biodistribution of activated brown adipose tissue.** 11-year-old female with history of localized osteosarcoma of the left femur presents for restaging 18F-FDG PET/CT after nine cycles of neoadjuvant chemotherapy. Anterior maximum intensity projection (MIP) image of the head and torso from 18F-FDG PET/CT of the whole-body demonstrates increased radiopharmaceutical uptake in activated brown adipose tissue located in the bilateral cervical, supraclavicular and paravertebral regions. Activated brown adipose tissue is also seen in the perirenal areas, right greater than left. The four main sites of activated brown fat, when present, are cervical/supraclavicular, mediastinal, paravertebral, and perirenal areas in decreasing order of frequency (From Ouellet et al. [183]). **B: Altered biodistribution of activated brown adipose tissue.** 15-year-old male with new diagnosis of right adrenal mass presents for staging evaluation. Anterior MIP image of the head and torso from 18F-FDG PET/CT of the whole body demonstrates a hypermetabolic right suprarenal mass (asterisk). There is a small hypermetabolic lesion in the left ischium (arrow) which corresponded to a small lytic lesion on the low-dose CT (not shown). There are multiple foci of activated brown fat in the mediastinum, retroperitoneum, and mesentery in the absence of cervical/supraclavicular and paravertebral activated brown adipose tissue. This atypical biodistribution of activated brown adipose tissue has been described in pheochromocytomas and paragangliomas (From Ogawa et al. [184]; Park et al. [185]; Hadi et al. [186].). The increased local adrenergic stimulation results in direct transformation of pure white adipocytes to brown adipocytes in the mesentery, omentum, or retroperitoneum (From Frontini et al. [187]) that results in an altered biodistribution of activated brown adipose tissue on 18F-FDG PET/CT (From Hadi et al. [186]; Iyer et al. [188]).

FIG. 17.30 ● **Hodgkin lymphoma.** 17-year-old female with mediastinal lymphadenopathy. Staging whole-body 18F-FDG PET/MR was performed. **A–D:** Anterior MIP image of the torso (A) and corresponding axial PET (B), post-contrast T1 fat-saturated MR (C), and fused PET/MR (D) images demonstrate hypermetabolic mediastinal lymphadenopathy. PET/MR after eight cycles of chemotherapy (not shown) demonstrated complete metabolic response.

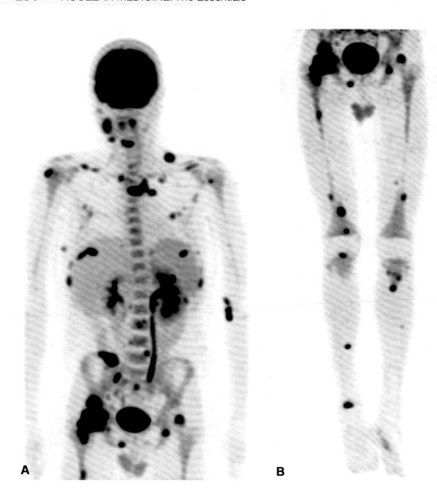

A

B

FIG. 17.31 ● **Non-Hodgkin lymphoma.** **A and B:** 13-year-old male presented with a 4-week history of right hip and knee pain, 2 weeks of daily fevers, chills, and night sweats, as well as a 7-pound weight loss. Radiograph of the pelvis (not shown) demonstrated permeative lesions in the right acetabulum and proximal femur. 18F-FDG PET/CT was performed for further evaluation. Anterior MIP images of the head and torso (A) and lower extremities (B) demonstrate multiple hypermetabolic osseous lesions in the axial and appendicular skeleton in addition to multiple hypermetabolic supra- and infra-diaphragmatic lymph nodes. Excisional biopsy of the left supraclavicular lymph node was consistent with anaplastic large cell lymphoma; stage III. There is retention of radiopharmaceutical in the left renal collecting system and ureter secondary to urinary stasis.

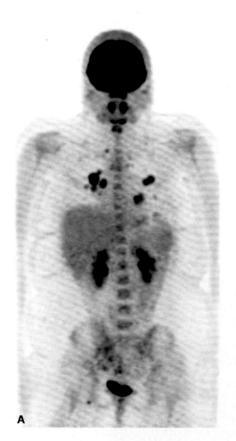

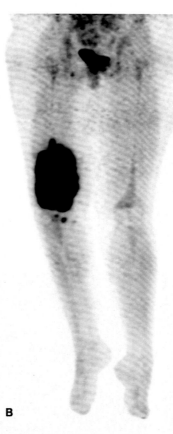

A

B

FIG. 17.32 ● **Osteosarcoma.** 16-year-old female with a newly identified aggressive lesion in the right distal femoral metadiaphysis, biopsy-proven osteosarcoma, undergoes staging whole-body 18F-FDG PET/CT. **A and B:** Frontal MIP of the torso (A) and lower extremities (B) demonstrates a markedly FDG-avid lesion in the right femoral metadiaphysis, numerous FDG-avid pulmonary metastases, and several small FDG-avid osseous metastases in the right tibial plateau and pelvis.

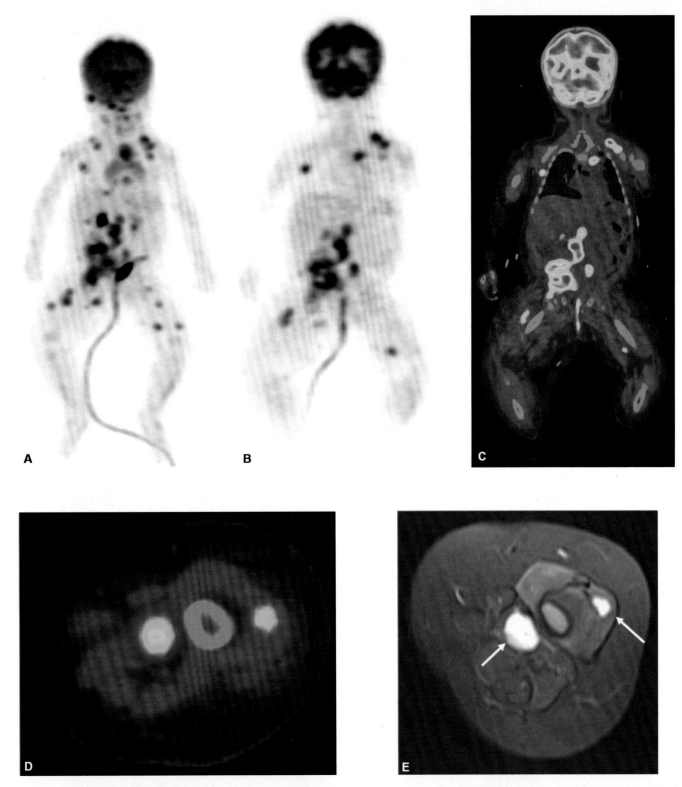

FIG. 17.33 ● Rhabdomyosarcoma. 4-month-old, previously healthy, female presents with palpable masses on her forehead and groin. MRI of the head, neck, chest, abdomen, and pelvis (not shown) demonstrated a primary retroperitoneal mass with multiple intramuscular metastases and extensive lymphadenopathy in the neck, chest, abdomen and pelvis. **A–C:** Anterior MIP (A), coronal PET (B), and coronal fused 18F-FDG PET/CT images of the whole-body demonstrate hypermetabolic primary retroperitoneal mass; hypermetabolic intramuscular metastases in the head, neck, torso, and lower extremities; and hypermetabolic cervical, mediastinal, and retroperitoneal lymphadenopathy. **D and E:** Axial fused PET/CT (D) and axial STIR MR (E) images demonstrate the hypermetabolic intramuscular metastases in the muscles in the anterior and posterior compartments of the left thigh. These lesions are hyperintense on STIR (arrows in E).

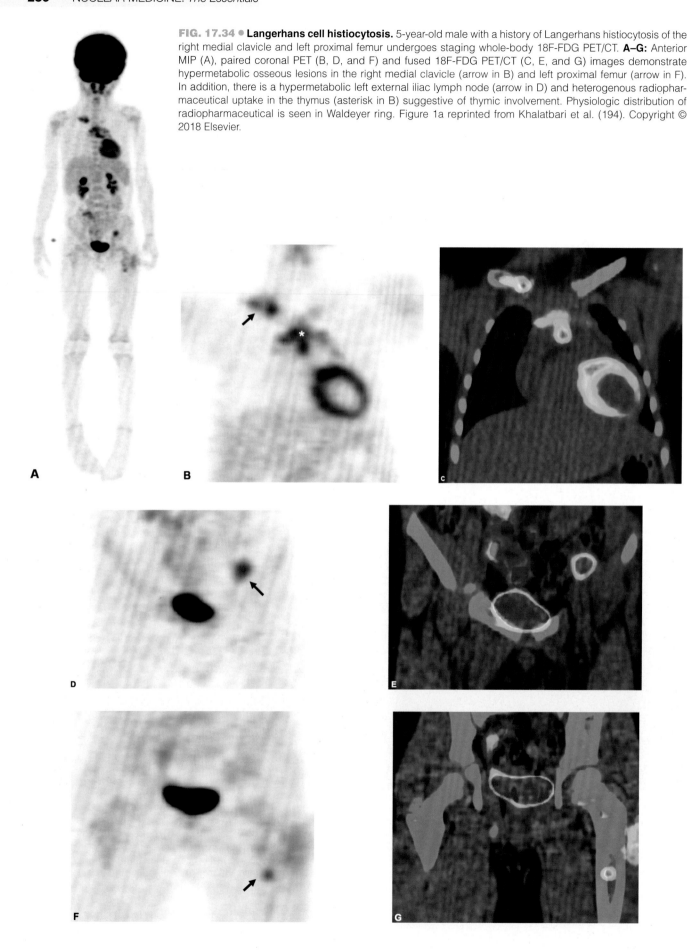

FIG. 17.34 ● **Langerhans cell histiocytosis.** 5-year-old male with a history of Langerhans histiocytosis of the right medial clavicle and left proximal femur undergoes staging whole-body 18F-FDG PET/CT. **A–G:** Anterior MIP (A), paired coronal PET (B, D, and F) and fused 18F-FDG PET/CT (C, E, and G) images demonstrate hypermetabolic osseous lesions in the right medial clavicle (arrow in B) and left proximal femur (arrow in F). In addition, there is a hypermetabolic left external iliac lymph node (arrow in D) and heterogenous radiopharmaceutical uptake in the thymus (asterisk in B) suggestive of thymic involvement. Physiologic distribution of radiopharmaceutical is seen in Waldeyer ring. Figure 1a reprinted from Khalatbari et al. (194). Copyright © 2018 Elsevier.

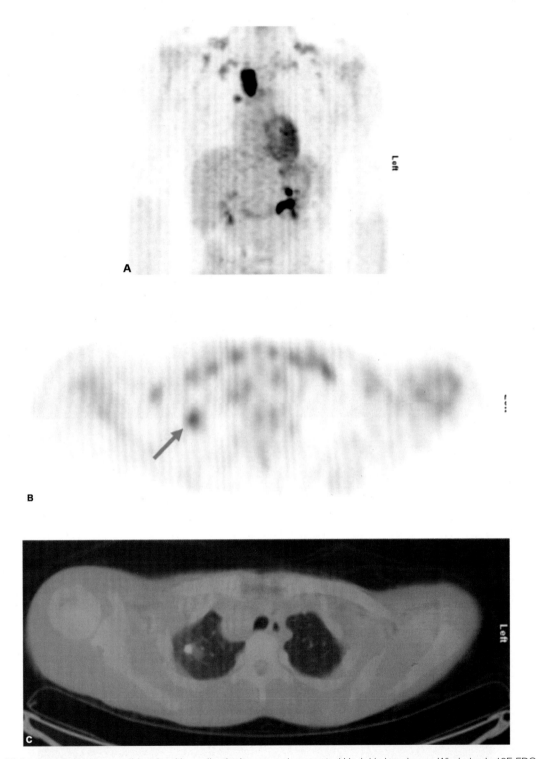

FIG. 17.35 ● Histoplasmosis. 14-year-old male with mediastinal mass and suspected Hodgkin lymphoma. Whole-body 18F-FDG PET/CT was performed. **A–G:** Anterior MIP (A) and paired axial PET (B, D, and F) and fused PET/CT (C, E, and G) images demonstrate hypermetabolic right paratracheal (arrow in D) and right hilar (arrow in F) lymphadenopathy as well as hypermetabolic ground glass opacity in the right upper lobe (arrow in B). Needle biopsy of the mediastinal lymphadenopathy demonstrated caseating granulomas and histoplasmosis antibodies were positive, findings consistent with a diagnosis of histoplasmosis.

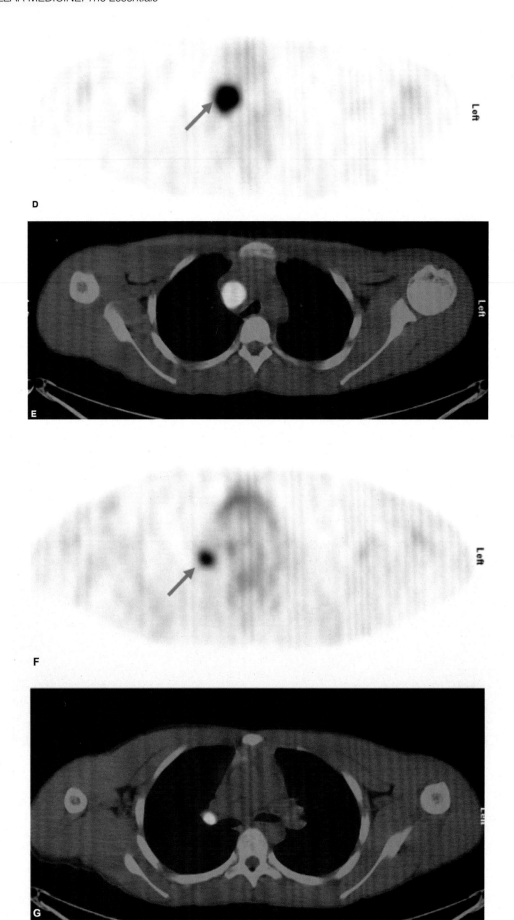

FIG. 17.35 ● (Continued)

CENTRAL NERVOUS SYSTEM

Epilepsy

Epilepsy is a common neurologic disorder in childhood. Approximately 30% of pediatric epilepsy is refractory to medical therapy and some of these patients are candidates for resection or functional surgery which may reduce or eliminate seizure activity (38,199,200). A wide range of cerebral abnormalities may cause epilepsy in pediatrics. The two most common are malformations of cortical development, such as focal cortical dysplasia (Fig. 17.36), hemimegalencephaly, and tuberous sclerosis, and benign or low-grade tumors (199,201–204). Other etiologies include hippocampal sclerosis, hypothalamic hamartoma, Rasmussen encephalitis, and vascular lesions (e.g., cavernomas) (199). Concurrent lesions (i.e., dual pathology) may be present in approximately 15% of patients (200).

Interictal 18F-FDG PET/CT or PET/MR and ictal/interictal SPECT compliment MRI in detecting epileptogenic lesions (38,205). The performance of 18F-FDG PET/CT or PET/MR is less labor intensive than ictal/interictal SPECT and is becoming more widely used for this indication. Electroencephalogram (EEG) monitoring during the procedure is required to confirm the absence of seizure activity. On interictal 18F-FDG PET, the epileptogenic substrate is seen as a hypometabolic lesion (38,200,206).

Nuclear medicine cerebrospinal fluid shunts

Management of hydrocephalus is the most common problem in pediatric neurosurgery. Therapeutic options for hydrocephalus include either addressing the underlying cause (such as resection of an intracranial mass or evacuation of an intracranial hematoma) or creating a temporary or permanent diversion of cerebrospinal fluid (CSF). CSF shunts are the most common option for permanent diversion of CSF to another compartment, typically the peritoneal cavity, that is capable of resorbing the fluid (207).

CSF shunts have a high failure rate. CT (preferably low dose) of the head or rapid MRI of the brain are used to evaluate the size of the ventricles and to look for other intracranial complications of CSF shunts (208). Radiographic shunt series evaluate the integrity of the CSF shunt components. NM CSF shunt studies are most commonly used to evaluate the flow of CSF from the ventricles to the peritoneal cavity. A normal CSF shunt study has several components including (i) adequate CSF flow to the needle hub and normal CSF opening pressure, (ii) absence of fracture or discontinuity in CSF shunt components, (iii) downsloping time-activity curve with emptying T1/2 of less than 5 to 7.5 min, and (iv) dispersion of the radiopharmaceutical in the peritoneal cavity by 15 to 20 min (Fig. 17.37) (209–219).

CONCLUSION

There are age-related developmental changes as well as physiologic variants in children that can be mistaken for pathology. Many of the disease processes encountered in the pediatric population are different from those in adults. Even when similar pathologies are encountered, the causes and the sites of involvement vary between adults and children. Awareness of these differences allows for improved accuracy of disease assessment when interpreting NM studies in children. In this chapter we have focused on the technical aspects of pediatric scintigraphy and the unique congenital and acquired pathologies that are less frequently seen in adults.

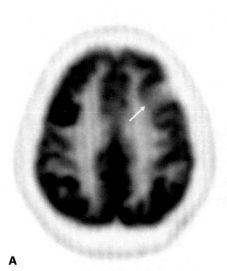
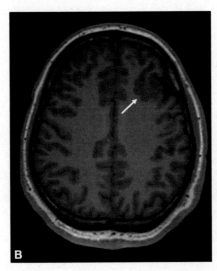
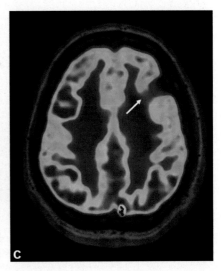

FIG. 17.36 ● **Focal cortical dysplasia.** 16-year-old male with medically refractory epilepsy. 18F-FDG PET/CT was performed and fused to MR images using a dedicated software program. **A–C:** Axial 18F-FDG PET (A), axial T1-weighted MR (B), and axial fused PET/MR (C) images demonstrate focal hypometabolism in the left frontal lobe (arrows in A and C) that corresponds to a focal area of thickened cortex on MRI (arrow in B). Fusion of the PET and MR images aid in the detection and localization of epileptogenic lesions. The patient underwent surgical resection of the epileptogenic substrate and pathology confirmed focal cortical dysplasia.

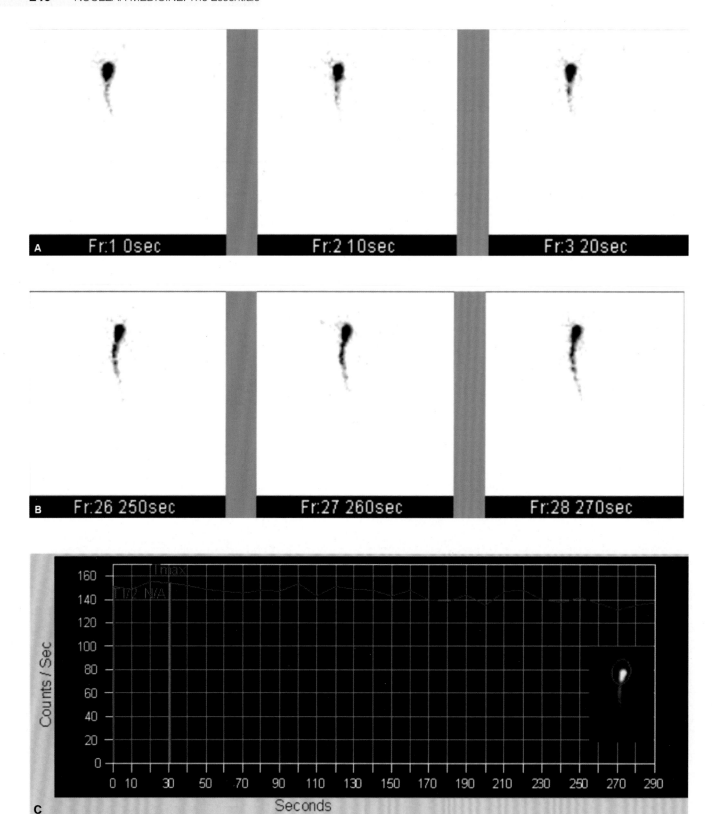

FIG. 17.37 ● NM CSF shunt study with partial obstruction of the ventricular catheter. 10-year-old female with a ventriculoperitoneal (VP) shunt placed shortly after birth that was last revised 7 years prior. Patient presents for routine follow-up after a 3-year hiatus. Rapid MRI of the brain (not shown) demonstrated interval increase in size of the ventricles compared to CT head performed 3 years ago. NM CSF shunt study is requested to evaluate CSF shunt function. **A–B:** The reservoir of the valve was accessed. CSF opening pressure was elevated, measuring 20 cm of H_2O. Using aseptic technique, radiopharmaceutical was instilled in the reservoir and dynamic images were obtained at 10 s/frame for a total of 5 min. Anterior frames 1 to 3 (A) and 26 to 28 (B) are shown. The radiopharmaceutical is in the valve and proximal peritoneal catheter. **C:** A region of interest was drawn around the valve (inset in the lower right corner) to generate a time-activity curve (TAC). The TAC plateaus and emptying half-time was not reached.

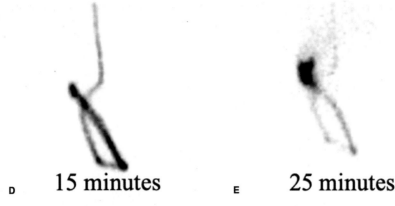

D **15 minutes** E **25 minutes**

FIG. 17.37 ● (Continued) **NM CSF shunt study with partial obstruction of the ventricular catheter. D and E:** Anterior static images of the chest and abdomen were obtained at 5 min (not shown) were repeated at 15 (D) and 25 (E) min; the patient sat upright between these two time points. There was slow flow of radiopharmaceutical into the peritoneal catheter with some spillage seen in the peritoneal cavity at 25 min. Constellation of findings of increased opening pressure, plateauing TAC, and delayed spillage of radiopharmaceutical in the peritoneal cavity are suggestive of partial obstruction of the ventricular catheter. This was confirmed at surgery and a new ventricular catheter was placed.

References

1. Lew DP, Waldvogel FA. Osteomyelitis. *N Engl J Med.* 1997;336(14):999–1007. doi:10.1056/NEJM199704033361406
2. Jaramillo D, Dormans JP, Delgado J, et al. Hematogenous osteomyelitis in infants and children: imaging of a changing disease. *Radiology.* 2017;283(3):629–643. doi:10.1148/radiol.2017151929
3. Schmitt SK. Osteomyelitis. *Infect Dis Clin North Am.* 2017;31(2):325–338. doi:10.1016/j.idc.2017.01.010
4. Majd M, Bar-Sever Z, Santos AI, et al. The SNMMI and EANM procedural guidelines for diuresis renography in infants and children. *J Nucl Med.* 2018;59(10):1636–1640. doi:10.2967/jnumed.118.215921
5. Blaufox MD, De Palma D, Taylor A, et al. The SNMMI and EANM practice guideline for renal scintigraphy in adults. *Eur J Nucl Med Mol Imaging.* 2018;45(12):2218–2228. doi:10.1007/s00259-018-4129-6
6. Mandell GA, Eggli DF, Gilday DL, et al. Procedure guideline for renal cortical scintigraphy in children. Society of Nuclear Medicine. *J Nucl Med.* 1997;38(10):1644–1646.
7. Brenner M, Bonta D, Eslamy H, et al. Comparison of 99mTc-DMSA dual-head SPECT versus high-resolution parallel-hole planar imaging for the detection of renal cortical defects. *AJR Am J Roentgenol.* 2009;193(2):333–337. doi:10.2214/AJR.08.1788
8. Cao X, Xu X, Grant FD, et al. Estimation of split renal function with (99m)Tc-DMSA SPECT: comparison between 3D volumetric assessment and 2D coronal projection imaging. *AJR Am J Roentgenol.* 2016;207(6):1324–1328. doi:10.2214/AJR.16.16307
9. Beslic N, Milardovic R, Sadija A, et al. Interobserver variability in interpretation of planar and SPECT Tc-99m-DMSA renal scintigraphy in children. *Acta Inform Med.* 2017;25(1):28–33.
10. Sarikaya I, Sarikaya A current status of radionuclide renal cortical imaging in pyelonephritis. *J Nucl Med Technol.* 2019;47(4):309–312. doi:10.2967/jnmt.119.227942
11. Fettich J, Colarinha P, Fischer S, et al. Guidelines for direct radionuclide cystography in children. *Eur J Nucl Med Mol Imaging.* 2003;30(5):B39–B44. doi:10.1007/s00259-003-1137-x
12. Treves ST, Gelfand MJ, Fahey FH, et al. 2016 Update of the North American consensus guidelines for pediatric administered radiopharmaceutical activities. *J Nucl Med.* 2016;57(12):15N–18N.
13. Lassmann M, Eberlein U, Lopci E, et al. Standardization of administered activities in paediatric nuclear medicine: the EANM perspective. *Eur J Nucl Med Mol Imaging.* 2016;43(13):2275–2278. doi:10.1007/s00259-016-3474-6
14. Leger J, Olivieri A, Donaldson M, et al. European society for paediatric endocrinology consensus guidelines on screening, diagnosis, and management of congenital hypothyroidism. *J Clin Endocrinol Metab.* 2014;99(2):363–384. doi:10.1210/jc.2013-1891
15. Keller-Petrot I, Leger J, Sergent-Alaoui A, et al. Congenital hypothyroidism: role of nuclear medicine. *Semin Nucl Med.* 2017;47(2):135–142. doi:10.1053/j.semnuclmed.2016.10.005
16. Ross DS, Burch HB, Cooper DS, et al. 2016 American thyroid association guidelines for diagnosis and management of hyperthyroidism and other causes of thyrotoxicosis. *Thyroid.* 2016;26(10):1343–1421. doi:10.1089/thy.2016.0229
17. Giovanella L, Avram AM, Iakovou I, et al. EANM practice guideline/SNMMI procedure standard for RAIU and thyroid scintigraphy. *Eur J Nucl Med Mol Imaging.* 2019;46(12):2514–2525. doi:10.1007/s00259-019-04472-8
18. Majd M, Reba RC, Altman RP. Effect of phenobarbital on 99mTc-IDA scintigraphy in the evaluation of neonatal jaundice. *Semin Nucl Med.* 1981;11(3):194–204. doi:10.1016/s0001-2998(81)80004-9
19. Kwatra N, Shalaby-Rana E, Narayanan S, et al. Phenobarbital-enhanced hepatobiliary scintigraphy in the diagnosis of biliary atresia: two decades of experience at a tertiary center. *Pediatr Radiol.* 2013;43(10):1365–1375. doi:10.1007/s00247-013-2704-3
20. Oates E, Austin JM, Becker JL. Technetium-99m-sulfur colloid SPECT imaging in infants with suspected heterotaxy syndrome. *J Nucl Med.* 1995;36(8):1368–1371.
21. Spottswood SE, Pfluger T, Bartold SP, et al. SNMMI and EANM practice guideline for meckel diverticulum scintigraphy 2.0. *J Nucl Med Technol.* 2014;42(3):163–169. doi:10.2967/jnmt.113.136242
22. Qutbi M, Neshandar Asli I. Pelvic Meckel's diverticulum mimicking bladder on meckel scan; the impact of quality control and technical issues. *J Nucl Med Technol.* 2017. doi:10.2967/jnmt.117.198531
23. Gelfand MJ, Wagner GG. Gastric emptying in infants and children: limited utility of 1-hour measurement. *Radiology.* 1991;178(2):379–381. doi:10.1148/radiology.178.2.1987596
24. Kwatra NS, Shalaby-Rana E, Andrich MP, et al. Gastric emptying of milk in infants and children up to 5 years of age: normative data and influencing factors. *Pediatr Radiol.* 2020;50(5):689–697. doi:10.1007/s00247-020-04614-3
25. Abell TL, Camilleri M, Donohoe K, et al. Consensus recommendations for gastric emptying scintigraphy: a joint report of the American neurogastroenterology and motility society and the society of nuclear medicine. *J Nucl Med Technol.* 2008;36(1):44–54. doi:10.2967/jnmt.107.048116
26. Farrell MB. Gastric emptying scintigraphy. *J Nucl Med Technol.* 2019;47(2):111–119. doi:10.2967/jnmt.117.227892
27. Heyman S, Respondek M .Detection of pulmonary aspiration in children by radionuclide "salivagram". *J Nucl Med.* 1989;30(5):697–699.

28. Van den Wyngaert T, Strobel K, Kampen WU, et al. The EANM practice guidelines for bone scintigraphy. *Eur J Nucl Med Mol Imaging.* 2016;43(9):1723–1738. doi:10.1007/s00259-016-3415-4

29. Bartel TB, Kuruva M, Gnanasegaran G, et al. SNMMI procedure standard for bone scintigraphy 4.0. *J Nucl Med Technol.* 2018;46(4):398–404.

30. Israel O, Pellet O, Biassoni L, et al. Two decades of SPECT/CT - the coming of age of a technology: an updated review of literature evidence. *Eur J Nucl Med Mol Imaging.* 2019;46(10):1990–2012. doi:10.1007/s00259-019-04404-6

31. Parisi MT, Iyer RS, Stanescu AL. Nuclear medicine applications in pediatric musculoskeletal diseases: the added value of hybrid imaging. *Semin Musculoskelet Radiol.* 2018;22(1):25–45. doi:10.1055/s-0037-1615782

32. Boellaard R, Delgado-Bolton R, Oyen WJG, et al. FDG PET/CT: EANM procedure guidelines for tumour imaging: version 2.0. *Eur J Nucl Med Mol Imaging.* 2015;42(2):328–354. doi:10.1007/s00259-014-2961-x

33. Bar-Sever Z, Biassoni L, Shulkin B, et al. Guidelines on nuclear medicine imaging in neuroblastoma. *Eur J Nucl Med Mol Imaging.* 2018;45(11):2009–2024. doi:10.1007/s00259-018-4070-8

34. Bombardieri E, Giammarile F, Aktolun C, et al. 131I/123I-metaiodobenzylguanidine (mIBG) scintigraphy: procedure guidelines for tumour imaging. *Eur J Nucl Med Mol Imaging.* 2010;37(12):2436–2446. doi:10.1007/s00259-010-1545-7

35. Fahey FH, Goodkind A, MacDougall RD, et al. Operational and dosimetric aspects of pediatric PET/CT. *J Nucl Med.* 2017;58(9):1360–1366. doi:10.2967/jnumed.116.182899

36. Parisi MT, Bermo MS, Alessio AM, et al. Optimization of pediatric PET/CT. *Semin Nucl Med.* 2017;47(3):258–274. doi:10.1053/j.semnuclmed.2017.01.002

37. Parisi MT, Otjen JP, Stanescu AL, et al. Radionuclide imaging of infection and inflammation in children: a review. *Semin Nucl Med.* 2018;48(2):148–165. doi:10.1053/j.semnuclmed.2017.11.002

38. Stanescu L, Ishak GE, Khanna PC, et al. FDG PET of the brain in pediatric patients: imaging spectrum with MR imaging correlation. *Radiographics.* 2013;33(5):1279–1303. doi:10.1148/rg.335125152

39. Fahey FH, Goodkind AB, Plyku D, et al. Dose estimation in pediatric nuclear medicine. *Semin Nucl Med.* 2017;47(2):118–125. doi:10.1053/j.semnuclmed.2016.10.006

40. Stabin MG, Gelfand MJ. Dosimetry of pediatric nuclear medicine procedures. *Q J Nucl Med.* 1998;42(2):93–112.

41. Little MP, Wakeford R, Tawn EJ, et al. Risks associated with low doses and low dose rates of ionizing radiation: why linearity may be (almost) the best we can do. *Radiology.* 2009;251(1):6–12. doi:10.1148/radiol.2511081686

42. Callahan MJ, MacDougall RD, Bixby SD, et al. Ionizing radiation from computed tomography versus anesthesia for magnetic resonance imaging in infants and children: patient safety considerations. *Pediatr Radiol.* 2018;48(1):21–30. doi:10.1007/s00247-017-4023-6

43. Queiroz MA, Delso G, Wollenweber S, et al. Dose optimization in TOF-PET/MR compared to TOF-PET/CT. *PLoS One.* 2015;10(7):e0128842. doi:10.1371/journal.pone.0128842

44. Kubo T. Vendor free basics of radiation dose reduction techniques for CT. *Eur J Radiol.* 2019;110:14–21. doi:10.1016/j.ejrad.2018.11.002

45. Jafari ME, Daus AM. Applying image gently SM and image wisely SM in nuclear medicine. *Health Phys.* 2013;104(2 Suppl 1):S31–S36. doi:10.1097/HP.0b013e3182764cd8

46. Zempsky WT. Pharmacologic approaches for reducing venous access pain in children. *Pediatrics.* 2008;122 Suppl 3(Supplement 3):S140–S153. doi:10.1542/peds.2008-1055g

47. Trottier ED, Dore-Bergeron M-J, Chauvin-Kimoff L, et al. Managing pain and distress in children undergoing brief diagnostic and therapeutic procedures. *Paediatr Child Health.* 2019;24(8):509–535.

48. Peters C, van Trotsenburg ASP, Schoenmakers N. Diagnosis of endocrine disease: congenital hypothyroidism: update and perspectives. *Eur J Endocrinol.* 2018;179(6):R297–R317. doi:10.1530/EJE-18-0383

49. Leung AKC, Leung AAC. Evaluation and management of the child with hypothyroidism. *Recent Pat Endocr Metab Immune Drug Discov.* 2018. doi:10.2174/1872214812666180508144513

50. Livett T, LaFranchi S. Imaging in congenital hypothyroidism. *Curr Opin Pediatr.* 2019;31(4):555–561. doi:10.1097/MOP.0000000000000782

51. Ruchala M, Szczepanek E, Szaflarski W, et al. Increased risk of thyroid pathology in patients with thyroid hemiagenesis: results of a large cohort case-control study. *Eur J Endocrinol.* 2010;162(1):153–160. doi:10.1530/EJE-09-0590

52. Szczepanek-Parulska E, Zybek-Kocik A, Wartofsky L, et al. thyroid hemiagenesis: incidence, clinical significance, and genetic background. *J Clin Endocrinol Metab.* 2017;102(9):3124–3137. doi:10.1210/jc.2017-00784

53. Smith TJ, Hegedus L. Graves' disease. *N Engl J Med.* 2017;376(2):185. doi: 10.1056/NEJMc1614624#SA3

54. Goichot B, Leenhardt L, Massart C, et al. Diagnostic procedure in suspected Graves' disease. *Ann Endocrinol (Paris).* 2018;79(6):608–617. doi:10.1016/j.ando.2018.08.002

55. Sharma A, Stan MN. Thyrotoxicosis: diagnosis and management. *Mayo Clin Proc.* 2019;94(6):1048–1064. doi:10.1016/j.mayocp.2018.10.011

56. Gupta A, Ly S, Castroneves LA, et al. A standardized assessment of thyroid nodules in children confirms higher cancer prevalence than in adults. *J Clin Endocrinol Metab.* 2013;98(8):3238–3245. doi:10.1210/jc.2013-1796

57. Parisi MT, Eslamy H, Mankoff D. Management of differentiated thyroid cancer in children: focus on the american thyroid association pediatric guidelines. *Semin Nucl Med.* 2016;46(2):147–164. doi:10.1053/j.semnuclmed.2015.10.006

58. Bauer AJ. Thyroid nodules in children and adolescents. *Curr Opin Endocrinol Diabetes Obes.* 2019;26(5):266–274. doi:10.1097/MED.0000000000000495

59. Francis GL, Waguespack SG, Bauer AJ, et al. Management guidelines for children with thyroid nodules and differentiated thyroid cancer. *Thyroid.* 2015;25(7):716–759. doi:10.1089/thy.2014.0460

60. Avram AM. Radioiodine scintigraphy with SPECT/CT: an important diagnostic tool for thyroid cancer staging and risk stratification. *J Nucl Med Technol.* 2014;42(3):170–180. doi:10.2967/jnumed.111.104133

61. Prasad PK, Mahajan P, Hawkins DS, et al. Management of pediatric differentiated thyroid cancer: an overview for the pediatric oncologist. *Pediatr Blood Cancer.* 2020;67(6):e28141. doi:10.1002/pbc.28141

62. Queisser-Luft A, Stolz G, Wiesel A, et al. Malformations in newborn: results based on 30,940 infants and fetuses from the Mainz congenital birth defect monitoring system (1990-1998). *Arch Gynecol Obstet.* 2002;266(3):163–167. doi:10.1007/s00404-001-0265-4

63. Sanna-Cherchi S, Ravani P, Corbani V, et al. Renal outcome in patients with congenital anomalies of the kidney and urinary tract. *Kidney Int.* 2009;76(5):528–533. doi:10.1038/ki.2009.220

64. Capone VP, Morello W, Taroni F, et al. Genetics of congenital anomalies of the kidney and urinary tract: the current state of play. *Int J Mol Sci.* 2017;18(4). doi:10.3390/ijms18040796

65. Murugapoopathy V, Gupta IR. A primer on congenital anomalies of the kidneys and urinary tracts (CAKUT). *Clin J Am Soc Nephrol.* 2020. doi:10.2215/CJN.12581019

66. Sanavi C, Dacher J-N, Caudron J, et al. Supranormal differential renal function in unilateral hydronephrotic kidney: insights from functional MR urography. *J Magn Reson Imaging.* 2014;40(3):577–582. doi:10.1002/jmri.24440

67. Assmus MA, Kiddoo DA, Hung RW, et al. Initially asymmetrical function on MAG3 renography increases incidence of adverse outcomes. *J Urolo.* 2016;195(4 Pt 2):1196–1202. doi:10.1016/j.juro.2015.11.011

68. European Association of Urology Guidelines. Chapter 3.12 Dilatation of the upper urinary tract (UPJ and UVJ obstruction). EAU Guidelines Office, Arnhem, The Netherlands. http://uroweb.org/guidelines/compilations-of-all-guidelines/. Accessed May 21, 2020.

69. Sussman RD, Blum ES, Sprague BM, et al. Prediction of clinical outcomes in prenatal hydronephrosis: importance of gravity assisted drainage. *J Urolo.* 2017;197(3):838–844. doi:10.1016/j.juro.2016.09.111

70. Sivakumar VN, Indiran V, Sathyanathan BP. Dynamic MRI and isotope renogram in the functional evaluation of pelviureteric junction obstruction: a comparative study. *Turk J Urol.* 2018;44(1):45–50.

71. De Palma D. Radionuclide tools in clinical management of febrile UTI in children. *Semin Nucl Med.* 2020;50(1):50–55. doi:10.1053/j.semnuclmed.2019.10.003

72. Okarska-Napierala M, Wasilewska A, Kuchar E. Urinary tract infection in children: diagnosis, treatment, imaging - Comparison of current guidelines. *J Pediatr Urol.* 2017;13(6):567–73. doi:10.1016/j.jpurol.2017.07.018

73. Silay MS, Spinoit A-F, Bogaert G, et al. Imaging for vesicoureteral reflux and ureteropelvic junction obstruction. *Eur Urol Focus.* 2016;2(2):130–138. doi:10.1016/j.euf.2016.03.015.

74. Karmazyn BK, Alazraki AL, Anupindi SA, et al. ACR Appropriateness Criteria((R)) urinary tract infection-child. *J Am Coll Radiology.* 2017;14(5S):S362–S371. doi:10.1016/j.jacr.2017.02.028

75. Arteaga MV, Caballero VM, Rengifo KM. Dosimetry of (99m)Tc (DTPA, DMSA and MAG3) used in renal function studies of newborns and children. *Appl Radiat Isot.* 2018;138:25–28. doi:10.1016/j.apradiso.2017.07.054

76. Duran C, Beltran VP, Gonzalez A, et al. Contrast-enhanced voiding urosonography for vesicoureteral reflux diagnosis in children. *Radiographics.* 2017;37(6):1854–1869. doi:10.1148/rg.2017170024

77. Ntoulia A, Back SJ, Shellikeri S, et al. Contrast-enhanced voiding urosonography (ceVUS) with the intravesical administration of the ultrasound contrast agent Optison for vesicoureteral reflux detection in children: a prospective clinical trial. *Pediatr Radiol.* 2018;48(2):216–226. doi:10.1007/s00247-017-4026-3

78. Mane N, Sharma A, Patil A, et al. Comparison of contrast-enhanced voiding urosonography with voiding cystourethrography in pediatric vesicoureteral reflux. *Turk J Urol.* 2018;44(3):261–267. doi:10.5152/tud.2018.76702

79. Torun N, Aktas A, Reyhan M, et al. Evaluation of cyclic direct radionuclide cystography findings with DMSA scintigraphy results in children with a prior diagnosis of vesicoureteral reflux. *Nucl Med Commun.* 2019;40(6):583–587. doi:10.1097/MNM.0000000000000994

80. Gelfand MJ, Koch BL, Elgazzar AH, et al. Cyclic cystography: diagnostic yield in selected pediatric populations. *Radiology.* 1999;213(1):118–120. doi:10.1148/radiology.213.1.r99oc14118

81. Joaquim AI, de Godoy MF, Burdmann EA. Cyclic direct radionuclide cystography in the diagnosis and characterization of vesicoureteral reflux in children and adults. *Clin Nucl Med.* 2015;40(8):627–631. doi:10.1097/RLU.0000000000000799

82. Haid B, Becker T, Koen M, et al. Lower radiation burden in state of the art fluoroscopic cystography compared to direct isotope cystography in children. *J Pediatr Urol.* 2015;11(1):35.e1–e6. doi:10.1016/j.jpurol.2014.08.015

83. Martin WG, Schneider K, Lauer O, et al. Investigations for vesicoureteric reflux in children: ultrasound vs. radionuclide voiding cystography. *Uremia Invest.* 1985;9(2):253–258. doi:10.3109/08860228509088217

84. Atala A, Ellsworth P, Share J, et al. Comparison of sonicated albumin enhanced sonography to fluoroscopic and radionuclide voiding cystography for detecting vesicoureteral reflux. *J Urolo.* 1998;160(5):1820–1822.

85. Pashankar D, Schreiber RA. Neonatal cholestasis: a red alert for the jaundiced newborn. *Can J Gastroenterol.* 2000;14 Suppl D:67D–72D. doi:10.1155/2000/657368

86. He J-P, Hao Y, Wang X-L, et al. Comparison of different noninvasive diagnostic methods for biliary atresia: a meta-analysis. *World J Pediatr.* 2016;12(1):35–43. doi:10.1007/s12519-015-0071-x

87. Wehrman A, Waisbourd-Zinman O, Wells RG. Recent advances in understanding biliary atresia. *F1000Res.* 2019;8(218):218. doi:10.12688/f1000research.16732.1

88. Sevilla A, Howman-Giles R, Saleh H, et al. Hepatobiliary scintigraphy with SPECT in infancy. *Clin Nucl Med.* 2007;32(1):16–23.

89. Yang J-G, Ma D-Q, Peng Y, et al. Comparison of different diagnostic methods for differentiating biliary atresia from idiopathic neonatal hepatitis. *Clin Imaging.* 2009;33(6):439–446. doi:10.1016/j.clinimag.2009.01.003

90. Camponovo E, Buck JL, Drane WE. Scintigraphic features of choledochal cyst. *J Nucl Med.* 1989;30(5):622–628.

91. Kao PF, Huang MJ, Tzen KY, et al. The clinical significance of gallbladder non-visualization in cholescintigraphy of patients with choledochal cysts. *Eur J Nucl Med.* 1996;23(11):1468–1472. doi:10.1007/BF01254470

92. Soares KC, Goldstein SD, Ghaseb MA, et al. Pediatric choledochal cysts: diagnosis and current management. *Pediatr Surg Int.* 2017;33(6):637–650. doi:10.1007/s00383-017-4083-6

93. William BM, Corazza GR. Hyposplenism: a comprehensive review. Part I: basic concepts and causes. *Hematology.* 2007;12(1):1–13. doi:10.1080/10245330600938422

94. Ashorobi D, Fernandez R. Asplenia. In: StatPearls [Internet]. *Treasure Island (FL)*: StatPearls Publishing; 2020. Accessed at https://www.ncbi.nlm.nih.gov/books/NBK538171/ on June 1, 2020.

95. El-Gohary Y, Khan S, Hodgman E, et al. Splenic function is not maintained long-term after partial splenectomy in children with sickle cell disease. *J Pediatr Surg.* 2020. doi:10.1016/j.jpedsurg.2019.12.006

96. Bakir M, Bilgic A, Ozmen M, et al. The value of radionuclide splenic scanning in the evaluation of asplenia in patients with heterotaxy. *Pediatr Radiol.* 1994;24(1):25–28. doi:10.1007/BF02017654

97. Cohen MS, Soper NJ, Underwood RA, et al. Laparoscopic splenopexy for wandering (pelvic) spleen. *Surg Laparosc Endosc.* 1998;8(4):286–290.

98. Chen JS, Lin CL, Tsai CC, et al. Giant ectopic pelvic spleen: report of a case and review of the literature. *Gaoxiong Yi Xue Ke Xue Za Zhi.* 1993;9(1):54–60.

99. Hardin VM, Morgan ME Thoracic splenosis. *Clin Nucl Med.* 1994;19(5):438–440. doi:10.1097/00003072-199405000-00014

100. Preece J, Phillips S, Sorokin V, et al. Splenogonadal fusion in an 18-month-old. *J Pediatr Urol.* 2017;13(2):214–215. doi:10.1016/j.jpurol.2016.06.005

101. Davies I, Burman-Roy S, Murphy MS. Gastro-oesophageal reflux disease in children: NICE guidance. *Bmj.* 2015;350:g7703. doi:10.1136/bmj.g7703

102. Vandenplas Y, Rudolph CD, Di Lorenzo C, et al. Pediatric gastroesophageal reflux clinical practice guidelines: joint recommendations of the North American Society for Pediatric Gastroenterology, Hepatology, and Nutrition (NASPGHAN) and the European Society for Pediatric Gastroenterology, Hepatology, and Nutrition (ESPGHAN). *J Pediatr Gastroenterol Nutr.* 2009;49(4):498–547. doi:10.1097/MPG.0b013e3181b7f563

103. Levin K, Colon A, DiPalma J, et al. Using the radionuclide salivagram to detect pulmonary aspiration and esophageal dysmotility. *Clin Nucl Med.* 1993;18(2):110–114. doi:10.1097/00003072-199302000-00003

104. Bar-Sever Z, Connolly LP, Treves ST. The radionuclide salivagram in children with pulmonary disease and a high risk of aspiration. *Pediatr Radiol.* 1995;25 Suppl 1:S180–S183.

105. Yang J, Codreanu I, Servaes S, et al. Radionuclide salivagram and gastroesophageal reflux scintigraphy in pediatric patients: targeting different types of pulmonary aspiration. *Clin Nucl Med.* 2015;40(7):559–563. doi:10.1097/RLU.0000000000000815

106. Irvine I, Doherty A, Hayes R. Bleeding meckel's diverticulum: a study of the accuracy of pertechnetate scintigraphy as a diagnostic tool. *Eur J Radiol.* 2017;96:27–30. doi:10.1016/j.ejrad.2017.09.008

107. Hong SN, Jang HJ, Ye BD, et al. Diagnosis of bleeding Meckel's diverticulum in adults. *PLoS One.* 2016;11(9):e0162615.

108. Vali R, Daneman A, McQuattie S, et al. The value of repeat scintigraphy in patients with a high clinical suspicion for Meckel diverticulum after a negative or equivocal first Meckel scan. *Pediatr Radiol.* 2015;45(10):1506–1514. doi:10.1007/s00247-015-3340-x

109. Wen Z, Salerno L, Zhuang H. Similar appearance on dynamic images of meckel scintigraphy caused by different etiologies: the value of lateral views. *Clin Nucl Med*. 2019;44(5):417–419. doi:10.1097/RLU.0000000000002479

110. Su T-P, Cheng N-M, Chuang H-C, et al. Potential false-positive meckel scan due to displaced kidney caused by recurrent retroperitoneal teratoma. *Clin Nucl Med*. 2014;39(10):e433–e435. doi:10.1097/RLU.0000000000000264

111. Kwatra N, Shalaby-Rana E, Majd M. Two-phase whole-body skeletal scintigraphy in children--revisiting the usefulness of the early blood pool phase. *Pediatr Radiol*. 2013;43(10):1376–1384. doi:10.1007/s00247-013-2650-0

112. Howard BA, Roy L, Kaye AD, et al. Utility of radionuclide bone scintigraphy in complex regional pain syndrome. *Curr Pain Headache Rep*. 2018;22(1):7. doi:10.1007/s11916-018-0659-7

113. Shalaby-Rana E, Majd M. (99m)Tc-MDP scintigraphic findings in children with leukemia: value of early and delayed whole-body imaging. *J Nucl Med*. 2001;42(6):878–883.

114. Mandell GA, Contreras SJ, Conard K, et al. Bone scintigraphy in the detection of chronic recurrent multifocal osteomyelitis. *J Nucl Med*. 1998;39(10):1778–1783.

115. Sato TS, Watal P, Ferguson PJ. Imaging mimics of chronic recurrent multifocal osteomyelitis: avoiding pitfalls in a diagnosis of exclusion. *Pediatr Radiol*. 2020;50(1):124–136. doi:10.1007/s00247-019-04510-5

116. Lusins JO, Elting JJ, Cicoria AD, et al. SPECT evaluation of lumbar spondylolysis and spondylolisthesis. *Spine (Phila Pa 1976)*. 1994;19(5):608–612. doi:10.1097/00007632-199403000-00018

117. Anderson K, Sarwark JF, Conway JJ, et al. Quantitative assessment with SPECT imaging of stress injuries of the pars interarticularis and response to bracing. *J Pediatr Orthop*. 2000;20(1):28–33.

118. Dunn AJ, Campbell RSD, Mayor PE, et al. Radiological findings and healing patterns of incomplete stress fractures of the pars interarticularis. *Skeletal Radiol*. 2008;37(5):443–450. doi:10.1007/s00256-008-0449-0

119. Trout AT, Sharp SE, Anton CG, et al. Spondylolysis and beyond: value of SPECT/CT in evaluation of low back pain in children and young adults. *Radiographics*. 2015;35(3):819–834. doi:10.1148/rg.2015140092

120. Kaeding CC, Miller T. The comprehensive description of stress fractures: a new classification system. *J Bone Joint Surg Am*. 2013;95(13):1214–1220. doi:10.2106/JBJS.L.00890

121. Franklyn M, Oakes B. Aetiology and mechanisms of injury in medial tibial stress syndrome: current and future developments. *World J Orthop*. 2015;6(8):577–589. doi:10.5312/wjo.v6.i8.577

122. Galbraith RM, Lavallee ME. Medial tibial stress syndrome: conservative treatment options. *Curr Rev Musculoskelet Med*. 2009;2(3):127–133. doi:10.1007/s12178-009-9055-6

123. Holder LE, Michael RH. The specific scintigraphic pattern of "shin splints in the lower leg": concise communication. *J Nucl Med*. 1984;25(8):865–869

124. Swischuk LE, Jadhav SP. Tibial stress phenomena and fractures: imaging evaluation. *Emerg Radiol*. 2014;21(2):173–177. doi:10.1007/s10140-013-1181-1

125. Fredericson M, Bergman AG, Hoffman KL, et al. Tibial stress reaction in runners. Correlation of clinical symptoms and scintigraphy with a new magnetic resonance imaging grading system. *Am J Sports Med*. 1995;23(4):472–481. doi:10.1177/036354659502300418

126. Nattiv A, Kennedy G, Barrack MT, et al. Correlation of MRI grading of bone stress injuries with clinical risk factors and return to play: a 5-year prospective study in collegiate track and field athletes. *Am J Sports Med*. 2013;41(8):1930–1941. doi:10.1177/0363546513490645

127. Zwas ST, Elkanovitch R, Frank G. Interpretation and classification of bone scintigraphic findings in stress fractures. *J Nucl Med*. 1987;28(4):452–457.

128. Ginsburg GM, Bassett GS. Back pain in children and adolescents: evaluation and differential diagnosis. *J Am Acad Orthop Surg*. 1997;5(2):67–78. doi:10.5435/00124635-199703000-00002

129. Bhatia NN, Chow G, Timon SJ, et al. Diagnostic modalities for the evaluation of pediatric back pain: a prospective study. *J Pediatr Orthop*. 2008;28(2):230–233. doi:10.1097/BPO.0b013e3181651bc8

130. Gennari JM, Themar-Noel C, Panuel M, et al. Adolescent spinal pain: the pediatric orthopedist's point of view. *Orthop Traumatol Surg Res*. 2015;101(6 Suppl):S247–S250. doi:10.1016/j.otsr.2015.06.012

131. Berger RG, Doyle SM. Spondylolysis 2019 update. *Curr Opin Pediatr*. 2019;31(1):61–68. doi:10.1097/MOP.0000000000000706

132. Cheung KK, Dhawan RT, Wilson LF, et al. Pars interarticularis injury in elite athletes - The role of imaging in diagnosis and management. *Eur J Radiol*. 2018;108:28–42. doi:10.1016/j.ejrad.2018.08.029

133. Campbell RSD, Grainger AJ, Hide IG, et al. Juvenile spondylolysis: a comparative analysis of CT, SPECT and MRI. *Skeletal Radiol*. 2005;34(2):63–73. doi:10.1007/s00256-004-0878-3

134. Child Abuse Prevention and Treatment Act. Available at: https://www.acf.hhs.gov/sites/default/files/cb/capta.pdf. Accessed May 22, 2020.

135. Christian CW. The evaluation of suspected child physical abuse. *Pediatrics*. 2015;135(5):e1337–e1354. doi:10.1542/peds.2015-0356

136. Wootton-Gorges SL, Soares BP, Alazraki AL, et al. ACR appropriateness criteria® suspected physical abuse-child. *J Am Coll Radiolo*. 2017;14(5S):S338–S349. doi:10.1016/j.jacr.2017.01.036

137. Harden RN, Bruehl S, Perez RSGM, et al. Validation of proposed diagnostic criteria (the "Budapest Criteria") for complex regional pain syndrome. *Pain*. 2010;150(2):268–274. doi:10.1016/j.pain.2010.04.030

138. Mackinnon SE, Holder LE. The use of three-phase radionuclide bone scanning in the diagnosis of reflex sympathetic dystrophy. *J Hand Surg Am*. 1984;9(4):556–563. doi:10.1016/s0363-5023(84)80110-0

139. Goldsmith DP, Vivino FB, Eichenfield AH, et al. Nuclear imaging and clinical features of childhood reflex neurovascular dystrophy: comparison with adults. *Arthritis Rheum*. 1989;32(4):480–485. doi:10.1002/anr.1780320419

140. Pachowicz M, Nocuń A, Postępski J, et al. Complex regional pain syndrome type I with atypical scintigraphic pattern--diagnosis and evaluation of the entity with three phase bone scintigraphy. A case report. *Nucl Med Rev Cent East Eur*. 2014;17(2):115–119. doi:10.5603/NMR.2014.0029

141. Laxer RM, Allen RC, Malleson PN, et al. Technetium 99m-methylene diphosphonate bone scans in children with reflex neurovascular dystrophy. *J Pediatr*. 1985;106(3):437–440. doi:10.1016/s0022-3476(85)80671-5

142. Johnsen JI, Dyberg C, Wickstrom M. Neuroblastoma-A neural crest derived embryonal malignancy. *Front Mol Neurosci*. 2019;12:9. doi:10.3389/fnmol.2019.00009

143. Park JR, Eggert A, Caron H. Neuroblastoma: biology, prognosis, and treatment. *Hematol Oncol Clin North Am*. 2010;24(1):65–86. doi:10.1016/j.hoc.2009.11.011

144. Vo KT, Matthay KK, Neuhaus J, et al. Clinical, biologic, and prognostic differences on the basis of primary tumor site in neuroblastoma: a report from the international neuroblastoma risk group project. *J Clin Oncol*. 2014;32(28):3169–3176. doi:10.1200/JCO.2014.56.1621

145. Angstman KB, Miser JS, Franz WB. 3 Neuroblastoma. *Am Fam Physician*. 1990;41(1):238–244.

146. Rudnick E, Khakoo Y, Antunes NL, et al. Opsoclonus-myoclonus-ataxia syndrome in neuroblastoma: clinical outcome and antineuronal antibodies-a report from the Children's Cancer Group Study. *Med Pediatr Oncol*. 2001;36(6):612–622. doi:10.1002/mpo.1138

147. Golden CB, Feusner JH. Malignant abdominal masses in children: quick guide to evaluation and diagnosis. *Pediatr Clin North Am*. 2002;49(6):1369–1392, viii. doi:10.1016/s0031-3955(02)00098-6

148. Swift CC, Eklund MJ, Kraveka JM, et al. Updates in diagnosis, management, and treatment of neuroblastoma. *Radiographics*. 2018;38(2):566–580. doi:10.1148/rg.2018170132

149. Park JR, Bagatell R, Cohn SL, et al. Revisions to the international neuroblastoma response criteria: a consensus statement from the national cancer institute clinical trials planning meeting. *J Clin Oncol*. 2017;35(22):2580–2587. doi:10.1200/JCO.2016.72.0177

150. Monclair T, Brodeur GM, Ambros PF, et al. The International Neuroblastoma Risk Group (INRG) staging system: an INRG Task Force report. *J Clin Oncol.* 2009;27(2):298–303. doi: 10.1200/JCO.2008.16.6876

151. Brodeur GM. Spontaneous regression of neuroblastoma. *Cell Tissue Res.* 2018;372(2):277–286. doi:10.1007/s00441-017-2761-2

152. Tolbert VP, Matthay KK. Neuroblastoma: clinical and biological approach to risk stratification and treatment. *Cell Tissue Res.* 2018;372(2):195–209. doi:10.1007/s00441-018-2821-2

153. Parisi MT, Eslamy H, Park JR, et al. (1)(3)(1)I-metaiodobenzylguanidine theranostics in neuroblastoma: historical perspectives; practical applications. *Semin Nucl Med.* 2016;46(3):184–202. doi:10.1053/j.semnuclmed.2016.02.002

154. Jacobson AF, Deng H, Lombard J, et al. 123I-metaiodobenzylguanidine scintigraphy for the detection of neuroblastoma and pheochromocytoma: results of a meta-analysis. *J Clin Endocrinol Metab.* 2010;95(6):2596–2606. doi:10.1210/jc.2009-2604

155. Pandit-Taskar N, Modak S. Norepinephrine transporter as a target for imaging and therapy. *J Nucl Med.* 2017;58(Suppl 2):39S–53S. doi:10.2967/jnumed.116.186833

156. Leung A, Shapiro B, Hattner R, et al. Specificity of radioiodinated MIBG for neural crest tumors in childhood. *J Nucl Med.* 1997;38(9):1352–1357.

157. Marachelian A, Shimada H, Sano H, et al. The significance of serial histopathology in a residual mass for outcome of intermediate risk stage 3 neuroblastoma. *Pediatr Blood Cancer.* 2012;58(5):675–681. doi:10.1002/pbc.23250

158. Nakajo M, Shapiro B, Copp J, et al. The normal and abnormal distribution of the adrenomedullary imaging agent m-[I-131]iodobenzylguanidine (I-131 MIBG) in man: evaluation by scintigraphy. *J Nucl Med.* 1983;24(8):672–682.

159. Sharp SE, Gelfand MJ, Shulkin BL. Pediatrics: diagnosis of neuroblastoma. *Semin Nucl Med.* 2011;41(5):345–353. doi:10.1053/j.semnuclmed.2011.05.001

160. Ady N, Zucker JM, Asselain B, et al. A new 123I-MIBG whole body scan scoring method--application to the prediction of the response of metastases to induction chemotherapy in stage IV neuroblastoma. *Eur J Cancer.* 1995;31A(2):256–261. doi:10.1016/0959-8049(94)00509-4

161. Messina JA, Cheng S-C, Franc BL, et al. Evaluation of semi-quantitative scoring system for metaiodobenzylguanidine (mIBG) scans in patients with relapsed neuroblastoma. *Pediatr Blood Cancer.* 2006;47(7):865–874. doi:10.1002/pbc.20777

162. Lewington V, Lambert B, Poetschger U, et al. (123)I-mIBG scintigraphy in neuroblastoma: development of a SIOPEN semi-quantitative reporting ,method by an international panel. *Eur J Nucl Med Mol Imaging.* 2017;44(2):234–241. doi:10.1007/s00259-016-3516-0

163. Matthay KK, Edeline V, Lumbroso J, et al. Correlation of early metastatic response by 123I-metaiodobenzylguanidine scintigraphy with overall response and event-free survival in stage IV neuroblastoma. *J Clin Oncol.* 2003;21(13):2486–2491. doi:10.1200/JCO.2003.09.122

164. Radovic B, Artiko V, Sobic-Saranovic D, et al. Evaluation of the SIOPEN semi-quantitative scoring system in planar simpatico-adrenal MIBG scintigraphy in children with neuroblastoma. *Neoplasma.* 2015;62(3):449–455. doi:10.4149/neo_2015_053

165. Suc A, Lumbroso J, Rubie H, et al. Metastatic neuroblastoma in children older than one year: prognostic significance of the initial metaiodobenzylguanidine scan and proposal for a scoring system. *Cancer.* 1996;77(4):805–811. doi:10.1002/(sici)1097-0142(19960215)77:4<805::aid-cncr29>3.0.co;2-3

166. Perel Y, Conway J, Kletzel M, et al. Clinical impact and prognostic value of metaiodobenzylguanidine imaging in children with metastatic neuroblastoma. *J Pediatr Hematol Oncol.* 1999;21(1):13–18. doi:10.1097/00043426-199901000-00004

167. Decarolis B, Schneider C, Hero B, et al. Iodine-123 metaiodobenzylguanidine scintigraphy scoring allows prediction of outcome in patients with stage 4 neuroblastoma: results of the Cologne interscore comparison study. *J Clin Oncol.* 2013;31(7):944–951. doi:10.1200/JCO.2012.45.8794

168. Ladenstein R, Lambert B, Potschger U, et al. Validation of the mIBG skeletal SIOPEN scoring method in two independent high-risk neuroblastoma populations: the SIOPEN/HR-NBL1 and COG-A3973 trials. *Eur J Nucl Med Mol Imaging.* 2018;45(2):292–305. doi:10.1007/s00259-017-3829-7

169. Frappaz D, Bonneu A, Chauvot P, et al. Metaiodobenzylguanidine assessment of metastatic neuroblastoma: observer dependency and chemosensitivity evaluation. The SFOP Group. *Med Pediatr Oncol.* 2000;34(4):237–241. doi:10.1002/(sici)1096-911x(200004)34:4<237::aid-mpo1>3.0.co;2-j

170. Yanik GA, Parisi MT, Shulkin BL, et al. Semiquantitative mIBG scoring as a prognostic indicator in patients with stage 4 neuroblastoma: a report from the Children's oncology group. *J Nucl Med.* 2013;54(4):541–548. doi:10.2967/jnumed.112.112334

171. Yanik GA, Parisi MT, Naranjo A, et al. Validation of postinduction curie scores in high-risk neuroblastoma: a children's oncology group and SIOPEN group report on SIOPEN/HR-NBL1. *J Nucl Med.* 2018;59(3):502–508. doi:10.2967/jnumed.117.195883

172. Katzenstein HM, Cohn SL, Shore RM, et al. Scintigraphic response by 123I-metaiodobenzylguanidine scan correlates with event-free survival in high-risk neuroblastoma. *J Clin Oncol.* 2004;22(19):3909–3915. doi:10.1200/JCO.2004.07.144

173. Schmidt M, Simon T, Hero B, et al. The prognostic impact of functional imaging with (123)I-mIBG in patients with stage 4 neuroblastoma >1 year of age on a high-risk treatment protocol: results of the German Neuroblastoma Trial NB97. *Eur J Cancer.* 2008;44(11):1552–1558. doi:10.1016/j.ejca.2008.03.013

174. Brodeur GM, Pritchard J, Berthold F, et al. Revisions of the international criteria for neuroblastoma diagnosis, staging, and response to treatment. *J Clin Oncol.* 1993;11(8):1466–1477. doi:10.1200/JCO.1993.11.8.1466

175. Cecchetto G, Mosseri V, De Bernardi B, et al. Surgical risk factors in primary surgery for localized neuroblastoma: the LNESG1 study of the European International Society of Pediatric Oncology Neuroblastoma Group. *J Clin Oncol.* 2005;23(33):8483–8489. doi:10.1200/JCO.2005.02.4661

176. McElroy KM, Binkovitz LA, Trout AT, et al. Pediatric applications of Dotatate: early diagnostic and therapeutic experience. *Pediatr Radiol.* 2020. doi:10.1007/s00247-020-04688-z

177. Shimada H, Ambros IM, Dehner LP, et al. The international neuroblastoma pathology classification (the Shimada system). *Cancer.* 1999;86(2):364–372.

178. Eisenhauer EA, Therasse P, Bogaerts J, et al. New response evaluation criteria in solid tumours: revised RECIST guideline (version 1.1). *Eur J Cancer.* 2009;45(2):228–247. doi:10.1016/j.ejca.2008.10.026

179. Cohn SL, Pearson ADJ, London WB, et al. The International Neuroblastoma Risk Group (INRG) classification system: an INRG Task Force report. *J Clin Oncol.* 2009;27(2):289–297. doi:10.1200/JCO.2008.16.6785

180. Colleran GC, Kwatra N, Oberg L, et al. How we read pediatric PET/CT: indications and strategies for image acquisition, interpretation and reporting. *Cancer Imaging.* 2017;17(1):28. doi:10.1186/s40644-017-0130-8

181. Voss SD. Functional and anatomical imaging in pediatric oncology: which is best for which tumors. *Pediatr Radiol.* 2019;49(11):1534–1544. doi:10.1007/s00247-019-04489-z

182. Chambers G, Frood R, Patel C, et al. (18)F-FDG PET-CT in paediatric oncology: established and emerging applications. *Br J Radiol.* 2019;92(1094):20180584. doi:10.1259/bjr.20180584

183. Ouellet V, Routhier-Labadie A, Bellemare W, et al. Outdoor temperature, age, sex, body mass index, and diabetic status determine the prevalence, mass, and glucose-uptake activity of 18F-FDG-detected BAT in humans. *J Clin Endocrinol Metab.* 2011;96(1):192–199. doi:10.1210/jc.2010-0989

184. Ogawa Y, Abe K, Sakoda A, et al. FDG-PET and CT findings of activated brown adipose tissue in a patient with paraganglioma. *Eur J Radiol Open.* 2018;5:126–130.

185. Park J, Byun BH, Jung CW, et al. Perirenal (18)F-FDG uptake in a patient with a pheochromocytoma. *Nucl Med Mol Imaging.* 2014;48(3):233–236.

186. Hadi M, Chen CC, Whatley M, et al. Brown fat imaging with (18)F-6-fluorodopamine PET/CT, (18)F-FDG PET/CT, and (123)I-MIBG SPECT: a study of patients being evaluated for pheochromocytoma. *J Nucl Med.* 2007;48(7):1077–1083. doi:10.2967/jnumed.106.035915

187. Frontini A, Vitali A, Perugini J, et al. White-to-brown transdifferentiation of omental adipocytes in patients affected by pheochromocytoma. *Biochim Biophys Acta.* 2013;1831(5):950–959. doi:10.1016/j.bbalip.2013.02.005

188. Iyer RB, Guo CC, Perrier N. Adrenal pheochromocytoma with surrounding brown fat stimulation. *AJR Am J Roentgenol.* 2009;192(1):300–301. doi:10.2214/AJR.08.1166

189. Wong KK, Sedig LK, Bloom DA, et al. 18F-2-fluoro-2-deoxyglucose uptake in white adipose tissue on pediatric oncologic positron emission tomography (PET)/computed tomography (CT). *Pediatr Radiol.* 2020;50(4):524–533. doi:10.1007/s00247-019-04574-3

190. Rosolen A, Perkins SL, Pinkerton CR, et al. Revised international pediatric non-hodgkin lymphoma staging system. *J Clin Oncol.* 2015;33(18):2112–2118. doi:10.1200/JCO.2014.59.7203

191. McCarten KM, Nadel HR, Shulkin BL, et al. Imaging for diagnosis, staging and response assessment of Hodgkin lymphoma and non-Hodgkin lymphoma. *Pediatr Radiol.* 2019;49(11):1545–1564. doi:10.1007/s00247-019-04529-8

192. Voss SD, Cairo MS. Surveillance imaging in pediatric lymphoma. *Pediatr Radiol.* 2019;49(11):1565–1573. doi:10.1007/s00247-019-04511-4

193. Harrison DJ, Parisi MT, Shulkin BL. The role of (18)F-FDG-PET/CT in pediatric sarcoma. *Semin Nucl Med.* 2017;47(3):229–241. doi:10.1053/j.semnuclmed.2016.12.004

194. Khalatbari H, Parisi MT, Kwatra N, et al. Pediatric musculoskeletal imaging: the indications for and applications of PET/computed tomography. *PET Clin.* 2019;14(1):145–174. doi:10.1016/j.cpet.2018.08.008

195. Schafer JF, Gatidis S, Schmidt H, et al. Simultaneous whole-body PET/MR imaging in comparison to PET/CT in pediatric oncology: initial results. *Radiology.* 2014;273(1):220–231. doi:10.1148/radiol.14131732

196. Muehe AM, Theruvath AJ, Lai L, et al. How to provide gadolinium-free PET/MR cancer staging of children and young adults in less than 1 h: the stanford approach. *Mol Imaging Biol.* 2018;20(2):324–335. doi:10.1007/s11307-017-1105-7

197. Daldrup-Link H. How PET/MR can add value for children with cancer. *Curr Radiol Rep.* 2017;5(3):1920. doi:10.1007/s40134-017-0207-y

198. Vaidyanathan S, Patel CN, Scarsbrook AF, et al. FDG PET/CT in infection and inflammation--current and emerging clinical applications. *Clin Radiol.* 2015;70(7):787–800. doi:10.1016/j.crad.2015.03.010

199. Jobst BC, Cascino GD. Resective epilepsy surgery for drug-resistant focal epilepsy: a review. *Jama.* 2015;313(3):285–293. doi:10.1001/jama.2014.17426

200. Engel JJ. The current place of epilepsy surgery. *Curr Opin Neurol.* 2018;31(2):192–197. doi:10.1097/WCO.0000000000000528

201. Shaker T, Bernier A, Carmant L. Focal cortical dysplasia in childhood epilepsy. *Semin Pediatr Neurol.* 2016;23(2):108–119. doi:10.1016/j.spen.2016.06.007

202. Guerrini R, Rosati A, Giordano F, et al. The medical and surgical treatment of tumoral seizures: current and future perspectives. *Epilepsia.* 2013;54 Suppl 9:84–90. doi:10.1111/epi.12450

203. Wong-Kisiel LC, Blauwblomme T, Ho M-L, et al. Challenges in managing epilepsy associated with focal cortical dysplasia in children. *Epilepsy Res.* 2018;145:1–17. doi:10.1016/j.eplepsyres.2018.05.006

204. Curatolo P, Nabbout R, Lagae L, et al. Management of epilepsy associated with tuberous sclerosis complex: updated clinical recommendations. *Eur J Paediatr Neurol.* 2018;22(5):738–748. doi:10.1016/j.ejpn.2018.05.006

205. Miller-Thomas MM, Benzinger TLS. Neurologic applications of PET/MR imaging. *Magn Reson Imaging Clin N Am.* 2017;25(2):297–313. doi:10.1016/j.mric.2016.12.003

206. Bernasconi A, Cendes F, Theodore WH, et al. Recommendations for the use of structural magnetic resonance imaging in the care of patients with epilepsy: a consensus report from the international league against epilepsy neuroimaging task force. *Epilepsia.* 2019;60(6):1054–1068. doi:10.1111/epi.15612

207. Kahle KT, Kulkarni AV, Limbrick DDJ, et al. Hydrocephalus in children. *Lancet.* 2016;387(10020):788–799. doi:10.1016/S0140-6736(15)60694-8

208. Hanak BW, Bonow RH, Harris CA, et al. Cerebrospinal fluid shunting complications in children. *Pediatr Neurosurg.* 2017;52(6):381–400. doi:10.1159/000452840

209. Bermo MS, Khalatbari H, Parisi MT. Two signs indicative of successful access in nuclear medicine cerebrospinal fluid diversionary shunt studies. *Pediatr Radiol.* 2018;48(8):1130–1138. doi:10.1007/s00247-018-4150-8

210. Thompson EM, Wagner K, Kronfeld K, et al. Using a 2-variable method in radionuclide shuntography to predict shunt patency. *J Neurosurg.* 2014;121(6):1504–1507. doi:10.3171/2014.8.JNS132898

211. Gok B, Batra S, Eslamy H, et al. Radionuclide shunt patency study for suspected ventriculoatrial shunt malfunction. *Clin Nucl Med.* 2013;38(7):527–533. doi:10.1097/RLU.0b013e31828da385

212. Feng F, Fu HL, Li JN, et al. Evaluation of radionuclide cerebrospinal fluid scintigraphy as a guide in the management of patients with hydrocephalus. *Clin Imaging.* 2009;33(2):85–89. doi:10.1016/j.clinimag.2008.06.033

213. Vassilyadi M, Tataryn ZL, Matzinger MA, et al. Radioisotope shuntograms at the Children's Hospital of Eastern Ontario. *Childs Nerv Syst.* 2006;22(1):43–49. doi:10.1007/s00381-005-1153-1

214. O'Brien DF, Taylor M, Park TS, et al. A critical analysis of "normal" radionucleotide shuntograms in patients subsequently requiring surgery. *Childs Nerv Syst.* 2003;19(5–6):337–341. doi:10.1007/s00381-003-0752-y

215. May CH, Aurisch R, Kornrumpf D, et al. Evaluation of shunt function in hydrocephalic patients with the radionuclide 99mTc-pertechnetate. *Childs Nerv Syst.* 1999;15(5):239–244, discussion 245. doi:10.1007/s003810050381

216. Vernet O, Farmer JP, Lambert R, et al. Radionuclide shuntogram: adjunct to manage hydrocephalic patients. *J Nucl Med.* 1996;37(3):406–410.

217. Uvebrant P, Sixt R, Bjure J, et al. Evaluation of cerebrospinal fluid shunt function in hydrocephalic children using 99mTc-DTPA. *Childs Nerv Syst.* 1992;8(2):76–80. doi:10.1007/bf00298444

218. Khalatbari H, Parisi MT. Management of hydrocephalus in children: anatomic imaging appearances of CSF shunts and their complication. *AJR Am J Roentgenol.* 2021 Jan;216(1):187–199.

219. Khalatbari H, Parisi MT. Complications of cerebrospinal fluid shunts. functional assessment with cerebrospinal fluid shunt scintigraphy: performance and interpretation. *AJR Am J Roentgenol.* 2020 Dec; 215(6):1474–1489 manuscript in press.

CHAPTER SELF-ASSESSMENT QUESTIONS

1. What is the most common extracranial solid tumor in pediatrics?

   A. Osteosvarcoma

   B. Neuroblastoma

   C. Ewing sarcoma

   D. Rhabdomyosarcoma

2. Five-week-old female with prenatal diagnosis of dilation of the left renal collecting system undergoes a Tc-99m MAG3 renogram with furosemide. Which of the following findings on the renogram is an indication that the patient will benefit from pyeloplasty?

   A. Complete emptying of the left renal collecting system after the administration of furosemide

   B. Differential function of 45% in the left kidney and 55% in the right kidney

   C. 60% emptying of the left renal collecting system on the gravity-assisted drainage images

   D. Differential function of 35% in the left kidney and 65% in the right kidney

Answers to Chapter Self-Assessment Questions

1. B   Neuroblastoma is the most common extracranial solid tumor in pediatrics. While neuroblastoma represents 8% to 10% of all childhood tumors, it accounts for approximately 15% of all pediatric cancer mortalities.

2. D   The main goal of the nuclear medicine renogram in infants with congenital dilation of the urinary tract is to identify that subset of patients that will benefit from surgical intervention. Such patients include those with (i) impaired split renal function (<40%), (ii) a decrease of split renal function of >10% in subsequent studies, or (iii) poor drainage after the administration of furosemide.

Quality Assurance of Nuclear Medicine Instrumentation

18

Kai Lee

LEARNING OBJECTIVES

1. Understand the rationale for each quality assurance procedure.
2. Learn the test procedures to monitor the equipment performance.
3. Familiarize with the results and abnormalities found in quality assurance tests.

INTRODUCTION

Accuracy and consistency are important goals for diagnostic nuclear medicine. Achievement of these goals requires artifact-free capable equipment appropriate for the patient's condition. Regulatory and accreditation agencies also require the equipment to be assured of functioning properly before administration of radiopharmaceutical to safeguard unnecessary radiation to the patient. A quality assurance (QA) program includes a set of test and evaluation procedures to evaluate the performance of the imaging or counting equipment such that it meets or exceeds established reference standards. For a QA program to be effective, the tests must be performed regularly at the appropriate frequencies, requiring only simple apparatus, a short time to perform, with critical analysis of the test results. This chapter presents an overview of QA tests for the imaging equipment, including the gamma cameras, single photon emission computed tomography (SPECT)/computed tomography (CT), and positron computed tomography (PET)/computed tomography (CT) (1,2). A summary of the frequency of the recommended QA tests is given in Table 18.2 at the end of the chapter for easy reference. The readers are encouraged to review the references for QA of the radiation safety survey and radioactivity assay instruments (3–5).

GAMMA CAMERA UNIFORMITY TEST

The intrinsic uniformity test is the most sensitive test to assure that the gamma camera is working properly. When exposed to a uniform source of radioactivity, the gamma camera should produce an image with uniform count density throughout the useful field of view. Due to the instability of photomultiplier tubes, variation in light production, and transmission in different crystal regions, gamma camera image nonuniformities may occur. Hot or cold spots in the field of view not only create a false impression of abnormal uptakes in the clinical images, but non-uniformity also causes linearity distortions, loss of resolution, and ring artifacts in SPECT images (6). One may simulate a uniform source of radioactivity or "flood" source by placing a small amount of radioactivity in a syringe and place it at a distance at least five times greater than the camera's useful field of view. For a typical gamma camera with a field of view of 50 × 40 cm, the point source must be 250 cm or farther away from the detector surface (7). An image is then acquired in a 256 × 256 or 512 × 512 matrix with the collimator removed. Field uniformity tests performed without the collimator are know as the intrinsic flood uniformity tests.

The gamma camera usually has a built-in software to measure integral and differential uniformities as indices of the field uniformity. A well-performing gamma camera should have values of integral and differential uniformities measuring <2.5%. However, gamma cameras having integral and differential uniformity <2.5% do not guarantee images free of artifacts. Careful inspection visually for any subtle hot or cold spots should always be performed. Linearity distortions in both the vertical and horizontal directions are shown in Figure 18.1, even though its integral and differential uniformities are <2.5%. Figure 18.2 shows a severe ring artifact in the SPECT image produced by a gamma camera whose integral and differential uniformity values met the manufacturer specifications; the ring artifact was caused by a small nonuniform spot in the location corresponding to the bull's-eye of the ring.

Another test for gamma camera uniformity is called the *extrinsic uniformity test*. It is done by placing a sealed sheet of Co-57 directly on the collimator. Co-57 ($t_{1/2}$ = 271.8 d) sheet sources are commercially available with 10, 15, or 20 mCi of Co-57 activity uniformity distributed better than 1% (8). The extrinsic uniformity test is not as sensitive as the intrinsic uniformity test for assessing the uniform response across the field of view of the gamma camera but is convenient to do daily and detects defects in the collimator. Most radioactive material licenses allow daily extrinsic uniformity test for its expediency, but a weekly intrinsic uniformity test has to be done to meet the QA test requirement. On annual basis, an extrinsic uniformity image is acquired using a 128 × 128 matrix for 120 million counts and stored on the computer for correction of subtle hot or cold spots in the projection images of a SPECT study. Such a high-count extrinsic uniformity image is called the uniformity correction matrix to correct for collimator defects and the nonuniform response of the sodium iodide and photomultiplier tube assembly.

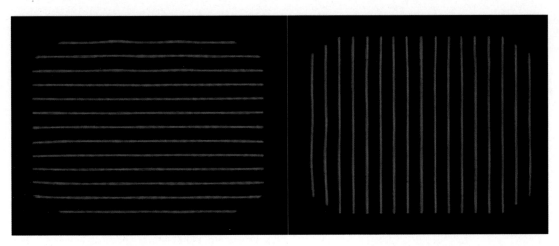

FIG. 18.1 • **The linearity distortions at the periphery were caused by nonuniformity.**

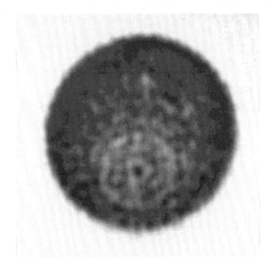

FIG. 18.2 • **A nonuniform spot produced a ring artifact in the single photon emission computed tomography (SPECT) image of a water phantom.** The ring artifact was not caused by the center-of-rotation error because it is not coinciding with the axis of rotation.

RESOLUTION AND LINEARITY

The radioactive material license in some states requires that a resolution and linearity test be done at least once a week. The test is done by placing a four-quadrant bar phantom (aka a quad phantom) in direct contact with the crystal surface after the intrinsic flood test. A quad phantom is a rectangular plate with rows of lead bars in each quadrant. The spacing of the parallel lead bars varies from 2.0 to 3.5 mm at 0.5 mm increment. A static image is then acquired into a 512 × 512 matrix for 5 million counts. The image should clearly show the lead bars spaced at 2.5 mm apart and appeared straight visually. Because of the difficulty in mounting the heavy quad phantom on the bare surface of the gamma camera, many users simply put the quad phantom on the collimator and then a Co-57 flood source on top of the quad phantom to acquire the image. In the author's opinion, the quad phantom test is not a sensitive test of the system's resolution and linearity. The system has to have badly deteriorated before an abnormal pattern is shown in the quad phantom image. The resolution and linearity of a gamma camera are strongly affected by its uniformity. Greater attention should be paid to the intrinsic uniformity test, and the SPECT system performance test to be described.

Center of rotation

The center of rotation (COR) is the center pixel in the computer image matrix corresponding to the mechanical axis of detector rotation. Gamma camera heads with the collimator on are heavy and can shift slightly on the mechanical support during rotation. Even a 1-pixel shift can produce an objectionable bull's-eye artifact in the center of the reconstructed image. The COR test measures the central pixel shift relative to the image matrix for each projection angle and makes the correction during image reconstruction. Shift correction is required to avoid bull's-eye artifacts in the center of a SPECT image. Latest generation gamma cameras are manufactured with great care to assure mechanical stability so users may perform the COR test once a month using the manufacturer-provided apparatus and software.

SPECT system performance evaluation

The filtered backprojection algorithm commonly used for image reconstruction is a noise amplification procedure. A slight shift in any number of variables can produce noticeable artifacts in a SPECT study. A SPECT phantom test is recommended at acceptance, and at least annually (9).

Figure 18.3 shows a typical SPECT three-section phantom. This includes a uniform activity section, a section with groups of plastic rods, and a section with spheres of different sizes and activities. The plastic rods section contains rods from about 5 to 13 mm in diameter. The spheres vary in diameter from 10 to 32 mm. Visual analysis of SPECT resolution is determined by the minimum size rods detectable in the reconstructed image. The ratio of counts per pixel in the spheres to counts per pixel in the surrounding water determines SPECT contrast. Visual assessment for SPECT uniformity is performed in the uniform activity section of the phantom, where the observer evaluates the evenness of count density and the absence of ring artifacts.

Quality assurance of CT scanners

QA for the CT scanner on a SPECT/CT or a PET/CT involves many complex procedures depending on whether it is a cone-beam CT or a thin-slice CT (10–12). However, the manufacturer provided phantom and software specifics for their system that are relatively easy for users to perform for daily QA. A mandatory procedure is tube warm-up. The CT control console flashes a warning message for the user to perform a tube warm-up if the CT has been idled for 2 h or longer. The kilovoltage (kV) and beam current (mA) in a cold x-ray tube are unsteady affecting

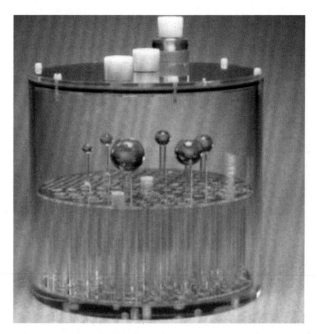

FIG. 18.3 ● **A commercially available single photon emission computed tomography (SPECT) phantom. Reprinted with permission from Lee (3).**

Table 18.1 **ACCEPTABLE COMPUTED TOMOGRAPHY NUMBERS**

	CT Number, HU
Polyethylene	−170 and −87
Water	−7 and 7
Acrylic	110 and 135
Teflon	850 and 970
Air	−1005 and −970

CT, computed tomography; HU, Hounsfield units.

the focal spot size and location, and emitted x-ray characteristics. The target in a cold x-ray tube could be damaged if a high exposure technique is applied to scan a large patient.

CT manufacturer-specific phantom and software are available for the technologist to perform daily measurements of CT numbers for water, image uniformity, image noise, resolution, and CT number linearity. The CT number for water is zero Hounsfield units (HU). In a well-calibrated system, the mean CT number for water should not vary from zero by more than 5 HU for the range of kV and slice thicknesses. The water-filled phantom section should be uniform and free of ring or streak artifacts by visual inspection. CT uniformity is quantitatively measured with region of interests (ROIs) at the center and at 12, 3, 6, and 9 o'clock in the periphery. The mean CT number of individual ROIs should agree to within 5 HU. Image noise is represented by the standard deviation of the CT numbers within an ROI in the central 70% of the uniform image and affected by kV, mA, rotation time, slice thickness, and reconstruction filter. There are no standardized procedural guidelines available for the acquisition of data and acceptable noise tolerance for CT images. The standard deviation of the CT number for water measured at the time of installation or after major repair is a reasonable reference value for daily QA. The manufacturer-provided phantoms usually have groups of bars at different spacing or some cylinders of different sizes. The CT resolution is checked by visual inspection of the smallest bar spacing or cylinder that can be seen on the reconstructed image.

CT number linearity can be evaluated by scanning the section of the American College of Radiology (ACR) accreditation phantom (10) that has a number of inserts of different densities. One of the inserts is a hollow air-filled tube while another insert is water filled. The other inserts include polyethylene, acrylic, and Teflon rods. Linearity check of the CT numbers evaluates if the measured CT numbers of the water, air, and plastic inserts are within acceptable ranges. The CT numbers shown in Table 18.1 are published by the American College of Radiology. Current CT scanners generally comply with these values.

Quality assurance of PET scanners

QA of PET scanners are manufacturer-specific involving different positron emitters and different jigs to position the source within the scanner. In spite of the variation of test procedures, the QA tests for PET can be classified into four general categories (9,13–15). The four general QA procedures for PET scanners are akin to the QA procedures for SPECT.

Blank scans

Blank scans are equivalent to the daily flood tests of a gamma camera to assure constancy of the tens of thousands of detectors in the PET scanner and to provide early warning of detector failure. Blank scans are done by having a sealed Ge-68 or a Na-22 source rotate around or placed in the center of the bore of the PET scanner. No other objects are placed in the bore so that each detector is exposed uniformly by the source. Results of the blank scan are presented as one or more sinograms. A normal sinogram should have an image pattern such as a spiral without drastic discontinuities or a band with a uniform shade of gray. Some scanners may have software to alert the user if the blank scan is out of tolerance.

Normalization scans

The normalization scan for a PET scanner is equivalent to the acquisition of the uniformity correction matrix for a gamma camera. When the tens of thousands of detectors are exposed to the same activity, one has to expect differences in the counting rates no matter how well each detector is tuned. The purpose of the normalization scan is to apply a correction factor to each detector so that every detector pair will give the same counting rate when exposed to the same activity. The correction factor applied to each detector pair is called the normalization factor. Normalization factors are typically obtained by acquiring counts from a Ge-68 source in the same manner as in the blank scan tests except that counts are acquired typically 5 to 10 h long to minimize the statistical noise. The normalization scan produces a table of correction factors for all possible pairs of detectors in the PET scanner. During image reconstruction, the correction factors are applied to normalize (i.e., correct) the counts in the corresponding detector pairs. For a normalized PET scanner, scan of a uniform source such as a cylinder with a well-mixed F-18 solution should yield a uniform tomographic image.

Radioactivity concentration calibration

The radioactivity concentration calibration is closely associated with computation of the standard uptake values (SUV). The SUV is computed as the ratio of the F-18 concentration in a region of interest, such as a spot in the liver with hypermetabolic activity, to the injected F-18 activity divided by the patient's body weight. A calibration factor is therefore needed to relate the number of counts in a voxel to the F-18 activity concentration in μCi/ml. The procedure for acquiring the calibration factor is manufacturer specific and has tradenames such as well-counter calibration, or SUV calibration.

Regardless of the manufacturer-specific procedures, the radioactivity concentration calibration factor involves putting an accurately measured quantity of F-18 in a phantom with a known volume of water. Typically, an accurately measured F-18 activity of about 1 mCi is mixed with an accurately known volume of water in a cylindrical phantom of about 5,000 ml. Since there is a known F-18 activity in a known volume of water, the activity concentration in the phantom is known. From the reconstructed image of the phantom, the number of counts and the number of voxels within a volume of interest are measured. The average voxel count density is obtained by dividing the total number of counts by the number of voxels within the chosen volume. The SUV calibration factor is obtained by dividing the voxel count density by the activity concentration. The radioactivity concentration calibration is simple to perform, but the quantitative measurements in each step must be precise. Unusual values of SUV are frequently due to an incorrect or outdated radioactivity concentration calibration factor. The calibration factor should be done at least once every quarter.

PET/CT performance evaluation

The ACR developed a protocol for assessing the overall performance of a PET/CT system (9). The ACR protocol uses a phantom, also known as the ACR PET accreditation phantom, which is a modification of the SPECT phantom shown in Figure 18.3. The PET accreditation phantom replaced the spheres in the SPECT phantom with seven cylinders attached to the cover plate. One of the cylinders is a solid Teflon cylinder to simulate bone. One cylinder is hollow with only air, and one cylinder is filled with water without any radioactivity. The other four cylinders are hollow with internal diameters varying from 8 to 25 mm. Depending on the dose of fluorodeoxyglucose (FDG) administered to the patient for PET scan, between 0.5 and 1.5 mCi of FDG is mixed into the main chamber of the phantom to simulate the background activity

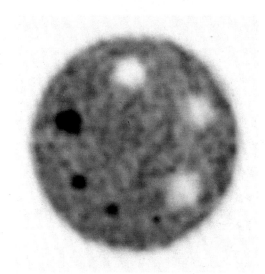

FIG. 18.4 ● Image of the ACR accreditation phantom produced by a well-calibrated positron computed tomography (PET)/computed tomography (CT). ACR, American College of Radiology; CT; PET.

in a patient of 70 kg. Another solution is mixed in a separate container to create an F-18 activity concentration approximately 2.5 times that of the concentration in the main chamber. The four hollow cylinders on the top plate are then filled with the concentrate FDG solution. Figure 18.4 shows an image produced from a scan of the phantom. The image may be visually assessed for the uniformity, artifacts, noise, hot lesion resolution, and adequacy of attenuation correction in the PET/CT system.

SUMMARY OF QUALITY ASSURANCE OF NUCLEAR MEDICINE INSTRUMENTATION

QA of the system performance starts after acceptance testing of the equipment and continues regularly. Table 18.2 summarizes the QA procedures that are recommended for each type of instrument and the test frequency.

Table 18.2 ROUTINE QUALITY ASSURANCE PROCEDURES

Test	Daily	Weekly	Monthly	Yearly
Gamma Camera/SPECT				
Extrinsic flood	√			
Intrinsic flood		√		
Linearity and resolution		√		
Center of rotation			√	
Uniformity correction matrix				√
Overall system performance				√
CT				
X-ray tube warm-up	√			
CT number of water	√			
Image uniformity	√			
Noise	√			
CT number linearity	√			
Image resolution	√			
PET				
Blank	√			
Normalization			6 months	
Radioactivity concentration				√
Overall performance, ACR				√

References

1. Sokole EB, Plachcinska A, Britten A. Routine quality control recommendations for nuclear medicine instrumentation. *Eur J Nucl Med Mol Imaging.* 2010;37:662–671.
2. Zanzonico P. Routine quality control of clinical nuclear medicine instrumentation: a brief review. *J Nucl Med.* 2008;49:1114–1131.
3. Lee, KH. *Basic science of Nuclear Medicine: The Bare Bones Essentials.* Society of Nuclear Medicine and Molecular Imaging; 2015.
4. IAEA, Quality assurance for Radioactivity Measurement in Nuclear Medicine, Safety reports series: ISSN 1020-6450; no. 16. International Atomic Energy Agency: Vienna; 2006.
5. IAEA. Calibration of Radiation Protection Monitoring Instruments, IAEA human health series: ISSN 2075-3772; no 6. International Atomic Energy Agency: Vienna; 2000.
6. IAEA. Quality assurance for SPECT systems, IAEA human health series: ISSN 2075-3772; no 6. International Atomic Energy Agency: Vienna; 2009.
7. National Electrical Manufacturers Association (NEMA). Standards Publication NU 1-2001. Performance Measurements of Scintillation Cameras.NEMA: Rosslyn, VA; 2001
8. Oswald B, Nardinger S. A review of common drawbacks inherent to Co-57 sheet sources. *J Nucl Med.* 2016;vol 57(Suppl 2):2613.
9. ACR. Site Scanning Instructions for the ACR Nuclear Medicine Phantom, American College of Radiology, Nuclear Medicine Accreditation Program, ACR. 2019.
10. ACR. Computed Tomography Quality Control Manual, American College of Radiology, Computed Tomography Accreditation Program, ACR. 2017.
11. IAEA. Quality Assurance Program for Computed Tomography: Diagnostic and Therapy Applications, IAEA human health series, ISSN 2075-3772; no.19. 2017.
12. EFOMP-ESTRO-IAEA. "Quality Control in Cone-beam Computed Tomography (CBCT)." http://dx.medra.org/10.19285/CBCTEFOMP.V1.0.2017.06
13. IAEA. Quality assurance for PET and PET/CT systems, IAEA human health series, ISSN 2075-3772; no 1. International Atomic Energy Agency: Vienna; 2009.
14. National Electrical Manufacturers Association (NEMA). Standards Publication NU 2-2007. Performance Measurements of Positron Emission Tomographs. NEMA: Rosslyn, VA; 2007.
15. National Electrical Manufacturers Association (NEMA). Standards Publication NU 4-2008. Performance Measurements of Small Animal Positron Emission Tomographs. NEMA: Rosslyn, VA; 2008.

CHAPTER SELF-ASSESSMENT QUESTIONS

1. Intrinsic uniformity test is useful for detecting potential problem with
   A. Center of rotation error
   B. Collimator defects
   C. Nonlinearity and ring artifacts

2. The QA test to assure consistency in the calculation of SUV is
   A. Normalization scan
   B. Radioactivity concentration
   C. PET and CT image alignment

3. Daily QA test of a CT scanner includes the following parameters
   A. CT number uniformity, CT number linearity, and noise
   B. X-ray tube kilovoltage, beam current, and temperature
   C. Radiation dose to the patient

Answers to Chapter Self-Assessment Questions

1. C Nonlinearity and ring artifacts.

2. B Radioactivity concentration.

3. A Measure the CT number uniformity, CT number linearity, and noise using the manufacturer-provided phantom and test procedure.

Nuclear Medicine Procedures in the Pregnant and Lactating Patient

19

Patrick M. Colletti

LEARNING OBJECTIVES

1. Describe the considerations for the use of radiopharmaceuticals in the pregnant patient.
2. Consult with the pregnant patients and their doctors regarding nuclear medicine procedures.
3. List nuclear medicine procedures never to perform during pregnancy.
4. Minimize the radiation exposure to the lactating patient and her child.

INTRODUCTION

It is of course reasonable to limit the use of radiopharmaceuticals in pregnant patients to situations where the potential benefits are greater than predicted fetal risks. Situations in pregnant patients arise in several scenarios. A patient may receive diagnostic or therapeutic radioisotope agents prior to the knowledge that she is pregnant, or she may receive a radioisotope scan to diagnose important conditions that occur during pregnancy. For example, the original use of placental scanning with ^{99m}Tc-human serum albumin was able to help locate the position of the placenta with the small estimated fetal dose <5 µGy (1). Nuclear medicine experts may be asked to estimate the risks for fetal injury associated with the radioisotopic procedure in question, including the possibility of consulting with the patient regarding potential recommendations for termination of the pregnancy.

WHAT ARE THE RISKS OF RADIATION IN PREGNANCY?

Potential risks for radiation to the fetus are difficult to differentiate from commonly occurring spontaneous fetal events. Table 19.1 summarizes the naturally occurring risks of common fetal adverse outcomes.

In addition to fetal loss, abnormal organogenesis, and intra-uterine growth retardation, fetal radiation may be associated with

postnatal malignancy. The background risk of childhood cancer mortality is 0.14%. The risk of childhood cancer death is thought to be 0.06% per 10 mGy in utero exposure (or 1/1700 additional cancers per 10 mGy). The lifetime risk of cancer is thought to be 0.4% per 10 mGy in utero exposure (3).

Recommendations regarding fetal radiation exposure

There are no convincing data linking medical imaging during pregnancy to adverse fetal outcomes. Brent (4) projected that diagnostic exposures to radiation presents a low risk, based on approximately 28.6% risk of spontaneous abortion, major malformation, mental retardation, and childhood malignancy among the general population that an exposure of 50 mSv (50 mGy) increases by approximately 0.17%.

Table 19.2 (5) presents recommendations for consulting with and advising pregnant patients regarding fetal risks associated with radiation exposure. In general, termination of pregnancy is not recommended unless there is reasonable documentation that an estimated fetal dose is greater than 150 mGy.

Radiopharmaceutical distribution and dosimetry in the pregnant patient

Fetal absorbed dose is the summation of external irradiation from maternal tissues as well as placental uptake and transplacental radiopharmaceutical transfer.

Table 19.1 **SPONTANEOUS ADVERSE OUTCOMES OF PREGNANCY FROM WILCOX 1988 (2)**

Period	Risk	Spontaneous Occurrence Rate	Estimated Threshold Dose
Day 1–10	Reabsorption	30%	50–100 mGy
Day 10–50	Abnormal Organogenesis	4%–6%	200 mGy
>Day 50	Intra-uterine Growth Retardation	4%	200–250 mGy

Table 19.2 RECOMMENDATIONS REGARDING FETAL IRRADIATION

Fetal Estimated Exposure (mGy)	Recommendation
<1 (Total gestation)	General public limit
<5 (0.50 per month)	Nuclear Regulatory Commission fetus exposure limit
Fetal dose <50	Fetal risk negligible
Fetal dose <100	Termination not justified
Fetal dose 100–150	Consider individual circumstances
Fetal dose >150	Possible fetal damage Termination should be seriously considered
Fetal dose >200	Termination generally recommended

From Colletti et al. (5). Copyright © 2013 American Roentgen Ray Society.

For radiopharmaceuticals excreted in urine, irradiation from maternal bladder may be the most important source. Hydration and frequent voiding may reduce the fetal absorbed dose significantly. Smaller administered dosages can significantly reduce the fetal absorbed dose at the expense of longer imaging times.

Lipophilic agents without significant albumin binding, with an molecular weight (MW) <500 to 1000 daltons (cut-off value 600 daltons) more likely cross the placental barrier. Large differences in amniotic structure and glucose transporter expression between animal models and the human placenta confound extrapolations of placental accumulation and transport. For reference, ^{18}F-fluorodeoxyglucose (FDG) is 181 daltons (0.7 nm). As most available positron emission tomography (PET) radiopharmaceuticals are typically small molecules; ^{18}F-FDG, Na[18]F, [82]Rb, and [18]F- Florbetapir would be expected to cross the placental barrier and directly irradiate the fetus.

Table 19.3 presents estimated fetal exposures associated with common routine dose nuclear medicine examinations (6–8). Table 19.4 correlates some of the limited newborn outcome data associated with nuclear medicine exams performed during pregnancy (9–13). Table 19.5 presents some of the case report information available regarding ^{18}F-FDG PET/computed tomography (CT) in pregnant patients (14–17).

Table 19.3 FETAL WHOLE-BODY DOSE FROM COMMON NUCLEAR MEDICINE EXAMINATIONS IN EARLY PREGNANCY AND AT TERM (6–8)

Isotope	Procedure/ Radiopharmaceutical	Dose (mCi/MBq)	Early Gestation (mGy)	Term (mGy)
Tc-99m	Bone scan (MDP)	20/750	4.6–4.7	1.8
Tc-99m	Lung perfusion (MAA)	5.4/200	0.4–0.6	0.8
Tc-99m	Lung ventilation (DTPA aerosol)	1.1/40	0.1–0.3	0.1
Tc-99m	Thyroid scan (pertechnetate)	11/400	3.2–4.4	3.7
Tc-99m	Red blood cell	25/930	3.6–6	2.5
Tc-99m	Liver colloid	8/300	0.5–0.6	1.1
Tc-99m	Renal DTPA	20/750	5.9–9.0	3.5
Ga-67	Abscess/tumor	5.1/190	14–18	25

Table 19.4 PREGNANCY OUTCOME AFTER NUCLEAR IMAGING PERFORMED IN PREGNANCY

Authors	Weeks of Gestation	Radiopharmaceutical	Imaging type	Estimated Dosimetry	Pregnancy Outcome
Zanotti-Fregonara et al., 2008 (9)	8 wk	^{18}F-FDG	PET/CT	18.9 mGy	Term healthy baby
Zanotti-Fregonara et al., 2009 (10)				19.35 mGy including SUV 2.5 placenta	
Marcus et al., 1985 (11)	10 wk	[99m]Tc	V/Q lung scan	0.50 mGy	Term healthy baby
Schaefer et al., 2009 (12)	First trimester	^{99m}Tc-MDP ^{99m}Tc-pertechnetate	Bone (n = 20) Thyroid (n = 102) Controls (n = 366)	→4.6 mGy →0.8 mGy	Major defects in 4/122 (3.7%) vs. controls 12/366 (3.7%)
Baker et al. 1987 (13)	15, 16, and 22 wk	^{99m}Tc-MDP	Bone scan	0.76 mGy	N/A

Table 19.5 **FETAL ESTIMATED IRRADIATION FROM ^{18}F-FDG PET/CT CASE REPORTS (18)**

	Maternal	Placental crossover	CT	Total
Zanotti-Fregonara et al. 2010 (14)	3.0 mGy	8.9 mGy	10 mGy	21.9 mGy
Takalkar et al. 2011 (15)	1.1–9.4 mGy (reported combined maternal plus placental crossover)		Negligible (^{68}Ge rod)	1.1–9.4 mGy
Hsieh et al. 2012 (16)	6.3 mGy (reported combined maternal plus placental crossover)		3.6 mGy	9.9 mGy
Drouet et al. 2020 (17)	6.7 mGy (reported combined maternal plus placental crossover)		3.9 mGy	10.6 mGy

Radiopharmaceuticals that cross the placenta can be retained in the amniotic circulation. From here, the agent may be swallowed by the fetus and passed back into the amniotic fluid from where it may be re-swallowed and adsorbed or passed through again into the amniotic fluid. For example, Stabin et al. predicted that fetal exposure from ^{18}F-FDG rises to 0.81 mGy/mCi up to 3 month and 0.61 mGy/mCi at 6 months to term when placental crossover is considered (18). Figure 19.1 demonstrates the mechanisms by which a fetus may receive radiation exposure. Figures 19.2 and 19.3 present an example of how PET/CT expose a fetus to radiation (17).

Imaging for suspected pulmonary embolism in pregnancy

Pregnant women are at two to four times the risk of pulmonary embolism (PE) compared with age-matched nonpregnant women. About 1 in 1000 pregnancies (19,20) may be complicated by PE, and PE is the cause of 20% of all maternal deaths (21). The clinical diagnosis of PE in a pregnant patient is particularly difficult because mild shortness of breath, elevated heart rate, and swollen legs are expected in late pregnancy, and Wells criteria and d-dimer levels may be unreliable in pregnancy (5). In view of the clinical problem of suspected PE in a pregnant patient, 2011 consensus guidelines from the American Thoracic Society and the Society of Thoracic Radiology along with the Society of Nuclear Medicine and Molecular Imaging and the American College of Obstetricians and Gynecologists recommend initial lower-extremity Doppler imaging and chest radiography followed by pulmonary CT angiography (CTA) if the chest radiographic findings are abnormal and ventilation–perfusion scintigraphy of the radiographic findings are normal (and in the absence of reactive airway disease). Follow-up is conducted with pulmonary CTA if the ventilation–perfusion findings are neither clearly positive nor clearly negative (22,23). Proceeding directly to pulmonary CTA is a credible alternative strategy (24–28).

Physiologic increased breast glandular tissue of pregnancy can cause increased breast radiosensitivity (28). CT strategies to reduce breast exposure should be considered (29).

Table 19.6 compares the advantages and disadvantages of pulmonary CTA and ventilation or perfusion scanning for pregnant

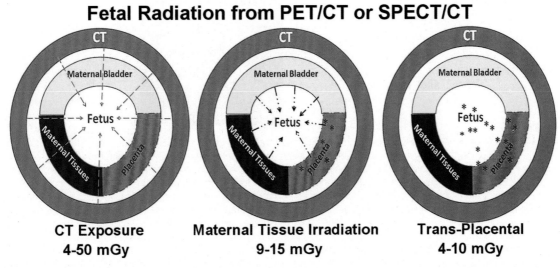

FIG. 19.1 ● Mechanisms of fetal radiation from PET/computed tomography (CT) or single photon emission computed tomography (SPECT)/computed tomography (CT). The total fetal radiation depends on radiation from isotope in placenta and surrounding tissues, radioactive urine in the maternal bladder, transplacental radiopharmaceutical transfer, and x-ray energy absorption associated with the CT. The relative exposures shown here may occur with typical fluorodeoxyglucose (FDG) positron emission tomography (PET)/computed tomography (CT).

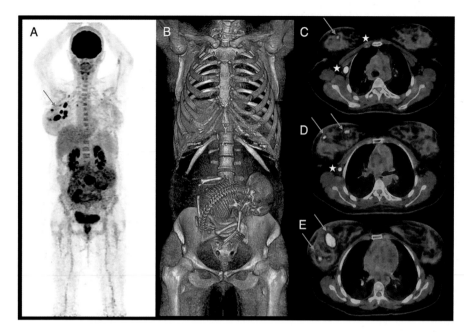

FIG. 19.2 • This 37-year-old woman underwent an fluorodeoxyglucose (FDG) positron emission tomography (PET)/computed tomography (CT) at 31 weeks of gestation for the staging of right breast cancer. The dose of FDG was reduced to 2 MBq/kg and the scan time per bed position was increased to 2 minutes. The patient was asked to drink water and void her bladder as needed between injection and acquisition. About 20 milligrams of furosemide were administered 30 minutes after the FDG infusion. The CT was obtained using a pitch of 1.375, 120 kV, and the available automatic tube current modulation with a noise index of 40 and a constrained maximum value of 150 mA. CT dose index (CTDIvol) given by the scanner was 3.1 mGy. Size-specific dose estimate was calculated as 3.9 mGy. The examination revealed multifocal hypermetabolic lesions of the right breast (**A**, **C**, **D**, **E**, arrows) with hypermetabolic right axillary and right internal mammary lymph nodes (**C**, **D**, stars) without distant metastases. The fetus had its head upward (**B**, CT volume rendering). Reprinted with permission from Drouet et al. (17).

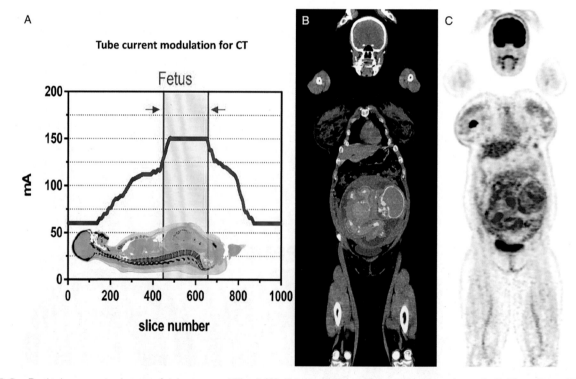

FIG. 19.3 • Real tube current value over fetal area was 150 mA (**A**). Fetal radiation dose from CT was estimated with VirtualDose CT software, which uses realistic anthropomorphic phantoms to compute organ doses. The 9-month pregnant female phantom was used, with a conservative tube current value of 150 mA over the whole body (i.e., neglecting automatic tube current modulation), to estimate an upper limit of 9.4 mGy for the fetal dose. FDG contribution was estimated using OLINDA/EXM 2.0.3 for a given radionuclide, OLINDA/EXM computes organ doses based on pharmacokinetic data and tabulated dose factors obtained from phantoms. Fetal activity was derived according to the methodology applied in Zanotti-Fregonara et al. (9), using the 9-month pregnant female phantom. Fetal volume delineation on CT and PET images (**B** and **C**, yellow area) yielded a fraction of injected activity of 0.052 in the fetus 75 minutes after injection. The fetal estimated time-integrated activity was 0.137 Bq × h/Bq. The estimated fetal dose from FDG was 1.15×10^{-2} mGy/MBq, leading to a total fetal dose estimate of 1.7 mGy. However, pharmacokinetics data do not model the effects of furosemide injection, which would tend to lower this value. Note that the dose coefficient obtained here (1.15×10^{-2} mGy/MBq) is higher than the one recommended by others at 9-month gestation (6.9×10^{-3} mGy/MBq) due to a higher fraction of injected activity measured in the fetus. In this case, as well as in others, the estimated fetal radiation dose is approximately 10 mGy, whereas the currently accepted threshold for deterministic effects is 100 mGy. This argues for reasonable use of fluorodeoxyglucose (FDG) positron emission tomography (PET)/computed tomography (CT) in pregnant women suffering from cancer, especially with new-generation digital PET/CT scanners that can provide high-quality CT and PET images while reducing patient's exposure. Reprinted with permission from Drouet et al. (17).

Table 19.6 **COMPARISON OF IMAGING STRATEGIES FOR PULMONARY EMBOLISM IN A PREGNANT PATIENT**

Characteristic	Pulmonary CT Angiography	Ventilation–Perfusion Scintigraphy
Accuracy	High	High (with pulmonary CT angiography backup)
Availability	High	Low
Expense	High	High
Efficiency	<1 h	Several hours
Reliability	High (may be reduced in pregnancy)	Moderate (3%–25% nondiagnostic)*
Risks	Iodinated contrast agent	
Fetal dose (mGy)	0.01–0.66	0.1–0.8
Maternal breast dose (mGy)	20–70	0.22–0.28

*Pulmonary CT angiography may be required if ventilation–perfusion scanning is nondiagnostic.

Reprinted with permission from Colletti et al. (5). Copyright © 2013 American Roentgen Ray Society.

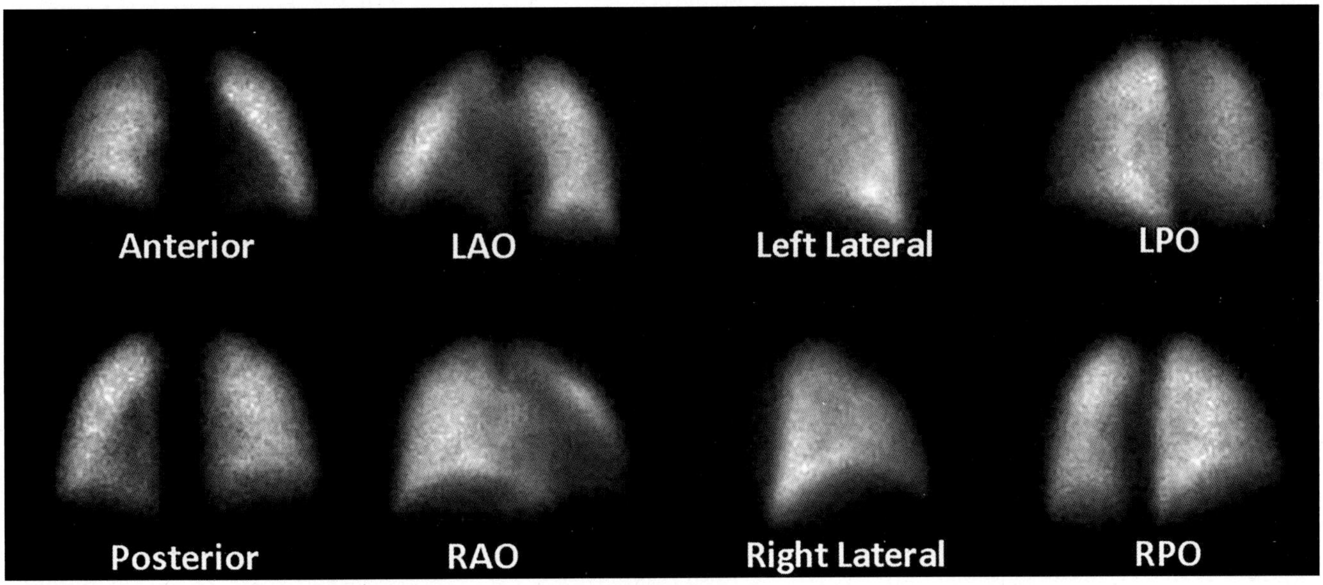

FIG. 19.4 ● Normal pulmonary perfusion scan in a 28-year-old woman with dyspnea at 16 weeks of pregnancy.

patients (5). Figure 19.4 shows a normal perfusion-only exam in a 28-year-old woman with dyspnea at 16 weeks of gestation. This is the most common result of perfusion-only scanning in a pregnant patient.

Radioiodine distribution and dosimetry in the pregnant patient

While the placental barrier prevents the passage of T3, T4, and thyroid stimulating hormone (TSH), radioiodine readily crosses to the fetus where it can be retained in the amniotic circulation. It is generally inappropriate to examine or treat a pregnant patient with radioiodine. Table 19.7 presents estimates of whole fetal exposure associated with radioiodine scanning during pregnancy.

While these estimated fetal exposures associated with diagnostic radioiodine imaging in pregnancy are likely without consequence, the same cannot be said for the likely deterministic effects

of radioiodine therapy in the pregnant patient. Table 19.8 presents some examples of fetal injury associated with therapeutic radioiodine administered during pregnancy (30,31).

The timing of fetal exposure to ^{131}I is important when predicting the risk of injury to the fetal thyroid. Prior to week 10, fetal thyroid injury is unlikely, whereas, after week 17, severe thyroid injury is likely.

The maturation of fetal thyroid function is presented in Table 19.9 (32). Fetal radiation exposure from ^{131}I depends on maternal dose, maternal thyroid physiology, and gestational age (Fig. 19.5). At 5 months, the fetal thyroid is significantly developed, and the ratio of thyroid/body size is maximal.

With hyperthyroidism, maternal thyroid uptake and retention reduces ^{131}I available to cross the placenta. Figure 19.6 is an example of maternal residual thyroid cancer and fetal thyroid ^{131}I uptake in a patient inadvertently treated with 100 mCi of ^{131}I at

Table 19.7 DIAGNOSTIC RADIOIODINE FETAL WHOLE BODY DOSE IN EARLY PREGNANCY AND AT TERM

Isotope	Procedure	Dose (mCi/MBq)	Early Gestation (mGy)	Term (mGy)
I-123	Thyroid uptake	0.8/30	0.4–0.6	0.3
I-131	Thyroid uptake	0.015/0.55	0.03–0.04	0.15
I-131	Metastases Imaging	1.1/40	2.0–2.9	11.0

Data from Russell et al. (6).

Table 19.8 PREGNANCY OUTCOME AFTER ^{131}I THERAPY DURING PREGNANCY (29, 30)

Authors	Weeks of Gestation	Treatment type	Estimated Dosimetry	Pregnancy Outcome
Stoffer et al., 1976 (30)	First trimester	[131]I Thyroid Rx for hyper-thyroidism or DTC	100–700 mGy	N = 237-55 (ToP) = 182 cases: 2 spontaneous abortions, 2 stillborn, 1 biliary atresia, 1 respiratory distress, 6 hypothyroid, and 4 "mentally deficient"
Berg et al. *Acta Oncol.* 2008 (31)	2 cases: 1. 20 wk 2. 20 wk	[131]I Thyroid Graves 15 mCi DTC 100 mCi	100 mGy 700 mGy	1. Hypothyroid at birth, at 8y Attention deficit, 1.3 SD < mean, and subnormal figurative memory 2. Did not survive

DTC, differentiated thyroid cancer; ToP, termination of pregnancy.

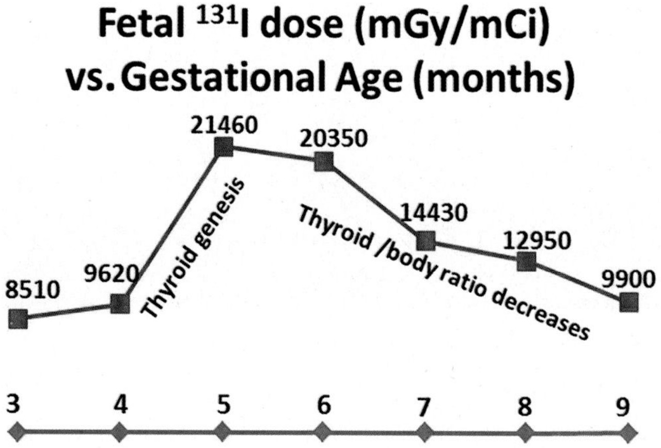

Fetal ^{131}I dose (mGy/mCi) vs. Gestational Age (months)

FIG. 19.5 ● Fetal ^{131}I dose in mGy/mCi versus gestational age in months. The relative radioiodine uptake in the thyroid increases as the thyroid develops over the first 5 months of gestation. After the fifth month, the fetal body grows more rapidly than the fetal head and neck, and thus the relative fetal thyroid uptake increases less than the remainder of the fetal body until term.

20 gestational weeks (31). Regarding the treatment of differentiated thyroid cancer (DTC) in pregnancy, higher doses and low maternal uptake significantly increase the amount of ^{131}I available to the maternal bladder and fetus and fetal thyroid.

Table 19.9 MATURATION OF THE FETAL THYROID

Weeks 7–9	Thyroid formation begins
Week 10	Thyroid follicles and TSH and T4 detectable
Week 17	Thyroid structural maturity
Week 20	Type II and III de-iodinases present
Weeks 18–40	Maturation of : fetal pituitary function and TRH production fetal thyroid response to TSH

EXAMPLE CASES OF ^{131}I TREATMENTS IN PREGNANT PATIENTS FROM THE UNITED STATES NUCLEAR REGULATORY COMMISSION OFFICE OF NUCLEAR MATERIAL SAFETY AND SAFEGUARDS

Case 1:

A patient was scheduled for RAI post surgery for DTC. She was interviewed by a certified nuclear medicine technologist (CNMT) and an authorized user (AU) physician, which included a discussion of pregnancy and breastfeeding status. The patient emphatically denied either. The patient was treated in the hospital with 5.75 GBq (155.2 mCi) of [131]I.

Unbeknownst to the licensee, the patient's referring physician had ordered a pregnancy test, in the belief that such a test was standard practice. About 4 h after the administration of the RAI, the results of the pregnancy test were forwarded to the nursing station.

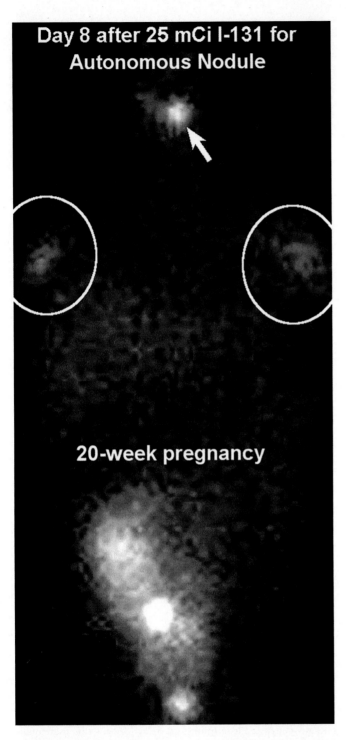

Day 8 after 25 mCi I-131 for Autonomous Nodule

20-week pregnancy

FIG. 19.6 ● This 28 year-old woman received 25 mCi of 131I as treatment for a hyperfunctioning autonomous thyroid nodule. Her torso scan at 8 days revealed the hyperfunctioning nodule (arrow) along with breast activity (circled). Incidentally noted is her 20 week pregnancy with prominent activity in the fetal thyroid. From Berg et al. (31). Reprinted by permission from Taylor & Francis Ltd., https://www.tandfonline.com.

1. DTC, differentiated thyroid cancer.

The test was positive and a subsequent ultrasound showed that at the time of the administration, the patient was approximately 13.5 weeks pregnant with twins. Total effective dose equivalent to each fetus was estimated to be 0.38 gray (38 rads) and the committed dose

equivalent to each of the fetal thyroids was estimated at 2,000 gray (200,000 rads). Before the ablation, the patient also underwent a metastatic scan, using 100 MBq (2.7 mCi) of ^{131}I, and two thyroidectomy surgeries, each within the period of time that she was pregnant.

As in the ablation procedure, licensee staff collected the patient's history, including the most recent menses. The patient emphatically denied the possibility of pregnancy.

NRC determined that this case did not constitute a misadministration (medical event), since the patient received the intended dosage, and the licensee had taken reasonable steps to ascertain the medical status of the patient, prior to the administration of radioiodine.

http://www.nrc.gov/reading-rm/doc-collections/gen-comm/info-notices/1999/in99011.html accessed 7/6/20.

Case 2:

A patient was scheduled for RAI for the treatment of thyroiditis, in accordance with an AU's written directive. Licensee staff interviewed the patient regarding pregnancy status and the patient certified that she was not pregnant and signed an informed consent form. The patient received 341 MBq (9.2 mCi) of [131]I. A month after the treatment, the patient discovered that she had been approximately 4 months pregnant at the time of RAI and notified the licensee. Licensee estimated that the dose to the fetal thyroid was 88 gray (8,800 rads) .

As in Case 1, Nuclear regulatory Commission (NRC) determined that this incident did not constitute a misadministration (medical event), since the patient received the intended dosage, and the licensee had taken reasonable steps to ascertain the medical status of the patient, before administration of radioiodine.

http://www.nrc.gov/reading-rm/doc-collections/gen-comm/info-notices/1999/in99011.html accessed July 6, 2010.

Case 3:

Event 070339 involved a thyroid cancer treatment to a patient that resulted in radiation exposure to an embryo or fetus.

On May 22, 2007, the AU performed a pregnancy test on the patient with negative results. The patient was advised not to get pregnant prior to the treatment.

On May 29, 2007, the patient received 4.64 GBq (125.5 mCi) of [131]I.

On May 30, 2007, the patient performed a home pregnancy test with positive results and notified the licensee. Licensee performed another test on May 30, 2007 with positive results. It was determined that the patient was 4 to 5 weeks pregnant at the time of RAI. This event was caused by a false-negative pregnancy test result (due to the early stage of pregnancy) and the patient's belief that she was not pregnant. The licensee estimated the dose to the embryo/fetus to be 25 to 34 cSv (rem).

The NRC contracted with a medical consultant to review the medical significance of this event.

The consultant concluded that the most likely outcome would be delivery of a normal infant with regard to thyroid function, however, there may be a slightly increased risk of childhood cancer. The licensee took no corrective actions because the cause of the event was beyond their control.

NRC Nuclear Material Events Database Annual Report Fiscal Year 2007

Case 4:

Item Number 100245—A pregnant patient received 1.11 GBq (30 mCi) of ^{131}I on March 16, 2010.

A blood serum pregnancy test was performed prior to the administration and results were negative. On April 26, 2010, the patient took a home urine pregnancy test that revealed positive results. Pregnancy was confirmed using a blood serum pregnancy test on April 27, 2010.

The patient's physician estimated that conception occurred on or around March 13, 2010. The fetal dose was estimated to be approximately 8 cSv (rem). The patient was notified. The Colorado Department of Health investigated the incident. A second medical physicist estimated the fetal whole-body dose to be between 5.3 and 9.2 cSv (rem). The hospital stated that all procedures were followed to prevent this incident.

The blood serum test does not detect a pregnancy until 7 to 12 days after conception.

NRC Nuclear Material Events Database Annual Report Fiscal Year 2010

Case 5:

Item Number 100400—A pregnant patient was administered 5.73 GBq (154.9 mCi) of ^{131}I for thyroid ablation on June 7, 2010. Prior to the administration, the patient received a blood serum pregnancy test to check for pregnancy and the results were negative. On 7/8/2010, the patient returned for a follow-up visit and informed the doctor that she was pregnant. An ultrasound estimated that the date of conception was 6/1/2010. A dose assessment conservatively estimated the fetal dose to be 41.27 cGy (rad).

Due to the age of the fetus, there was no thyroid present and no acute effect to the fetus is expected. The patient was informed of these results on 8/11/2010. Corrective actions included updating the patient consent form to explain that the pregnancy test may not show a positive result until 7 to 10 days after conception and reinforcing with staff the need to inform patients of the potential for false-negative results from the pregnancy test and advise the patient to refrain from actions that may lead to pregnancy.

NRC Nuclear Material Events Database Annual Report Fiscal Year 2010

Case 6:

Item Number 100319—A pregnant patient was administered 3.81 GBq (102.9 mCi) of ^{131}I as a treatment for reoccurring cancer associated with a previous thyroidectomy conducted in 2006. The treatment was administered on May 1, 2007 and the patient was 25 to 27 weeks pregnant. The patient had received ^{131}I following the thyroidectomy in 2006 and was treated a second time with ^{131}I on May 1, 2007. The doctor stated that when he asked the patient if she was pregnant, she replied that she was not. No independent test was conducted.

The doctor was contacted on June 11, 2007 by the physician's obstetrician, who advised that she was 32 weeks pregnant. Calculations were performed by the Illinois Emergency Management Agency resulted in an estimated dose to the fetus of 86 cGy (rad). The child was delivered after a full-term pregnancy and is receiving thyroid hormone therapy.

NRC Nuclear Material Events Database Annual Report Fiscal Year 2010

In summary, it is advisable to acquire a pregnancy test prior to treating a woman of childbearing age with unsealed radioisotopes.

Pregnancy tests may be unreliable in the first 1 to 2 weeks after ovulation (33).

DECISION-MAKING REGARDING IMAGING WITH RADIOPHARMACEUTICALS IN THE PREGNANT PATIENT

There are a series of questions to consider when considering nuclear medicine imaging in a woman of childbearing age:

Decision 1: Is imaging required?
Decision 2: Is the patient pregnant?
Decision 3: Is imaging with ionizing radiation required?
Decision 4: Is scintigraphy required?
Decision 5: Can scintigraphy be delayed?
Decision 6: Can scintigraphy be performed with reduced dose and increased maternal hydration?

Figure 19.7 presents a nuclear medicine decision flow chart demonstrating the logical choices required to make optimal choices when considering nuclear medicine procedures in a pregnant or potentially pregnant patient.

Radioisotopes and the lactating patient

There are three considerations regarding the lactating patient. These include direct radiation due to biodistribution in the lactating breast, gamma radiation to the child from maternal breast and other tissues, and radiation to the child due to swallowed secreted radioisotope in the breast milk (Fig. 19.8).

Lactating breast tissue may accumulate radioiodine where it may be secreted in breast milk. Lactation is controlled by prolactin and can be inhibited by cessation of breast feeding or by the introduction of dopamine agonists such as bromocriptine or longer-acting dopamine agonists such as cabergoline (34,35). Thus, if a breastfeeding woman is under consideration for treatment with ^{131}I for hyperthyroidism or DTC, she must of course discontinue breastfeeding for her current child. As per the Advisory Committee on Medical Uses of Isotopes Sub-Committee on Nursing Mother Guidelines for the Medical Administration of Radioactive Materials, this should allow "…at least six weeks prior to the anticipated radioiodine procedure…" (36).

The relative amount of radioiodine distribution to the recently lactating breast may be predicted with ^{123}I imaging (37–39). While the typical breast radioiodine uptake may be relatively modest many weeks after lactation (Fig. 19.9), some increased accumulation may continue (Fig. 19.10). Figure 19.11 suggests that the 6-week delay post-cessation of lactation prior to ^{131}I therapy suggested as a minimum delay (36) may be inadequate without pharmaceutical intervention.

Simplified recommendations regarding breastfeeding after receiving radiopharmaceuticals are presented in Table 19.10 (36,37).

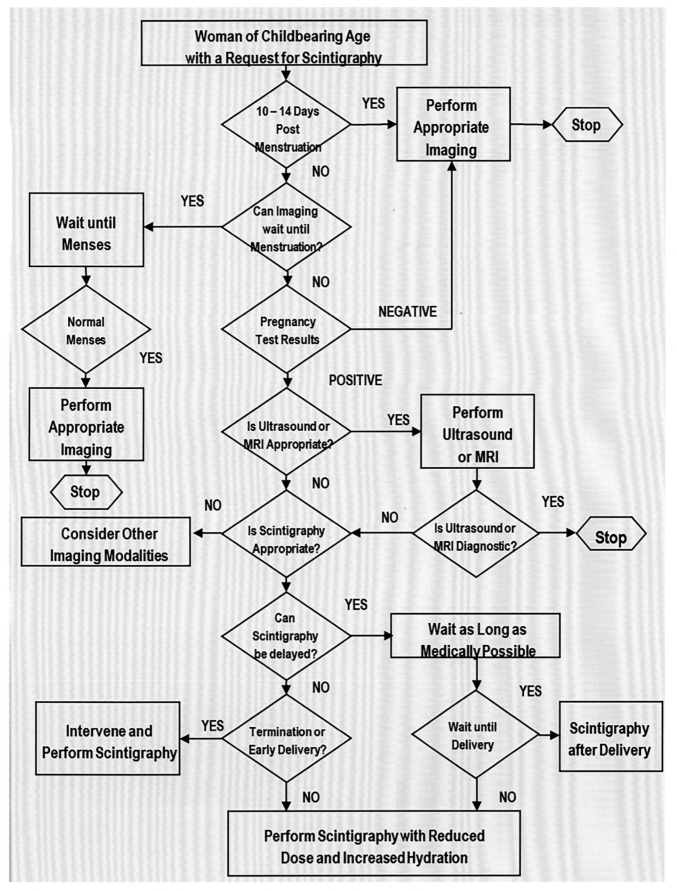

FIG. 19.7 ● Decision Flowchart for the use of nuclear medicine and positron emission tomography (PET) in the pregnant patient.

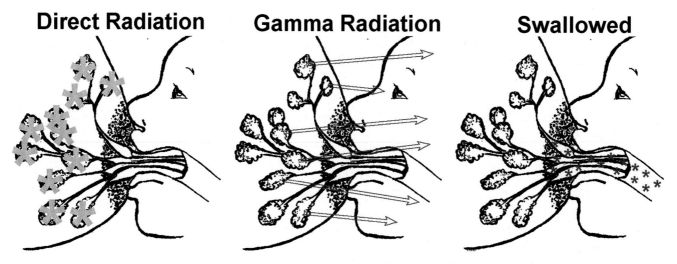

FIG. 19.8 ● Mechanisms of radiation associated with breastfeeding and the lactating breast. The lactating breast is a vascular secretory tissue that accumulates most radiopharmaceuticals with likelihood for direct breast tissue radiation (left), gamma radiation to the feeding baby (center), and inclusion of radioactivity into the milk with potential internal radiation in the feeding baby.

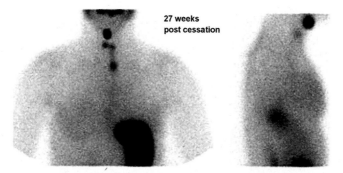

FIG. 19.9 ● Anterior and lateral views of ^{123}I scan 27 weeks after cessation of breastfeeding showing typical mild breast tissue uptake. Reprinted with permission from Brzozowska and Roach (37).

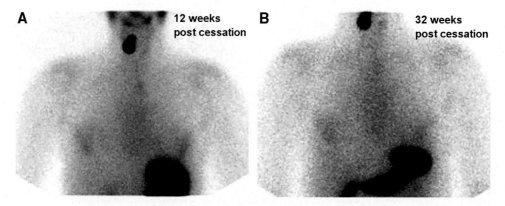

FIG. 19.10 ● (**A**) ^{123}I scan 12 weeks after breastfeeding showing moderate uptake of tracer in breast tissue. (**B**) ^{123}I scan 32 weeks after cessation of breastfeeding, also showing moderate uptake of tracer in breast tissue. Reprinted with permission from Brzozowska and Roach (37).

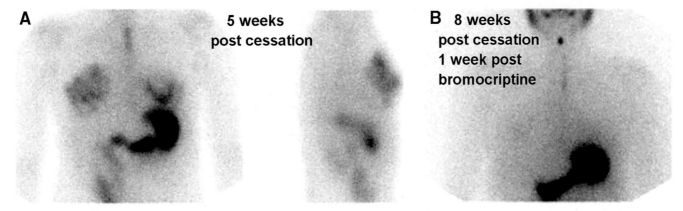

FIG. 19.11 ● (**A**) Anterior and lateral views of ^{123}I scan 5 weeks after cessation of breastfeeding showing marked uptake of tracer in breast tissue. (**B**) Anterior view of ^{123}I scan 8 weeks after cessation of breastfeeding showing negligible uptake of tracer in breast tissue. Reprinted with permission from Brzozowska and Roach (37).

Table 19.10 **NRC SUBCOMMITTEE RECOMMENDATIONS FOR THE NURSING MOTHER JUNE 26, 2018 (36, 37)**

Radiopharmaceutical	Breastfeeding Discontinuation to Achieve 0.1 rad to the Limiting Tissue
^{15}O and ^{82}Rb	No discontinuation
^{11}C and ^{13}N	1 h
^{18}F and ^{68}Ga	4 h
^{99m}Tc	24 h (especially MAA, RBCs, and pertechnetate)
^{123}I-NaI	3 days*
^{201}Tl-chloride	4 days*
^{111}In-white blood cells and ^{111}In-OCTREOTATE	6 days*
^{67}Ga and ^{89}Zr	28 days#
^{124}I-NaI, ^{131}I-NaI	Stop breast feeding
^{177}Lu-OCTREOTATE—diagnostic or therapeutic	
^{223}Ra and all alpha emitters	

*Can pump and store, possibly obtain breast milk sample radioactivity measurement.

#For practical purposes, stop breastfeeding.

References

1. Secker Walker RH, Kohorn EI, Morris J. Placental localization by isotope and ultrasound scanning. *Proc R Soc Med.* 1969 May;62(5): 446–448.
2. Wilcox A, Weinberg C, O'Connor J, et al. Incidence of early loss of pregnancy. *New Engl J Med.* 1988;319:189–194.
3. Wieseler KM, et al. Imaging in pregnant patients: examination appropriateness. *Radio-Graphics.* 30:1215–1229.
4. Brent RL. Utilization of developmental basic science principles in the evaluation of reproductive risks from pre- and post-conception environmental radiation exposure. *Teratology.* 1999;59:182–204.
5. Colletti PM, Lee KH, Elkayam U. Cardiovascular imaging of the pregnant patient. *AJR Am J Roentgenol.* 2013;200:515–521.
6. Russell JR, Stabin MG, Sparks RB. Radiation absorbed dose to the embryo/fetus from radiopharmaceuticals. *Health Phys.* 1997;73: 756–769.
7. Bural GG, Laymon CM, Mountz JM. Nuclear imaging of a pregnant patient: should we perform nuclear medicine procedures during pregnancy? *Mol Imaging Radionucl Ther.* 2012;21(1):1–5. doi:10.4274/ Mirt.123
8. Wagner LK, Lester RG, Saldana LR. Exposure of the pregnant patient to diagnostic radiations: a guide to medical management, 2nd Ed. Medical Physics Publishing: Madison WI; 1997.
9. Zanotti-Fregonara P, Champion C, Trebossen R, Maroy R, Devaux JY, Hindie E. Estimation of the b1 dose to the embryo resulting from 18F-FDG administration during early pregnancy. *J Nucl Med.* 2008;49:679–682.
10. Zanotti-Fregonara P, Jan S, Champion C, et al. In vivo quantification of 18F-FDG uptake in human placenta during early pregnancy. *Health Phys.* 2009;97:82–85.
11. Marcus CS, Mason GR, Kuperus JH, Mena I. Pulmonary imaging in pregnancy. Maternal risk and fetal dosimetry. *Clin Nucl Med.* 1985;10(1):1–4.
12. Schaefer, C, Meister, R, Wentzeck, R, et al. Fetal outcome after technetium scintigraphy in early pregnancy. *Reprod Toxicol.* 2009;28:161–166.
13. Baker J, Ali A, Groch MW, Fordham E, Economou SG. Bone scanning in pregnant patients with breast carcinoma. *Clin Nucl Med.* 1987;12:519–524.
14. Zanotti-Fregonara P, Jan S, Taieb D, et al. Absorbed 18F-FDG dose to the fetus during early pregnancy. *J Nucl Med.* 2010;51:803–805.

15. Takalkar AM, Khandelwal A, Lokitz S, Lilien DL, Stabin MG. 18F-FDG PET in pregnancy and fetal radiation dose estimates. *J Nucl Med.* 2011;52:1035–1040.

16. Hsieh T-C, Wu Y-C, Sun S-S, et al. FDG PET/CT of a late-term pregnant woman with breast cancer. *Clin Nucl Med.* 2012;37:489–491.

17. Drouet C, Vrigneaud J-M, Desmoulins I, Cochet A. FDG PET/CT in a pregnant woman with breast cancer. *Clin Nucl Med.* 2020;45:e339–e341.

18. Stabin MG. Proposed addendum to previously published fetal dose estimate tables for ^{18}F-FDG. *J Nucl Med.* 2004 Apr;45(4):634–635.

19. Elliott CG. Evaluation of suspected pulmonary embolism in pregnancy. *J Thoracic Imaging.* 2012; 27:3–4.

20. Schaefer-Prokop C, Prokop M. CTPA for the diagnosis of acute pulmonary embolism during pregnancy. *Eur Radiol.* 2008;18:2705–2708.

21. Abele JT, Sunner P. The clinical utility of a diagnostic imaging algorithm incorporating low-dose perfusion scans in the evaluation of pregnant patients with clinically suspected pulmonary embolism. *Clin Nucl Med.* 2013;38:29–32.

22. Leung AN, Bull TM, Jaeschke R, et al. An official American Thoracic Society/Society of Thoracic Radiology clinical practice guideline: evaluation of suspected pulmonary embolism in pregnancy. *Am J Respir Crit Care Med.* 2011;184:1200–1208.

23. Pahade JK, Litmanovich D, Pedrosa I, et al. Imaging pregnant patients with suspected pulmonary embolism: what the radiologist needs to know. *RadioGraphics.* 2009;29:639–654.

24. Remy-Jardin M, Pistolesi M, Goodman LR, et al. Management of suspected acute pulmonary embolism in the era of CT angiography: a statement from the Fleischner Society. *Radiology.* 2007;245:315–329.

25. Kallen JA, Coughlin BF, O'Loughlin MT, Stein B. Reduced Z-axis coverage multidetector CT angiography for suspected acute pulmonary embolism could decrease dose and maintain diagnostic accuracy. *Emerg Radiol.* 2010;17:31–35.

26. Atalay MK, Walle NL, Egglin TK. Prevalence and nature of excluded findings at reduced scan length CT angiography for pulmonary embolism. *J Cardiovasc Comput Tomogr.* 2011;5:325–332.

27. Wang PI, Chong ST, Kielar AZ, et al. Imaging of pregnant and lactating patients. Part 2. Evidence based review and recommendations. *AJR.* 2012;198:785–792.

28. Chen J, Lee RJ, Tsodikov A, Smith L, Gaffney DK. Does radiotherapy around the time of pregnancy for Hodgkin's disease modify the risk of breast cancer? *Int J Radiat Oncol Biol Phys.* 2004;58:1474–1479.

29. Litmanovich D, Boiselle PM, Bankier AA, Kataoka ML, Pianykh O, Raptopoulos V. Dose reduction in computed tomographic angiography of pregnant patients with suspected acute pulmonary embolism. *J Comput Assist Tomogr.* 2009;33:961–966.

30. Stoffer SS, Hamburger JI. Inadvertent 131I therapy for hyperthyroidism in the first trimester of pregnancy. *J Nucl Med.* 1976;17(02):146–149.

31. Berg G, Jacobsson L, Nyström E, Gleisner KS, Tennvall J. Consequences of inadvertent radioiodine treatment of Graves' disease and thyroid cancer in undiagnosed pregnancy. Can we rely on routine pregnancy testing? *Acta Oncol.* 2008;47(1):145–149.

32. Leung AM. Thyroid function in pregnancy. *J Trace Elem Med Biol.* 2012;26(2–3):137–140.

33. Johnson S, Godbert S, Perry P, et al. Accuracy of a home-based device for giving an early estimate of pregnancy duration compared with reference methods. *Fertility Sterility.* 100(6),:1635–1641.

34. Verhelst J, Abs R, Maiter D, et al. Cabergoline in the treatment of hyperprolactinemia: a study in 455 patients. *J Clin Endocrinol Metab.* 1999;84:2518–2522.

35. Webster J, Piscitelli G, Polli A, et al. A comparison of cabergoline and bromocriptine in the treatment of hyperprolactinemic amenorrhea. Cabergoline Comparative Study Group. *N Engl J Med.* 1994;331:904–909.

36. Advisory Committee on Medical Uses of Isotopes (ACMUI) Sub-Committee on Nursing Mother Guidelines for the Medical Administration of Radioactive Materials. https://www.nrc.gov/docs/ML1817/ML18177A451.pdf#:~:text=Breast%2Dfeeding%20is%20not%20regulated,5%20mSv%20(0.5%20rem). Viewed July 7, 2020.

37. Brzozowska M, Roach PJ. Timing and Potential Role of Diagnostic I-123 Scintigraphy in assessing radioiodine breast uptake before ablation in postpartum women with thyroid cancer A case series. *Clin Nucl Med.* 2006;31:683–687.

38. Hsiao E, Huynh T, Mansberg R, et al. Diagnostic I-123 scintigraphy to assess potential breast uptake of I-131 prior to radioiodine therapy in a post-partum woman with thyroid cancer. *Clin Nucl Med.* 2004;29:498–501.

39. Stabin MG, Breitz HB. Breast milk excretion of radiopharmaceuticals: mechanisms, findings, and radiation dosimetry. *J Nucl Med.* 2000;41(5):863–873.

CHAPTER SELF-ASSESSMENT QUESTIONS

1. What is the greatest risk of radiation in the first 10 days of gestation?

   A. Embryo reabsorption

   B. Hypothyroidism

   C. Malformation

   D. Neoplasm

2. Why is it difficult to demonstrate fetal injury related to radiation from diagnostic imaging?

   A. Abnormalities are naturally common.

   B. Anomalies are often misdiagnosed.

   C. Doses are difficult to estimate.

   D. Pregnancy may be unsuspected.

3. What is the largest radiopharmaceutical moiety size that is likely to achieve placental–fetal transfer?

   A. 5 to 10 nm

   B. 50 to 100 nm

   C. 500 to 1000 daltons

   D. 5000 to 10000 daltons

4. After what gestational age is fetal thyroid accumulation of ^{131}I likely?

   A. 8 weeks

   B. 12 weeks

   C. 16 weeks

   D. 20 weeks

5. A 25-year-old woman with shortness of breath (SOB) has a 2 mCi ^{99m}Tc macroaggregated albumin (MAA) lung scan. It is later determined she was 6 weeks pregnant. Fetal estimated dose is 0.5 mGy. What will be your advice to the patient?

   A. Risk is negligible.

   B. Fetal injury risk is very low and discussion of termination is unwarranted.

   C. Fetal injury risk is possible but unlikely and discussion of termination is optional.

   D. Fetal injury is a significant possibility and termination recommended.

6. Which radiopharmaceuticals would least likely be recycled in the amniotic circulation?

   A. ^{123}I and ^{131}I

   B. ^{18}FDG and ^{18}F-flouride

   C. diethylene-triamine-pentaacetate (DTPA), mercapto-acetyltriglycine (MAG3), and methylene diphosphonate (MDP)

   D. Sulfur colloid, MAA, ^{111}In-WBCs, and ^{99m}Tc-RBCs

7. At what gestational age in months is fetal ^{131}I dose in mGy/mCi the greatest?

   A. 3

   B. 5

   C. 7

   D. 9

8. What maternal hyperthyroid radioactive iodine uptake (RIU) pattern would deliver the greatest fetal ^{131}I dose?

   A. 4 h, 80%; 24 h, 50%

   B. 4 h, 80%; 24 h, 85%

   C. 4 h, 40%; 24 h, 25%

   D. 4 h, 40%; 24 h, 50%

9. At what stage of gestation is fetal radiation associated with computed tomography pulmonary angiogram (CTPA) greatest?

   A. Implantation

   B. First trimester

   C. Second trimester

   D. Third trimester

10. A woman age 32 has just been given 15 mCi of ^{131}I for hyperthyroidism. The lab calls to report a transcription error, and in fact the patient is pregnant. She has not menstruated for 3 months. What should you do?

    A. Prescribe 0.1 mg levothyroxine tabs for 3 days

    B. Give 130 mg potassium iodide as soon as possible

    C. Induce vomiting with ipecac

    D. Perform gastric lavage

11. Which therapeutic use of radioisotopes does not affect lactation and breastfeeding?

    A. ^{90}Y-TheraSpheres for hepatocellular carcinoma

    B. ^{131}I for thyroid cancer

    C. ^{177}Lu-Lutathera for neuroendocrine tumor

    D. ^{223}RaCl for bone metastases

12. Based on 2018 NRC Subcommittee Recommendations for the Nursing Mother, what is the minimum preparation for ^{131}I therapy in a lactating breastfeeding mother?

    A. Discontinue breastfeeding for 24 h and give radioiodine.

    B. Discontinue breastfeeding and apply an estradiol patch for one week prior to radioiodine.

    C. Discontinue breastfeeding for 8 days prior to radioiodine.

    D. Discontinue breastfeeding for at least 6 weeks prior to radioiodine.

Answers to Chapter Self-Assessment Questions

1. A   It is unlikely that the patient would be aware of the pregnancy and embryo loss.

2. A   Abnormalities are naturally common. Up to 6% of fetuses have some abnormality and 0.6% of live births have anomalies.

3. C   Molecules between 500 to 1,000 are the largest moieties likely to penetrate the placental barrier. Presumably, antibodies, sulfur colloid, RBCs, WBCs, and MAA will not pass. ^{18}F-FDG at ~181 daltons about 0.7 nm passes readily. Large moieties (>4 nm) including antibodies, sulfur colloid, RBCs, WBCs, and MAA will not pass the placental barrier.

4. B   By 10 weeks, thyroid follicles, TSH and T4 are detectable. Fetal thyroid accumulation of ^{131}I is likely at 12 weeks.

5. A   0.5 mGy is less than the NRC recommended maximum total gestational dose of 1.0 mGy.

6. D   Particles and cells would not cross the intact placenta; other listed agents cross the placenta and would be excreted into the amniotic fluid space, swallowed and absorbed (e.g., iodine) or passed again to the amniotic fluid.

7. B   At 5 months, the fetal thyroid is significantly developed and the ratio of thyroid/body size is maximal.

8. C   Lower maternal uptakes and greater washout increase the amount of ^{131}I available for fetal uptake and maternal bladder activity.

9. D   Fetal radiation exposure related to chest CT should be entirely caused by Compton scatter. The larger third trimester fetus is significantly closer to the radiation scattering maternal tissues.

10. B   Gastric removal of ^{131}I is awkward and unlikely to help as iodine is rapidly absorbed. T4 (MW 800) does not easily traverse the placenta and could in fact release more ^{131}I to the fetus. Potassium iodide (KI) crosses the placenta and blocks ^{131}I uptake.

11. A ^{90}Y is entirely retained within the glass spheres and so it does not migrate to the lactating breast. The majority of ^{90}Y radiation is bremsstrahlung, though there is sufficient ^{90}Zr produced to perform satisfactory PET images of ^{90}Y. The other agents produce far greater gamma radiation and ^{131}I and ^{223}Ra would cross the placental barrier.

12. D   In the absence of bromocriptine or cabergoline, the other choices are much too short. The use of estradiol patches has not been shown to be helpful in reliably reducing lactation.

INDEX

Note: Page numbers followed by *f* and *t* indicate figures and tables respectively.

Spill, radioactive materials, 8
Spleen, 215–216
Splenic pathologies, 215–216
Splenic scintigraphy, 133–134, 134f
Splenosis, 219f
Spondylolysis, 221, 223
Squamous cell carcinoma (SCC), 151
Standard uptake values (SUV), 250
Standardized uptake value (SUV), 140, 145
Staphylococcus aureus bioprosthetic aortic valve endocarditis, 105f
Stress fracture, 79, 221, 227f
Stress reactions, 221
Systemic Infection and inflammation, 87–89

T
Targeted radionuclide therapy (TRT), 184, 185
Tc^{99m}-MDP, 186
Technetium-99m diethylenetriaminepentaacetic acid (^{99m}Tc-DTPA), 136
Tertiary hyperparathyroidism (tHPT), 48, 52f
Thiol group, 16
Thomson's atomic model, 11
Thoracic malignancies, 155
Thyroglobulin (Tg), 39
Thyroid cancer

background, 37
congenital hypothyroidism, 196–200
graves' disease, 200
nodules of, 200–202
non-iodine avid disease, 43–44
nuclear imaging/therapy, role, 40, 41f
post-therapy scans, 43
radioiodine scans, 41–42
radioiodine therapy, 42–43
side effects/radiation precautions, 43
treatment overview, 37–40
Thyroid Cancer Association (ThyCa.org), 42
Thyroid imaging and therapy
hyperthyroidism, 34–37
overview, 34
thyroid cancer, 37–44
Thyroiditis, 34
Technetium-99m dimercaptosuccinic acid (^{99m}Tc-DMSA), 136
Technetium-99m mercaptoacetyltriglycine (^{99m}Tc-MAG3), 136
Thyroid-stimulating hormone (TSH), 187, 196, 257
Time of flight (TOF) PET/CT, 31
Timeactivity curve (TAC), 202, 240f
Tl-201, decays electron capture, 4f
Toddler fracture, 225f
Top–down approach, 73f

Total lesion glycolysis (TLG), 146
Tracer distribution, 110
Transient equilibrium, 4
Transthyretin amyloid cardiomyopathy, 107f
Trauma, 79
Typical gas detectors, 23f

U
Universal decay table, 3–4
Uranium atoms fission, 13
Ureteropelvic junction obstruction, 208f–210f
Urinary tract infection (UTI), 202

V
Vascular graft infections, 90
Ventriculoperitoneal (VP), 69
Vesicoureteral reflux (VUR), 202
Voiding cystography, 213, 215
Voiding cystourethrogram (VCUG), 213

W
Wall motion, 103
Warburg effect, 146
Waste disposal, 7–8

Y
Y-90, 143
Yukawa, 12